Selected Topics in Pediatrics

Selected Topics in Pediatrics

Edited by Alice Kunek

hayle
medical

New York

Hayle Medical,
750 Third Avenue, 9th Floor,
New York, NY 10017, USA

Visit us on the World Wide Web at:
www.haylemedical.com

ISBN: 978-1-63241-516-5

Cataloging-in-Publication Data

Selected topics in pediatrics / edited by Alice Kunek.
    p. cm.
Includes bibliographical references and index.
ISBN 978-1-63241-516-5
1. Pediatrics. 2. Children--Diseases. I. Kunek, Alice.
RJ45 .S45 2018
618.92--dc23

Table of Contents

Preface

I am honored to present to you this unique book which encompasses the most up-to-date data in the field. I was extremely pleased to get this opportunity of editing the work of experts from across the globe. I have also written papers in this field and researched the various aspects revolving around the progress of the discipline. I have tried to unify my knowledge along with that of stalwarts from every corner of the world, to produce a text which not only benefits the readers but also facilitates the growth of the field.

The branch of medicine which focuses on the physical, mental and emotional well being of children and adolescents is known as pediatrics. It has a number of sub-fields such as child abuse pediatrics, pediatric endocrinology, pediatric hematology, pediatric oncology, pediatric emergency medicine and sports pediatrics. Those in search of information to further their knowledge will be greatly assisted by this book. For someone with an interest and eye for detail, this book covers the most significant topics in the field of pediatrics.

Finally, I would like to thank all the contributing authors for their valuable time and contributions. This book would not have been possible without their efforts. I would also like to thank my friends and family for their constant support.

Editor

SGA Children with Moderate Catch-Up Growth Are Showing the Impaired Insulin Secretion at the Age of 4

Ivana Milovanovic[1]*, Falucar Njuieyon[1], Samia Deghmoun[1], Didier Chevenne[2], Claire Levy-Marchal[1], Jacques Beltrand[3,4,5]

1 INSERM CIE 05 – Unité d'épidémiologie clinique, Hôpital Robert Debré, Paris, France, 2 Service de biochimie et hormonologie, Hôpital Robert Debré, Paris, France, 3 Endocrinologie et diabétologie pédiatrique, Hôpital Necker, Paris, France, 4 Université Paris 5, René Descartes, Paris, France, 5 INSERM U845, Imagine Affiliated, Paris, France

Abstract

Background: Being born small for gestational age (SGA) is a risk factor for later development of type 2 diabetes. The development of glucose tolerance disorders in adults involves insulin resistance and impaired insulin secretion.

Objective: To evaluate insulin secretion and insulin sensitivity in a 4-yr old cohort of SGA.

Methods: 85 children were prospectively followed from mid-gestation to 4 years of age. Fetal growth velocity (FGV) was measured using ultrasound measurements. Body composition and hormonal profile were measured at birth, 1 and 4 years.

Results: 23 SGA babies had lower birth weight compared to 62 AGA (-1.9 ± 0.3 vs. -0.6 ± 0.8 z-score; p<0.0001) and they were thinner at birth (ponderal index 24.8 ± 1.8 vs. 26.3 ± 3.1 kg/m3; p = 0.01 and fat mass 11 ± 2.6 vs. $12.9\pm3.1\%$; p = 0.01). No significant differences in other measured metabolic and hormonal parameters were observed between two groups at birth. SGA infants experienced an early catch-up growth in weight (mean gain of 1.1 ± 0.6 SD) during the first year of life. At 4 years, SGA children remain lighter than AGA, but with weight z-score in the normal range (-0.1 ± 1.3 vs. 0.5 ± 1.3 z-score; p = 0.05). No excess of fat mass was observed (19 ± 4.8 vs. $19.7\pm4.1\%$; p = 0.45). 120-min plasma glucose was significantly higher (6.2 ± 1.1 vs. 5.6 ± 0.9 mmol/l; p = 0.006) and insulinogenic index was significantly lower (0.28 ± 0.15 vs. 0.40 ± 2.4; p = 0.02) in the SGA group at 4-yrs of life contrasting with a preserved insulin sensitivity (QUICKI 0.47 ± 0.09 vs. 0.43 ± 0.05; p = 0.06).

Conclusion: SGA children with compensatory catch-up growth in first year of life show mild disturbances of glucose tolerance associated to a lower insulinogenic index at 4-yrs of age suggesting impairment of β-cell function.

Editor: Melania Manco, Scientific Directorate, Bambino Hospital, Italy

Funding: This work was supported by a grant from the "Institut National de la Santé et de la Recherche Médicale (INSERM)", a grant from the «Programme Hospitalier de Recherche Clinique» (AOM 06-136, 2006) and from Pfizer Inc. Jacques Beltrand was supported by a fellowship from the "Institut Appert" (France, 2006) and by INSERM (Poste d'accueil, 2007). Ivana Milovanovic was supported by a fellowship SFP 2011. Falucar Njuieyon was supported by a fellowship SFEDP 2009. Claire Levy-Marchal was awarded a Contrat d'Interface de Recherche Hospitalière 2007–2012 from Assistance Publique-Hôpitaux de Paris. The funders had no role in study design, data collection and analysis, decision to publish, or preparation of the manuscript.

Competing Interests: The authors have declared that no competing interests exist.

* Email: ivana.milovanovic@inserm.fr

Introduction

The association between a low birth weight and development of type 2 diabetes has been consistently reported in numerous publications [1,2] ; this association is strengthened after adjusting for adult BMI [3]. The pathway leading from small size at birth as a result of the exposure to an adverse fetal environment, to metabolic diseases later in life is not clear. The development of glucose tolerance disorders in adults involves insulin resistance and impaired insulin secretion. The early appearance of insulin resistance without obesity in SGA subjects is a well-known phenomenon. Thinness at birth (apart from birth weight itself) and the magnitude of the compensatory postnatal catch-up growth, which in turn induces abnormal growth of the adipose

tissue, are two components that are associated with later insulin resistance [4,5].

In animal models it has been demonstrated that in utero malnutrition affects pancreatic β-cell development leading to impaired β-cell function later in life [6,7]. In contrast, insulin secretion in SGA born children has been poorly studied and yield conflicting results in adults [8–10]. Our understanding of fetal programming events in the human endocrine pancreas is then limited.

The aim of this study was to evaluate insulin secretion and insulin sensitivity in a cohort of SGA born children in whom both prenatal and postnatal growth have been monitored in a prospective study in order to determine whether changes in insulin secretion and/or insulin sensitivity can be detected early in life.

Materials and Methods

CASyMIR cohort

The CASyMIR cohort (**C**roissance **A**nténatale **Sy**ndrome **M**étabolique et **I**nsulino-**R**ésistance) is a French prospective cohort exploring the metabolic consequences in early infancy of being born SGA. The infants were born to women of Caucasian origin recruited during their first or second trimester of pregnancy in the maternity of the Robert Debré Hospital in Paris.

Ethical statements

The Ethics Committee Ile-de-France 4 approved the study and written consent was obtained from both parents for all children.

Inclusion and exclusion criteria

Inclusion criteria were the presence of one of the risk factors of delivering an SGA baby : preexisting hypertension, smoking more than five cigarettes per day, history of small for gestational age baby either in a previous pregnancy or among parents, a history of pregnancy-induced hypertensive disorder, maternal height less than 152 cm corresponding to −2SD of the mean height for French women, uterine malformations, abnormal uterine or umbilical artery Doppler and small fetal size at second trimester ultrasound examination (abdominal circumference and/or femoral length at 22 weeks of gestation). All newborns were evaluated at birth. Newborns with fetal or congenital diseases that could affect fetal growth were excluded (TORCH infections: Toxoplasmosis, Other (syphilis, varicella-zoster, parvovirus B19), Rubella, Cytomegalovirus (CMV), Herpes infections, and congenital malformation). Gestational age below 34 weeks of gestation (WG) or newborns presenting with a severe neonatal condition were also not included in the post-natal follow-up.

Study population

Results of obstetrical, anthropometric and metabolic assessments were obtained at the age of 4 for 85 children included at birth in the CASyMIR cohort. The number of participating children was decreasing during the follow-up (at 1 year, 162 children had the anthropometric and hormonal evaluation; this number decrease to 122 children at 2 years and 104 at 3 years of life), but the data on body size and hormonal levels at birth and at age of 1 year did not differ significantly between subjects who completed the 4 year follow-up and those who did not. We could observe a difference regarding the risk factors among mothers. The children of mothers with short stature or placental vascular problems were more likely to complete the follow-up.

Assessment of fetal growth

Fetal growth was assessed every 4 weeks by ultrasound from 22 to 36 week of gestation. All four ultrasound scans were performed by the same observer for each woman under a standardized protocol. Estimated fetal weight (EFW) was calculated using the second Hadlock formula, which includes abdominal, head circumferences, and femur length measurements [11].

One way to understand whether smallness is due to a pathological condition is the utilisation of individually adjustable, customized standards. In addition to gestational age and gender, other pregnancy characteristics, such as maternal height and weight before pregnancy, parity, and ethnicity, count for a considerable part of the variation in fetal growth velocity and weight at birth [12]. A computer program, named "Customized birth weight standards" (Gestation related optimal weight program. Software version 5.15 and Centile calculator software v5.12.1 March 2007, www.gestation.net) has been created by Gardosi et al. in which estimated fetal weight (EFW) centiles are adjusted for all these variables [13]. Using this program we were able to identify the children who reached their "optimal fetal development" and those who did not due to growth restriction.

All the babies were classified at birth as SGA or AGA. For the purpose of the study, SGA was defined as birth weight ≤ -1.5 SD and AGA > -1.5 SD according to the French reference curves for gender and gestational age [14].

Measurements

A trained midwife or pediatrician performed the clinical measurements in all children at birth. Weight was measured using an electronic scale to the nearest 10 grams. Supine length was measured to the nearest 0.5 cm with a standardized length board consisting of a fixed board for the infant's head and a movable board allowing feet to be placed perpendicular to the longitudinal axis of the infant. Body mass index (BMI = weight/length^2) at 1and 4 years of age were calculated. Weight, length and BMI were converted into z-scores to adjust for age and sex using the French references curves [15,16]. Skinfold thickness measurements were recorded at birth, at 1 and 4 years of age, on the left side of the body at four different sites (biceps, triceps, subscapular and suprailliacal), by the same trained pediatrician dedicated to the study. Two separate measurements were performed with a skinfold caliper (Harpenden skinfold caliper, Baty international, England) and the mean was recorded [17]. Total subcutaneous fat mass was evaluated using the sum of the four skinfold thicknesses. Percentage of body fat was derived from four skinfold measurements from the equations of Brook and Siri [18,19].

Body composition at 4 years of age (fat mass, lean mass, and bone mineral density) was assessed by dual X-ray absorptiometry (DEXA) scan (LunaR Prodigy DXP, GE Medical Systems, Madison, WI, USA), with a specific program for small body weight [20,21].

Blood pressure was measured on the right arm of seated subjects after 5 min of rest, using an automated device (Dinamap, Critikon, Neuilly-Plaisance, France) and a cuff of recommended size for the mid-upper arm circumference.

At 4 years of age, glucose tolerance was assessed using an oral glucose tolerance test (OGTT) performed with the administration of 1.75 g of glucose solution per kilogram of body weight, after an overnight fast. Blood samples were drawn at 0, 30 and 120 min for measurements of glucose and insulin.

Assays

Hormonal analyses were performed at birth on a mixed venous and arterial cord blood sample. At 1 and 4 years of age, a venous sample was obtained after an overnight fast. Glucose was measured immediately whereas samples for hormonal analysis were quickly centrifuged and serum was separated and stored at −80°C until analysis. Serum insulin was measured by an IRMA kit (BI-INS-IRMA) from Cis Bio international (Gifsur-Yvette, France). Cross-reactivity with pro insulin and derived metabolites was less than 1%. Assay sensitivity was 3.0 pmol/L. Serum leptin was measured using a specific radioimmunoassay (Linco research, St Charles, USA). Sensitivity of the assay is 0.4 ng/ml. Intra- and inter- assay coefficients of variation are 5.2% and 8.7% respectively at 2.3 ng/ml.

Insulin sensitivity was assessed from fasting insulin and glucose levels using the index QUICKI (Quantitative insulin sensitivity check index) as 1/(log (fasting insulin)+log (fasting glucose) [22].

Insulinogenic index, calculated as the ratio of the increment of plasma insulin to that of plasma glucose during the first 30 min of

OGTT, was used to assess beta cell function. : insulinogenic index = (insulin 30 − insulin 0)/(glucose 30 − glucose 0) [23,24].

The disposition index describes the capacity of the pancreatic b-cells to secrete additional insulin to compensate over time for alterations in insulin sensitivity. It is calculated as the product of insulin secretion and sensitivity derived from OGTT (ΔI30/ΔG30×ISI).

Insulin sensitivity index (ISI Index) proposed by Matsuda and DeFronzo [25] was calculated as follows: ISI = 10,000/square root of [fasting glucose×fasting insulin] ×[mean glucose×mean insulin during OGTT]

Statistical analysis

Statistical analyses were performed using the SAS software version 9.1.3 for Windows (SAS statistical package, SAS institute, Meylan France).

Data are given as mean ± SD. Univariate analyses were performed for the comparison between the 2 groups using the Chi-2 test for qualitative variables and the Student's t-test, or nonparametric tests when appropriate, for quantitative variables.

For hormonal parameters, the comparisons between 2 groups of newborns were made by using general linear model with fat mass as covariate.

Results

The anthropometric and hormonal characteristics between groups SGA and AGA children at birth, 1 and 4 years are given in Table 1. Figure 1A shows fetal weight changes from 22 weeks of gestation to birth. From 30 weeks of gestation, EFW was significantly lower in SGA subjects (14.8±17.9 vs. 44.6±32.2 percentiles, p<0.0001 at 30 weeks of gestation; 11.4±16.6 vs. 42.7±33.4 percentiles, p<0.0001 at 36 weeks of gestation) showing that SGA babies slowed down fetal growth during the 3rd trimester of pregnancy.

The SGA babies were thinner at birth with significantly lower ponderal index (24.8±1.8 vs. 26.3±3.1 kg/m3; p = 0.01) and lower total subcutaneous fat mass assessed by the sum of skin folds (11±2.6 vs. 12.9±3.1%; p = 0.01). No other significant differences in any of the measured metabolic and hormonal parameters were observed between SGA and AGA subjects at birth.

The time-course of weight (expressed in z-scores - Figure 1B) illustrates that only SGA infants had experienced an early catch-up growth with a mean gain of 1.1±0.6 SD during the first year of life, correcting for the loss seen at birth. Height z-scores followed the same pattern of catch-up growth so that, although the mean height z-score was significantly lower at 1 yr of age in SGA, none of the SGA children presented with a short stature (height z-score < −2SD) at that age. Catch-up growth was not associated with excessive fat mass measured by the sum of skin folds (Figure 1C). Accordingly, leptin levels were lower in SGA children (2.9±1vs. 3.7±1.9; p = 0.05). By contrast, there was no difference in any other measured metabolic and hormonal parameters at 1 year of age.

At 4 years of age, even if SGA children were somewhat lighter than AGA children, weight z-score were in the normal range (−0.1±1.3 vs. 0.5±1.3 z-score; p = 0.05) and no significant difference in fat mass measured by either the sum of skin fold or by DEXA, was observed. Lean mass was also similar between SGA and AGA children at the age of 4 years (11741.8±932.1 vs. 12319.2±1889.2; p = 0.09). Surprisingly, OGTT data attested for mild glucose tolerance disorders in the SGA group: indeed, plasma glucose 2 hours after the oral glucose load was significantly higher in the SGA group (6.2±1.1 vs. 5.6±0.9 mmol/l; p = 0.006)

despite lower fasting plasma glucose (4.2±0.8 vs. 4.6±0.5 mmol/l; p = 0.02) (Figure 2A). Insulinogenic index was significantly lower in the SGA group than in the AGA group (0.28±0.15 vs. 0.40±2.4; p = 0.02) at 4 years of life (Figure 2C) contrasting with a preserved insulin sensitivity (QUICKI 0.47±0.09 vs. 0.43±0.05; p = 0.06) (Figure 2B).

No significant difference in lipid results was observed between two groups of children at the age of 4.

To note, calorie intake was similar in both groups at all ages (data not shown). In our study, at the age of four months (data not shown) we observed a difference in the type of feeding between the two groups of children with the AGA children that were more likely to be exclusively breast fed. But weight gain was still significantly different between children born small and those born with a normal weight, even after adjustment for type of feeding.

No type 1 or type 2 diabetes was found on the mother's side in the two groups of children. On the father's side one case (4.3%) of type 1 diabetes was noted in the SGA group, and one of type 2 diabetes in each group of children (data not shown).

Discussion

Our study is the first prospective one that studied insulin secretion in young healthy children born SGA in relationship with fetal and postnatal growth and associated changes in body composition. We found that SGA children do not have changes in insulin sensitivity but have lower glucose stimulated insulin secretion by comparison with AGA children at the age of four.

Furthermore, we found that catch-up growth following fetal growth restriction does not induce changes in insulin resistance or fat mass excess. The lack of these confounding factors that can affect insulin sensitivity and then increase fasting and stimulated insulin secretion allowed us to show that SGA children had defect in stimulated insulin secretion, suggesting that the exposure to an adverse nutritional environment during fetal life may affect pancreatic β-cell development, leading to impaired β-cell function later in the life.

Numerous animal studies already pointed that fetal growth restriction alters the endocrine function of the pancreas. For example, in sheep, chronic restriction of nutrient supply due to poor placental growth induces an intrauterine growth restriction (IUGR) associated to a reduced β-cell replication, and consequently, a reduced β-cell mass. Such changes were associated with changes in beta cell genes expression and then to a decreased pancreatic insulin content which reduced the capacity for insulin secretion [26]. The same defects were observed in fetal growth restricted rats, which also developed significant β-cell hypoplasia [27–29].

Human studies mostly reported that children with restricted fetal growth leading to thinness at birth were these who experienced catch up growth during the first months of life. Numerous clinical data also suggested that catch-up growth was a risk factor of developing excessive central fat mass and insulin resistance, both contributing to favor the development of metabolic diseases later in life [30–35]. Few studies reported an impaired insulin secretion in SGA subjects and mostly in adults [36]. Cook and al. [37] reported a reduced beta cell function in a small number of adult subjects born with low birth weight and having a family history of type 2 diabetes. One may ask whether this decrease was explained by the birth weight or by genetic factors. In our study, no family history of type 1 or type 2 diabetes was found in SGA children, so the lower glucose stimulated insulin secretion can be a consequence of intra uterine growth restriction and of consecutively impaired β-cell function.

Table 1. Estimated fetal weight (EFW) from 22 weeks of pregnancy until birth and anthropometric and hormonal characteristics at birth, 1 and 4 years of life between SGA and AGA babies.

Variable	SGA	AGA	p
	n = 23	n = 62	
Percentiles of EFW			
22 weeks of gestation	23.7±27.4	38.6±28.6	0.05
26 weeks of gestation	35.3±33.2	52±32.4	0.08
30 weeks of gestation	14.8±17.9	44.6±32.2	*<0.0001*
36 weeks of gestation	11.4±16.6	42.7±33.4	*<0.0001*
Birth percentiles	3.3±2.6	36.6±24.5	*<0.0001*
Birth			
Female gender (%)	13 (56.5)	34 (54.8)	0.89
Gestational age (wk)	38.8±2	38.9±1.7	0.8
Birth weight (g)	2363.3±384.3	2929.5±507.6	*<0.0001*
Birth weight (z-score)	−1.9±0.3	−0.6±0.8	*<0.0001*
Birth Lenght (cm)	45.5±2.9	48±2.3	*<0.0001*
Birth Lenght (z-score)	−1.9±0.8	−0.6±1	*<0.0001*
Cranial perimeter (cm)	32.6±1.7	33.8±1.6	*0.006*
Ponderal index (kg/m3)	24.8±1.8	26.3±3.1	*0.01*
Sum of folds (mm)	14.2±2.3	16.7±3.5	*0.001*
Fat Mass - sum of folds (%)	11±2.6	12.9±3.1	*0.01*
Glucose (mmol/l)	4.7±1.1	4.5±1.1	0.9
Triglyceride (mg/dl)	0.69±0.4	0.5±0.2	0.22
Cord insulin (mUI/l)	4.1±3.5	4.5±5.3	0.87
Cord leptin (ng/ml)	5.5±6.3	6.9±8.2	0.47
QUICKI	0.48±0.1	0.47±0.1	0.89
1 year of age			
Weight (kg)	8.7±6	9.3±0.9	*0.0006*
Weight (z-score)	−0.8±0.6	−0.2±0.8	*0.0005*
Height (cm)	72.7±1.9	73.9±2.3	*0.02*
Height (z-score)	−0.4±0.7	0.08±0.9	*0.02*
BMI (kg/m^2)	16.4±1.1	17±1.1	*0.04*
BMI (z-score)	−0.7±0.9	−0.2±0.8	*0.04*
Cranial perimeter (cm)	45.7±1.7	45.9±1.5	0.57
Delta weight 1 yr-birth	1.1±0.6	0.4±0.9	*0.002*
Sum of folds (mm)	28.8±5	30.5±6.5	0.27
Fat Mass - sum of folds (%)	19.5±3.3	20.1±3.4	0.49
Glucose (mmol/l)	4.4±0.5	4.6±0.4	0.14
Insulin (mUI/l)	2.1±1.8	2.3±2.3	0.75
Leptin (ng/ml)	2.9±1	3.7±1.9	0.05
QUICKI	0.51±0.1	0.54±0.2	0.38
4 years of age			
Weight (kg)	15.2±1.8	16.3±1.9	*0.02*
Weight (z-score)	−0.1±1.3	0.5±1.3	*0.05*
Height (cm)	100.3±3.1	102.1±3.6	*0.03*
Height (z-score)	0.4±1	0.8±1.1	0.1
BMI (kg/m^2)	15.1±1.3	15.6±1.2	0.08
BMI (z-score)	−0.4±1.1	0.01±1	0.08
Cranial perimeter (cm)	50±1.5	50.3±1.7	0.26
Sum of folds (mm)	28.3±9.2	30±7.3	0.40
Fat Mass - sum of folds (%)	19±4.8	19.7±4.1	0.45
Systolic BP (mmHg)	101.4±10.8	100.4±10.6	0.71

Table 1. Cont.

Variable	SGA	AGA	p
	n = 23	n = 62	
Diastolic BP(mmHg)	51±10.5	55.3±12.7	0.14
Lean Mass (g)	11741.8±932.1	12319.2±1889.2	0.09
Fat Mass (g)	2519.6±1338.2	2723.4±1075	0.5
Bone mineral content (g/cm)	419.2±58	512.4±79.3	0.21
Triglyceride (mg/dl)	0.6±0.1	0.6±0.2	0.95
Total cholesterol (mmol/l)	4.1±0.6	4.1±0.8	0.94
HDL cholesterol (mmol/l)	41.3±24.6	35.1±25	0.36
Leptin (ng/ml)	4.3±3.8	3.8±1.8	0.22
Glucose t0 (mmol/l)	4.2±0.8	4.6±0.5	*0.01*
Glucose t30 (mmol/l)	7.9±1.6	8.3±1.8	0.38
Glucose t120 (mmol/l)	6.2±1.1	5.6±0.9	*0.006*
Insulin t0 (mUI/l)	2.4±1.5	3±1.7	0.2
Insulin t30 (mUI/l)	21±15.1	28.1±16.2	0.11
Insulin t120 (mUI/l)	10.2±5.3	9.1±5.1	0.36
QUICKI	0.47±0.09	0.43±0.05	0.06
Insulinogenic index	0.28±0.15	0.40±0.24	*0.02*
Disposition Index	8.3±5.3	10.2±6.3	0.29

Ong et al. examined associations between size at birth, postnatal weight gain, circulating IGF-I levels and insulin sensitivity and secretion in 8 years old children. They found that the association between low birth weight and insulin resistance may be dependent on rapid weight gain during the early postnatal years. But, irrespective of postnatal weight gain, smaller size at birth, lower IGF-I levels and lower childhood height predicted reduced compensatory insulin secretion [38].

Mericq and al. [39] studied insulin secretion and sensitivity at the age of 3 years in SGA and AGA children. They found that the development of insulin resistance occurred in early postnatal life in case of rapid catch-up growth. Moreover, they observed a reduced compensatory beta cell secretion independent of postnatal catch-up growth.

In the present study, SGA children did not show excessive weight gain, neither changes in fat mass nor insulin resistance at the age of 4. We previously reported that early catch-up growth following fetal growth restriction promoted restoration of fat storage but did not induce excess of fat mass or unfavorable changes either in body composition or in insulin sensitivity at one year of age. This catch-up growth was then an adaptive and "physiological" phenomenon [40]. So, we could conclude that catch-up growth was not deleterious for infants and was an adaptive phenomenon to compensate for fetal growth restriction. By the contrast, an excessive one could promote an excess of fat mass and the appearance of IR and then the risk of type 2 diabetes later in the life.

In our study catch-up growth was symmetrical in weight and height (even slightly more important in height) and independent of postnatal feeding or later caloric intake explaining the lack of IR or excess in fat mass at the age of 4. In case of asymmetric catch-up growth, we could think that the insulin resistance is rather a consequence of excessive postnatal weight gain then of the catch-up growth itself.

In the present study, subjects born SGA showed a reduction in early phase insulin secretion with normal insulin levels in the late phase. Because early phase insulin secretion is important in priming the liver and inhibiting endogenous glucose production during OGTT [41], this defect may reasonably account for the highest glucose levels we observed in OGTT late values in the SGA group.

Children in our study did not show any difference in insulin sensitivity but they had a lower glucose stimulated insulin secretion at 4 years of age. We calculated the Disposition index in order to characterize β-cell function according to the insulin sensitivity and we founded it to be lower in the SGA group but without statistically significant difference. We believe that this absence of significance is more reflecting the lack of statistical power then a real lack of difference.

Changes in pancreatic function seem dependent on the model and timing of fetal growth restriction. Early gestation was identified long time ago as a critical window. In a recent Indian study, the authors did not find an effect of maternal under nutrition in mid-pregnancy pregnancy on human fetal pancreas morphology [42]. By the contrast, in our study, SGA children experienced fetal growth restriction in the 3rd trimester of pregnancy and were thinner at birth, so we believe that they were not "constitutionally small babies" and we can argue for an effect of fetal growth restriction during that moment of pregnancy on pancreas development. The time of beginning of follow-up (22 weeks) did not allow us to know if fetal growth restriction also occurred in the early pregnancy.

Some limits must be taken into account in our study. First, we did not study insulin sensitivity with the gold standard of the euglycemic hyperinsulinemic clamp. Indeed this is a rather complicated method that involves the hospitalization and continuous intravenous administration of insulin and glucose over a period of 3 hours. The use of euglycemic clamp would have been complicated in such young children and ethically doubtable as

A) Estimated fetal weight (EFW) converted to customized percentiles of SGA and AGA fetuses from 22 to 36 weeks of gestation

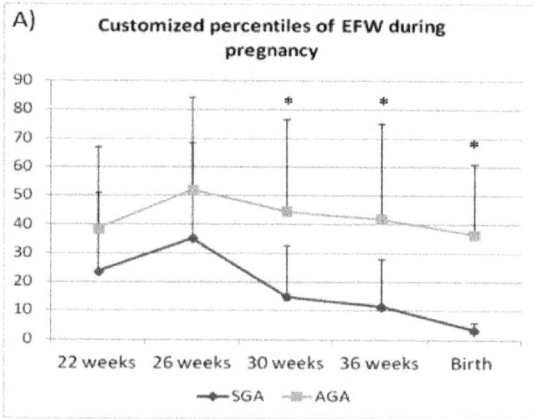

B) Weight z-scores of SGA and AGA babies from birth to 4 years of age

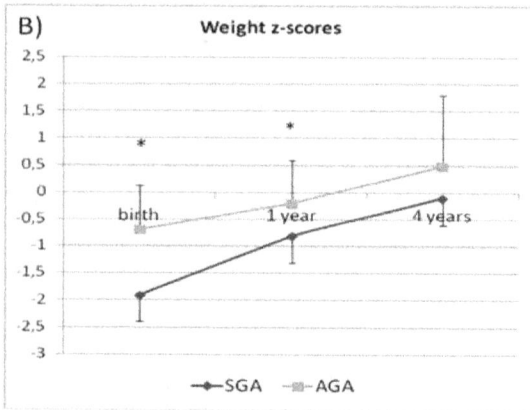

C) Percentage of fat mass between SGA and AGA babies from birth to 4 years of age

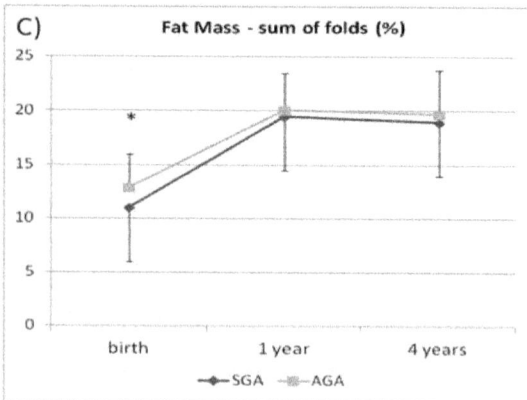

Figure 1. A) Estimated fetal weight (EFW) converted to customized percentiles of SGA and AGA fetuses from 22 to 36 weeks of gestation. B) Birth weight z-scores of SGA and AGA babies from birth to 4 years of age. C) Percentage of fat mass between SGA and AGA babies from birth to 4 years of age.

most of the children in our study were healthy. Another limit of our study is the lack of an independent control group i.e children without risk factors of being born SGA. This kind of comparison would have strengthened our results.

All longitudinal studies are subject to selection bias caused by difficulties to include and keep the children until the end of the follow-up. This raises the question of lack of statistical power of the study, and demands a careful interpretation of our results and confirmation studies. The small number of subjects in our case can be explained by the fact that children were followed prospectively including the fetal period and measurement of fetal growth. Such cohorts are still exceptional and very difficult to organize.

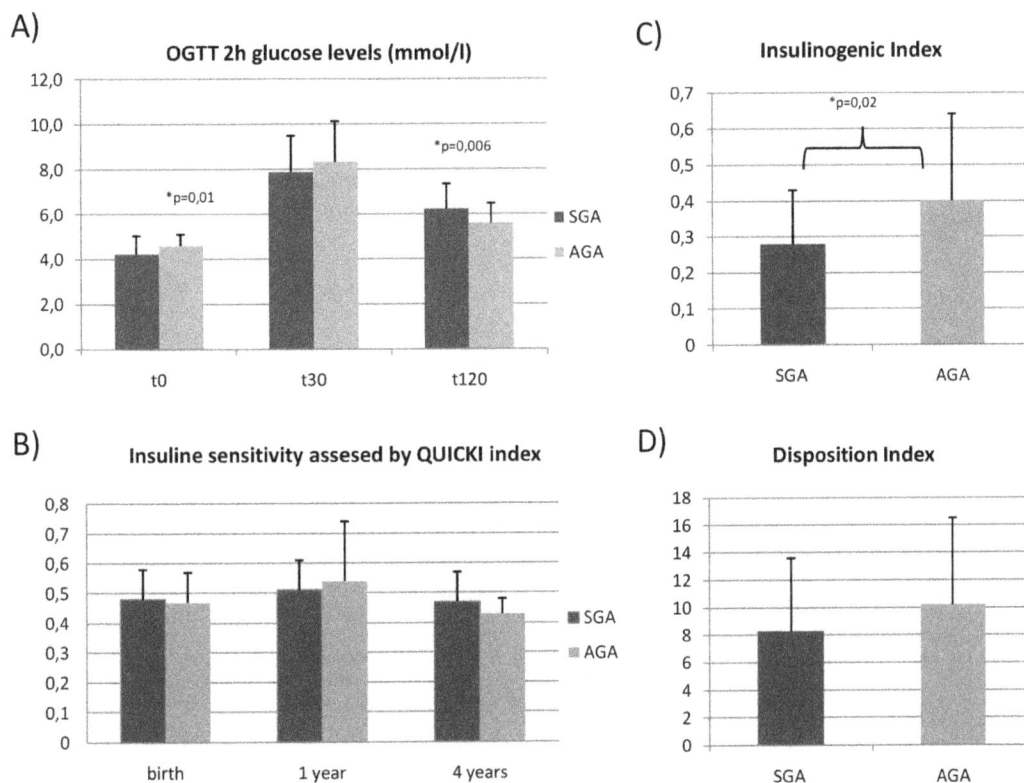

Figure 2. A) Changes in glucose levels during the OGTT between SGA and AGA children at 4 years of age. B) Changes in insulin sensitivity assessed by Quicki Index from birth to 4 years of age between SGA and AGA children. C) Insulinogenic index values between SGA and AGA children at 4 years of age. D) Disposition index values between SGA and AGA children at 4 years of age.

In conclusion, healthy SGA children that experience a compensatory catch-up growth, leading to the restoration of their body composition at the age of four without relative fat mass excess, show mild disturbances of glucose tolerance associated to a lower glucose stimulated insulin secretion at 4-yrs of age suggesting impairment of β-cell function in line with the already described predisposition to type 2 diabetes later in life.

Author Contributions

Conceived and designed the experiments: CL-M. Performed the experiments: JB FN IM. Analyzed the data: IM JB CL-M. Contributed reagents/materials/analysis tools: DC. Wrote the paper: IM JB CL-M. Clinical trial assistant: SD.

References

1. Meas T, Deghmoun S, Alberti C, Carreira E, Armoogum P, et al. (2010) Independent effects of weight gain and fetal programming on metabolic complications in adults born small for gestational age. Diabetologia May;53(5):907–13.

2. Beltrand J, Verkauskiene R, Nicolescu R, Sibony O, Gaucherand P, et al. (2008) Adaptive changes in neonatal hormonal and metabolic profiles induced by fetal growth restriction. J Clin Endocrinol Metab Oct;93(10):4027–32.

3. Whincup PH, Kaye SJ, Owen CG, Huxley R, Cook DG, et al. (2008) Birth weight and risk of type 2 diabetes: a systematic review. JAMA J Am Med Assoc Dec 24;300(24):2886–97.

4. Jaquet D, Gaboriau A, Czernichow P, Levy-Marchal C (2000) Insulin resistance early in adulthood in subjects born with intrauterine growth retardation. J Clin Endocrinol Metab Apr;85(4):1401–6.

5. Ezzahir N, Alberti C, Deghmoun S, Zaccaria I, Czernichow P, et al. (2005) Time course of catch-up in adiposity influences adult anthropometry in individuals who were born small for gestational age. Pediatr Res Aug;58(2):243–7.

6. Garofano A, Czernichow P, Bréant B (1999) Effect of ageing on beta-cell mass and function in rats malnourished during the perinatal period. Diabetologia Jun;42(6):711–8.

7. Garofano A, Czernichow P, Bréant B (1998) Beta-cell mass and proliferation following late fetal and early postnatal malnutrition in the rat. Diabetologia Sep;41(9):1114–20.

8. Jensen CB, Storgaard H, Dela F, Holst JJ, Madsbad S, et al. (2002) Early differential defects of insulin secretion and action in 19-year-old caucasian men who had low birth weight. Diabetes Apr;51(4):1271–80.

9. Stefan N, Weyer C, Levy-Marchal C, Stumvoll M, Knowler WC, et al. (2004) Endogenous glucose production, insulin sensitivity, and insulin secretion in normal glucose-tolerant Pima Indians with low birth weight. Metabolism Jul;53(7):904–11.

10. Schou JH, Pilgaard K, Vilsbøll T, Jensen CB, Deacon CF, et al. (2005) Normal secretion and action of the gut incretin hormones glucagon-like peptide-1 and glucose-dependent insulinotropic polypeptide in young men with low birth weight. J Clin Endocrinol Metab Aug;90(8):4912–9.

11. Hadlock FP, Harrist RB, Sharman RS, Deter RL, Park SK (1985) Estimation of fetal weight with the use of head, body, and femur measurements–a prospective study. Am J Obstet Gynecol Feb 1;151(3):333–7.

12. Gardosi J, Chang A, Kalyan B, Sahota D, Symonds EM (1992) Customised antenatal growth charts. Lancet Feb 1;339(8788):283–7.

13. Gardosi J, Mongelli M, Wilcox M, Chang A (1995) An adjustable fetal weight standard. Ultrasound Obstet Gynecol Off J Int Soc Ultrasound Obstet Gynecol Sep;6(3):168–74.

14. Leroy B, Lefort F (1971) The weight and size of newborn infants at birth. Rev Fr Gynécologie Obstétrique Jul;66(6):391–6.

15. Rolland-Cachera MF, Cole TJ, Sempé M, Tichet J, Rossignol C, et al. (1991) Body Mass Index variations: centiles from birth to 87 years. Eur J Clin Nutr Jan;45(1):13–21.

16. Sempé M (1977) Study of growth from birth to 18 months. Arch Fr Pédiatrie Sep;34(7):687–8.

17. Rodríguez G, Samper MP, Olivares JL, Ventura P, Moreno LA, et al. (2005) Skinfold measurements at birth: sex and anthropometric influence. Arch Dis Child Fetal Neonatal Ed May;90(3):F273–275.

18. Brook CG (1971) Determination of body composition of children from skinfold measurements. Arch Dis Child Apr;46(246):182–4.

19. Siri WE (1956) The gross composition of the body. Adv Biol Med Phys 4:239–80.

20. Rigo J, Nyamugabo K, Picaud JC, Gerard P, Pieltain C, et al.(1998) Reference values of body composition obtained by dual energy X-ray absorptiometry in preterm and term neonates. J Pediatr Gastroenterol Nutr Aug;27(2):184–90.

21. Picaud J-C, Duboeuf F, Vey-Marty V, Delams P, Claris O, et al. (2003) First all-solid pediatric phantom for dual X-ray absorptiometry measurements in infants. J Clin Densitom Off J Int Soc Clin Densitom 6(1):17–23.

22. Katz A, Nambi SS, Mather K, Baron AD, Follmann DA, et al. (2000) Quantitative insulin sensitivity check index: a simple, accurate method for assessing insulin sensitivity in humans. J Clin Endocrinol Metab Jul;85(7):2402–10.

23. Phillips DI, Clark PM, Hales CN, Osmond C (1994) Understanding oral glucose tolerance: comparison of glucose or insulin measurements during the oral glucose tolerance test with specific measurements of insulin resistance and insulin secretion. Diabet Med J Br Diabet Assoc Apr;11(3):286–92.

24. Hanson RL, Pratley RE, Bogardus C, Narayan KM, Roumain JM, et al. (2000) Evaluation of simple indices of insulin sensitivity and insulin secretion for use in epidemiologic studies. Am J Epidemiol Jan 15;151(2):190–8.

25. Matsuda M, DeFronzo RA (1999) Insulin sensitivity indices obtained from oral glucose tolerance testing: comparison with the euglycemic insulin clamp. Diabetes Care Sep;22(9):1462–70.

26. Limesand SW, Jensen J, Hutton JC, Hay WW Jr (2005) Diminished beta-cell replication contributes to reduced beta-cell mass in fetal sheep with intrauterine growth restriction. Am J Physiol Regul Integr Comp Physiol May;288(5):R1297–1305.

27. Garofano A, Czernichow P, Bréant B (1997) In utero undernutrition impairs rat beta-cell development. Diabetologia Oct;40(10):1231–4.

28. Holness MJ (1996) Impact of early growth retardation on glucoregulatory control and insulin action in mature rats. Am J Physiol Jun;270(6 Pt 1):E946–954.

29. Yuan Q, Chen L, Liu C, Xu K, Mao X, et al. (2011) Postnatal pancreatic islet β cell function and insulin sensitivity at different stages of lifetime in rats born with intrauterine growth retardation. PloS One 6(10):e25167.

30. Soto N, Bazaes RA, Peña V, Salazar T, Avila A, et al. (2003) Insulin sensitivity and secretion are related to catch-up growth in small-for-gestational-age infants at age 1 year: results from a prospective cohort. J Clin Endocrinol Metab Aug;88(8):3645–50.

31. Eriksson JG, Forsén T, Tuomilehto J, Winter PD, Osmond C, et al. (1999) Catch-up growth in childhood and death from coronary heart disease: longitudinal study. BMJ Feb 13;318(7181):427–31.

32. Fagerberg B, Bondjers L, Nilsson P (2004) Low birth weight in combination with catch-up growth predicts the occurrence of the metabolic syndrome in men at late middle age: the Atherosclerosis and Insulin Resistance study. J Intern Med Sep;256(3):254–9.

33. Beltrand J, Lévy-Marchal C (2008) Pathophysiology of insulin resistance in subjects born small for gestational age. Best Pract Res Clin Endocrinol Metab Jun;22(3):503–15.

34. Ong KK, Ahmed ML, Emmett PM, Preece MA, Dunger DB (2000) Association between postnatal catch-up growth and obesity in childhood: prospective cohort study. BMJ Apr 8;320(7240):967–71.

35. Kerkhof GF, Leunissen RWJ, Hokken-Koelega ACS (2012) Early origins of the metabolic syndrome: role of small size at birth, early postnatal weight gain, and adult IGF-I. J Clin Endocrinol Metab Aug;97(8):2637–43.

36. Silva AAM, Santos CJN, Amigo H, Barbieri MA, Bustos P, et al. (2012) Birth weight, current body mass index, and insulin sensitivity and secretion in young adults in two Latin American populations. Nutr Metab Cardiovasc Dis NMCD Jun;22(6):533–9.

37. Cook JT, Levy JC, Page RC, Shaw JA, Hattersley AT, et al. (1993) Association of low birth weight with beta cell function in the adult first degree relatives of non-insulin dependent diabetic subjects. BMJ Jan 30;306(6873):302–6.

38. Ong KK, Petry CJ, Emmett PM, Sandhu MS, Kiess W, et al. (2004) Insulin sensitivity and secretion in normal children related to size at birth, postnatal growth, and plasma insulin-like growth factor-I levels. Diabetologia Jun;47(6):1064–70.

39. Mericq V, Ong KK, Bazaes R, Peña V, Avila A, et al. (2005) Longitudinal changes in insulin sensitivity and secretion from birth to age three years in small- and appropriate-for-gestational-age children. Diabetologia Dec;48(12):2609–14.

40. Beltrand J, Nicolescu R, Kaguelidou F, Verkauskiene R, Sibony O, et al. (2009) Catch-up growth following fetal growth restriction promotes rapid restoration of fat mass but without metabolic consequences at one year of age. PloS One 4(4):e5343.

41. Abdul-Ghani MA, Williams K, DeFronzo RA, Stern M (2007) What is the best predictor of future type 2 diabetes? Diabetes Care Jun;30(6):1544–8.

42. Kumar PU, Ramalaxmi BA, Venkiah K, Sesikeran B (2013) Effect of maternal undernutrition on human foetal pancreas morphology in second trimester of pregnancy. Indian J Med Res Feb;137(2):302–7.

2

IGF-IR Signal Transduction Protein Content and Its Activation by IGF-I in Human Placentas: Relationship with Gestational Age and Birth Weight

Germán Iñiguez[1]*, Juan José Castro[1], Mirna Garcia[2], Elena Kakarieka[2], M. Cecilia Johnson[1], Fernando Cassorla[1], Verónica Mericq[1]

1 Institute of Maternal and Child Research, University of Chile, Santiago, Chile, 2 Hospital Clínico San Borja-Arriarán, University of Chile, Santiago, Chile

Abstract

Introduction: The human placenta expresses the IGF-I and IGF-IR proteins and their intracellular signal components (IRS-1, AKT and mTOR). The aim of this study was to assess the IGF-IR content and activation of downstream signaling molecules in placentas from newborns who were classified by gestational age and birth weight. We studied placentas from 25 term appropriate (T-AGA), 26 term small (T-SGA), 22 preterm AGA (PT-AGA), and 20 preterm SGA (PT-SGA) newborns. The total and phosphorylated IGF-IR, IRS-1, AKT, and mTOR contents were determined by Western Blot and normalized by actin or with their respective total content. The effect of IGF-I was determined by stimulating placental explants with recombinant IGF-I 10^{-8} mol/L for 15, 30, and 60 minutes.

Results: The IGF-IR content was higher in T-SGA compared to T-AGA placentas, and the IRS-1 content was higher in PT-placentas compared with their respective T-placentas. The effect of IGF-I on the phosphorylated forms of IGF-IR was increased in T-SGA (150%) and PT-SGA (300%) compared with their respective AGA placentas. In addition, AKT serine phosphorylation was higher in PT-SGA compared to PT-AGA and T-SGA placentas (90% and 390% respectively).

Conclusion: The higher protein content and response to IGF-I of IGF-IR, IRS-1, and AKT observed in SGA placentas may represent a compensatory mechanism in response to fetal growth restriction.

Editor: Ana Claudia Zenclussen, Medical Faculty, Otto-von-Guericke University Magdeburg, Medical Faculty, Germany

Funding: This work was supported by FONDECYT Grant 111 0240. The funders had no role in study design, data collection and analysis, decision to publish, or preparation of the manuscript.

Competing Interests: The authors have declared that no competing interests exist.

* Email: giniguez@med.uchile.cl

Introduction

Fetal growth is under the control of genetic, environmental, and nutritional factors. Intrauterine growth restriction (IUGR) is an important obstetrical problem and refers to a fetus that has not reached its growth potential [1]. This condition may be the consequence of maternal, fetal, or placental factors. Growth-restricted fetuses/newborns are characterized by increased fetal and neonatal mortality and morbidity [2,3], as well as preterm birth and risk of chronic disorders in adult life [4,5].

Recent advances in neonatal care have led to an improvement in the clinical outcome of premature infants (gestational age <37 weeks). Unfortunately, some of these infants develop both [6] early and late morbidities, which may include motor, cognitive, visual, hearing, social-emotional, growth and metabolic problems [7].

The insulin-like growth factors (IGFs) have potent mitogenic activity and appear to be major determinants of fetal growth [8,9,10]. These factors are expressed both in the fetus and placenta in most species[11,12,13].

IGF-I initiates its biological effects by binding to its cell surface receptor, i.e., IGF-IR [14]. This tyrosine kinase receptor is composed of two heterodimers, which consist of an α- and a β-subunit. Ligand binding to IGF-IR leads the endogenous tyrosine kinase activation resulting in the autophosphorylation of tyrosine residues located in the cytoplasmic regions of the receptor β-subunit, followed by phosphorylation of downstream signaling pathways. One of the most important families of proteins which are phosphorylated by activated IGF-IR are the insulin receptor substrate (IRS) proteins [15,16]. The activated IRS proteins serve as docking proteins for several signaling molecules, which become activated upon binding. This ultimately results in the activation of at least two main signaling pathways: the Ras/Raf/mitogen-activated protein kinase (MAPK) pathway and the phosphoinositide-3 kinase (PI3K)/AKT/mTOR/p70S6K pathway [17]. Upon activation, these downstream molecules mediate a wide variety of intracellular signals in many cells and tissues, including those regulating glucose transport, protein synthesis, cell proliferation, and survival [17].

The aim of this study was to assess whether IGF-IR and downstream signaling molecules content and activation induced by IGF-I have differences in placentas of different gestational ages and according to birth weight. We also analyzed the associations between the placental protein content and IGF-I induction with birth length and placental weight.

Materials and Methods

Sample collection

The placental tissue was collected immediately after delivery. We selected placentas from full term (T: 37–40 weeks of gestation) and preterm newborns (PT: 32–36 weeks of gestation). The newborns were delivered by cesarean section in approximately one third of the cases and their Apgar scores were normal. The newborns with a birth weight between the 10th and the 90th percentiles for gestational age were defined as appropriate for gestational age (AGA), and the newborns with a birth weight below the 10th percentile as small for gestational age (SGA) using Chilean birth weight references [18]. Exclusion criteria were maternal hypertension, diabetes, or a reduced amount of amniotic fluid at delivery. We studied 93 gestations; 25 T-AGA placentas, 26 T-SGA placentas, 22 PT-AGA placentas and 20 PT-SGA placentas. The clinical characteristics of the T-AGA, T-SGA, PT-AGA and PT-SGA neonates are shown in Table 1. All mothers gave their written informed consent and this protocol was approved by the Institutional Review Boards of the San Borja Arriarán Clinical Hospital and the School of Medicine of the University of Chile in Santiago, Chile.

Each placenta was inspected by a pathologist (EK) for any possible abnormalities. Placental villous tissue was collected from preterm and term pregnancies, 30–50 g villous tissue was dissected and quickly washed thoroughly in cold sterile saline solution (NaCl 0.154 mol/L). To study total protein content, placental tissue was dissected free of chorion and decidua into 80–100 mg pieces, washed in sterile saline solution and immediately frozen in liquid nitrogen and stored at $-80°C$.

Placental explant cultures

Small fragments of placental tissue (10–20 mg) were dissected from the placenta and washed in ice-cold sterile saline solution. Three fragments per well were placed and cultured at $37°C$ in 12-well plates for 1 hour in 2.0 ml of DMEM/F-12 (Invitrogen, Life Technologies; Carlsbad, CA, USA) medium containing 100 U/ml penicillin100 µg/ml streptomycin and 0.25 µg/ml amphotericin (Invitrogen, Life Technologies). Subsequently, the medium was changed by fresh DMEM/F-12 medium and the explants were stimulated with 10^{-8} mol/L IGF-I (Austral Biologicals, San Ramon, CA, USA) during 0 (basal), 15, 30 or 60 minutes; this dose of IGF-I was previously determined in our laboratory by testing IGF-I concentrations ranging from 10^{-9} to 10^{-6} mol/L in human placental explants; we selected 10^{-8} M because at this concentration we observed a significant increase in Tyr-IGF-IR (data not shown); in addition this concentration has been employed in previous studies [19]. At each time point the explants were removed, frozen in liquid nitrogen and stored at $-80°C$.

Protein extraction

Frozen placental tissue was powdered in a ceramic mortar with liquid N_2 and homogenized for 30 seconds with a mechanical homogenizer (Kontes Glass Company, Vineland, NJ, USA) in ice-cold Tissue Extraction Reagent 1 (Biosource International, Inc, Camarillo, CA, USA) supplemented with 1% Triton X-100 (Sigma-Aldrich, St Louis, MO, USA) and anti-proteases [Complete, Mini, EDTA-free Protease Inhibitor Cocktail Tablets, Roche Applied Science, Basel, Switzerland)].

The tissue homogenate was incubated for 30 minutes at $4°C$ with gentle stirring and centrifuged at 10,000 x g for 30 minutes.

Table 1. Anthropometric data for T-SGA, T-AGA, PT-SGA and PT-AGA newborns.

	T-SGA (26)	T-AGA (25)	PT-SGA (20)	PT-AGA (22)
Gestational age (weeks)	38.3±0.2	39.4±0.2	34.1±0.6	34.9±0.3
Gender: males/females	10/16	11/14	11/9	13/9
Birth weight (g)	2621±28*	3418±75	1755±124*	2449±75
Birth weight (SDS)	-1.66±0.07*	-0.07±0.16	-2.12±0.19*	-0.46±0.13
Birth length (cm)	47.2±0.3*	50.2±0.3	40.1±1.2*	45.0±0.8
Birth Length (SDS)	-1.66±0.15*	-0.17±0.17	-2.83±0.51*	-0.79±0.36
Placental Weight (SDS)	531±19*	654±23	405±47*	596±34

Data are expressed as mean ± SEM. * A p value of less than 0.05 was considered statistically significant.

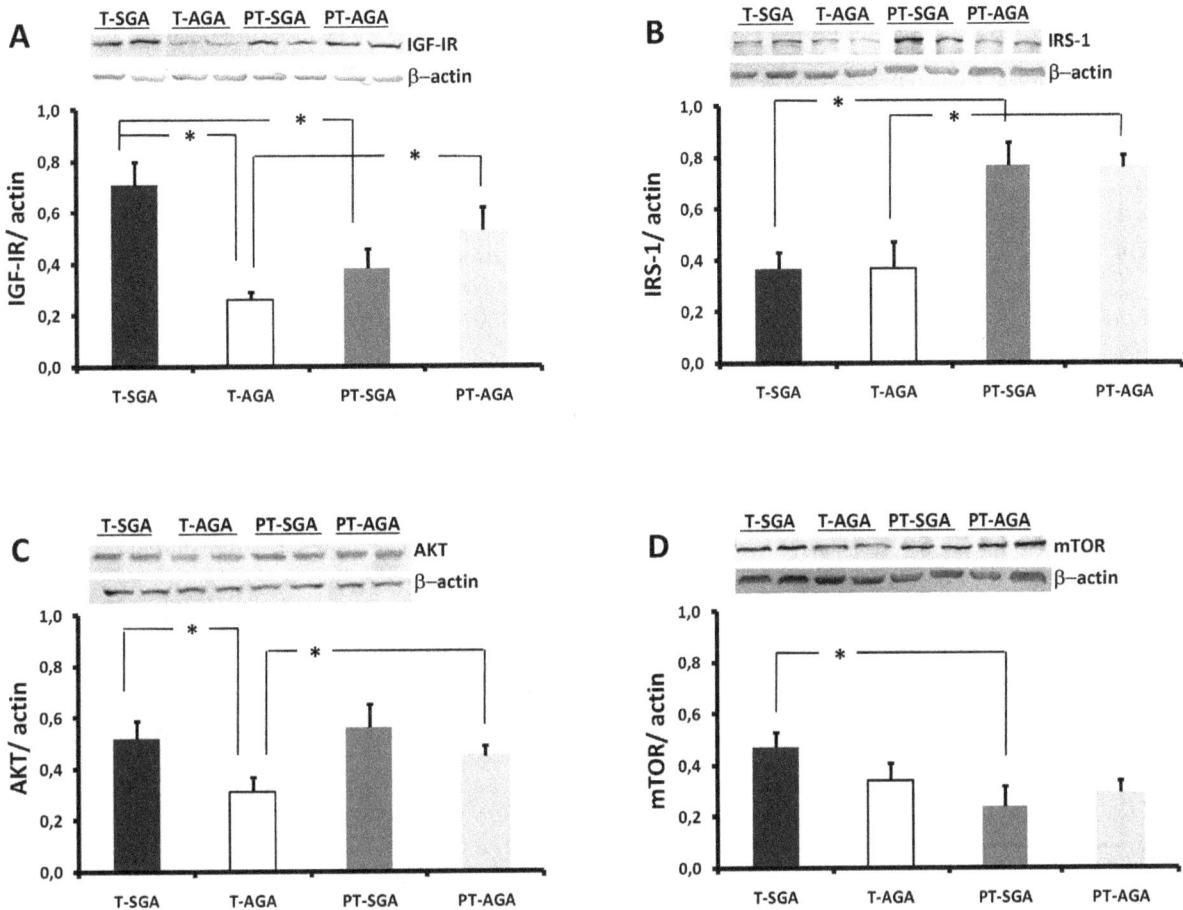

Figure 1. Placental IGF-IR (A), IRS-1 (B), AKT (C), and mTOR (D) obtained from T-SGA (n = 26), T-AGA (n = 25), PT-SGA (n = 20) and PT-AGA (n = 22) pregnancies. Representative electrophoretic gel for each protein is included in each graph. A p value of less than 0.05 was considered statistically significant.

The resulting supernatant was collected and assayed for protein concentration using the BCA protein assay kit (Pierce, Rockford, IL, USA) with bovine serum albumin (BSA) as standard.

Western blot analysis

Equal amounts (25 µg) of placental proteins were resolved by electrophoresis using 8% SDS-polyacrylamide gels and then transferred to nitrocellulose membranes (BioRad Laboratories, Hercules, CA). The membranes were blocked with 5% BSA in TBS-T (20 mmol/L Tris pH 7.2, 137 mmol/L, NaCl, 0.1% (v/v) and Tween-20) for 1 h at room temperature. Blots were probed with antibodies against total IGF-IRβ, IRS-I and AKT [Santa Cruz Biotechnology, Santa Cruz, CA, USA]; mTOR (Cell Signaling, Danvers, MA, USA), phospho-IGF-IR-Tyr1161, (Abcam,Cambridge, England), phospho-IRS-1- tyr1229, AKT-Ser473 and AKT-Thr308 (Santa Cruz Biotechnology,) and phospho-mTOR-Ser2481 (Cell Signaling). Anti β-actin (Sigma-Aldrich) was used to normalize the different placental protein content. After extensive washing, bands were detected with the appropriate horseradish peroxidase-conjugated secondary antibodies (Rockland Immunochemical Research, Gilbertsville, PA, USA), followed by enhanced chemiluminescence (ECL plus Western Blotting Detection System, Amersham Biosciences, Bucking Hanshire, UK).

The images were acquired and evaluated by scanning densitometry using the UltraQuant Image Acquisition and Analysis Software (Ultralum Incorporated, Claremont, CA, USA); specific times of exposure and settings were established for each protein. Total protein content band intensity was expressed in arbitrary units (optic densitometry units, AU) and normalized relative to β-actin content. The activation induced by IGF-I of each protein was obtained by the ratio of phosphorylated-protein/total protein content at each time point.

Statistical analysis

Results are shown as mean ± SEM. Differences within each group (T-AGA, T-SGA, PT-AGA and PT-SGA) were assessed by one-way ANOVA or Kruskall-Wallis, followed by the Bonferroni test for multiple comparisons. According to the distribution of the data, correlations were established using the Pearson or Spearman test. Statistics were performed using SPSS v21, and a value of $p < 0.05$ was considered significant.

Results

Clinical data of the subjects studied and placental weight are shown in Table 1. As expected, birth weight, birth length and placental weight from SGA newborns was significantly lower than their AGA counterparts.

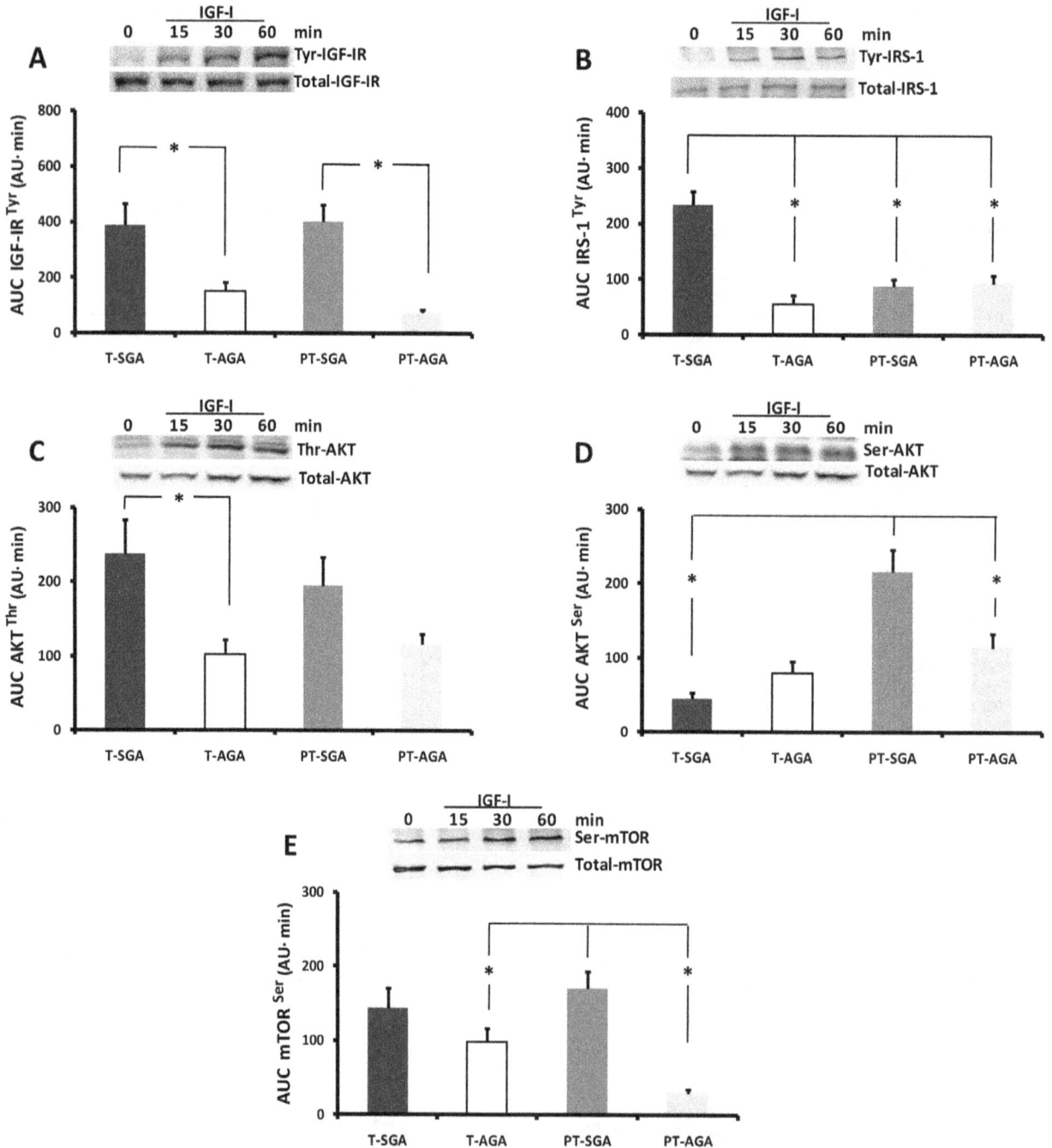

Figure 2. Activation of Tyr-IGF-IR (A), Tyr-IRS-1(B), Thr-AKT (C), Ser-AKT (D) and Ser-mTOR (E) with IGF-I 10-8 mol/L in placental explants from T-SGA, T- AGA, PT-SGA and PT-AGA newborns. Representative electrophoretic gel for each protein is included in each graph. The activation is expressed as area under the curve AUC. A p value of less than 0.05 was considered statistically significant.

Ex vivo Placental Total protein content

The total protein contents of IGF-IR, IRS, AKT and mTOR from SGA and AGA placentas is shown in Figure 1. The protein content of IGF-IR was higher in T-SGA placentas compared with T-AGA (170%; p<0.001) and PT-SGA placentas (82%; p = 0.014); we also observed a higher IGF-IR content in PT-AGA compared with T-AGA placentas (103%; p = 0.027) (Figure 1A).

The content of IRS-1 content was higher in PT-SGA compared with T-SGA placentas (110%; p<0.001) and in PT-AGA compared with T-AGA placentas (105%; p<0.001) (Figure 1B).

The AKT placental content was higher in T-SGA compared to T-AGA placentas (67%; p = 0.047), but not between preterm placentas. We also observed a higher AKT content in the PT-AGA compared to T-AGA placentas (45%; p = 0.012) (Figure 1C).

The mTOR content was similar in SGA and AGA placentas from term and preterm newborns. However, we found higher

Table 2. Correlations between: birth weight, birth length and placental weight with placental protein content.

	Birth Weight (SDS)	Birth Length (SDS)	Placental Weight (g)
IGF-IR	−0.272*	−0.214*	−0.161
IRS-1	−0.056	−0.127	−0.126
AKT	−0.284*	−0.335*	−0.247*
mTOR	−0.054	0.015	0.031

* A p value of less than 0.05 was considered statistically significant.

mTOR protein content in T-SGA compared with PT-SGA (105%; p = 0.008) (Figure 1D).

Effect of IGF-I on IGF-IR, AKT and mTOR activation.

We studied the effect of stimulation with IGF-I 10^{-8} mol/L for 60 min on the phosphorylation of IGF-IR, AKT, and mTOR in explants from term and preterm placentas. The integrated activation of each protein is shown in the Figure 2 as the area under the curve (AUC), calculated by the trapezoidal rule.

The activation of IGF-IR was higher in T-SGA (155%; p = 0.047) compared with T-AGA and in PT-SGA compared with PT-AGA (300%; p<0.001) placentas (Figure 2A). The tyrosine IRS-1 activation induced by IGF-I was higher in T-SGA compared with T-AGA placentas (314%; p<0.001) and compared with PT-SGA (165%; p<0.001) placentas, but it was lower in T-AGA when compared with PT-AGA placentas (68%; p = 0.013) (Figure 2B).

AUC phosphorylation of placental threonine AKT after one hour of incubation with IGF-I was higher in placentas from SGA compared to AGA newborns (131%; p = 0.033) (Figure 2C). The AUC for serine-AKT was higher in PT-SGA compared with PT-AGA (90%; p = 0.012) and with T-SGA placentas (390%; p<0.001) Figure 2D).

There were no differences in the activation of placental mTOR induced by IGF-I (Figure 2E) in the placentas from term newborns, but it was higher in PT-SGA compared with PT-AGA placentas (470%; p<0.001), and in T-AGA compared to PT-AGA placentas (230%; p = 0.001).

Correlation of placental protein contents and IGF-I responses with birth weight, birth length and placental weight

The correlations between IGF-IR protein content and signaling molecules with birth weight, birth length and placental weight are shown in Table 2, and the correlations between the activation of these proteins after stimulation with IGF-I with birth weight, birth

length and placental weight are shown in Table 3. We observed an inverse correlation between the content and activation of IGF-IR, IR and AKT with birth weight and birth length (SDS).

Discussion

To our knowledge this is the first study that investigates the IGF-IR signal transduction pathway in human preterm and term placentas from SGA and AGA newborns. In addition, we studied the activation of these placental proteins induced by IGF-I. We observed differences in the protein content and activation of the IGF-IR signal transduction pathway according to gestational age and birth weight.

The increased IGF-IR content observed in T-SGA compared with T-AGA placentas has been previously described by our group [20]. However, this difference was not found in the preterm group, perhaps due to a maturational compensatory process to enhance growth that it is not ongoing at that gestational age. The higher IGF-IR protein content observed in SGA placentas is in concordance with some studies but not with others [21,22,23]. These differences are probably related to the different etiologies of the SGA newborns studied in each series, but in particular, by their length of gestation as suggested by our results. In one of these studies, they compared preterm SGA with term AGA placentas [22] and in another study [23] the authors analyzed placentas from comparable gestational ages of approximately 36 weeks. The *in vitro* IGF-IR activation induced by IGF-I showed a similar behavior, with both T-SGA and PT-SGA placentas showing a higher activation compared with their respective AGA placentas. These findings suggest that the higher receptor content and activation induced by IGF-I represent a possible compensatory mechanism of the placenta in response to fetal growth restriction in both term and preterm gestations.

In addition, our study showed a higher IRS-1 protein content in placentas from premature newborns. However, we observed a higher tyrosine activation of IRS-1 in response to IGF-I in T-SGA compared with the other groups of placentas, Two studies have

Table 3. Correlations between birth weight, birth length and placental weight with activated proteins in placental explants.

	Birth Weight (SDS)	Birth Length (SDS)	Placental Weight (g)
AUC Tyr-IGF-IR	−0.239*	−0.250*	−0.106
AUC Tyr-IRS-1	−0.420*	−0.380*	−0.243
AUC Thr-AKT	−0.377*	−0.277*	−0.177
AUC Ser-AKT	−0.244*	−0.179	−0.068
AUC Ser-mTOR	−0.442*	−0.235	−0.196

* A p value of less than 0.05 was considered statistically significant. [AUC] = area under curve).

described a higher basal (*ex vivo*) IRS-1 phospho protein in AGA compared to SGA placentas [22,23]. The increased basal phosphorylation of IRS reported by these authors in placenta, does not necessarily represent the responsiveness of the placental tissue to stimulation with IGF-I. It is interesting to consider the significant differences in IRS-1 protein content observed in the placentas from preterm compared with term pregnancies. We also observed an increased activation of tyrosine-IRS-1 in SGA placentas, particularly from term newborns, suggesting that following acute IGF-I stimulation, IRS-1 is phosphorylated on tyrosine residues to propagate IGF-I signaling, as has been observed in other experimental models [24,25,26].

The AKT activation by IGF-I is a multistep process involving translocation and phosphorylation. Two phosphorylation sites, Thr308 and Ser473, appear to be critical for the activation of AKT induced by growth factors [27]. Phosphorylation of Thr308 in the activation loop by PDK1 is essential for AKT activation, and of Ser473 at the C-terminal tail by either autophosphorylation, or by PDK2 for maximal activation of kinase activity [27].

Although total protein placental AKT and Thr-AKT phosphorylation were higher in T-SGA compared to T-AGA placentas, we observed an increased Ser-AKT in PT-SGA, compared to T-SGA and PT-AGA placentas, suggesting another possible compensatory placental mechanism in response to fetal growth restriction. As mentioned, the Thr308 phosphorylation activates partially AKT, but for complete activation, the phosphorylation of Ser473 is required for regulating the function of several cellular proteins involved in glucose [28] and amino acid [29] metabolism, survival/apoptosis, cell differentiation and proliferation [30]. The fully Ser-AKT phosphorylated form induced by IGF-I in PT-SGA placentas, suggests that this placental compensatory mechanism is probably more important in preterm pregnancies.

The mTOR protein is an evolutionarily conserved serine/threonine kinase that integrates signals from multiple pathways [31], including nutrients (amino acids and glucose) [32], growth factors [29] (insulin and IGF-I), hormones [33] (e.g., leptin), and different stresses [34] (e.g., starvation, hypoxia, and DNA damage). It regulates a wide variety of eukaryotic cellular functions, such as transcription, translation, transcription, protein turnover, cell growth, differentiation, metabolism, energy balance,

and stress response [35]. This suggests that mTOR is involved in the uptake of amino acids during pregnancy for fetal development. We did not find differences in placental mTOR contents between T-SGA and PT-SGA compared with their respective AGA placentas, but the mTOR content was higher in T-SGA compared to PT-SGA placentas. The greater activation of mTOR induced by IGF-I in PT-SGA placentas suggests that this molecule is more sensitive to IGF-I in preterm SGA placentas. The fact that no differences were observed in the activation of mTOR in placentas from term newborns indicates that this molecule is a key component of placental IGF-I signaling during early gestation and may regulate fetal growth.

Interestingly, most protein contents and their activation by IGF-I were inversely related with birth weight and birth length, suggesting that this placental signal transduction pathway plays an important role in fetal growth. The inverse relationship between fetal weight with IGF-IR, IRS-1, AKT and mTOR placental content and with the activation of these proteins induced by IGF-I, suggest that this placental signal transduction pathway plays an important role in fetal growth.

In conclusion, we describe for the first time that the IGF-IR/IRS-1/AKT/mTOR protein contents, as well as their activation induced by IGF-I in human placental explants are up-regulated in term and preterm SGA compared to AGA placentas. In addition, we observed an inverse correlation between birth weight and the placental content, as well as the activation of these proteins. These findings may represent a compensatory placental mechanism in response to fetal growth restriction.

Acknowledgments

We are grateful for the generous contribution of all the patients who donated the placentas.

Author Contributions

Conceived and designed the experiments: GI MG EK MCJ FC VM. Performed the experiments: GI JJC MCJ. Analyzed the data: GI EK MCJ FC VM. Contributed reagents/materials/analysis tools: GI MG EK. Wrote the paper: GI MG EK MCJ FC VM. Obtained the placentas MG. Inspected the placentas EK.

References

1. Resnik R (2002) Intrauterine growth restriction. Obstet Gynecol; 99:490–496.
2. Low JA, Handley-Derry MH, Burke SO, Peters RD, Pater EA, et al. (1992) Association of intrauterine fetal growth retardation and learning deficits at age 9 to 11 years. Am J Obstet Gynecol 167:1499–1505.
3. Kramer MS, Olivier M, McLean FH, Willis DM, Usher RH (1990) Impact of intrauterine growth retardation and body proportionality on fetal and neonatal outcome. Pediatrics 86:707–713.
4. Hattersley AT, Tooke JE (1999) The fetal insulin hypothesis: an alternative explanation of the association of low birth weight with diabetes and vascular disease. Lancet 353:1789–1792.
5. Barker DJ (2004) The developmental origins of well-being. Philos Trans R Soc Lond B Biol Sci 359:1359–1366.
6. Ge WJ, Mirea L, Yang J, Bassil KL, Lee SK, et al. (2013) Prediction of neonatal outcomes in extremely preterm neonates. Pediatrics. 132(4):e876–85.
7. Institute of Medicine (US) Committee on Understanding Premature Birth and Assuring Healthy Outcomes, Behrman RE, Butler AS (2007) Preterm Birth: Causes, Consequences, and Prevention. Washington, DC: National Academies Press.
8. DeChiara TM, Efstratiadis A, Robertson EJ (1990) A growth-deficiency phenotype in heterozygous mice carrying an insulin-like growth factor II gene disrupted by targeting. Nature; 345:78–80.
9. Baker J, Liu JP, Robertson EJ, Efstratiadis A (1993) A role of insulin-like growth factors in embryonic and postnatal growth. Cell 75:73–82.
10. Liu JP, Baker J, Perkins AS, Robertson EJ, Efstratiadis A (1993) Mice carrying null mutations of the genes encoding insulin-like growth factor I (Igf-1) and type 1 IGF receptor (Igf1r). Cell 75:59–72.
11. Fowden AL (2003) The insulin-like growth factors and feto-placental growth. Placenta 24:803–812.
12. Han VK, Carter AM (2000) Spatial and temporal patterns of expression of messenger RNA for insulin-like growth factors and their binding proteins in the placenta of man and laboratory animals. Placenta 21:289–305.
13. Iñiguez G, Argandoña F, Medina P, González C, San Martin S, et al. (2011) Acid-labile subunit (ALS) gene expression and protein content in human placentas: differences according to birth weight. J Clin Endocrinol Metab 96(1):187–91.
14. Bornfeldt KE, Raines EW, Nakano T, Graves LM, Krebs EG, et al. (1994) Insulin-like growth factor-I and platelet-derived growth factor-BB induce directed migration of human arterial smooth muscle cells via signaling pathways that are distinct from those of proliferation. J Clin Invest 93: 1266–1274.
15. White MF (1997) The insulin signalling system and the IRS proteins. Diabetologia (Suppl. 2):S2–S17.
16. White MF (2002) IRS proteins and the common path to diabetes. Am. J. Physiol. Endocrinol. Metab. 283:E413–E422.
17. Foulstone E, Prince S, Zaccheo O, Burns JL, Harper J, et al. (2005) Insulin-like growth factor ligands, receptors, and binding proteins in cancer. J. Pathol. 205:145–153.
18. Milad M, Novoa JM, Fabres J, Samame MM, Aspillaga C (2010) Recomendación sobre Curvas de Crecimiento Intrauterino. Rev. Chil. Pediatr. 81 (3): 264–274.
19. Harris LK, Crocker IP, Baker PN, Aplin JD, Westwood M (2011) IGF2 actions on trophoblast in human placenta are regulated by the insulin-like growth factor 2 receptor, which can function as both a signaling and clearance receptor. Biol Reprod. 84(3):440–6.

20. Iñiguez G, González CA, Argandoña F, Kakarieka E, Johnson MC, et al., (2010) Expression and protein content of IGF-I and IGF-I receptor in placentas from small, adequate and large for gestational age newborns. Horm Res Paediatr 73(5):320–7.

21. Abu-Amero SN, Ali Z, Bennett P, Vaughan JI, Moore GE (1998) Expression of the insulin-like growth factors and their receptors in term placentas: a comparison between normal and IUGR births. Mol Reprod Dev. 49:229–35.

22. Laviola L, Perrini S, Belsanti G, Natalicchio A, Montrone C, et al. (2005) Intrauterine growth restriction in humans is associated with abnormalities in placental insulin-like growth factor signaling. Endocrinology. 146(3):1498–1505.

23. Street ME, Viani I, Ziveri MA, Volta C, Smerieri A, et al. (2011) Impairment of insulin receptor signal transduction in placentas of intra-uterine growth-restricted newborns and its relationship with fetal growth. Eur J Endocrinol. 164(1):45–52.

24. Boura-Halfon S, Zick Y (2009) Phosphorylation of IRS proteins, insulin action, and insulin resistance. Am J Physiol Endocrinol Metab. 6(4):E581–91.

25. Peres SB, de Moraes SM, Costa CE, Brito LC, Takada J, et al. (2005) Endurance exercise training increases insulin responsiveness in isolated adipocytes through IRS/PI3-kinase/Akt pathway. J Appl Physiol (1985) 98(3):1037–43.

26. Wang CC, Adochio RL, Leitner JW, Abeyta IM, Draznin B, et al. (2013) Acute effects of different diet compositions on skeletal muscle insulin signalling in obese individuals during caloric restriction. Metabolism 62(4):595–603.

27. Ji P, Osorio JS, Drackley JK, Loor JJ (2012) Overfeeding a moderate energy diet prepartum does not impair bovine subcutaneous adipose tissue insulin signal transduction and induces marked changes in peripartal gene network expression. J Dairy Sci. 95(8):4333–4351.

28. Chen R, Kim O, Yang J, Sato K, Eisenmann KM, et al. (2001) Regulation of Akt/PKB activation by tyrosine phosphorylation. J Biol Chem. 276(34):31858–62.

29. Ma Y, Zhu MJ, Uthlaut AB, Nijland MJ, Nathanielsz PW, et al. (2011) Upregulation of growth signaling and nutrient transporters in cotyledons of early to mid-gestational nutrient restricted ewes. Placenta. 32(3): 255–263.

30. Aye IL, Jansson T, Powell TL (2013) Interleukin-1β inhibits insulin signaling and prevents insulin-stimulated system A amino acid transport in primary human trophoblasts. Mol Cell Endocrinol. 381(1-2):46–55.

31. Hasson SP, Rubinek T, Ryvo L, Wolf I (2013) Endocrine Resistance in Breast Cancer: Focus on the hosphatidylinositol 3-Kinase/Akt/Mammalian Target of Rapamycin Signaling Pathway. Breast Care (Basel). 8(4):248–255.

32. Watanabe R, Wei L, Huang J (2011) mTOR Signaling, Function, Novel Inhibitors, and Therapeutic TargetsJ Nucl Med 52 (4): 497–500.

33. Wullschleger S, Loewith R, Hall MN (2006) TOR signaling in growth and metabolism. Cell. 124:471–484.

34. Harlan SM, Guo DF, Morgan DA, Fernandes-Santos C, Rahmouni K (2013) Hypothalamic mTORC1 signaling controls sympathetic nerve activity and arterial pressure and mediates leptin effects. Cell Metab. 17(4): 599–606.

35. Sengupta S, Peterson TR, Sabatini DM (2010) Regulation of the mTOR complex 1 pathway by nutrients, growth factors, and stress. Mol Cell. 40(2):310–22.

3

POPI (Pediatrics: Omission of Prescriptions and Inappropriate Prescriptions): Development of a Tool to Identify Inappropriate Prescribing

Sonia Prot-Labarthe[1][*][¶], Thomas Weil[1,2][¶], François Angoulvant[3], Rym Boulkedid[4,5], Corinne Alberti[4,5,6], Olivier Bourdon[1,2,7]

1 Pharmacie, AP-HP Hôpital Robert-Debré, Paris, France, 2 Pharmacie Clinique, Université Paris Descartes, Paris, France, 3 Service d'Accueil des Urgences, AP-HP Hôpital Robert-Debré, Paris, France, 4 Unité d'Epidémiologie Clinique, AP-HP Hôpital Robert Debré, Paris, France, 5 Inserm U 1123 et CIC 1426, Paris, France, 6 Sorbonne Paris Cité UMRS 1123, Université Paris Diderot, Paris, France, 7 Laboratoire Educations et Pratiques de Santé, Université Paris XIII, Bobigny, France

Abstract

Introduction: Rational prescribing for children is an issue for all countries and has been inadequately studied. Inappropriate prescriptions, including drug omissions, are one of the main causes of medication errors in this population. Our aim is to develop a screening tool to identify omissions and inappropriate prescriptions in pediatrics based on French and international guidelines.

Methods: A selection of diseases was included in the tool using data from social security and hospital statistics. A literature review was done to obtain criteria which could be included in the tool called POPI. A 2-round-Delphi consensus technique was used to establish the content validity of POPI; panelists were asked to rate their level of agreement with each proposition on a 9-point Likert scale and add suggestions if necessary.

Results: 108 explicit criteria (80 inappropriate prescriptions and 28 omissions) were obtained and submitted to a 16-member expert panel (8 pharmacists, 8 pediatricians hospital-based −50%- or working in community −50%-). Criteria were categorized according to the main physiological systems (gastroenterology, respiratory infections, pain, neurology, dermatology and miscellaneous). Each criterion was accompanied by a concise explanation as to why the practice is potentially inappropriate in pediatrics (including references). Two round of Delphi process were completed via an online questionnaire. 104 out of the 108 criteria submitted to experts were selected after 2 Delphi rounds (79 inappropriate prescriptions and 25 omissions).

Discussion Conclusion: POPI is the first screening-tool develop to detect inappropriate prescriptions and omissions in pediatrics based on explicit criteria. Inter-user reliability study is necessary before using the tool, and prospective study to assess the effectiveness of POPI is also necessary.

Editor: Imti Choonara, Nottingham University, United Kingdom

Funding: The authors have no support or funding to report.

Competing Interests: The authors have declared that no competing interests exist.

* Email: sonia.prot-labarthe@rdb.aphp.fr

¶ These authors are joint senior authors on this work

Introduction

Rational use of medicines refers to the correct, proper and appropriate use of medicines. The WHO estimates that over 50% of medications are prescribed, dispensed or sold inappropriately and that more than 50% of all countries do not implement basic policies to promote rational use of medicines [1]. In developing countries, less than 40% of patients in the public sector and 30% in the private sector are treated according to clinical guidelines [1]. The use of medication in pediatrics should be based on established recommendations from well-conducted clinical trials, however in the absence of such trials, recommendations are often based on clinical experience. Rational prescribing for children is an issue for all countries and has been inadequately studied [2,3].

The Medical Subject Headings (MeSH) tool is a thesaurus integrated into the PubMed search engine that allows access to the MEDLINE database. In 2011, it introduced the term '*Inappropriate Prescribing*' [4]. The use of a medication for which the associated risks outweigh the expected benefits can be considered as inappropriate, especially if an alternative treatment has been shown to be safer and more effective. According to a report published by the French National Authority for Health, both prescription of medication for excessively long periods and the failure to prescribe recommended medications can be classified as inappropriate prescribing [5]. In addition, the prescription of medications that have a high risk to interact with other drugs, or with the disease can also be considered as inappropriate. All of these examples will be herein described as inappropriate prescription (IP).

Many tools have been developed to detect IP in the elderly. This is largely due to the susceptibility of the elderly to disease and the prevalence of polypharmacy in this population. The *Beers Criteria for Potentially Inappropriate Medication Use in Older Adults* [6] were the first criteria to be proposed and are also the most well-known. However, one major disadvantage of this tool is that it includes many medications that are not sold in Europe. In 2008, Gallagher *et al.* developed a tool called STOPP/START (*Screening Tool of Older Person's Prescriptions/Screening Tool to Alert doctors to Right Treatment*) that comprises two medication lists [7]. The 'STOPP' list includes prescriptions that should be stopped and the 'START' list includes prescriptions that should be initiated, in the absence of any contra-indication. This system is particularly useful because it classifies drugs according to various medical conditions that are commonly found in the elderly. In a study in 2008, the use of the STOPP list identified IPs in 35% of a cohort of elderly patients and one third of these IPs were associated with an adverse drug event [8]. Another study involving randomized hospitalized patients showed that the occurrence of IP was 35% lower in patients who were prescribed drugs according to STOPP/START criteria than in patients for who usual pharmaceutical criteria were used [9]. However, so far no tool has been created to the pediatric population.

Our objective was to create the first IP tool in pediatrics, which we called POPI (Pediatrics: Omission of Prescriptions and Inappropriate prescriptions) [10]. Our objective was to raise awareness about this tool and to validate its content through a network of medical professionals working in pediatrics.

Materials and Methods

POPI should contain around 100 propositions that were classified according to biological system and classified according to whether they involve an omitted or an inappropriate prescription. The propositions were further divided within these two lists according to the major biological systems (as this was done for other geriatric tools [6,8]). We decided to include around 100 propositions: this was a good compromise between the number of major biological systems to explore, the number of items in the geriatric lists and the maximum number of items compatible with a tool easy use.

This project began in the Robert-Debré University Hospital, AP-HP (Assistance Publique-Hôpitaux de Paris) in Paris, France. POPI is comprised of a list of health problems frequently encountered in pediatrics. These problems were chosen in 2010 according to the following criteria, as concerns pediatrics: their frequency in the general population, the reasons for hospitalization (listed in the French hospital system's medico-administrative database in 2011 'programme de médicalisation des systèmes d'information' [PMSI] at the Robert-Debré University Hospital), and their prevalence according to data from the French National Health Insurance Fund for Employees (la caisse nationale de l'assurance maladie des travailleurs salariés [CNAMTS]) of long-term illnesses [11]. According to these criteria, we selected health problems requiring either drug intervention, or no pharmacological intervention whatsoever (i.e. treatment in such cases would be considered as inappropriate).

For each disease, we considered the recommended pharmacological treatments, the risks of errors, contra-indications, drug-drug interactions, drug-disease interactions, and issues associated with dose and route.

For each of the chosen themes (or diseases), we established a literature search strategy to retrieve management recommendations. We selected only recommendations that were both backed up by evidence and were published after 2000. Recommendations were weighted according to their publication date. Data was obtained from learned or professional societies or agencies in France, the United States, or Great Britain: the French Health Products Safety Agency (ANSM or *Agence Française de Sécurité Sanitaire des Produits de Santé*), the French National Authority for Health (*Haute Autorité de Santé Française*), the French Society for Pediatricians (*Société Française de Pédiatrie*), the American Academy of Pediatrics (National Guideline Clearing House), and finally the National Institute for Health and Clinical Evidence, Cochrane Library (UK). We used the following databases for the origin of pharmacological agents, the commercially available forms, and potential drug-drug interactions: Thériaque [12], Micromedex [13], Lexi-Comp's Pediatric & Neonatal Dosage Handbook [14], and the French medical journal 'La Revue Prescrire' [15]. We also used the MEDLINE database to search for examples of medication error and inappropriate prescription.

We validated the propositions included in POPI by a two round Delphi method [16,17]. The aim of the Delphi method is to achieve a convergence of opinion and a general consensus on a particular topic, by questioning experts through successive questionnaires. The experts were chosen according to their area of expertise, and included pediatricians most of who are members of the French Society of Pediatricians, and pharmacists mostly members of the French Society of Clinical Pharmacy. Each expert has disclosed his conflicts of interest.

The fisrt round questionnaire comprised all of the propositions included in POPI draft, which were graded according to a nine-point Likert scale for agreement. A score of 1 indicates 'total disagreement' whereas a score of 9 'total agreement', with intermediate values indicating degrees of agreement between these two extremes. The experts were also encouraged to make suggestions about the dose, the frequency, and the duration of treatment, provided that they could cite appropriate references to back up these suggestions. The experts could also comment on the propositions. The questionnaire was available online via the website 'SurveyMonkey', which is a tool designed to conduct web-based surveys [18].

Each of the panelists who had participated in the first round was sent the second-round questionnaire. These panelists were also given feedback on the results of the first round (their own previous individual ratings, median panel rating, and frequency distribution of the agreement rating). The panelists were then asked to re-rate each proposition based on both their own opinion and the group response to the previous round.

Only the propositions that obtained a median score in the upper tertile (between 7 and 9) with an agreement of more than 65% of participants in the first round of Delphi were retained. These propositions were modified according to the experts' comments, and were subjected to a second round of questioning. Only the propositions that obtained a median score between 7 and 9 with an agreement of more than 75% of participants in this second round were retained. The experts had two weeks to reply to the questionnaire. For both the first and second questionnaire, a reminder was sent out one and two weeks before the deadline.

Experts characteristics were also noted, including their age, their place of work, and their number of years of experience.

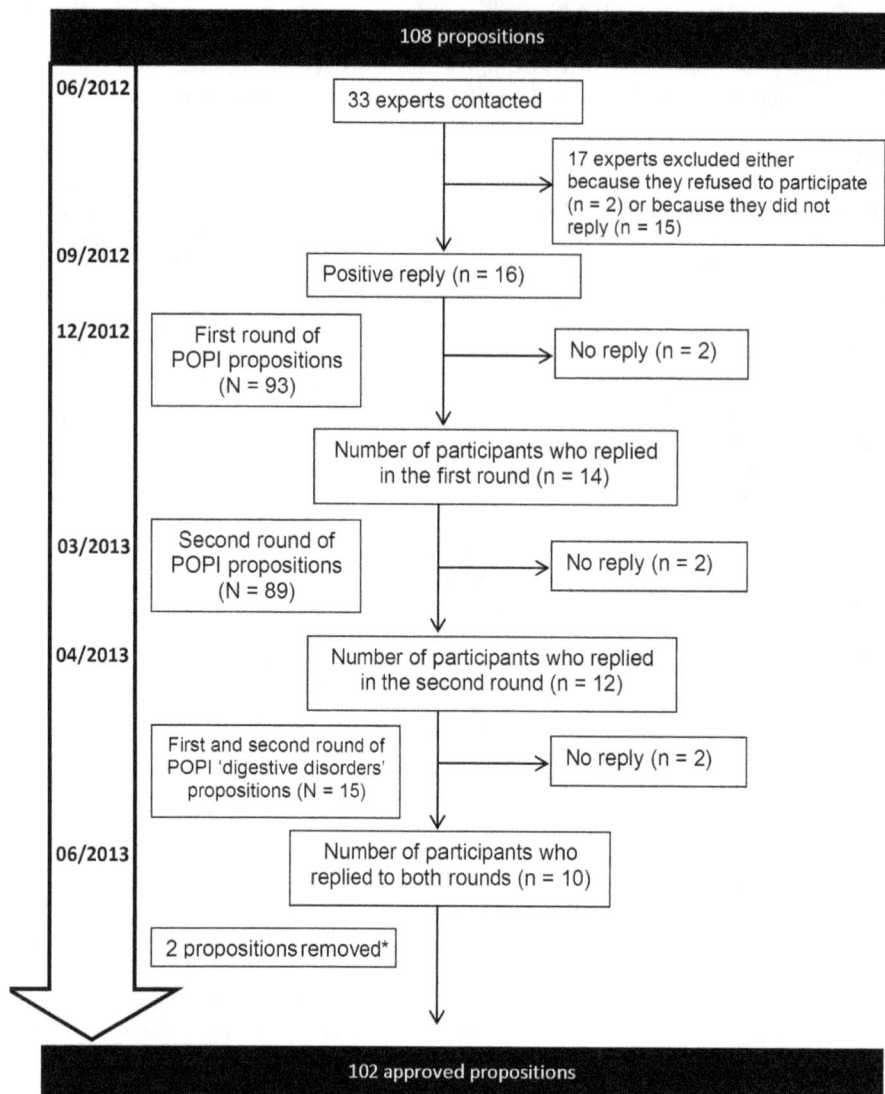

Figure 1. Workflow for the validation of POPI.*An item involving codeine was removed subsequent to the validation of the propositions included in POPI, following the revelation of new contraindications for this drug in children under 12 years old [22]. N: Number of items; n: number of panelists.

Qualitative data are expressed as numbers (percentages) and quantitative data as median (quartiles) and minima, maxima. SAS software (VERSION 9.3) was used for statistical analysis.

The study was reviewed and approved by the Robert-Debré institutional review board.

Results

The first draft of POPI contained 108 propositions: 80 propositions of Inappropriate Prescription (IP) and 28 propositions of Omission of Prescription (OP). These propositions were classified into five broad categories: digestive problems (n = 15); Ear, Nose and Throat (ENT) problems or pulmonary problems (n = 23); dermatological problems (n = 30); neuropsychiatric disorders (n = 16); and diverse illnesses (n = 24). Each category was further divided into several medical conditions. We contacted 33 experts between June and September 2012. Sixteen experts agreed to participate in the development of the POPI tool. The median expert age was 49 years, range [32–66 years] and their median

number of years of experience was 25 years, range [3–40 years]. The ratio of pediatricians to pharmacists was 1:1. Half were working in a hospital environment and the other half were working in the community. Each physician working within a hospital environment was specialized in a particular medical domain: endocrinology, hematology, nephrology, cancerology, or pulmonology.

Figure 1 shows the workflow of the study. The first round questionnaire was sent to the 16 experts at the start of December 2012 and the replies were collected by the start of January 2013; 14 (14/16, 87.5%) participants responded to the first round of questions. Two propositions received 13 replies because one expert did not use the answer grid properly. More than 65% of the panelists gave top-tertile (7–9) agreement to 93 propositions. Ten propositions were modified according to the experts' comments during this first round of questions producing 93 propositions for the second round.

Table 1. Propositions validated for use in POPI.

DIVERSE ILLNESSES	PAIN AND FEVER
	Inappropriate prescriptions
	Prescription of two alternating antipyretics as a first-line treatment
	Prescription of a medication other than paracetamol as a first line treatment (except in the case of migraine)
	Rectal administration of paracetamol as a first-line treatment
	The combined use of two NSAIDs
	Oral solutions of ibuprofen administered in more than three doses per day using a graduated pipette of 10mg/kg (other than Advil)
	Opiates to treat migraine attacks
	Omissions
	Failure to give sugar solution to new-born babies and infants under four months old two minutes prior to venipuncture
	Failure to give an osmotic laxative to patients being treated with morphine for a period of more than 48 hours
	URINARY INFECTIONS
	Inappropriate prescriptions
	Nitrofurantoin used as a prophylactic
	Nitrofurantoin used as a curative agent in children under six years of age, or indeed any other antibiotic if avoidable
	Antibiotic prophylaxis following an initial infection without complications (except in the case of uropathy)
	Antibiotic prophylaxis in the case of asymptomatic bacterial infection (except in the case of uropathy)
	VITAMIN SUPPLEMENTS AND ANTIBIOTIC PROPHYLAXIS
	Inappropriate prescriptions
	Fluoride supplements prior to six months of age
	Omissions
	Insufficient intake of vitamin D. Minimum vitamin D intake: Breastfed baby = 1 000 to 1 200 IU/day; Infant <18 months of age (milk enriched in vitamin D) = 600 to 800 IU/day; Child aged between 18 months and five years, and adolescents aged between 10 and 18 years: two quarterly loading doses of 80 000 to 100 000 IU/day in winter (adolescents can take this dose in one go)
	Antibiotic prophylaxis with phenoxymethylpenicillin (Oracilline) starting from two months of age and lasting until five years of age for children with sickle-cell anemia: 100 000 IU/kg/day (in two doses) for children weighing 10kg or less and 50 000 IU/kg/day for children weighing over 10kg (also in two doses)
	MOSQUITOS
	Inappropriate prescriptions
	The use of skin repellents in infants less than six months old and picardin in children less than 24 months old
	Citronella (lemon grass) oil (essential oil)
	Anti-insect bracelets to protect against mosquitos and ticks
	Ultrasonic pest control devices, vitamin B1, homeopathy, electric bug zappers, sticky tapes without insecticide
	Omissions
	DEET: "30%" (max) before 12 years old; "50%" (max) after 12 years old
	IR3535: "20%" (max) before 24 months old; "35%" (max) after 24 months old
	Mosquito nets and clothes treated with pyrethroids
DIGESTIVE PROBLEMS	**NAUSEA, VOMITTING, OR GASTROESOPHAGEAL REFLUX**
	Inappropriate prescriptions
	Metoclopramide
	Domperidone
	Oral administration of an intravenous proton pump inhibitor (notably by nasogastric tube)
	Gastric antisecretory drugs to treat gastroesophageal reflux, dyspepsia, the crying of new-born babies (in the absence of any other signs or symptoms), as well as faintness in infants
	The combined use of proton pump inhibitors and NSAIDs, for a short period of time, in patients without risk factors
	The use of type H2 antihistamines for long periods of treatment
	Erythromycin as a prokinetic agent
	The use of setrons (5-HT3 antagonists) for chemotherapy-associated nausea and vomiting
	Omissions
	Oral rehydration solution
	DIARRHEA

Table 1. Cont.

	Inappropriate prescriptions
	Loperamide before 3 years of age
	Loperamide in the case of invasive diarrhea
	The use of Diosmectite (Smecta) in combination with another medication
	The use of Saccharomyces boulardii (Ultralevure) in powder form, or in a capsule that has to be opened prior to ingestion, to treat patients with a central venous catheter or an immunodeficiency
	Intestinal antiseptics
	Omissions
	Oral rehydration solution
–ENT-PULMONARY PROBLEMS	**COUGH**
	Inappropriate prescriptions
	Pholcodine
	Mucolytic drugs, mucokinetic drugs, or helicidine before two years of age
	Alimemazine (Theralene), oxomemazine (Toplexil), promethazine (Phenergan, and other types)
	Terpene-based suppositories
	Omissions
	Failure to propose a whooping cough booster vaccine for adults who are likely to become parents in the coming months or years (only applicable if the previous vaccination was more than 10 years ago). This booster vaccination should also be proposed to the family and entourage of expectant parents (parents, grand-parents, nannies/child minders)
	BRONCHIOLITIS IN INFANTS
	Inappropriate prescriptions
	Beta2 agonists, corticosteroids to treat an infant's first case of bronchiolitis
	H1-antagonists, cough suppressants, mucolytic drugs, or ribavirin to treat bronchiolitis
	Antibiotics in the absence of signs indicating a bacterial infection (acute otitis media, fever, etc.)
	Omissions
	0.9% NaCl to relieve nasal congestion (not applicable if nasal congestion is already being treated with 3% NaCl delivered by a nebulizer)
	Palivizumab in the following cases: (1) babies born both at less than 35 weeks of gestation and less than six months prior to the onset of a seasonal RSV epidemic; (2) children less than two years old who have received treatment for bronchopulmonary dysplasia in the past six months; (3) children less than two years old suffering from congenital heart disease with hemodynamic abnormalities
	ENT INFECTIONS
	Inappropriate prescriptions
	An antibiotic other than amoxicillin as a first-line treatment for acute otitis media, strep throat, or sinusitis (provided that the patient is not allergic to amoxicillin). An effective dose of amoxicillin for an pneumoncoccal infection is 80–90 mg/kg/day and an effective dose for a streptococcal infection is 50 mg/kg/day
	Antibiotic treatment for a sore throat, without a positive rapid diagnostic test result, in children less than three years old
	Antibiotics for nasopharyngitis, congestive otitis, sore throat before three years of age, or laryngitis; antibiotics as a first-line treatment for acute otitis media showing few symptoms, before two years of age
	Antibiotics to treat otitis media with effusion (OME), except in the case of hearing loss or if OME lasts for more than three months
	Corticosteroids to treat acute suppurative otitis media, nasopharyngitis, or strep throat
	Nasal or oral decongestant (oxymetazoline (Aturgyl), pseudoephedrine (Sudafed), naphazoline (Derinox), ephedrine (Rhinamide), tuaminoheptane (Rhinofluimicil), phenylephrine (Humoxal))
	H1-antagonists with sedative or atropine-like effects (pheniramine, chlorpheniramine), or camphor; inhalers, nasal sprays, or suppositories containing menthol (or any terpene derivatives) before 30 months of age
	Ethanolamine tenoate (Rhinotrophyl) and other nasal antiseptics
	Ear drops in the case of acute otitis media
	Omissions
	Doses in mg for drinkable (solutions of) amoxicillin or josamycin
	Paracetamol combined with antibiotic treatment for ear infections to relieve pain
	ASTHMA
	Inappropriate prescriptions
	Ketotifen and other H1-antagonists, sodium cromoglycate
	Cough suppressants
	Omissions

Table 1. Cont.

	Asthma inhaler appropriate for the child's age
	Preventative treatment (inhaled corticosteroids) in the case of persistent asthma
DERMATOLOGICAL PROBLEMS	**ACNE VULGARIS**
	Inappropriate prescriptions
	Minocycline
	Isotretinoin in combination with a member of the tetracycline family of antibiotics
	The combined use of an oral and a local antibiotic
	Oral or local antibiotics as a monotherapy (not in combination with another drug)
	Cyproterone+ethinylestradiol (Diane 35) as a contraceptive to allow isotretinoin per os
	Androgenic progestins (levonorgestrel, norgestrel, norethisterone, lynestrenol, dienogest, contraceptive implants or vaginal rings)
	Omissions
	Contraception (provided with a logbook/diary) for menstruating girls taking isotretinoin
	Topical treatment (benzoyl peroxide, retinoids, or both) in combination with antibiotic therapy
	SCABIES
	Inappropriate prescriptions
	The application of benzyl benzoate (Ascabiol) for periods longer than eight hours for infants and 12 hours for children or for pregnant girls
	Omissions
	A second dose of ivermectin two weeks after the first
	Decontamination of household linen and clothes and treatment for other family members
	LICE
	Inappropriate prescriptions
	The use of aerosols for infants, children with asthma, or children showing asthma-like symptoms such as dyspnea
	RINGWORM
	Inappropriate prescriptions
	Treatment other than griseofulvin for Microsporum
	Omissions
	Topical treatment combined with an orally-administered treatment
	Griseofulvin taken during a meal containing a moderate amount of fat
	IMPETIGO
	Inappropriate prescriptions
	The combination of locally applied and orally administered antibiotic
	Fewer than two applications per day for topical antibiotics
	Any antibiotic other than mupirocin as a first-line treatment (except in cases of hypersensitivity to mupirocin)
	HERPES SIMPLEX
	Inappropriate prescriptions
	Topical agents containing corticosteroids
	Topical agents containing acyclovir before six years of age
	Omissions
	Paracetamol during an outbreak of herpes
	Orally administered acyclovir to treat primary herpetic gingivostomatitis
	ATOPIC ECZEMA
	Inappropriate prescriptions
	A strong dermocorticoid (clobetasol propionate 0.05% Dermoval, betamethasone dipropionate Diprosone) applied to the face, the armpits or groin, and the backside of babies or young children
	More than one application per day of a dermocorticoid, except in cases of severe lichenification
	Local or systemic antihistamine during the treatment of outbreaks
	Topically applied 0.03% tacrolimus before two years of age
	Topically applied 0.1% tacrolimus before 16 years of age
	Oral corticosteroids to treat outbreaks

Table 1. Cont.

NEUROPSYCHIATRIC EPILEPSY
DISORDERS

    Inappropriate prescriptions

      Carbamazepine, gabapentin, oxcarbazepine, phenytoin, pregabalin, tiagabine, or vigabatrin in the case of myoclonic epilepsy

      Carbamazepine, gabapentin, oxcarbazepine, phenytoin, pregabaline, tiagabine, or vigabatrin in the case of epilepsy with absence seizures (especially for childhood absence epilepsy or juvenile absence epilepsy)

      Levetiracetam, oxcarbazepine in mL or in mg without systematically writing XX mg per Y mL

    DEPRESSION

    Inappropriate prescriptions

      An SSRI antidepressant other than fluoxetine as a first-line treatment (in the case of pharmacotherapy)

      Tricyclic antidepressants to treat depression

    NOCTURNAL ENURESIS

    Inappropriate prescriptions

      Desmopressin administered by a nasal spray

      Desmopressin in the case of daytime symptoms

      An anticholinergic agent used as a monotherapy in the absence of daytime symptoms

      Tricyclic agents in combination with anticholinergic agents

      Tricyclic agents as a first-line treatment

    ANOREXIA

    Inappropriate prescriptions

      Cyproheptadine (Periactin), clonidine

    ATTENTION DEFICIT DISORDER WITH OR WITHOUT HYPERACTIVITY

    Inappropriate prescriptions

      Pharmacological treatment before age six (before school), except in severe cases

      Antipsychotic drugs to treat attention deficit disorder without hyperactivity

      Slow release methylphenidate as two doses per day, rather than only one dose

    Omissions

      Recording a growth chart (height and weight) if the patient is taking methylphenidate

The second questionnaire was submitted at the end of March 2013 and the replies were collected within one month. During this second round of questions, 85.5% (12/14) of participants replied. More than 75% of the panelists gave top-tertile agreement to all the 93 propositions submitted.

The propositions involving the category 'digestive problems' (n = 15) were submitted separately in April 2013 for 2 rounds rating. All of these propositions were unanimously accepted during two rounds of questions that took place between April and May 2013. Ten experts participated in these rounds of questions (i.e. 71.5% of the 14 experts who replied in the initial survey carried out between December 2012 and January 2013.

Table 1 shows the 102 propositions that were validated for use in POPI. A proposition involving codeine was removed subsequent to the validation of POPI, following the revelation of new contraindications for this drug in children under 12 years old [19]. Another proposition about the use of permethrin for lice was removed because of new recommendation to use dimeticone first (lack of resistance) [20]. Table 2 summarizes the references justification for each table 1 pathology.

Discussion

POPI (Pediatrics: Omission of Prescriptions and Inappropriate prescriptions) is the first tool that has been designed to detect the omission of prescriptions or inappropriate prescriptions specifically in pediatric patients [21]. If polymedication is unusual for children, there are however multiple health care professional who prescribe or counsel drug for children: general practitioner, paediatricians, pharmacists, nurses, midwives etc.

The POPI criteria are based on the same classification system as the STOPP/START criteria, (i.e. according to the major biological systems [8]). We selected this form because such lists have been successfully used to detect preventable adverse drug events [8,9,22]. The Beers criteria were updated in 2012 to incorporate this classification system [6]. Our tool, which was developed using a Delphi method, was validated by 14 health care professionals. The Delphi method is one of the main method used for the development of tools designed to detect inappropriate prescriptions in geriatric patients [6,8,22–26]. The number of experts to develop geriatric tools vary between 11 and 32 and their specialties include pharmacy, psychopharmacology, pharmacology, pharmacoepidemiology, internal medicine or geriatrics [6,7,23,24,26]. For the validation of POPI, the number of experts in each category was equal so as to ensure that hospital and community environments were equally represented. There is currently no consensus regarding the composition of such panels of experts; there are no recommendations about the numbers or qualifications of experts to be included. More pharmacists were involved in the validation of the POPI criteria than in the validation of similar criteria that were developed for geriatrics.

Table 2. References justification for each POPI statement.

Pain and Fever

Mise au point sur la prise en charge de la fièvre chez l'enfant – **AFSSAPS** –2005

Fever and Antipyretic use in children – American Academy of Pediatrics (AAP) –2011

Feverish illness in children – **NICE** –2007

Prise en charge médicamenteuse de la douleur aiguë et chronique chez l'enfant - **AFSSAPS** –2009

Prevention and Management of Pain in the Neonate - **AAP** –2006

Urinary Infections

Nitrofurantoïne et risque de survenue d'effets indésirables hépatiques et pulmonaires lors de traitements prolongés – **AFSSAPS** –2011

Urinary tract infection in children – **NICE** –2007

Vitamin Supplements and Antibiotic Prophylaxis

Utilisation du fluor dans la prévention de la carie dentaire avant l'âge de 18 ans – **AFSSAPS** –10/2008

Dents et fluor chez les enfants – **Idées-Forces Prescrire** – Novembre 2011

Alimentation du nourrisson et de l'enfant en bas âge. Réalisation pratique – **SFP** (Société Française de Pédiatrie) –2003

La Vitamine D : une vitamine toujours d'actualité chez l'enfant et l'adolescent. Mise au point par le Comité de nutrition de la Société française de pédiatrie – **SFP** – 2012

Prise en charge de la drépanocytose chez l'enfant et l'adolescent – **HAS** –09/2005

Mosquitos

Protection Antivectorielle RBP – **Société Française de Parasitologie** –2010

BEH –29 mai 2012– n°20–21

Prévention des piqûres de moustiques ou des morsures de tiques – **Idées-Forces Prescrire** – Juin 2012

Nausea, Vomitting, or Gastroesophageal Reflux

Contre-indication des spécialités à base de métoclopramide (Primpéran et génériques) chez l'enfant et l'adolescent et renforcement des informations sur les risques neurologiques et cardiovasculaires – **AFSSAPS** - Lettre aux professionnels de santé –08/02/2012

Antisécrétoires gastriques chez l'enfant – **AFSSAPS** –06/2008

Pediatric Gastroesophageal Reflux Clinical Practice Guidelines – **NASPGHAN** –2009

Traitement médicamenteux des diarrhées aiguës infectieuses du nourrisson et de l'enfant - **SFP** –2002

Managing Acute Gastroenteritis Among Children: Oral Rehydration, Maintenance, and Nutritional Therapy - Centers for Disease Control and Prevention – **AAP** –2003

Diarrhoea and vomiting in children under 5– **NICE** –2009

Diarrhea

Diarrhoea and vomiting in children under 5– **NICE** –2009

Traitement médicamenteux des diarrhées aiguës infectieuses du nourrisson et de l'enfant – **SFP** –2002

Managing Acute Gastroenteritis Among Children: Oral Rehydration, Maintenance, and Nutritional Therapy - Centers for Disease Control and Prevention – **AAP** –2003

Cough

Pholcodine – **AFSSSAPS** –2011

Toux aiguë chez les enfants de moins de 2 ans – AFSSAPS –2010

BHE – Calendrier vaccinal –10 avril 2012– n°14–15

Bronchiolotis in Infants

Diagnosis and Management of Bronchiolitis – **AAP** –2006

Bronchiolite du nourrisson – Conférence de consensus – HAS –2000

Bronchiolite chez les nourrissons – Traitement – **Idées-Forces Prescrire** – Septembre 2011

Ear Infections

Antibiothérapie dans les infections respiratoires hautes – **SFP** –12/2011

Respiratory tract infections – **NICE** –2011

Rhume : traitements – **Idées-Forces Prescrire** – Avril 2011

Otite moyenne aiguë : traitement antibiotique – **Idées-Forces Prescrire** – Janvier 2011

Diagnosis and Management of Acute Otitis Media – **AAP** –2004

Asthma

Global Initiative for Asthma –2011

Asthme de l'enfant de moins de 36 mois : diagnostic, prise en charge et traitement en dehors des épisodes aigus – **HAS** – Mars 2009

Managing Asthma Long Term In Children 0–4 and 5–11 Years of Age – **NHLBI** –2007

Acne Vulgaris

Recommandations de bonne pratique – **AFSSAPS**–2007

Table 2. Cont.

Minocycline : restriction d'utilisation en raison d'un risque de syndromes d'hypersensibilité graves et d'atteintes auto-immunes – Lettre aux professionnels de santé – **ANSM** –2012

Isotrétinoïne orale – Renforcement du Programme de Prévention des Grossesses et rappel sur la survenue éventuelle de troubles psychiatriques – **AFSSAPS** –05/ 2009

Scabies

Sexually Transmitted Diseases Treatment Guidelines – **CDC** –2010

Gale – **Avis du conseil supérieur d'hygiène publique de France** –2003

Lice

Poux du cuir chevelu – **La Revue Prescrire N°365**–2014

Ringworm

Guidelines for the Management of Tinea Capitis in Children – **ESPD** –2010

Impetigo

Prescription des antibiotiques par voie locale dans les infections cutanées bactériennes primitives et secondaires – **AFSSAPS** –2004

Herpes Simplex

Prise en charge de l'herpès cutanéo-muqueux chez le sujet immunocompétent – **SFD** –2001

Atopic Eczema

Prise en charge de la dermatite atopique de l'enfant – **Société Française de Dermatologie** –2005

Atopic eczema in children – **NICE** –2007

Protopic – **HAS** – Commission transparence –2011

Epilepsy

Epilepsy – **NICE** –2012

Epilepsies graves – **HAS** –07/2007

Depression

Bon usage des antidépresseurs au cours de la dépression de l'enfant et de l'adolescent – **AFSSAPS** – Janvier 2008

Depression in children and young people – **NICE** –2009

Nocturnal Enuresis

Utilisation de la desmopressine (Minirin) dans l'énurésie nocturne isolée chez l'enfant – **AFSSAPS** –2006
Nocturnal enuresis – **NICE** –2010

Anorexia

Anorexie : recommandation pour la pratique clinique – **HAS** – Juin 2010

Attention Deficit Disorder with or withou Hyperactivity

Attention deficit hyperactivity disorder Diagnosis and management of ADHD in children, young people and adults – **NICE** –2008

ADHD : Clinical Practice Guideline for the Diagnosis, Evaluation, and Treatment of Attention-Deficit/Hyperactiviy Disorder in Children and Adolescents – **AAP** –2010

This strong representation is partly because the initial project was developed by hospital pharmacists. One limitation of our study in the absence of general practitioners from our panel of experts. Indeed, these doctors regularly deliver health care to children in the community and hence could greatly benefit from the use of POPI.

Few data about inappropriate prescriptions have been published in pediatric patients. Although studies have investigated medication errors [27–29], not one study has examined the link between the rate of medication errors and the rate of adverse drug events in pediatrics. In adults, it is estimated that around one adverse drug occurs for every 100 medication errors [30,31]. There is increasing recognition that rational prescribing is an important issue in children [2].

The different propositions included in POPI were based on recommendations from recognized learned and academic societies and were preselected by the initial working group. Of the 108 propositions, 104 were validated by experts in the first round of Delphi, and all of the propositions submitted in the second round were subsequently validated. The final version of the POPI criteria contains 79 examples of inappropriate prescription and 25 examples of omission of prescription. The modifications that were made during the first and second rounds of Delphi involved refinements in the phrasing and exact details of the propositions. Overall, the experts were very responsive, and we collected around 80% of replies within three weeks of sending the questionnaires. The feedback of the experts was very positive and many of them commented that they were very interested in the development of POPI. The STOPP/START criteria contained as many propositions to validate as the POPI criteria. For STOPP/START, a consensus was obtained for 77 out of 80 propositions that were submitted in the first round [7]. For the criteria developed by Laroche *et al.* a consensus was reached for 33 out of 37 criteria during the first round [26]. This illustrates the importance of preselecting the propositions prior to their submission to experts, to ensure that a consensus will be reached on the largest possible number of propositions. The time that experts were given to reply to questionnaires during the development of criteria similar to POPI is often not stated, with the exception of STOPP/START, in which all answers were obtained within two months [7]. We estimated that one month (a minimum of two weeks with two reminders) was a reasonable amount of time for the completion of the questionnaire. This time constraint was applied to both rounds of questions.

Our criteria contain more propositions than the STOPP/START criteria (83 propositions vs. 102 for POPI) and more than the updated 2012 Beers criteria (85 propositions). The classification of these propositions by biological system makes the POPI criteria fast to use, and POPI considers only those medical conditions that require prescriptions. The categories that we used are not the same as those in the STOPP/START criteria or the updated 2012 Beers criteria because diseases that affect children are not the same as those that affect the elderly. Indeed, in most criteria designed for use in geriatrics, psychiatry and cardiology constitute major categories [6,7,26], whereas the categories that contain the most propositions in POPI are respiratory problems, gastroenterology, and dermatology.

The POPI criteria have not yet been tested in the setting of routine prescriptions and needs validating clinically. Two studies will be carried out with this objective in mind. One study will examine the degree of inter-rater agreement of the various propositions of POPI, by assessing the percentage of concordance corrected for chance agreement, termed κ (Kappa). This will provide a measure of the precision of the POPI criteria. A second study will examine the capacity of the POPI criteria to identify medication errors and evaluate the safety of drug used (involved drugs, indication) prospectively.

Conclusion

We created the first set of criteria for the detection of inappropriate prescriptions and the omission of prescriptions in pediatrics. The resulting tool, named POPI, is available to all medical professionals (clinicians, pharmacists, in hospital or community working environment) liable to prescribe or dispense medication to children.

Acknowledgments

Thanks to our panelists: F Amouroux, R Assathiany, JP Blanc, V Breant, D Cau, L Cret, N Davoust, M Detavernier, N Duval-Ehrenfeld, A Lecoeur, F Netzer, L Priqueler, H Sarda, E Séror, B Virey, C Wehrle.

Thanks to the PMSI unit at the Robert-Debré University Hospital for the data concerning the patients' reasons for hospitalizations.

Thanks to S Auvin, E Bourrat, A Hubert, MF Le Heuzey, C Madre.

Author Contributions

Conceived and designed the experiments: SPL TW FA OB. Performed the experiments: SPL TW FA OB. Analyzed the data: TW RB CA. Contributed reagents/materials/analysis tools: SPL TW FA RB CA OB. Contributed to the writing of the manuscript: SPL TW FA RB CA OB.

References

1. WHO | Medicines: rational use of medicines (n.d.). WHO. Available: http://www.who.int/mediacentre/factsheets/fs338/en/. Accessed 2014 May 12.
2. Choonara I (2013) Rational prescribing is important in all settings. Arch Dis Child 98: 720–720. doi:10.1136/archdischild-2013-304559.
3. Risk R, Naismith H, Burnett A, Moore SE, Cham M, et al. (2013) Rational prescribing in paediatrics in a resource-limited setting. Arch Dis Child 98: 503–509. doi:10.1136/archdischild-2012-302987.
4. Inappropriate Prescribing - MeSH - NCBI (n.d.). Available: http://www.ncbi.nlm.nih.gov/mesh?term = inappropriate%20prescription. Accessed 2012 June 18.
5. Legrain S, others (2005) Consommation médicamenteuse chez le sujet âgé. Consomm Prescr Iatrogénie Obs. Available: http://has-sante.fr/portail/upload/docs/application/pdf/pmsa_synth_biblio_2006_08_28_16_44_51_580.pdf. Accessed 2012 June 17.
6. Fick D, Semla T, Beizer J, Brandt N (2012) American Geriatrics Society Updated Beers Criteria for Potentially Inappropriate Medication Use in Older Adults - J Am Geriatrics Society - 2012.pdf. J Am Geriatr Soc 60: 616–631. doi:10.1111/j.1532-5415.2012.03923.x.
7. Gallagher P, Ryan C, Kennedy J, O'Mahony D (2008) STOPP (Screening Tool of Older Person's Prescriptions) and START (Screening Tool to Alert doctors to Right Treatment). Consensus validation. Int J Clin Pharmacol Ther 46: 72–83.
8. Gallagher P, O'Mahony D (2008) STOPP (Screening Tool of Older Persons' potentially inappropriate Prescriptions): application to acutely ill elderly patients and comparison with Beers' criteria. Age Ageing 37: 673–679. doi:10.1093/ageing/afn197.
9. Gallagher P, O'Connor M, O'Mahony D (2011) Prevention of Potentially Inappropriate Prescribing for Elderly Patients: A Randomized Controlled Trial Using STOPP/START Criteria. Clin Pharmacol Ther 89: 845–854. doi:10.1038/clpt.2011.44.
10. Prot-Labarthe S, Vercheval C, Angoulvant F, Brion F, Bourdon O (2011) «POPI; pédiatrie: omissions et prescriptions inappropriées». Outil d'identification des prescriptions inappropriées chez l'enfant. Arch Pédiatrie Organe Off Société Fr Pédiatrie 18: 1231–1232. doi:10.1016/j.arcped.2011.08.019.
11. ameli.fr - Affection de longue durée (ALD) (n.d.). Available: http://www.ameli.fr/l-assurance-maladie/statistiques-et-publications/donnees-statistiques/affection-de-longue-duree-ald/index.php. Accessed 2012 June 18.
12. Thériaque (n.d.). Available: http://www.theriaque.org. Accessed: 2012 July 3.
13. Thomson Healthcare Products (n.d.). Available: http://www.thomsonhc.com/home/dispatch. Accessed: 2012 July 3.
14. Taketomo CK, Hodding JH, Kraus DM (2011) Pediatric & neonatal dosage handbook: a comprehensive resource for all clinicians treating pediatric and neonatal patients. Hudson, Ohio; [United States]: Lexi-Comp; American Pharmacists Association.
15. La Revue Prescrire (n.d.). Rev Prescrire. Available: http://www.prescrire.org/fr/. Accessed Accessed: 2012 July 12.
16. Bourrée F, Michel P, Salmi LR (2008) Methodes de consensus: Revue des méthodes originales et de leurs grandes variantes utilisées en santé publique. Rev Epidémiologie Santé Publique 56.
17. Hsu CC, Sandford BA (2007) The Delphi technique: Making sense of consensus. Pract Assess Res Eval 12: 1–8.
18. SurveyMonkey (n.d.) SurveyMonkey. SurveyMonkey. Available: http://fr.surveymonkey.net/home/. Accessed: 2012 Sept 12.
19. ANSM (2013) Médicaments à base de tétrazépam, d'almitrine, de ranélate de strontium et de codéine (chez l'enfant) - Retour d'information sur le PRAC - ANSM. Médicam À Base Tétrazépam Almitrine Ranélate Strontium Codéine Chez Enfant - Retour Inf Sur Pr - ANSM. Available: http://ansm.sante.fr/S-informer/Du-cote-de-l-Agence-europeenne-des-medicaments-Retours-d-information-sur-le-PRAC/Medicaments-a-base-de-tetrazepam-d-almitrine-de-ranelate-de-strontium-et-de-codeine-chez-l-enfant-Retour-d-information-sur-le-PRAC/(language)/fre-FR. Accessed 2013 June 23.
20. La Revue Prescrire (2014) Poux du cuir chevelu - Diméticone, substance pédiculicide de premier choix. Rev Prescrire 34: 198–202.
21. Kaufmann CP, Tremp R, Hersberger KE, Lampert ML (2013) Inappropriate prescribing: a systematic overview of published assessment tools. Eur J Clin Pharmacol. Available: http://link.springer.com/10.1007/s00228-013-1575-8. Accessed 2013 Dec 16.
22. Levy HB, Marcus EL, Christen C (2010) Beyond the beers criteria: A comparative overview of explicit criteria. Ann Pharmacother 44: 1968–1975.
23. Beers MH, Ouslander JG, Rollingher I, Reuben DB, Brooks J, et al. (1991) Explicit Criteria for Determining Inappropriate Medication Use in Nursing Home Residents. Arch Intern Med 151: 18255–32.
24. McLeod PJ, Huang AR, Tamblyn RM, Gayton DC (1997) Defining inappropriate practices in prescribing for elderly people: a national consensus panel. Can Med Assoc J 156: 385.
25. Waller JL, Maclean JR (2003) Updating the Beers Criteria for potentially inappropriate medication use in older adults. Arch Intern Med 163: 2716–2724.
26. Laroche M-L, Charmes J-P, Merle L (2007) Potentially inappropriate medications in the elderly: a French consensus panel list. Eur J Clin Pharmacol 63: 725–731. doi:10.1007/s00228-007-0324-2.
27. Kaushal R, Bates DW, Landrigan C, McKenna KJ, Clapp MD, et al. (2001) Medication errors and adverse drug events in pediatric inpatients. JAMA J Am Med Assoc 285: 2114.
28. Kaushal R, Goldmann DA, Keohane CA, Abramson EL, Woolf S, et al. (2010) Medication errors in paediatric outpatients. Qual Saf Health Care 19: 1–6. doi:10.1136/qshc.2008.031179.
29. Davis T (2010) Paediatric prescribing errors. Arch Dis Child 96: 489–491. doi:10.1136/adc.2010.200295.
30. Bates DW, Boyle DL, Vliet MBV, Schneider J, Leape L (1995) Relationship between medication errors and adverse drug events. J Gen Intern Med 10: 199–205.
31. Schmitt E (1999) Le risque médicamenteux nosocomial: circuit hospitalier du médicament et qualité des soins. Masson. IX–287 p.

4

Cost-Effectiveness of the "Helping Babies Breathe" Program in a Missionary Hospital in Rural Tanzania

Corinna Vossius[1]*, Editha Lotto[2], Sara Lyanga[2], Estomih Mduma[2], Georgina Msemo[3], Jeffrey Perlman[4], Hege L. Ersdal[1,2]

1 SAFER (Stavanger Acute Medicine Foundation for Education and Research), Stavanger University Hospital, Stavanger, Norway, 2 Research Institute, Haydom Lutheran Hospital, Haydom, Tanzania, 3 Ministry of Health and Social Welfare, Dar es Salaam, Tanzania, 4 Department of Pediatrics, Weill Cornell Medical College, New York, New York, United States of America

Abstract

Objective: The Helping Babies Breathe" (HBB) program is an evidence-based curriculum in basic neonatal care and resuscitation, utilizing simulation-based training to educate large numbers of birth attendants in low-resource countries. We analyzed its cost-effectiveness at a faith-based Haydom Lutheran Hospital (HLH) in rural Tanzania.

Methods: Data about early neonatal mortality and fresh stillbirth rates were drawn from a linked observational study during one year before and one year after full implementation of the HBB program. Cost data were provided by the Tanzanian Ministry of Health and Social Welfare (MOHSW), the research department at HLH, and the manufacturer of the training material Lærdal Global Health.

Findings: Costs per life saved were USD 233, while they were USD 4.21 per life year gained. Costs for maintaining the program were USD 80 per life saved and USD 1.44 per life year gained. Costs per disease adjusted life year (DALY) averted ranged from International Dollars (ID; a virtual valuta corrected for purchasing power world-wide) 12 to 23, according to how DALYs were calculated.

Conclusion: The HBB program is a low-cost intervention. Implementation in a very rural faith-based hospital like HLH has been highly cost-effective. To facilitate further global implementation of HBB a cost-effectiveness analysis including government owned institutions, urban hospitals and district facilities is desirable for a more diverse analysis to explore cost-driving factors and predictors of enhanced cost-effectiveness.

Editor: Craig Rubens, Seattle Childrens Hospital, United States of America

Funding: The study was partly funded by the Lærdal Foundation for Acute Medicine (grant number 40023; http://www.laerdal.com/no/doc/311/Laerdals-Fond-for-Akuttmedisin), that provided travel expenses for Corinna Vossius and Hege L. Ersdal and a reserach grant for Hege L. Ersdal. Further, the research was funded by the municipaility of Stavanger, Norway and the research department of Haydom Lutheran Hospital, Tanzania. No funding bodies had any role in study design, data collection, decision or preparation of the manuscript.

Competing Interests: Corinna Vossius has received project support from the Lærdal Foundation for Acute Medicine. Hege L. Ersdal has received project support and research grants from the Lærdal Foundation for Acute Medicine. Jeffrey Perlman has received travel support from the Lærdal Foundation for Acute Medicine to facilitate implementation of the HBB program in Tanzania. The other authors have indicated they have no financial relationships relevant to this article to disclose. Lærdal Global Health A/S, a nonprofit sister company of Lærdal Medical A/S, designs, develops and manufactures low cost training equipment and therapeutic devices, including those used in the HBB program.

* Email: c.vossius@hotmail.com

Introduction

Neonatal mortality is defined as death before one month of age and recent global estimates range from 2.9 to 3.6 million deaths per year [1–4]. Of these, as much as 50–70 percent may occur within the first day of life [1,5–8]. Almost 99% of all neonatal deaths take place in resource-poor settings [1,9–12]. A major factor contributing to the high mortality is a global lack of trained providers in neonatal stabilization and/or resuscitation. This is most acute in Sub-Saharan Africa with the highest neonatal mortality [13]. The context of "Helping Babies Breathe" (HBB) is based on the International Liaison Committee on Resuscitation (ICLOR) Consensus in Science recommendations. The program includes an evidence-based curriculum in basic neonatal care and resuscitation, utilizing simulation-based training to educate large numbers of birth attendants in low-resource countries [14]. The program was developed by the Global Implementation Task Force of the American Academy of Pediatrics. In September 2009, the Tanzanian Ministry of Health and Social Welfare (MOHSW) launched the National HBB program by implementing HBB training and data collection at eight study-sites in Tanzania. Haydom Lutheran Hospital (HLH) was the only rural site, located in the in the Manyara region in Northern Tanzania.

An evaluation of the HBB program with pooled data of all eight sites showed that early neonatal mortality (within the first 24 hours, ENM) was reduced significantly during the first year with a relative risk reduction of 42%, and that this reduction was sustained during the second year at 47%. Fresh stillborn (FSB) rates were significantly reduced in the second year, with a relative risk reduction of 24% [15].

The HBB program is especially developed for low resource settings. Recently, the United Nations promoted HBB as one of ten breakthrough innovations in order to close the Millennium Development Goal 4 gap before 2015 [16], and the HBB program will be implemented in many low-resourced countries around the world within the next years. However, a proper cost-effectiveness analysis (CEA) is missing. The implementation of the HBB program at HLH was closely linked to a descriptive observational open cohort study in the delivery room, initiated in August 2009 [17,18]. In addition, it has been possible to obtain detailed cost information from the MOHSW and the research unit at HLH. Thus, we aimed at a CEA of the HBB program in a rural hospital in Tanzania by presenting the total costs to society per live saved and per life year gained and the separate cost factors.

Methods

The "Helping Babies Breathe" Training Program

HBB is an evidence-based curriculum in basic neonatal care and resuscitation, utilizing simulation-based training to educate large numbers of birth attendants in low-resource countries [14]. The course methodology focuses on hands-on practice using a simulator mannequin, emphazising the very first basic steps: drying, stimulation, suction, warmth, and initiation of bag mask ventilation within the "Golden Minute" after birth if indicated. The teaching tools are developed for efficient dissemination, and the educational kit contains a set of flip-over illustrations, an action plan, a neonatal simulator (NeoNatalie, Laerdal Medical), a student handbook, a manual resuscitator (Laerdal Medical), and a suction device (Pinguin, Laerdal Medical). The materials and equipment are left behind to facilitae re-training and dissemination.

Haydom Lutheran Hospital HLH is a faith-based organization (FBO), located in Northern Tanzania, at the Southern border of Mbulu district in the Manyara region, 300 km west of Arusha, which is the nearest urban center. The immediate catchment area includes about 500 000 people, while the greater reference area covers more than two million people. HLH is a missionary hospital. About 60% of the total funding is provided by the Norwegian government. In addition to a Norwegian managing medical director there is also a varying number of staff from Western countries working there in long-term or short-term appointments. The hospital is a 420-bed hospital owned by the Mbulu Diocese of the Evangelical Lutheran Church in Tanzania, and is fully incorporated in the national health plan under the MOHSW. The hospital provides surgical, medical, gynecological, comprehensive emergency obstetric, and basic emergency newborn care. Since 2009, HLH has offered free transport service for delivering women with an increase in annual number of deliveries from 3000 in 2008 to 5000 in 2011.

Implementation of the HBB Training Program at HLH

National implementation of HBB in Tanzania started in September 2009 and has been facilitated by a Health Ministry Commitment and integration into the Health Care System. The program was launched with two days HBB trainings of 40 Master Instructors selected from University and Referral hospitals [15] to start a cascade model where Master Instructors could train Trainers of Trainees (ToTs) who again would train health care providers. In April 2010 the initial one-day HBB course was held at HLH. Only half of the birth attendants were able to attend and no local Master Instructors were trained to facilitate continuation of HBB re-trainings. An evaluation of data from HLH revealed no improvements in mortality during the first months after the initial

HBB course [19]. An additional study, testing skills and knowledge among birth attendants at HLH showed that both knowledge and technical skills were improved when rated in a simulated setting seven months after the initial one-day HBB course as compared to before, but this improvement did not transfer into clinical practice. The number of babies being suctioned and/or ventilated at birth did not change, and the use of immediate stimulation decreased after the initial HBB training [20]. Therefore, in February 2011, a Master Instructor, representative from the MOHSW, returned to HLH and trained six ToTs who started in-situ low-dose-high-frequency (LDHF) HBB trainings in the labor ward: The newborn simulator (NeoNatalie, Lærdal, Norway) was placed in the labor ward easily accessible for frequent practicing in addition to weekly training sessions conducted by ToTs of about 30 minutes during working hours. Finally, a second full-day HBB course took place in May 2011 where most of the staff from Maternity participated. Consequently to the establishment of LDHF-training the number of infants being stimulated increased and the need for bag mask ventilation decreased with a corresponding decline in ENM [19].

Data collection – ENM and FSB

In August 2009, closely linked to the national HBB program, an ongoing descriptive observational open cohort study was initiated in the delivery room at HLH [17,18]. Fourteen research assistants/observers were trained to observe the birth attendants' performances related to delivery, newborn management, and perinatal outcome. The findings are recorded on a data collection form following every delivery. The observers work in three shifts over 24 hours. Three observers cover each shift; two are always located in the labour ward or in the theatre during caesarean sections; one in the adjacent neonatal area.

The HBB program was fully implemented at HLH in February 2011, when the LDHF training was initiated by local ToT. To calculate the effectiveness of the training program, we compared ENM and FSB during the 12 months before the complete implementation (01.02.2010–31.01.2011) and the 12 months after (01.02.2011–31.01.2012). We hypothesized that without the training program the rate of ENM and FSB would be the same during both years. No other interventions were implemented and the number of deliveries and staff were stable. The number of lives saved was thus calculated by the estimated number of deaths during the 12 months after the HBB implementation given the same mortality as during the 12 months before implementation minus the observed number of deaths during this period.

Data collection – costs

Costs for the initial one-day HBB course in April 2010 were borne by the Tanzanian MOHSW, and cost information was provided by the Principle Investigator for the National HBB program (GM) in the MOHSW. Costs for the second one-day HBB course in May 2011 and the LDHF HBB re-trainings were borne by HLH, and the number of participants, number of trainers and cost details were provided by the research department at HLH. Costs for training material were given by Lærdal Global Health.

The initial training of 40 Master Instructors in 2009 did not include personnel from HLH, therefore Master Instructors form this pool had to travel to HLH to conduct the first HBB course. These Master Instructors have delivered HBB courses in their own hospitals but also around the country. The cost of training these 40 initial Master Instructors were not included.

All costs are expressed in USD with an exchange rate of 1 USD = 1350 TZS for April 2010 and of 1 USD = 1510 TZS for May 2011.

For the evaluation of the cost-effectiveness in an international context, total costs were converted to International Dollars (ID) based on the purchasing power parity (PPP) as given by the World Health Organization (WHO) for 2005 [21].

Statistics

The software program PASW 20.0 (SPSS Inc; Chicago, USA) was used for statistical analysis. Independent-samples t-test was used to compare means of continuous parametric variables. The relation between categorical variables was explored by Chi-square tests. Two-sided p-values lower than 0.05 were considered statistically significant. The number of live years gained was based on the number of lives saved and the life expectancy at birth in Tanzania of 55.4 years as given by UN-DESA [22]. Disease adjusted life years (DALYs) were calculated based on the calculations outlined by Fox-Rushby and Hansons [23]. As recommended there, calculations are based on the life expectancy in the observed population (55.44 years). We calculated DALYs based on two assumptions: i) Discounting rate (r) = 0.03 per year (implying that years that might be gained in the future have less value than years gained right now) and age weighting with K = 1 and β = 0.04 (assigning a lower number of DALYs to years lived at young and older ages); ii) no discounting, no age weighting (equivalent to life years gained).

Ethics statement

The ongoing observational study at the delivery room at Haydom Lutheran hospital that forms the basis for the measurement of effectiveness in the present study, received the following approval by The Regional Committee for Medical and Health Research Ethics, Western Norway: The committee considers the project (reference number 2009/302) to be "an evaluation program among certified health care workers with standardized anonymous collection of related routine data on patient outcomes." Formal approval from a Norwegian ethical committee is thus not required. Informed consent was not obtained. The National Institute for Research in Tanzania approved of the observational study as part of the research project "Towards: MDG 4&5: Implementing "Helping Babies Breathe" and "Helping Mothers Survive" to improve perinatal and maternal outcome at Haydom Lutheran Hospital (reference number NIMR/HQ/R.6a/Vol IX/1247).

As the presented cost-effectiveness analysis does not involve any confidential or personal data, an ethics statement from the Regional Committee for Medical and Health Research Ethics, Western Norway was not required and thus not applied for. The National Institute for Research in Tanzania was informed about the extension of the research project and approved the study (reference number NIMR/HQ/R.6c/Vol II/172) and as well of the publication of the results (reference number NIMR/HQ/R.12/Vol XIV/15).

All authors participated in the collection of the cost data: Costs borne by the Tanzanian Ministry of Health and Welfare were provided by Georgina Msemo and Jeffrey Perlman. Costs borne by Haydom Lutheran Hospital were provided by Editha Lotto, Sara Lyanga, Estomih Mduma and Hege L.Ersdal. Costs for the training material were collected by Corinna Vossius, who also coordinated the collection of cost data.

Results

Lives saved and live years gained

As shown in table 1 there were 4876 deliveries during the 12-month observation period before full HBB implementation, and 4734 deliveries during the 12-month period after full implementation, for a total of 9610 deliveries. The ENM decreased significantly from 11.1 to 7.2 deaths per 1000 deliveries (p = 0.047) in the period after full HBB implementation, while the decrease in FSB was not statistically significant.

Based on the ENM of 11.1/1000 the expected number of deaths during the post-implementation period was 53 deaths, while the observed number was 34. As the difference in FSB was not significant, we assumed that no lives were saved due to averted FSB. Hence, the total number of lives saved was 19.

Based on a live expectancy at birth of 55.4 years the total number of potential life years gained was 1052.6 years.

Costs

Costs for the initial one-day HBB training in April 2010 were USD 2084, while it was USD 1515 for the one-day HBB re-training in May 2011. The training of four local ToT in February 2011 was linked to research activity. Therefore, only costs for one day accommodation amounted to USD 20. Table 2 presents details about the different costs factors. Costs for training material amounted to USD 812. Once implemented, the LDHF re-training incurred no direct costs as it was done during working hours and with the existing training material.

Hence, the total costs for the full HBB implementation was USD 4431.

Costs per life saved, per life year gained and per DALY averted

Costs per live saved were USD 233, while it was USD 4.21 per life year gained (table 3).

We regard costs for the initial HBB course and the training of local Master Instructors as pure implementation costs, while the LDHF training and one HBB refresher course per year are regarded crucial for maintaining knowledge, skills, and commitment to the HBB program. As the LDHF incurs no direct costs, expenses arise only for the one-day HBB refresher course of USD1515 per year. Thus, once the program is implemented costs are USD80 per life saved and USD 1.44 per life year gained.

The total number of DALYs averted was 578 DALYs if age weighting and discounting was applied and 1053 without age weighting and discounting. Converted to ID, the costs would amount to ID 22.75 per DALY averted and ID 12.49 per DALY averted, respectively for the two scenarios (table 3). To range the costs of an intervention per DALY, the WHO discerns three categories of cost-effectiveness: Highly cost-effective (less than gross domestic product (GDP) per capita); Cost-effective (between one and three times GDP per capita); and Not cost-effective (more than three times GDP per capita) [WHO-CHOICE; 23]. As the GDP per capita in Tanzania is ID 2154 the HBB program can be ranged as highly cost-effective.

Sensitivity analysis (Table 4)

At HLH, no substitutes were hired to replace the staff participating in the full-day HBB courses. However, we assume that this might be necessary at other sites. Alternatively, participants may attend the course in their spare time and have to be paid extra. Therefore, the sensitivity analysis includes wages for one working day per participant (64 participants in 2010 and 53 in 2011) in addition to the LDHF training of 30 minutes per week, increasing costs by 53%.

On the other hand, as HLH is a very rural and remote hospital. Travel expenses amounted to almost half of the total costs as trainers had to come from larger hospitals like Bugando in

Table 1. Comparison of the 12-months observation period before and after full HBB implementation.

Time Period	01.02.10–29.01.11	01.02.11–31.01.12	P-value*
Deliveries	N = 4876	N = 4734	
ENM/1000	11.1/1000 (n = 54)	7.2/1000 (n = 34)	0.047
FSB/1000	16.0/1000 (n = 78)	14.4/1000 (n = 68)	0.517
Stimulation	N = 704 (14.4%)	N = 758 (16.0%)	0.032
BMV	N = 352 (7.2%)	N = 259 (5.7%)	0.003

*Pearson Chi-Square analysis, 2-sided.
ENM = Early neonatal mortality; BMV = Bag mask ventilation.

Table 2. Total direct costs and cost factors of HBB training at HLH.

	Total costs and cost factors in USD		Payer
Initial HBB training April 2010	**Total costs**	**2084**	**MHSW**
	Travel expenses[a]	1248	
	Trainers' allowance	89	
	Participants' allowance	474	
	Administration[b]	273	
	Substitutes; 64 participants, one working day[c]	0	
Training of four local Trainers of Trainees February 2011	**Total costs**	**20**	**HLH**
	Travel expenses[a]	20	
	Trainers' allowance	0	
	Participants' allowance	0	
	Administration[b]	0	
	Substitutes; four participants, one working day[c]	0	
Refresher HBB course May 2011	**Total costs**	**1515**	**HLH**
	Travel expenses[a]	790	
	Trainers' allowance	139	
	Participants' allowance	331	
	Administration[b]	255	
	Substitutes, 53 participants, one working day[c]	0	
LDHF training	**Total costs**	**0**	**HLH**
	Trainers' allowance	0	
	Working time 30 minutes once per week[c]	0	
Material	**Total costs**	**812**	**Donation**
	8 NeoNatalies à USD 70	560	
	8 Resuscitators à USD 15	120	
	8 Penguin suctions à USD 3	24	
	4 Flip charts à USD 27	108	
	Maintenance	0	
Overall costs (%)	**Total costs**	**4431 (100)**	
	Travel expenses[a]	2048 (46)	
	Trainers' allowance	228 (5)	
	Participants' allowance	805 (18)	
	Administration[b]	528 (12	
	Material	812 (18)	

[a]Travel expenses include transport, accommodation and per diems.
[b]Administration includes as well refreshments during the course.
[c]Courses took place during normal working hours and no extra staff was hired during the courses.
MHSW = Tanzanian Ministry of Health and Social Welfare; HLH = Haydom Lutheran Hospital; LDHF = Low-dose-high-frequency.

Table 3. Costs per life saved, life year gained and DALY averted.

Unit	n	Costs per unit
Implementation and maintenance costs included		
Lives saved	16	USD 233
Life years gained	1053	USD 4.21
Only maintenance costs included		
Lives save	|19	USD 80
Life years gained	1053	USD 1.44
DALYs averted [0.03,1,0.04]	578	ID 22.75
DALYs averted [0,0,0]	1053	ID 12.49

DALYs [r, K, β] = Disability adjusted life years [discounting rate, age weighting constant K, age weighting constant β].

Mwanza, about 400 kilometers away. Avoiding travel expenses in a more urban setting and without the need to provide competent instructors from out of state would thus reduce costs by 46%.

We assumed a number of 19 lives saved, based on a risk reduction of ENM of 35.1%. In the sensitivity analysis we present as well a cost-effectiveness analysis with a risk reduction of 20% and 10%, respectively. However, even assumed a risk reduction of only 10%, costs per DALY averted (including discounting and age weighting) would amount to ID 87 and thus still be in the range of highly cost-effective measures.

Discussion

A retrospective evaluation of the costs-effectiveness of the HBB program in a rural FBO hospital in Northern Tanzania revealed costs of USD 233 per life saved and USD 4.21 per life year gained. However, costs for maintaining the program were significantly lower and are estimated to be USD 80 per life saved and USD 1.44 per life year gained.

With costs of about 12 to 23 ID per DALY averted, the HBB program can be considered highly cost-effective. These costs per DALY are comparable to a number of other measurements for maternal and neonatal health listed by WHO-CHOICE for Sub-Saharan countries such as the community newborn care package (8 ID per DALY averted) or support for breast feeding mothers (ID 10 per DALY) [24]. It is also comparable to the Essential Newborn Care Course that focuses on the first 7 days after birth. A CEA of this course in urban Zambia states costs per live saved of USD 208 and USD5.24 per life year gained, while costs for maintaining the program were USD1.84 per life year gained [25].

However, comparisons across various CEAs might be impaired by different methodologies regarding items included or not included into the cost analysis.

The implementation of the HBB program at HLH started with a one-day HBB course. Though this led to an improved performance in simulation of skills and knowledge [20], a decrease in ENM was first seen only after full implementation with systemized LDHF [19]. We therefore assume that there is a certain threshold for training input – both resource and money-wise - before the implementation of new health measurements pays off, while any training below this threshold might not yield much benefit. However, maintenance costs for the training program are significantly lower than the initial implementation.

We describe the costs as they presented in realtime at HLH. Importantly, in contrary to the WHO CHOICE guidelines [26], these costs did not comprise wages, as the courses were attended during working hours and no substitutes were hired. However, the need for substitutes might raise the costs by about 50 percent, and even more in an urban setting where wages are higher. On the other hand, HLH is a rural hospital, and the Master Instructors had to travel far distances and be accommodated. Thus, travel expenses were the biggest cost driver. In an urban setting where competence is more readily available, costs are likely to be significantly lower.

The major strengths of this study are its linkage to the observational study in the delivery room, securing reliable outcome data, and the meticulous registration of training activities and costs by the research department of the hospital. On the other

Table 4. Sensitivity analysis.

	Costs	Costs per life saved	Costs per life year gained
Presented costs*	**4431**	**231**	**4,21**
Staff salary included	+2384	345	6,22
Travel costs excluded	−2048	125	2,26
	Lives saved		
Presented risk reduction for ENM of 35.1%	19	**231**	4,21
Risk reduction of ENM 20%	10	443	8,06
Risk reduction of ENM 10%	5	886	16,11

*All costs in USD.

hand, the single center design is a limitation of the study. About five thousand births per year might not yield enough statistical power to prove changes due to the program. The rural setting at a missionary FBO hospital might not be transferrable to other sites, and a CEA at a public urban hospital might yield quite different results. In addition, we are not aware of any other interventions during the observation period, however, there might be confounding factors contributing to a decrease in ENM that are not captured in this study. ENM and FSB during the pre-implementation phase were lower than the national average [15], possibly resulting in a lower reduction in ENM and FSB and thus lower effectiveness. Furthermore, we had no data about morbidity. The calculation of DALYs is solely based on mortality data, not taking into account that an increased resuscitation activity might lead to an increased number of children with hypoxic brain damage. However, data from both the observational study and the national study reveal a significant decrease in the need of bag mask ventilation, indicating that the increase in immediate stimulation prevented development of severe asphyxia. In addition, at HLH a 40% reduction in 24 hour mortality was noted, without a corresponding increase in deaths beyond 24 hours and with a 50% reduction in admissions to neonatal area after full HBB implementation [27]. We therefore assume that morbidity due to hypoxic brain damage was not increased.

Conclusions

The number of children five years and younger dying worldwide has been reduced from 12 million per year in 1990 to seven to eight million in 2011. Vaccination programs have played an important role in this progress. However, to reduce mortality further early newborn mortality has to be addressed. The HHB program has been proven highly effective with a reduction of ENM of nearly fifty percent at eight sites in Tanzania. This study of a rural missionary FBO hospital reveals that the program is as well highly cost-effective measures in a low-resource setting. However, to facilitate further global implementation of the program an analysis of the cost-effectiveness in a multi-center setting including urban and government owned hospitals, is necessary, exploring cost-driving factors and predictors for enhanced cost-effectiveness.

Acknowledgments

This study was made possible by the help of research assistants, data quality controllers, data clerks, and the health providers working at Haydom Lutheran Hospital. We thank the Hospital Management for their approval and collaboration and Erling Svensen (Centre for International Health, University of Bergen) for his help with data collection. We thank the municipality of Stavanger, Norway for the funding of research for Corinna Vossius. We want to acknowledge Jurate Saltyte-Benth for her kind assistance in calculating DALYs.

Author Contributions

Conceived and designed the experiments: CV EL SL EM GM JP HLE. Analyzed the data: CV EL EM HLE. Contributed with cost data or provided information about the organization of the clinical work at the delivery room: CV EL SL EM GM JP HLE. Contributed to the writing of the manuscript: CV EL SL EM GM JP HLE.

References

1. Lozano R, Wang H, Foreman KJ, Rajaratnam JK, Naghavi M, et al. (2011) Progress towards Millennium Development Goals 4 and 5 on maternal and child mortality: an updated systematic analysis. Lancet 378(9797):1139–1165.
2. Black RE, Cousens S, Johnson HL, Lawn JE, Rudan I, et al. (2010) Global, regional, and national causes of child mortality in 2008: a systematic analysis. Lancet 375(9730):1969–1978.
3. Rajaratnam JK, Marcus JR, Flaxman AD, Wang H, Levin-Rector A, et al. (2010) Neonatal, postneonatal, childhood, and under-5 mortality for 187 countries, 1970–2010: a systematic analysis of progress towards Millennium Development Goal 4. Lancet 375(9730):1988–2008. Epub 2010/06/16.
4. Oestergaard MZ, Inoue M, Yoshida S, Mahanani WR, Gore FM, et al. (2011) Neonatal mortality levels for 193 countries in 2009 with trends since 1990: a systematic analysis of progress, projections, and priorities. PLoS medicine 8(8):e1001080. Epub 2011/09/16.
5. UNICEF(2011) UNICEF report 2011: Levels and Trend in Child Mortality. New York: UNICEF, 2011.
6. The World Health Report 2005 (2005): making every mother and child count. [database on the Internet]. World Health Organization. 2005.
7. UNICEF (2004) State of World's Children Report 2005. New York: 2004.
8. WHO (2006) Neonatal and perinatal mortality:country, regional and global estimates. Geneva: World Health Organization, 2006.
9. WHO (2006)Working together for health. Geneva: World Health Organization.
10. UN. (1994) International Conference on Population and Development 5.–13.September 1994. Summary of the Programme of Action: United Nations; 1994.
11. Countdown Coverage Writing Group (2008) Countdown to 2015 for maternal, newborn, and child survival: the 2008 report on tracking coverage of interventions. Lancet 371(9620):1247–1258.
12. WHO (2009) The National Roadmap Strategic Plan Tanzania 2010–2015. Available: http://www.afro.who.int/index.php?option = com_docman&task = doc_download&gid = 3349&Itemid = 2111-572k. Accessed 9 December 2013.
13. Save The Children (2009) Situation Analysis of Newborn Health in Tanzania. March 2009. Available: http://events.maildirect.se/30/Show.aspx?AccountId = 984400ac-d9e4-4f7a-b5d4-4f87249280e6&IssueId = 03704252-4538-45d3-8bd3-4a268bcdd0c6&ContactId = 29761fac-3d50-4ff0-b07f-50d9886445f8. Accessed 9 December 2013.
14. The American Academy of Pediatrics (2009) Helping Babies Breathe. Available: http://www.helpingbabiesbreathe.org/ Accessed 9 December 2013.
15. Msemo G, Massawe A, Mmbando D, Rusibamayila N, Manji K, et al. (2013) Newborn mortality and fresh stillbirth rates in Tanzania after Helping Babies Breathe training. Pediatrics Feb;131(2):e353–360.
16. United Nations (2013) Breakthrough innovations that can save mothers and children now. https://dub110.mail.live.com/mail/ViewOfficePreview. aspx?messageid = 3ce4a811-28ea-11e3-979d-00215ad6a710&folderid = 42a0b4b5 -cdf2-453f-9764-a2a02042b84f&attindex = 0&cp = -1&attdepth = 0&n = 1245908249. Accessed 24.03.2014.
17. Ersdal HL, Mduma E, Svensen E, Perlman JM (2012) Birth Asphyxia: A Major Cause of Early Neonatal Mortality in a Tanzanian Rural Hospital. Pediatrics 129:1238–1243.
18. Ersdal HL, Mduma E, Svensen E, Perlman JM (2012) Early initiation of basic resuscitation interventions including face mask ventilation may reduce birth asphyxia related mortality in low-income countries. Resuscitation 83:869–873.
19. Mduma E, Ersdal HL, Svensen E, Perlman J (2013) Low-dose-high- frequency simulation training reduces Early Neonatal Mortality in an African Hospital. Oral presentation PAS 2013, US.
20. Ersdal HL, VossiusC, Bayo E, Mduma E, Perman J, et al. (2013) A one-day "Helping Babies Breathe" course improves simulated performance but not clinical management of neonates. Resuscitation Oct;84(10):1422–1427.
21. World Health Organization (2005) Choosing Interventions that are Cost-Effective (WHO-Choice); Purchasing power parity 2005. Available: http:// www.who.int/choice/costs/ppp/en/. Accessed 9 December 2013.
22. United Nations Department of Economic and Social Affairs (UN DESA) (2011) Population Division, World Population Prospects, The 2010 Revision. Table A 28. Available: http://esa.un.org/unpd/wpp/Documentation/pdf/WPP2010_ Volume-I_Comprehensive-Tables.pdf. Accessed 9 December 2013.
23. Fox-Rushby JA, Hanson K (2001) Health policy and planning. Oxford University Press 16(3):326–331.
24. World Health Organization (2005) Choosing Interventions that are Cost-Effective (WHO-Choice); Cost-Effectiveness Results for AFR E. Available: http://www.who.int/choice/results/mnh_afroe/en/index.html. Accessed 9 December 2013.
25. Manasyan A, Chomba E, McClure EM, Wright LL, Krzywanski S, et al. (2011) Cost-effectiveness of essential newborn care training in urban first-level facilities. Pediatrics May;127(5):e1176–1181.
26. Johns B, Balthussen R, Hutubessy R (2003) Programme costs in the economic evaluation of health interventions. Available: http://www.resource-allocation. com/content/1/1/1. Accessed 7 June 2014.
27. Ersdal HL, Mduma E, Perlman JM (2013) Helping Babies Breathe (HBB) Training is Associated with Decreased Early Neonatal Mortality (ENM); This Positive Benefit is Reduced Due to Late Deaths (LD). Abstracts, presented at PAS 2013, US.

5

The Vitamin D Status in Inflammatory Bowel Disease

Lauren Elizabeth Veit[1], Louise Maranda[2], Jay Fong[1], Benjamin Udoka Nwosu[1]*

1 Department of Pediatrics, University of Massachusetts Medical School, Worcester, Massachusetts, United States of America, **2** Department of Quantitative Health Sciences, University of Massachusetts Medical School, Worcester, Massachusetts, United States of America

Abstract

Context: There is no consensus on the vitamin D status of children and adolescents with inflammatory bowel disease (IBD).

Aim: To determine the vitamin D status of patients with IBD by comparing their serum 25(OH)D concentration to that of healthy controls.

Hypothesis: Serum 25(OH)D concentration will be lower in patients with IBD compared to controls.

Subjects and Methods: A case-controlled retrospective study of subjects with IBD (n = 58) of 2–20 years (male n = 31, age 16.38±2.21 years; female n = 27, age16.56±2.08 years) and healthy controls (n = 116; male n = 49, age 13.90±4.59 years; female n = 67, age 15.04±4.12years). Study subject inclusion criteria: diagnosis of Crohn's disease (CD) or ulcerative colitis (UC). Vitamin D deficiency was defined as 25(OH)D of (<20 ng/mL) (<50 nmol/L), overweight as BMI of ≥85th but <95th percentile, and obesity as BMI ≥95th percentile. Data were expressed as mean ± SD.

Results: Patients with CD, UC, and their controls had mean serum 25(OH)D concentrations of 61.69±24.43 nmol/L, 53.26±25.51, and 65.32±27.97 respectively (ANOVA, p = 0.196). The overweight/obese controls had significantly lower 25(OH)D concentration compared to the normal-weight controls (p = 0.031); whereas 25(OH)D concentration was similar between the normal-weight and overweight/obese IBD patients (p = 0.883). There was no difference in 25(OH)D between patients with UC and CD, or between subjects with active IBD and controls. However, IBD subjects with elevated ESR had significantly lower 25(OH)D than IBD subjects with normal ESR (p = 0.025), as well as controls (65.3±28.0 nmol/L vs. 49.5±25.23, p = 0.045).

Conclusion: There is no difference in mean serum 25(OH)D concentration between children and adolescents with IBD and controls. However, IBD subjects with elevated ESR have significantly lower 25(OH)D than controls. Therefore, IBD subjects with elevated ESR should be monitored for vitamin D deficiency.

Editor: Andrzej T. Slominski, University of Tennessee, United States of America

Funding: This work was funded in part by the Faculty Diversity Scholars Program, and the Department of Pediatrics, University of Massachusetts Medical School, Worcester, Massachusetts, USA. The funders had no role in study design, data collection and analysis, decision to publish, or preparation of the manuscript.

Competing Interests: The authors have declared that no competing interests exist.

* Email: Benjamin.Nwosu@umassmemorial.org

Introduction

There is no consensus on the vitamin D status of children and adolescents with inflammatory bowel disease (IBD).The composite term IBD refers to two diseases, Crohn's disease (CD) and ulcerative colitis (UC), which are characterized by chronic inflammation of the gastrointestinal tract, marked by recurrent periods of remission and exacerbation [1]. Pediatric CD is characterized by discontinuous, transmural inflammation of the gastrointestinal tract with preferential involvement of the ileo-colonic segment, while UC is characterized by a more superficial, continuous inflammation that extends proximally from the rectum to variable areas of the large intestine [1].

Prolonged vitamin D deficiency could lead to poor health, as strong associations between vitamin D deficiency and increased risk for several diseases such as type 1 and type 2 diabetes,

cardiovascular diseases, rheumatoid arthritis, infectious diseases, depression, and cancers of the breast, prostate, colon, and pancreas, have been reported [2–4]. Though there is an ongoing debate on the significance of these extra-skeletal functions of vitamin D in humans [5,6], there is a universal consensus on its skeletal functions, as vitamin D has been demonstrated to be vital for bone mineralization, maintenance of bone strength, and the prevention of fractures and consequent immobilization [6,7].

The lack of consensus on the vitamin D status of children and adolescents with IBD stems from two primary reasons: first, the studies that investigated the vitamin D status of children and adolescents with IBD [8–12] focused primarily on determining the prevalence of vitamin D deficiency in IBD, and secondarily on comparing the vitamin D status of patients with the subtypes of

IBD, i.e., UC and CD, but failed to compare their results directly to a local control group of healthy children and adolescents.

Secondly, only one study has directly compared the vitamin D status of children and adolescents with IBD to the vitamin D status of age- and gender-matched peers [13]. This cross-sectional study of 60 children with newly-diagnosed IBD and 56 controls found that 25(OH)D level was significantly lower in children with IBD compared to the controls. However, no subsequent studies have been performed to confirm these findings. Furthermore, to our knowledge, there has been no case-controlled study examining the vitamin D status of patients with established IBD of more than one year duration. This lack of clarity on the vitamin D status of children and adolescents with IBD compared to their peers has made it difficult to propose a coherent recommendation for vitamin D supplementation in patients with IBD [9,14].

We designed this study to explore the hypothesis that serum 25(OH)D concentration is significantly lower in patients with IBD compared to controls. The primary aim of this study was to characterize the vitamin D status of patients with IBD by directly comparing their mean serum 25(OH)D concentration to that of a local group of healthy children.

Materials and Methods

Ethics statement

The study protocol was approved by the University of Massachusetts Institutional Review Board. All patient records and information were anonymized and de-identified prior to analysis.

Subjects

All data were sourced from the Children's Medical Center Database of the UMassMemorial Medical Center, Worcester, Massachusetts, USA. The medical records of children and adolescents of ages 2–20 years with a confirmed diagnosis of Crohn's disease or ulcerative colitis from January 1, 2007 through June 30, 2013, were reviewed. Study subjects (n = 58; 31 males) were included if they had a diagnosis of Crohn's disease or ulcerative colitis. Subjects' height, weight, gender, race, IBD diagnosis, date of endoscopic IBD diagnosis, and any history of vitamin D supplementation were recorded.

A group of healthy peers served as controls. The controls were identified from the same database as the subjects. Subjects were included in the control group (n = 116; 49 males) if they carried no diagnosis of Crohn's disease or ulcerative colitis. Subjects' height, weight, gender, race, and history of vitamin D supplementation were similarly recorded.

Patients were excluded from this study if they carried a concurrent diagnosis of any disease that affects calcium or vitamin D metabolism. Subjects with a malabsorption syndrome, other than IBD, were excluded. Further exclusion criteria included patients with a history of vitamin D or calcium supplementation prior to the date of 25(OH)D measurement, subjects on continuous doses of oral corticosteroids for the management of any disease other than IBD, pregnant or lactating subjects, and patients with chronic liver disease.

We identified 76 children and adolescents of ages 2–20 years with a diagnosis of IBD. Eighteen subjects were excluded based on the above exclusion criteria. Fifty-eight subjects were included in the study. The control group consisted of 116 non-IBD peers who were randomly drawn from the same database using a systematic sampling scheme. For this method, we alphabetized the list of control patients then selected every 5th patient for inclusion in our control group, thereby preserving randomization.

The ages of both the study subjects and their controls were determined by the date of 25(OH)D measurement. The duration of disease was designated as the interval from the date of endoscopic diagnosis of IBD to the date of 25(OH)D measurement. The percentages of subjects from the various ethnic/racial groups for the control group were as follows: Non-Hispanic 75%, African American 8%, White Hispanic 5%, Multi-ethnicity 5%, Unknown 4%. Similarly, the percentages from the various ethnic/racial groups for the IBD groups were: Non-Hispanic white 85%, African American 3%, White Hispanic 3%, Multi-ethnicity 3%, Unknown 5%.

Because vitamin D status varies with sunlight exposure and the seasons, we categorized each subject's date of vitamin D draw according to the seasons as follows: fall (September 22–December 21), winter (December 22–March 21), spring (March 22–June 21), and summer (June 22–September 21)[15].

Anthropometry

Height was measured to the nearest 0.1 cm using a wall-mounted stadiometer (Holtain Ltd, Crymych, Dyfed, UK) that was calibrated daily. Weight was measured to the nearest 0.1 kg using an upright scale. BMI was derived using the formula weight/height^2 (kg/m^2), and expressed as standard deviation score (SDS) for age and gender based on National Center for Health Statistics (NCHS) data [16]. Overweight was defined as BMI of $\geq 85^{th}$ but $< 95^{th}$ percentile, while obesity was defined as a BMI of $\geq 95^{th}$ percentile for age and gender.

Assay

Serum 25(OH)D concentration was analyzed using 25-hydroxy chemiluminescent immunoassay (DiaSorin Liaison; Stillwater, Minnesota), which has a 100% cross-reactivity with both metabolites of 25(OH)D namely, 25(OH)D$_2$ and 25(OH)D$_3$ and thus measures total serum 25(OH)D content. Its functional sensitivity is 10 nmol/L, and its intra- and inter-assay coefficients of variation are 5% and 8.2%, respectively. Vitamin D status was defined using 25(OH)D values based on criteria by The Endocrine Society Clinical Practice Guideline as follows: vitamin D deficiency<20 ng/mL (50 nmol/L), insufficiency 20–29.9 ng/mL (50–74.5 nmol/L), and sufficiency≥ 30 ng/mL (75 nmol/L)[5], which is similar to the classification of vitamin D status by the American Academy of Pediatrics and the Institutes of Medicine criteria which denote vitamin D deficiency as 25(OH)D <50 nmol/L; and sufficiency as 25(OH)D >50 nmol/L [6,17].

Statistical analyses

Statistical analyses were performed using the SPSS Predictive Analytics SoftWare v.21 (IBM Corporation, Armonk, NY) and Microsoft Excel (2007). Means and standard deviations were calculated for descriptive summary statistics and 25(OH)D measurements. Multivariate and univariate comparisons on anthropometrics, 25(OH)D, and other variables were conducted using ANOVA and two-tailed student's t-test respectively. Specifically, ANOVA was used to compare the differences in the parameters of interests between the controls, UC, and CD subjects. Height, weight, and BMI data were expressed as z-scores. Race, gender proportionality, and seasons of blood draw were compared using Fisher's exact test. Data were expressed as mean ± standard deviation (SD).

Table 1. A Comparative Analysis of the Characteristics of Subjects with Ulcerative Colitis, Crohn's Disease, and Healthy Controls.

Parameter	CD	95% CI	UC	95% CI	Controls	95% CI	p
Total	40	-	18	-	116	-	-
Age (years)	16.61±2.20	(15.91, 17.32)	16.13±1.99	(15.14, 17.12)	14.56±4.35	(13.76, 15.36)	0.008
Height z-score	−0.63±1.18	(−1.01, −0.25)	0.00±0.98	(−0.49, 0.49)	−0.02±1.42	(−0.28, 0.24)	0.040
Weight z-score	−0.31±1.45	(−0.77, 0.16)	0.30±1.11	(−0.26, 0.85)	0.40±1.60	(0.11, 0.70)	0.041
BMI z-score	−0.08±1.35	(−0.51, 0.35)	0.28±0.99	(−0.21, 0.78)	0.48±1.38	(0.23, 0.74)	0.076
Sex (% males)	24/40 (60.0%)	-	7/18 (38.9%)	-	49/116 (42.2%)	-	0.124
Race (% white)	36/40 (90.0%)	-	15/18 (83.3%)	-	87/116 (75.0%)	-	0.118
Season (%Winter-Spring)	17/40 (42.5%)	-	8/18 (44.4%)	-	51/116 (44.0%)	-	0.985
BMI status (% overweight/obese)	11/40 (27.5%)	-	2/18 (11.1%)	-	45/116 (38.8%)	-	0.046
Disease duration (years)	2.61±2.76	(1.68, 3.54)	2.76±2.54	(1.49, 4.02)	-	-	0.854
Mean serum 25(OH)D (nmol/L)	61.69±24.43	(53.88, 69.50)	53.26±25.51	(40.57, 65.94)	65.32±27.97	(60.18, 70.46)	0.196
25(OH)D ≤15 ng/mL (%)	6/40 (15.0%)	-	5/18 (27.8%)	-	12/116 (10.3%)	-	0.118
25(OH)D ≤20 ng/mL (%)	16/40 (40.0%)	-	9/18 (50.0%)	-	31/116 (26.7%)	-	0.070
25(OH)D ≤30 ng/mL (%)	29/40 (72.5%)	-	15/18 (83.3%)	-	87/116 (75%)	-	0.671

SDS standard deviation score; 25(OH)D 25-hydroxyvitamin D.

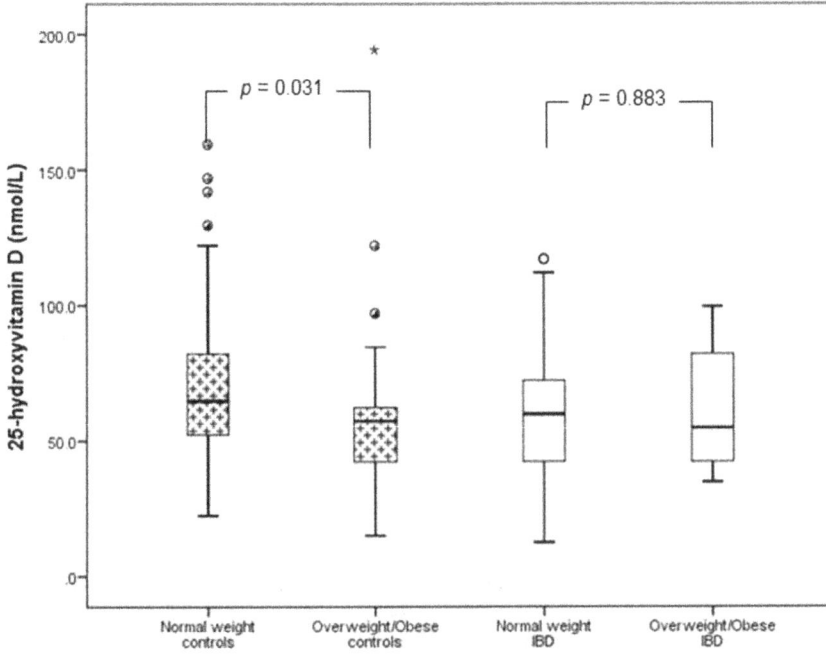

Figure 1. Box plots of the comparison of 25-hydroxyvitamin D concentration of patients with inflammatory bowel disease (IBD) and normal controls stratified by body mass index. This figure shows that the overweight/obese controls had significantly lower value for 25(OH)D than the normal weight controls (58.32±27.63 vs. 69.76±27.45, p=0.031), while there was no significant difference in 25(OH)D value between the normal weight and overweight/obese IBD patients (59.71±26.44 vs. 60.91±23.26, p=0.883). Note: 50 nmol/L=20 ng/mL.

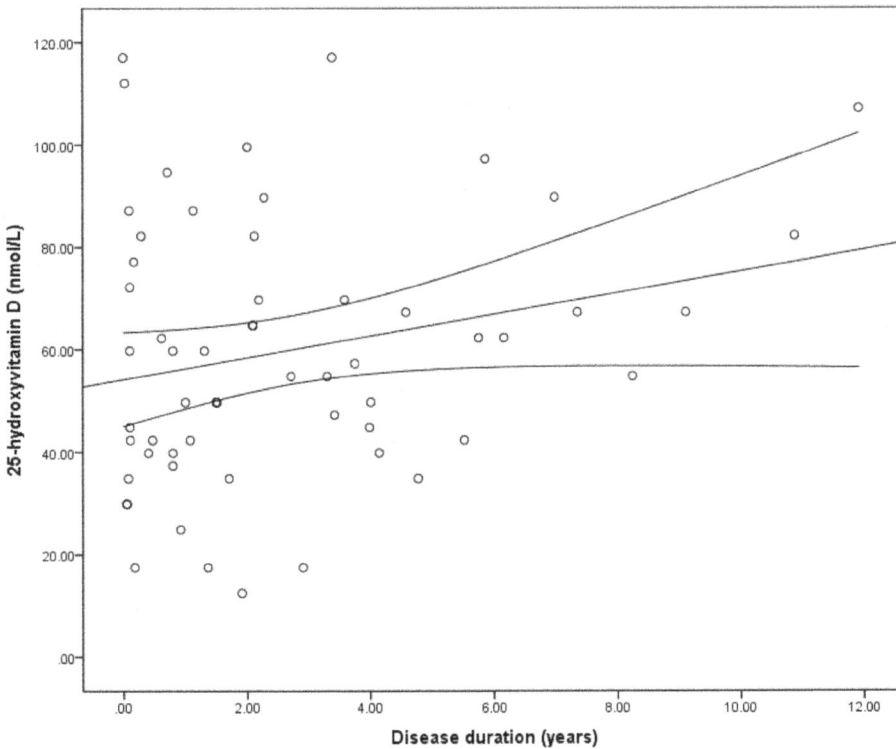

Figure 2. Scatterplot of the comparison of the 25-hydroxyvitamin D concentration and the duration of disease in inflammatory bowel disease. This figure shows a non-significant positive relationship between serum 25(OH)D concentration and the duration of disease ($r^2=0.054$, $\beta=0.23$, p=0.08).

Results

Comparative analysis of the characteristics of subjects with UC, CD, and their controls

Table 1 shows the analysis of the characteristics of the subjects with UC, CD, and controls using a one-way ANOVA. The controls were younger, had higher value for weight SDS, and a higher prevalence of overweight/obese status compared to the UC and CD groups. There was no difference in mean serum 25(OH)D concentration (p = 0.196) between the groups. There was a non-significantly higher prevalence of vitamin D deficiency as defined by a 25(OH)D value of <50 nmol/L (20 ng/mL) in both the UC and CD compared to controls (p = 0.070).

Comparison of the characteristics of the subjects with UC vs. CD

When the IBD cohort was stratified by IBD sub-types, UC vs. CD, there were no significant differences in age, gender, weight, BMI, disease duration, or season of vitamin D measurement. Subjects with CD were non-significantly shorter than the UC patients (p = 0.05). There was no difference in mean serum 25(OH)D concentration between groups (53.3±25.4 vs. 61.8±24.4, p = 0.24). Subjects with UC had a non-significantly higher prevalence of vitamin D deficiency compared to the CD subjects (50% vs. 40%, p = 0.53).

The effect of adiposity on serum 25(OH)D in IBD vs. controls

To investigate the effect of adiposity on 25(OH)D concentration in IBD vs. controls, the subjects were stratified into normal-weight vs. overweight/obese groups (Figure 1). The overweight/obese controls had significantly lower 25(OH)D concentration compared to the normal-weight controls (p = 0.031), whereas 25(OH)D concentration was similar between the normal-weight and overweight/obese IBD patients (p = 0.883). Further stratification of the IBD cohort into UC and CD showed no difference in 25(OH)D concentration between the normal-weight and overweight/obese groups for CD (p = 0.98) or UC (p = 0.70). These data suggest that adiposity has no effect on serum 25(OH)D concentration of patients with IBD.

The relationship between the duration of IBD and serum 25(OH)D concentration

We first compared the mean 25(OH)D concentration of the control group to 13 patients with IBD who had serum 25(OH)D estimation at the time of diagnosis of IBD, i.e. during active disease, and found no significant difference in their mean 25(OH)D concentration (65.3±28.0 vs. 63.8±30.1 nmol/L, p = 0.86). Next, we investigated the relationship between the duration of disease and serum concentration of 25(OH)D (Figure 2). There was a non-significant, positive relationship between serum 25(OH)D concentration and the duration of disease (r^2 = 0.054, β = 0.23, p = 0.08).

The relationship between the severity of IBD and serum 25(OH)D concentration

Using the Pediatric Crohn's Disease Activity Index (PCDAI)[18] and Lichtiger Colitis Activity Index (LCAI)[19], to quantify the severity of IBD, we investigated the differences in serum 25(OH)D concentration in the three groups: controls, n = 116; quiescent IBD cases n = 22; active IBD cases n = 8. There was no difference in serum 25(OH)D concentration between three groups: [controls, 65.3±27.7 nmol/L; quiescent IBD cases

61.3±28.3; active IBD cases 54.5±22.5, ANOVA p = 0.498. Post hoc comparisons detected no significant difference in 25(OH)D levels between the groups.

We then stratified the IBD cohort using ESR as a marker of inflammation and compared their serum 25(OH)D level to the controls. Within the IBD cohort, serum 25(OH)D concentration was significantly lower in patients with elevated ESR levels (ESR of >21 mm/hr) compared to those with normal ESR values (49.5±25.2 nmol/L vs. 65.6±22.1, p = 0.025).

Subsequent analysis of the mean serum 25(OH)D concentrations of the 3 groups: controls (n = 116), IBD with elevated ESR (n = 19), and IBD with normal ESR (n = 37), showed a near-significant difference in 25(OH)D between the groups (ANOVA p = 0.052). Post hoc comparisons showed a significant difference in 25(OH)D concentration between the controls and IBD subjects with elevated ESR (65.3±28.0 nmol/L vs. 49.54±25.23, p = 0.045), but not between the controls and the IBD subjects with normal ESR (65.3±28.0 vs. 65.6±22.1, p = 0.998).

Discussion

This study found no significant difference in the serum concentration of 25(OH)D in children and adolescents with IBD compared to normal controls. The normal-weight controls had significantly higher 25(OH)D concentration compared to the overweight/obese controls as well as the normal-weight IBD subjects. There was no difference in 25(OH)D between the normal-weight IBD and the overweight/obese IBD subjects. In contrast, subjects with IBD and elevated ESR had significantly lower serum 25(OH)D concentration compared to the healthy controls, and subjects with IBD and normal ESR level.

This is the second study to directly compare the vitamin D status of children and adolescents with IBD to healthy controls. Our finding, however, is contrary to the report by El-Matary et al [13] who described lower 25(OH)D concentration in a cross-sectional study of children with newly-diagnosed IBD compared to controls. Our report differed from the above-referenced study in that our study included subjects with more established IBD, with mean disease duration of thirty-two months. However, our sub-analysis found no difference in the mean 25(OH)D concentration measure at the time of IBD diagnosis compared to the mean 25(OH)D of the controls. Thus, this study found no evidence for subnormal vitamin D status in patients with newly-diagnosed IBD compared to controls in our cohort.

This study's findings on the 25(OH)D levels of established IBD are consistent with the report of a case-controlled study that reported no significant difference in serum 25(OH)D in adult patients with established IBD [20].

The effect of disease duration on vitamin D deficiency is unclear, as some studies report longer disease duration as a risk factor for vitamin D deficiency [20], while others found a positive correlation between disease duration and serum 25(OH)D concentration [8]. This study's findings are in agreement with the above report of a positive relationship between disease duration in IBD and 25(OH)D concentration (Figure 2). One explanation for this association is that the initiation of treatment in patients with IBD results in some degree of healing of the mucosal damage and consequent improvement in the absorption of vitamin D. It is also possible that the phenomenon of compensation which has been described in celiac disease, also occurs in IBD and leads to increased vitamin D absorptive capacity by the unaffected mucosal surfaces [21].

Additional case-controlled studies are warranted to accurately characterize the vitamin D status of patients with IBD at various phases of the disease. This is necessary because the other studies that have examined the vitamin D status of patients with IBD lacked control groups, focused primarily on either the prevalence rate of vitamin D deficiency in IBD, or limited their comparison of vitamin D status to patients with the subtypes of IBD, i.e., UC and CD. For example, one study found normal 25(OH)D concentration in children with CD [12], while another study reported lower 25(OH)D concentration in children with CD compared to those with UC, even though the mean 25(OH)D concentration was normal for the two IBD sub-types [11]. Two studies that defined vitamin D deficiency using a cut-off value of 37.4 nmol/L (15 ng/mL) reported prevalence rates of 16% for children with CD [10] and 10.8% for children and adolescents with IBD [8]. Three studies have investigated the vitamin D status of children and adolescents using a 25(OH)D cut-off value of 50 nmol/L (20 ng/mL), similar to the current study. The first of these studies which was conducted in Australia [22] reported a 19% prevalence of vitamin D deficiency while the other two studies from the same center in New England, USA, reported prevalence rates of 34.6% [8] and 14.3%[9]. A similar study in healthy adolescents in New England that used a cut-off value of 50 nmol/L to define vitamin D deficiency reported a prevalence of 42.0% [23]. An analysis of the prevalence of vitamin D deficiency in the subtypes of IBD detected no significant differences between UC and CD at 25(OH)D cut-off values of 38 nmol/L or 50 nmol/L [8]. Thus, the results of studies investigating the vitamin D status of children and adolescents with IBD are limited and discordant.

Though the studies that characterized the prevalence of vitamin D deficiency in IBD have provided important information in this field, they have not proven that vitamin D deficiency is a feature of IBD as they did not compare their vitamin D data to those of healthy children and adolescents in a case-controlled research design. This is expressed in a recent call for more studies comparing the vitamin D status of patients with IBD to those of healthy controls [9].

The lack of a demonstration of subnormal vitamin D status in IBD compared to controls may be explained by the fact that in addition to oral intake, this prohormone is synthesized in the skin through exposure to ultra-violet radiation. Hence, dietary intake of vitamin D is not necessarily required to maintain normal vitamin D status in individuals who maintain adequate exposure to sunlight.

There was neither a significant difference in serum 25(OH)D concentration between IBD subjects and controls, nor between IBD subjects with active vs. quiescent disease.

In contrast, IBD subjects with elevated ESR had significantly lower 25(OH)D concentration than IBD subjects with normal ESR values. When compared to controls, subjects with IBD and normal ESR level had similar 25(OH)D concentration as controls, whereas subjects with IBD and elevated ESR had significantly lower 25(OH)D than controls (65.3±28.0 nmol/L vs. 49.54±25.23, p = 0.045). This finding supports previous reports of an independent association between ESR and lower 25(OH)D concentration in IBD [8,14]. However, to the best of our knowledge, this is the first study to report significantly lower 25(OH)D concentration in patients with IBD and elevated ESR compared to healthy controls.

Adiposity and 25-hydroxyvitamin D

Obesity occurs in IBD despite the strong association between IBD and growth retardation [24]. A recent study of nearly 1600 children reported an obesity rate of 20% in children with IBD; and a rate for overweight status that is similar to that of the general population at nearly 30% [25]. The control group in this study had a non-significantly higher BMI z-score than the subjects with IBD. To determine the effect of adiposity on 25(OH)D concentration, we stratified the subjects and controls into normal-weight and overweight/obese groups based on BMI criteria(Figure 1). Even though there was no difference in mean serum 25(OH)D between the IBD patients and controls (Table 1), upon stratification into BMI sub-groups, the normal-weight controls had significantly higher 25(OH)D concentration compared to the overweight/obese IBD patients (p = 0.031). In contrast, serum 25(OH)D concentration was similar between the normal-weight IBD and the overweight/obese IBD patients (p = 0.883). The normal-weight controls had significantly higher 25(OH)D concentration compared to the normal-weight IBD subjects (p = 0.023), but there was neither a difference in serum 25(OH)D concentration between the overweight/obese controls vs. the overweight/obese IBD subjects, nor between normal-weight IBD vs. overweight/obese IBD.

We and others have shown that increased adiposity is associated with vitamin D deficiency [26,27]. The mechanism of this association is unclear, however, proposed causative factors include poor nutrition, inadequate exposure to sunlight, and the sequestration of vitamin D in fat stores in overweight/obese individuals [28]. Interestingly, adiposity had no effect on the vitamin D status of our IBD cohort. More research is needed to determine the adiposity threshold necessary to induce significant reduction in serum 25(OH)D concentration [9] through processes such as the sequestration of vitamin D in fat stores in patients with IBD [28].

Strengths and limitations

This study has some limitations. First, the cross-sectional study design limits causal inference on the effects of seasons, race, and adiposity on vitamin D status. Second, we did not administer a food-recall to accurately determine dietary vitamin D intake. Third, we did not exhaustively evaluate the components of the complex vitamin D metabolic pathway, such as parathyroid hormone (PTH), 1,25-dihydroxyvitamin D, 24,25-dihydroxyvitamin D, and vitamin D receptor activity. This is important because PTH could be elevated in states of vitamin D deficiency and hypocalcemia, while 24,25-dihyroxyvitamin D could be elevated in states on increased vitamin D degradation. However, 25(OH)D is the major circulation form of vitamin D and its stability in plasma, and a long half-life of >15 days makes it a highly sensitive and specific marker of vitamin D status [29]. Fourth, our control group was younger than the IBD cohort: such a difference could potentially influence our results, however, earlier studies found no relationship between age and 25(OH)D concentration in children and adolescents with IBD [8,13]. Fifth, we did not adjust for the effect of pubertal maturation on 25(OH)D concentration, however, others have shown that pubertal maturation does not influence vitamin D concentration in IBD [30]. Finally, our results were derived from a single tertiary care center in the northern United States located at latitude 42°N. Therefore, we are uncertain that our results are generalizable to other centers, countries, and geographical latitudes.

The unique strength of this study is its case-controlled design which enabled us to evaluate a large cohort of patients with IBD and compare their results to a control group. This large sample size enabled us to detect subtle differences between the groups of interest. Our sample contained a fair representation of the fractional composition of each of the major racial groups in Central Massachusetts, thus enabling us to analyze the effects of differential insolation on racial groups. The control group was randomly selected using a structured randomization scheme. This study was conducted exclusively amongst subjects living in the same geographical latitude (42°N), thus ensuring uniformity of exposure to solar radiation. Phlebotomy was performed at different seasons of the year, thus ensuring that seasonality did not confound our results. Furthermore, the relationship between duration of IBD and 25(OH)D was analyzed, and effect of disease severity on 25(OH)D concentration in IBD was analyzed and compared to controls. All anthropometric data were expressed as z-score, and the analyses were adjusted for covariates.

Conclusions

There was no difference in mean serum 25(OH)D concentration between children and adolescents with IBD and controls. IBD subjects with elevated ESR had significantly lower serum 25(OH)D concentration compared to the healthy controls, and subjects with IBD and normal ESR level. This finding of vitamin

D deficiency in subjects with IBD and elevated ESR suggests that inflammation is a risk factor for vitamin D deficiency in IBD. Therefore, it may be prudent to closely monitor patients with IBD and elevated ESR for vitamin D deficiency.

Acknowledgments

We thank Francis M. Wanjau for his assistance with data management, and Jessica L. Kowaleski for her clerical assistance.

Author Contributions

Conceived and designed the experiments: BUN. Performed the experiments: LV BUN LM JF. Analyzed the data: LM LV BUN. Contributed reagents/materials/analysis tools: LM JF. Contributed to the writing of the manuscript: BUN LV LM JF.

References

1. Day AS, Ledder O, Leach ST, Lemberg DA (2012) Crohn's and colitis in children and adolescents. World J Gastroenterol 18: 5862–5869.
2. Stewart R, Hirani V (2010) Relationship between vitamin D levels and depressive symptoms in older residents from a national survey population. Psychosom Med 72: 608–612.
3. Holick MF (2007) Vitamin D deficiency. N Engl J Med 357: 266–281.
4. Bikle D (2009) Nonclassic actions of vitamin D. J Clin Endocrinol Metab 94: 26–34.
5. Holick MF, Binkley NC, Bischoff-Ferrari HA, Gordon CM, Hanley DA, et al. (2011) Evaluation, treatment, and prevention of vitamin D deficiency: an Endocrine Society clinical practice guideline. J Clin Endocrinol Metab 96: 1911–1930.
6. Ross AC, Manson JE, Abrams SA, Aloia JF, Brannon PM, et al. (2011) The 2011 report on dietary reference intakes for calcium and vitamin D from the Institute of Medicine: what clinicians need to know. J Clin Endocrinol Metab 96: 53–58.
7. Cranney A, Horsley T, O'Donnell S, Weiler H, Puil L, et al. (2007) Effectiveness and safety of vitamin D in relation to bone health. Evid Rep Technol Assess (Full Rep): 1–235.
8. Pappa HM, Gordon CM, Saslowsky TM, Zholudev A, Horr B, et al. (2006) Vitamin D status in children and young adults with inflammatory bowel disease. Pediatrics 118: 1950–1961.
9. Pappa HM, Langereis EJ, Grand RJ, Gordon CM (2011) Prevalence and risk factors for hypovitaminosis D in young patients with inflammatory bowel disease. J Pediatr Gastroenterol Nutr 53: 361–364.
10. Sentongo TA, Semaeo EJ, Stettler N, Piccoli DA, Stallings VA, et al. (2002) Vitamin D status in children, adolescents, and young adults with Crohn disease. Am J Clin Nutr 76: 1077–1081.
11. Gokhale R, Favus MJ, Karrison T, Sutton MM, Rich B, et al. (1998) Bone mineral density assessment in children with inflammatory bowel disease. Gastroenterology 114: 902–911.
12. Issenman RM, Atkinson SA, Radoja C, Fraher L (1993) Longitudinal assessment of growth, mineral metabolism, and bone mass in pediatric Crohn's disease. J Pediatr Gastroenterol Nutr 17: 401–406.
13. El-Matary W, Sikora S, Spady D (2011) Bone mineral density, vitamin D, and disease activity in children newly diagnosed with inflammatory bowel disease. Dig Dis Sci 56: 825–829.
14. Pappa HM, Mitchell PD, Jiang H, Kassiff S, Filip-Dhima R, et al. (2012) Treatment of vitamin D insufficiency in children and adolescents with inflammatory bowel disease: a randomized clinical trial comparing three regimens. J Clin Endocrinol Metab 97: 2134–2142.
15. Svoren BM, Volkening LK, Wood JR, Laffel LM (2009) Significant vitamin D deficiency in youth with type 1 diabetes mellitus. J Pediatr 154: 132–134.
16. Kuczmarski RJ, Ogden CL, Guo SS, Grummer-Strawn LM, Flegal KM, et al. (2002) 2000 CDC Growth Charts for the United States: methods and development. Vital Health Stat 11: 1–190.
17. Sacheck J, Goodman E, Chui K, Chomitz V, Must A, et al. (2011) Vitamin D deficiency, adiposity, and cardiometabolic risk in urban schoolchildren. J Pediatr 159: 945–950.
18. Hyams JS, Ferry GD, Mandel FS, Gryboski JD, Kibort PM, et al. (1991) Development and validation of a pediatric Crohn's disease activity index. J Pediatr Gastroenterol Nutr 12: 439–447.
19. Lichtiger S, Present DH, Kornbluth A, Gelernt I, Bauer J, et al. (1994) Cyclosporine in severe ulcerative colitis refractory to steroid therapy. N Engl J Med 330: 1841–1845.
20. Suibhne TN, Cox G, Healy M, O'Morain C, O'Sullivan M (2012) Vitamin D deficiency in Crohn's disease: prevalence, risk factors and supplement use in an outpatient setting. J Crohns Colitis 6: 182–188.
21. Semeraro LA, Barwick KW, Gryboski JD (1986) Obesity in celiac sprue. J Clin Gastroenterol 8: 177–180.
22. Levin AD, Wadhera V, Leach ST, Woodhead HJ, Lemberg DA, et al. (2011) Vitamin D deficiency in children with inflammatory bowel disease. Dig Dis Sci 56: 830–836.
23. Gordon CM, DePeter KC, Feldman HA, Grace E, Emans SJ (2004) Prevalence of vitamin D deficiency among healthy adolescents. Arch Pediatr Adolesc Med 158: 531–537.
24. Zwintscher NP, Horton JD, Steele SR (2014) Obesity has minimal impact on clinical outcomes in children with inflammatory bowel disease. J Pediatr Surg 49: 265–268; discussion 268.
25. Long MD, Crandall WV, Leibowitz IH, Duffy L, del Rosario F, et al. (2011) Prevalence and epidemiology of overweight and obesity in children with inflammatory bowel disease. Inflamm Bowel Dis 17: 2162–2168.
26. Vimaleswaran KS, Berry DJ, Lu C, Tikkanen E, Pilz S, et al. (2013) Causal relationship between obesity and vitamin D status: bi-directional Mendelian randomization analysis of multiple cohorts. PLoS Med 10: e1001383.
27. Setty-Shah N, Maranda L, Candela N, Fong J, Dahod I, et al. (2013) Lactose intolerance: lack of evidence for short stature or vitamin D deficiency in prepubertal children. PLoS One 8: e78653.
28. Liel Y, Ulmer E, Shary J, Hollis BW, Bell NH (1988) Low circulating vitamin D in obesity. Calcif Tissue Int 43: 199–201.
29. Jones G (2008) Pharmacokinetics of vitamin D toxicity. Am J Clin Nutr 88: 582S–586S.
30. Pappa HM, Grand RJ, Gordon CM (2006) Report on the vitamin D status of adult and pediatric patients with inflammatory bowel disease and its significance for bone health and disease. Inflamm Bowel Dis 12: 1162–1174.

6

Disgust Sensitivity Is Not Associated with Health in a Rural Bangladeshi Sample

Mícheál de Barra[1]*, **M. Sirajul Islam**[2], **Val Curtis**[1]

1 Environmental Health Group, London School of Hygiene and Tropical Medicine, London, United Kingdom, **2** Environmental Microbiology Lab, ICDDR,B, Dhaka, Bangladesh

Abstract

Disgust can be considered a psychological arm of the immune system that acts to prevent exposure to infectious agents. High disgust sensitivity is associated with greater behavioral avoidance of disease vectors and thus may reduce infection risk. A cross-sectional survey in rural Bangladesh provided no strong support for this hypothesis. In many species, the expression of pathogen- and predator-avoidance mechanisms is contingent on early life exposure to predators and pathogens. Using childhood health data collected in the 1990s, we examined if adults with more infectious diseases in childhood showed greater adult disgust sensitivity: no support for this association was found. Explanations for these null finding and possible directions for future research are discussed.

Editor: Christine A Caldwell, University of Stirling, United Kingdom

Funding: This research was supported by a grant from Hindustan Unilever Ltd to Valerie A. Curtis. The funders had no role in study design, data collection and analysis, decision to publish, or preparation of the manuscript.

Competing Interests: This research was supported by a grant from Hindustan Unilever Ltd to Valerie A. Curtis.

* Email: mdebarra@gmail.com

Introduction

The emotion disgust is characterized by behavioral avoidance or rejection. A broad range of stimuli including body wastes, deformity, spoilage and certain immoral and sexual acts elicit the emotion [1]. People vary in the degree to which they experience disgust in response to these things, and this variation is known as disgust sensitivity. Disgust often motivates avoidance of things that carry an infection risk; this overlap between infective substances and disgust elicitors suggests that disgust may play a functional role in preventing infection [2]. Over evolutionary timescales the costs associated with parasitism have been an important selection pressure and have sculpted several host defense mechanisms, including behavioral strategies [3–5]. Functionally speaking, our feeling of revulsion and the associated avoidance behavior can be considered a psychological arm of the broader immune system [6].

One implication of the parasite-avoidance model is that people prone to strong feelings of disgust will be exposed to pathogens less frequently. Disgust sensitivity is associated with unwillingness to approach/touch things that can cause infection [7] and this reduced exposure could translate into fewer bouts of infectious disease. Consistent with this, Stevenson et al. found that people who were both highly sensitive to disgusting stimuli and inclined to make inferences about spreading contamination reported less recent infections [8]. While the health benefits of disgust were modest, these results suggest that disgust sensitivity can influence health in a high-income population where public health infrastructure is well developed and where infectious disease is rare. In this paper, we examine if individual variation in disgust sensitivity influences infection rates in rural Bangladesh. In this environment, people are exposed to diseases uncommon in high-income settings [9]. If disgust does indeed provide a protective effect, the relationship between infection rate and disgust sensitivity should be clear in this population.

Another prediction derived from the parasite-avoidance model is that disgust sensitivity will be higher where the threat of infection is greater. Systems that protect organisms from pathogens or predators often entail trade-offs: the individual benefits from fewer infections or reduced risk of predation but must pay a cost to develop or maintain the system. The costs of disgust may include rejected food and social partners, or an increased risk of psychopathology [10]. In other species, the costs of disease avoidance can be considerable. For example, Hutchings and colleagues found that sheep with conservative foraging behavior also had lower weight because avoiding pathogens also entailed avoiding high quality forage [11]. Finding the right balance of cost and benefit is an important problem, and one solution lies in facultative expression of the protective system. In humans, food disgust sensitivity appears to decline when the costs of rejection increase, i.e., when people are hungry [12]. Conversely, when the immune system is weakened by pregnancy, there is a compensatory increase in disgust sensitivity [13]. In other species, adjustment to local pathogen/predator risk often occurs in during development and is relatively stable over the lifespan; the organism can use early-life cues to estimate the current threat and develop accordingly [14]. In humans, many life history parameters such as age-at-first birth and age-at-marriage appear to be influenced by early life cues indicative of a risky environment [15,16]. Local infection risk depends on factors like immunocompetence, sanitation and water infrastructure, local hygiene practices, animal husbandry, and climate. These factors change relatively slowly (i.e., over decades) and so childhood infection rates should provide a reliable medium-term measure of local infection risk and could

Table 1. Illness among the 284 participants in the year prior to data collection.

Disease	Number of participants experiencing disease
Flu	118 (42%)
Gastric Pain	105 (37%)
Cough	82 (29%)
Vomiting	70 (25%)
Diarrhea	61 (21%)
Eye Infection	33 (12%)
Tooth Ache	28 (10%)
Skin Infection	27 (10%)
Fever	9 (3%)
Ear Ache	8 (3%)
Sinus Infection	8 (2%)
Dysentery	7 (0%)
Tuberculosis	0 (%)

thus be used to benchmark a locally appropriate level of disgust sensitivity. Consistent with this, we previously found that childhood exposure to disease is associated with a greater preference for opposite sex faces with exaggerated sex typical characteristics, a putative health cue [17]. In other words, people sick more often as children prioritize health cues in partner choice as adults. Thus, our second hypothesis was that people with more

infections in childhood would show greater disgust sensitivity in adulthood. We tested this hypothesis using disgust sensitivity data collected in 2010 and longitudinal childhood health data collected in the 1990s.

Materials and Methods

The data was collected as part of a broader study on health, hygiene and psychology in rural Bangladesh. Participants, all of whom were 16 years of age or older, saw an information sheet, had the aims and methods explained, and were given the opportunity to ask questions. Participants gave written consent before data collection began. Informed consent from participants' next of kin, caretaker or guardian was not sought. The London School of Hygiene and Tropical Medicine Review Board approved the research, including the information sheets, consent forms, and consent procedure.

Sample

Sample size calculation was based on hypothesis one; that disgust sensitivity will correlate negatively with recent infection frequency. We anticipated that the correlation between disgust and health in the present study would be of small or medium magnitude ($r \approx .2$). A sample size calculation with $r = .2$, significance threshold $= .05$, and power $= .9$ indicated that 258 participants were needed.

Participants were randomly selected from a list of people born between July 1990 and August 1997 and living in one of 13 villages familiar to the field workers (i.e., in regions where they had previously conducted field work). The wording of childhood health questions and the frequency of interview remained constant for

Table 2. Exploratory factor analysis of disgust items: two factor solution.

Back Translated Item	Factor 1	Factor 2	Communality
Picking your nose	.80		.51
Touching the inside of a toilet	.65	.32	.75
Skin with scabies	.59		.35
Eating from dirty plate	.55		.38
Spit on the road	.54		.26
Accidentally using other persons toothbrush	.50		.25
Sour milk	.50		.26
Dead animal	.45		.44
Eating something with left hand	.45		.36
Small acne	.43		.29
Person who never washes himself	.36		.33
Infected eye	.35		.24
Hand without a finger		.79	.64
Deformed body		.67	.56
Perished/decomposed fish		.66	.38
Animal feces in yard		.66	.34
Touching an animal		.53	.52
Eating last nights food		.50	.30
Unkempt beggar		.49	.40
Child with diarrhoea		.38	.23
Very obese man		.31	.22

Note: Items are ordered according to loading on relevant factor. Loadings less than .3 are omitted for clarity.

children born within this period. The sample included 113 men and 171 women and had an average age of 18 years (SD = 1.3). Most participants were unmarried (88%) and Muslim (87%).

Data collection

Participants were interviewed by one of four FWs (field workers). All four FWs had worked as enumerators in two or more previous research projects. Before data collection began, FWs underwent one week of training that included mock interviews and group discussion. During data collection, progress and evaluation meetings were held every third day. Interviews were conducted in Bengali and took place in the participants' homes in the afternoon or evening. Matlab is the site of a long-term health and demographic research project and people are accustomed to visits from field workers and researchers.

Measures

The Disgust Scale [18] (revised in [19]) and the Three Domain Disgust Scale [20] are the most commonly used measures of disgust sensitivity. However, neither has been translated into Bengali, and both contain include items with little relevance to a rural, low-income Bangladeshi sample (e.g., "eating vanilla ice cream with ketchup", "seeing some mold on old leftovers in your refrigerator"). In order to measure disgust sensitivity we designed a simple measure with locally relevant items modeled on these two measures and our previous work on disgust sensitivity in the UK [21]. Consistent with the disease-avoidance model discussed above, these were items related to infectious disease transmission. Hence, this disgust measure focused on what Tybur et al. have termed 'pathogen disgust' [20] and what Haidt et al. have referred to as 'core' or 'contagion' disgust [19]. It is this pathogen related disgust that is most likely to influence participant health and is therefore most relevant to the current analysis. Items were first written in English, then translated into Bengali by a native speaker, and then back translated into English by a second translator who was fluent in both English and Bengali. Minor discrepancies between the versions were resolved through discussion with the translators. Participants were read each item and asked to rate it from 0 ('not at all disgusting') to 4 ('extremely disgusting'). The

Bengali and English versions of the questionnaire, as well as the individual-level response data, are available on the Figshare data repository [22].

Participants' current health (i.e. health as adults) was measured using a Benagli- language questionnaire adapted from the 1996 Matlab Health and Socio-Economic Survey [23]. Participants were asked whether or not they had a list of ailments/diseases in the previous twelve months, how many bouts of the illness they experienced, and the recency of the last bout. 73% of participants reported experiencing an infectious disease in the previous 12 months; see Table 1 for more detailed health information. In our analysis *number of infectious diseases* refers to the total number of different infectious diseases experienced in the year before data collection. Following Stevenson et al. [8] we coded the recency of each disease as '4' if the illness was current, '3' if it occurred within the past week, '2' if it occurred in the past month, '1' if it occurred in the past year, and '0' for all other values. By summing the recency score for each disease, an illness recency score was calculated for each participant.

The health of participants during their childhood was estimated using data collected by the ICDDR,B in the early nineties [24]. During this period, all mothers of children under 5 years were visited each month and asked if their children had experienced diarrhea in the past fortnight or pneumonia in the past month. These two diseases are the major causes of child mortality in rural Bangladesh [25]. On average, 6.1 (SD: 4.8) bouts of diarrhea and 1.8 (SD: 1.4) bouts were recorded per child. There was a marginal association between childhood diarrhoea and current number of infectious diseases (Spearman's $\rho = .11$, p = .06) and no association between childhood pneumonia and number of infectious diseases (Spearman's $\rho = .06$, p = .4). Childhood diarrhea and pneumonia correlate positively (Spearman's $\rho = .22$, p<.001).

Results

The raw data and analysis code are available from figshare.com [22]. Disgust responses were first analyzed using exploratory factor analysis. We used the ordinary least squared method to find the solution with minimum residuals. A parallel analysis [26] indicated that the data was best summarized with two factors: The first five

Table 3. A multilevel model of number of infections over past year and disgust sensitivity (two disgust factors).

	Model 1		Model 2		Model 3	
	Estimate	95% CI	Estimate	95% CI	Estimate	95% CI
Fixed effects						
Intercept	2.18	[1.45, 2.91]	3.06	[1.51, 4.63]	2.87	[0.02, 5.75]
disgust1			−0.19	[−0.73, 0.35]	−0.18	[−0.73, 0.36]
disgust2			−0.13	[−0.64, 0.39]	−0.13	[−0.64, 0.40]
sex					0.03	[−0.32, 0.38]
age					0.01	[−0.13, 0.14]
Random effects						
Intercept	0.52		0.39		0.40	
Residual	2.07		2.08		2.10	
Model fit statistics						
Deviance	1023		1022		1022	
Model AIC	1030		1034		1043	
Model AIC – minimum AIC	-		4		13	

Table 4. A multilevel model of illness recency and disgust sensitivity (two disgust factors).

	Model 1		Model 2		Model 3	
	Estimate	95% CI	Estimate	95% CI	Estimate	95% CI
Fixed effects						
Intercept	3.32	[2.50, 4.14]	5.28	[2.77, 7.89]	6.33	[0.93, 11.72]
disgust1			−0.51	[−1.48, 0.45]	−0.49	[−1.46, 0.48]
disgust2			−0.17	[−1.11, 0.78]	−0.15	[−1.10, 0.80]
sex					0.21	[−0.48, 0.90]
age					−0.07	[−0.33, 0.19]
Random effects						
Intercept	0.58		0.32		0.32	
Residual	7.99		8.03		8.06	
Model fit statistics						
Deviance	1402		1400		1399	
Model AIC	1408		1410		1416	
Model AIC – minimum AIC	-		2		8	

eigenvalues were 7.42, 1.76, 1.26, 1.01, and 0.98 while the first three average eigenvalues from 1,000 randomly generated datasets with the same dimensions were 1.59, 1.48, 1.40, 1.33, and 1.29. (95th percentile: 1.68, 1.54, 1.46, 1.38, and 1.31). A scree plot similarly indicated a two-factor solution. For eight of the disgust items, these two latent variables explained less than 20% of the variance and therefore these items were removed and the analysis was repeated [26]. Two items that cross-loaded weakly on both factor 1 and factor 2 were also excluded. To allow for correlation between factors, a direct oblimin rotation was performed. Factor loadings and communality for the surviving items are shown in Table 2. Factor one was primarily associated with unhygienic behavior while several items about people and food loaded on factor two. By averaging the items that loaded most strongly on factor 1 and factor 2 we created two variables, *disgust1* and *disgust2*. These two disgust measures were positively correlated ($r = .67$, $p < .001$). Cronbach's alpha for disgust1 and disgust2 were .85 and .81, respectively.

Men rated disgust1 items ($M = 3.15$ versus 2.96, $t(282) = 2.74$, $p = .007$, Cohen's $d = .33$) and disgust2 items ($M = 2.62$ versus 2.47, $t(282) = 2.18$, $p = .03$, Cohen's $d = .26$) as more disgusting than women did. Disgust sensitivity differed according to which field worker conducted the interview (disgust1 ANOVA: $F(3,280) = 173$, $p < .001$; disgust2: $F(3, 280) = 149$, $p < .001$). These interview effects – i.e., measurement error attributable to characteristics of the interviewer [27] – were accommodated in the analysis using multilevel (mixed) models [28]. Field worker group was modeled as a random effect while disgust, age, and sex were modeled as fixed effects. Using the AIC [29] we compared the fit of different models to the data. In the case of number of infections, a model with no fixed effects (i.e. without disgust, sex or age) fit the data better than a model including disgust, see Table 3. A similar analysis was conducted to investigate the relationship between disgust and recency of infection. As Table 4 indicates, disgust sensitivity had no strong relationship with illness recency.

Childhood health was measured by a different team of FWs and so interviewer effects and the associated correlated error are not

Table 5. Adult disgust sensitivity and childhood health: multiple regression analyses.

	Disgust1		Disgust2		Disgust: Single factor	
	Beta	95% CI	Beta	95% CI	Beta	95% CI
Intercept	2.64***	[2.06, 3.22]	1.17***	[1.55, 2.79]	2.28***	[1.72, 2.85]
Childhood Diarrhea	0.00	[−0.01, 0.01]	0.00	[−0.01, 0.01]	0.00	[−0.00, 0.01]
Childhood Pneumonia	0.02	[−0.01, 0.05]	0.01	[−0.03, 0.04]	0.02	[−0.01, 0.05]
Field Worker 1 (ref)						
2	0.90***	[0.79, 1.01]	0.31***	[0.20, 0.43]	0.87***	[0.76, 0.98]
3	0.78***	[0.68, 0.90]	1.03***	[0.92, 1.15]	1.26***	[1.16, 1.37]
4	−0.27***	[−0.39, −0.14]	−0.16**	[−0.30, −0.03]	−0.13*	[−0.26, −0.01]
Age	0.00	[−0.03, 0.03]	0.00	[−0.03, 0.04]	0.01	[−0.03, 0.03]
Sex (female)	−0.11*	[−0.20, −0.04]	−0.11*	[−0.20, −0.02]	−0.10**	[−0.18, −0.02]

Note: *** indicates $p < .001$, ** indicates $p < .01$ and * indicates $p < .05$.

Table 6. Exploratory factor analysis of disgust items: one factor solution.

Back Translated Item	Factor Loading	Communality
Touching the inside of a toilet	0.83	0.68
A stranger touching your things	0.74	0.55
Eating dropped sweet	0.73	0.53
Touching an animal	0.72	0.52
Deformed body	0.69	0.47
Hand without a finger	0.68	0.46
Dead animal	0.68	0.46
Eating something with left hand	0.62	0.38
Unkempt beggar	0.6	0.36
Person who never washes himself	0.59	0.35
Eating from dirty plate	0.57	0.33
Picking your nose	0.53	0.29
Eating last nights food	0.52	0.27
Sour milk	0.51	0.26

Note: Items ordered according to factor loading

relevant in the analysis of childhood health and disgust sensitivity. The data were analyzed using multiple regression. As Table 5 shows, there was no relationship between disgust1 (adjusted $R^2 = .65$, $F(7,276) = 77.3$, $p<.001$) or disgust2 (adjusted $R^2 = .61$, $F(7,276) = 65.22$, $p<.001$) and childhood diarrhea or pneumonia.

Although the parallel analysis and scree plot indicated that disgust sensitivity is best measured by two variables, disgust1 and disgust2, these two factors do correlate strongly and have some overlap in content (e.g., items that could be considered hygiene related load on both factors). Thus disgust sensitivity might be better measured as a single variable. Following a reviewer's recommendation, we reexamined the relationship between disgust sensitivity and health with a single disgust variable. The factor analysis was repeated, items with a communality $<.2$ were excluded, and all items with a loading of .5 or higher that factor

were averaged to created a general disgust score (Cronbach's alpha $= .9$; see Table 6). The multivariate analyses results were broadly consistent with those presented above. Number of infectious diseases was best predicted by a simple model excluding disgust (see Table 7). Results displayed in Table 8 indicate that people higher in disgust sensitivity were sick less recently than people lower in disgust. However, this effect was not statistically significant and the AIC statistic indicates that a model excluding disgust provides a better fit. Finally, we found no relationship between disgust and childhood diarrhea or pneumonia (Table 5). To summarize, disgust, when measured as a single construct, is unrelated to the number of infections in childhood or adulthood, or the recency of disease.

Table 7. A multilevel model of number of infections over past year and disgust sensitivity (single disgust factor).

	Model 1		Model 2		Model 3	
	Estimate	95% CI	Estimate	95% CI	Estimate	95% CI
Fixed effects						
Intercept	2.18	[1.45, 2.91]	2.78	[1.41, 4.16]	2.60	[0.20, 5.40]
disgust			−0.22	[−0.68, 0.23]	−0.21	[−0.68, 0.24]
sex					0.04	[−0.31, 0.40]
age					0.01	[−0.13, 0.14]
Random effects						
Intercept	0.52		0.39		0.37	
Residual	2.07		2.08		2.09	
Model fit statistics						
Deviance	1023		1022		1022	
Model AIC	1030		1032		1040	
Model AIC – minimum AIC	-		2		10	

Table 8. A multilevel model of illness recency and disgust sensitivity (single disgust factor).

	Model 1		Model 2		Model 3	
	Estimate	95% CI	Estimate	95% CI	Estimate	95% CI
Fixed effects						
Intercept	3.32	[2.50, 4.14]	5.00	[3.01, 6.98]	6.14	[0.96, 11.31]
disgust			−0.62	[−1.32, 0.08]	−0.60	[−1.31, 0.11]
sex					0.23	[−0.46, 0.92]
age					−0.07	[−0.33, 0.19]
Random effects						
Intercept	0.58		0.23		0.22	
Residual	7.99		8.00		8.04	
Model fit statistics						
Deviance	1402		1400		1399	
Model AIC	1408		1409		1414	
Model AIC – minimum AIC	-		1		6	

Discussion

Contrary to our hypotheses, we found no relationship between disgust sensitivity and childhood health, or between disgust sensitivity and recent health. Below we discuss theoretical and methodological explanations for these null findings

One possible explanation is that disgust sensitivity is unrelated to infection risk. A number of different processes, enumerated below, may weaken the association between disgust and health. (1) Disease exposure depends on community and family behavior as well as individual behavior. If the role of these other people is relatively strong, we are unlikely to detect and relationship between individual psychology and health. Most of our participants were young adults still living at home and their health may therefore be more dependent on parents' and siblings' precautionary behavior. (2) Removing pathogen risks from the one's environment often involves interaction with disgust elicitors and in some circumstances high disgust sensitivity may inhibit actions that benefit health. (3) There is good evidence that people socially learn what constitutes a disgust elicitor [30]. It may be the case that the overlap of disgust elicitors and disease risks is a more important determinant of health than disgust sensitivity itself. In other words, high disgust sensitivity may prevent infection only in individuals who are disgusted by the locally important disease threats. (4) As the findings of Stevenson *et al.* [8] suggests, the interaction of disgust and the tendency to make strong inferences about the spread of contamination may be more important than disgust sensitivity alone. (5) Stevenson *et al.* also suggest that disease exposure results in an increase in disgust sensitivity. Such an effect may mask the protective effects of disgust in a cross-sectional study. Longitudinal data on both disgust sensitivity and health would help to resolve this question.

Our results do not support the hypothesis that adult disgust sensitivity is calibrated by childhood disease exposure. We estimated childhood health using incidence of diarrhea and pneumonia. Although these are important causes of childhood mortality, they kill relatively few adults. Moreover, data from this sample suggests a weak relationship between diarrhea and adult health, and no relationship between pneumonia and adult health. It may be the case the there are other diseases/pathogens that are better predictors of adult pathogen stress and consequently adult disease avoidance behavior.

A more general point is that in some circumstances, a more risky environment can counter-intuitively favor individuals who invest *less* in precautionary behavior [31]. E.g., consider how a solider likely to die in battle gains little in life expectancy from not smoking compared to a general who can expect to survive the war. Unavoidable risks make precautionary behavior for avoidable risks less worthwhile. We have assumed that disease risk is, by in large, an avoidable risk which can be mitigated through precautionary behavior. If, however, a large proportion of infection risk is unavoidable, then individuals in high-risk environments are unlikely to invest more. More research on the extent to which disease risks are avoidable – and are *perceived* to be avoidable – would be help to clarify this issue.

An alternative explanation for these null results is that the measures of health and/or disgust were lacking in validity or reliability. Measuring psychological constructs like disgust sensitivity in a low-income, non-English speaking population is not straightforward. Although Bengali is the 6th most commonly spoken language, few, if any, psychological measures have been translated and validated in Bengali. Our disgust measure followed the format of some commonly used and well-validated measures and was well understood by participants and field workers. However, there are two causes for concern. Contrary to several published studies [2,32,33], male participants rated the items more disgusting that women. This indicates that either sex differences in pathogen related disgust are not as consistent as previously argued, or that the measure is biased in some way. However, there are some reasons to think that sex differences in disgust play out differently in this population. In Matlab there is an uneven exposure to disgust-relevant stimuli; women do almost all cleaning and cooking, and they care for infants and the infirm. Rozin has argued that repeated interaction with disgust cues reduces sensitivity [34] and thus this may account for the reversal of sex differences. Another point of concern with the disgust measure was that sensitivity appeared to vary according to field worker. Some interviewer effects are inevitable in this kind of study, and the effects were statistically controlled for in the analysis, but nevertheless they may have weakened our ability to detect a real relationship. Future research on disgust sensitivity may benefit from asking participants to rate pre-recorded audio versions of the items or to rate images of disgust stimuli instead. Another possible explanation for this null result is health was not accurately measured. In particular, our measure of recent health was relatively crude; participants may have forgotten disease events or misremembered the exact timing. However, the positive correlation between childhood and adult disease frequency does suggest these measures have some validity.

We argued that high disgust sensitivity would be associated with fewer infections because more sensitive individuals have less contact with infectious matter. However, actual sickness is a relatively poor measure of pathogen exposure. Most exposure events (e.g., eating contaminated food, being coughed upon) do not result in disease because the pathogenic organisms are destroyed by the immune system or because the infection remains 'latent' [35]. Morcover, people differ in the extent to which they can prevent disease occurring, given exposure. A more direct way

to study the protective effects of disgust may be to examine immunological markers of disease exposure. By measuring specific antibody levels, researchers may be able to estimate the frequency of pathogen exposure more accurately [36,37]. Such a study should have a more power to detect the relationship between disgust and pathogen exposure, if one does indeed exist.

Acknowledgments

We thank Dr Zahid Hayat, Mr Zakir Hossain and Mr Rashed Zaman for their support during fieldwork.

Author Contributions

Conceived and designed the experiments: MDB VC SI. Performed the experiments: MDB SI. Analyzed the data: MDB. Wrote the paper: MDB VC.

References

1. Curtis V, Biran A (2001) Dirt, disgust, and disease: Is hygiene in our genes? Perspect Biol Med 44: 17–31.
2. Curtis V, Aunger R, Rabie T (2004) Evidence that disgust evolved to protect from risk of disease. Proc Biol Sci 271 Suppl: S131–3. doi:10.1098/rsbl.2003.0144.
3. Curtis V, de Barra M, Aunger R (2011) Disgust as an adaptive system for disease avoidance behaviour. Philos Trans R Soc B 366: 389–401. doi:10.1098/rstb.2010.0117.
4. Wisenden BD, Goater CP, James CT (2003) Behavioral Defenses against Parasites and Pathogens. In: Zaccone C, Perriere A, Mathis A, Kapoor G, editors. Fish Defenses. Vol 2 Enfield, USA. pp. 151–168.
5. Hart BL (2011) Behavioural defences in animals against pathogens and parasites: parallels with the pillars of medicine in humans. Philos Trans R Soc B 366: 3406–3417. doi:10.1098/rstb.2011.0092.
6. Oaten M, Stevenson RJ, Case TI (2009) Disgust as a disease-avoidance mechanism. Psychol Bull 135: 303–321. doi:10.1037/a0014823.
7. Rozin P, Haidt J, McCauley C, Dunlop L, Ashmore M (1999) Individual Differences in Disgust Sensitivity: Comparisons and Evaluations of Paper-and-Pencil versus Behavioral Measures. J Res Pers 33: 330–351.
8. Stevenson RJ, Case TI, Oaten MJ (2009) Frequency and recency of infection and their relationship with disgust and contamination sensitivity. Evol Hum Behav 30: 363–368. doi:10.1016/j.evolhumbehav.2009.02.005.
9. Lozano R, Naghavi M, Foreman K, Lim S, Shibuya K, et al. (2012) Global and regional mortality from 235 causes of death for 20 age groups in 1990 and 2010: a systematic analysis for the Global Burden of Disease Study 2010. Lancet 380: 2095–2128. doi:10.1016/S0140-6736(12)61728-0.
10. Davey GCL, Bond N (2006) Using controlled comparisons in disgust psychopathology research: The case of disgust, hypochondriasis and health anxiety. J Behav Ther Exp Psychiatry 37: 4–15.
11. Hutchings MR, Judge J, Gordan IJ, Athanasiadou S, Kyriazakis I (2006) Use of trade-off theory to advance understanding of herbivore-parasite interactions. Mamm Rev 36: 1–16. doi:10.1111/j.1365-2907.2006.00080.x.
12. Hoefling A, Likowski KU, Deutsch R, Mu A, Weyers P, et al. (2009) When hunger finds no fault with moldy corn: food deprivation reduces food-related disgust. Emotion 9: 50–58. doi:10.1037/a0014449.
13. Fessler DMT, Navarrete CD (2003) Domain-specific variation in disgust sensitivity across the menstrual cycle. Evol Hum Behav 24: 406–417. doi:10.1016/S1090-5138(03)00054-0.
14. Lively C (1986) Predator-induced shell dimorphism in the acorn barnacle Chthamalus anisopoma. Evolution (N Y) 40: 232–242.
15. Nettle D, Coall DA, Dickins TE (2011) Early-life conditions and age at first pregnancy in British women. Proc R Soc B 278: 1721–1727. doi:10.1098/rspb.2010.1726.
16. Waynforth D (2012) Life-history theory, chronic childhood illness and the timing of first reproduction in a British birth cohort. Proc R Soc B 279: 2998–3002. doi:10.1098/rspb.2012.0220.
17. De Barra M, DeBruine LM, Jones BC, Mahmud ZH, Curtis VA (2013) Illness in childhood predicts face preferences in adulthood. Evol Hum Behav 24: 384–389. doi:10.1016/j.evolhumbehav.2013.07.001.
18. Haidt J, McCauley C, Rozin P (1994) Individual differences in sensitivity to disgust: A scale sampling seven domains of disgust elicitors. Pers Individ Dif 16: 701–713. doi:10.1016/0191-8869(94)90212-7.
19. Olatunji BO, Cisler JM, Deacon BJ, Connolly K, Lohr JM (2007) The Disgust Propensity and Sensitivity Scale-Revised: psychometric properties and specificity in relation to anxiety disorder symptoms. J Anxiety Disord 21: 918–930. doi:10.1016/j.janxdis.2006.12.005.
20. Tybur JM, Lieberman D (2009) Microbes, mating, and morality: Individual differences in three functional domains of disgust. J Pers Soc Psychol 97: 103–22.
21. Curtis V (2013) Don't Look, Don't Touch: The Science Behind Revulsion. Chicago: University of Chicago Press.
22. De Barra M (2013) Infectious disease and disgust sensitivity in Bangladesh. Figshare. doi:10.6084/m9.figshare.839646.
23. Rahman O, Menken J, Foster A, Peterson CE, Khan MN, et al. (1999) The 1996 Matlab Health and Socioeconomic Survey. RAND Corporation.
24. Rahman MM, Alam MN, Razzaque A, Streatfield PK (2012) Health and Demographic Surveillance System–Matlab, v. 44. Registration of health and demographic events 2010. Dhaka.
25. Baqui AH, Black RE, Arifeen SE, Hill K, Mitra SN, et al. (1998) Causes of childhood deaths in Bangladesh: results of a nationwide verbal autopsy study. Bull World Health Organ 76: 161–171.
26. Hayton JC, Allen DG, Scarpello V (2004) Factor Retention Decisions in Exploratory Factor Analysis: a Tutorial on Parallel Analysis. Organ Res Methods 7: 191–205. doi:10.1177/1094428104263675.
27. Freeman J, Butler E (1976) Some sources of interviewer variance in surveys. Public Opin Q 40: 79–91.
28. Hox J (1994) Hierarchical regression models for interviewer and respondent effects. Sociol Methods Res 22: 300–318.
29. Akaike H (1974) A new look at the statistical model identification. Autom Control IEEE Trans.
30. Bayliss AP, Frischen A, Fenske MJ, Tipper SP (2006) Affective evaluations of objects are influenced by observed gaze direction and emotional expression. Cognition 104: 644–663. doi:10.1016/j.cognition.2006.07.012.
31. Nettle D (2010) Why are there social gradients in preventative health behavior? A perspective from behavioral ecology. PLoS One 5: e13371. doi:10.1371/journal.pone.0013371.
32. Tybur JM, Bryan AD, Lieberman D, Caldwell Hooper AE, Merriman L a. (2011) Sex differences and sex similarities in disgust sensitivity. Pers Individ Dif 51: 343–348. doi:10.1016/j.paid.2011.04.003.
33. Olatunji BO, Moretz MW, McKay D, Bjorklund F, de Jong PJ, et al. (2009) Confirming the Three-Factor Structure of the Disgust Scale–Revised in Eight Countries. J Cross Cult Psychol 40: 234–255. doi:10.1177/0022022108328918.
34. Rozin P (2008) Hedonic "adaptation": Specific habituation to disgust/death elicitors as a result of dissecting a cadaver. Judgm Decis Mak 3: 191–194.
35. Janeway CA, Travers P, Walport M, Shlomchik MJ (2001) Immunobiology. 5th ed. New York: Garland Science.
36. Albers R, Antoine J-M, Bourdet-Sicard R, Calder PC, Gleeson M, et al. (2007) Markers to measure immunomodulation in human nutrition intervention studies. Br J Nutr 94: 452. doi:10.1079/BJN20051469.
37. Drakeley CJ, Corran PH, Coleman PG, Tongren JE, McDonald SLR, et al. (2005) Estimating medium- and long-term trends in malaria transmission by using serological markers of malaria exposure. Proc Natl Acad Sci U S A 102: 5108–5113. doi:10.1073/pnas.0408725102.

7

The Cost-Effectiveness of Different Feeding Patterns Combined with Prompt Treatments for Preventing Mother-to-Child HIV Transmission in South Africa: Estimates from Simulation Modeling

Wenhua Yu[9], **Changping Li**[9], **Xiaomeng Fu**[9], **Zhuang Cui, Xiaoqian Liu, Linlin Fan, Guan Zhang, Jun Ma***

Department of Health Statistics, College of Public Health, Tianjin Medical University, Tianjin, China

Abstract

Objectives: Based on the important changes in South Africa since 2009 and the Antiretroviral Treatment Guideline 2013 recommendations, we explored the cost-effectiveness of different strategy combinations according to the South African HIV-infected mothers' prompt treatments and different feeding patterns.

Study Design: A decision analytic model was applied to simulate cohorts of 10,000 HIV-infected pregnant women to compare the cost-effectiveness of two different HIV strategy combinations: (1) Women were tested and treated promptly at any time during pregnancy (Promptly treated cohort). (2) Women did not get testing or treatment until after delivery and appropriate standard treatments were offered as a remedy (Remedy cohort). Replacement feeding or exclusive breastfeeding was assigned in both strategies. Outcome measures included the number of infant HIV cases averted, the cost per infant HIV case averted, and the cost per life year(LY) saved from the interventions. One-way and multivariate sensitivity analyses were performed to estimate the uncertainty ranges of all outcomes.

Results: The remedy strategy does not particularly cost-effective. Compared with the untreated baseline cohort which leads to 1127 infected infants, 698 (61.93%) and 110 (9.76%) of pediatric HIV cases are averted in the promptly treated cohort and remedy cohort respectively, with incremental cost-effectiveness of $68.51 and $118.33 per LY, respectively. With or without the antenatal testing and treatments, breastfeeding is less cost-effective ($193.26 per LY) than replacement feeding ($134.88 per LY), without considering the impact of willingness to pay.

Conclusion: Compared with the prompt treatments, remedy in labor or during the postnatal period is less cost-effective. Antenatal HIV testing and prompt treatments and avoiding breastfeeding are the best strategies. Although encouraging mothers to practice replacement feeding in South Africa is far from easy and the advantages of breastfeeding can not be ignored, we still suggest choosing replacement feeding as far as possible.

Editor: Julian W. Tang, Alberta Provincial Laboratory for Public Health/University of Alberta, Canada

Funding: This study was not only supported by the grants from China's ministry of health, bureau of education of science and technology (201202017), and China's Ministry of Education, Humanities and Social Sciences Project (11YJCZH022, 11YJCZH080), but also partially sponsored by National Natural Science Foundation of China (NSFC, 71373175). The funders had no role in study design, data collection and analysis, decision to publish, or preparation of the manuscript.

Competing Interests: The authors have declared that no competing interests exist.

* Email: junma@tijmu.edu.cn

9 These authors contributed equally to this work.

Introduction

Identification of human immunodeficiency virus (HIV) infection is critical from both clinical and public health perspectives. Antenatal HIV testing is undertaken primarily to offer interventions to reduce the risk of HIV transmission from mother to child. Globally, about 40% of pregnant women in low- and middle-income countries received HIV testing and counseling in 2012, up from 26% in 2009 [1].These prevention of Mother-to-child transmission (PMTCT) services in low- and middle-income countries have prevented approximately 409,000 children from acquiring HIV [2]. Around 330,000 children were HIV-infected

prenatally in 2011, which represented a decline of 24% since 2009 in sub-Saharan Africa [2]. Especially the implementation of South Africa's massive HIV testing and counseling campaign between April 2010 and June 2011,which urged everyone in 12–60 years old to be tested [3], caused the national testing coverage to exceed 95% in 2012 [2].

However, there are the persons who are tested late or are unaware of their infection until relatively late in their disease course, as a result, missing the opportunity of getting prompt intervention. A World Health Organization (WHO) study of HIV diagnoses in Georgia in 2009–2011 found that 64% of new HIV diagnoses could be considered 'late' and that the reasons for the high rates of late diagnosis included lack of access to acceptable HIV testing and counseling services [2]. An interview study of 760 HIV-infected persons in Los Angeles County suggested that many persons reported with Acquired Immune Deficiency Syndrome (AIDS) were unaware of their infection until relatively late in their disease course. Of particular concern is that almost half (46%) of the reported respondents did not seek testing until they were ill [4]. A study based in two Durban clinics found most patients were tested at a late stage of infection with over 60% of CD4 counts below 200 cells/mm^3.Of those who were eligible for treatment, more than a fifth died, mostly before any treatment [5]. A survey had suggested that late HIV diagnosis may lead to accelerted progression and that some of the patients in the survey developed AIDS within a year of HIV infection[6]. These findings are in excellent agreement with those reported by other researchers [7].

Since the first report of transmission of HIV through breastfeeding was published in 1985 [8], avoidance of breastfeeding has remained an important component of efforts to prevent mother-to-child transmission (MTCT) of HIV [9]. There is no doubt that breastfeeding is risky for MTCT [8,10] and approximately 5%-20% of babies infected through MTCT acquire HIV infection via breastfeeding [2], but breastfeeding may be associated with other factors. Breastfeeding is particularly important in resource-poor regions of the world, where limited access to clean water increases the risk of diarrhea if replacement feeding is used, and many mothers do not have the means to afford the cost of formula [11]. Infant morbidity and mortality rates are generally decreased by breastfeeding, which provides optimal nutrition and partially protects against common childhood infections [11–13,20].

On account of realistic public health considerations, in 2010, WHO issued its first guidelines [14] that allowed new recommendations on antiretroviral (ARV) prophylaxis to either the mother or infant during breastfeeding in areas where breastfeeding was judged to be the most appropriate choice of infant feeding for HIV-infected women. In addition, guidelines were developed to provide international standards to reduce the risk of MTCT from a background risk of 35% to less than 5% (or even lower) in breastfeeding populations [14]. Exclusive breastfeeding for the first few months of life can be successfully supported in HIV-infected women [2] and if replacement feeding is not available [15], one alternative is to provide antiretroviral prophylaxis (ART) to the mother or child during breastfeeding [16–19].

HIV/AIDS in South Africa is a prominent health concern [21]. The Joint United Nations Programme on HIV and AIDS (UNAIDS) report estimated that 5,700,000 South Africans had HIV/AIDS, with HIV prevalence in pregnant women at 28% [22], or just under 12% of South Africa's population of 48 million in 2007 [23]. However, important changes have occurred in the country since 2009 [24]. Government funding in South Africa increased for expansion of antiretroviral therapy, scaling up of PMTCT programmes, promotion of HIV and tuberculosis treatment integration, and increased investments in HIV prevention [25]. South Africa now has the world's largest programme of antiretroviral therapy, with about 1.8 million people estimated to be taking antiretroviral. HIV prevention has received increasing attention [24].

Breastfeeding is the norm in South Africa, but the percentage of exclusive breastfeeding for 6 months among South African HIV infected mothers is one of the lowest in the world, at 8% in 2003 [26,27]. However, the situations have been changed since 2010 when the infants feeding patterns shifted the emphasis to exclusive breastfeeding [24], and as a result, South Africa has had one of the sharpest declines in new infections among children [28]. Yearly infections in children have dropped from 56,500 in 2009 to 29,100 in 2011. [29] A cohort study of 1032 HIV-infected mothers showed that 40% of women reported to exclusive breastfeeding [30].There were approximately 45% of HIV mothers reported as exclusive breastfeeding in another Kesho Bora study [16].

It should be noted that the cost of drugs to HIV are usually borne by the government, whereas formula is usually paid for by the individual. Meanwhile, encouraging HIV mothers to practice exclusive breastfeeding is also far from easy. Breast milk provides all of the fluids and nutrients that a young baby requires, so it means that even water should be avoided [31,32]. However, in many societies, it is normal for a baby to be given water, tea, porridge or other foods as well as breast milk, even during the first few weeks of life [33,34]. The HIV-infected mothers assigned to the formula feeding often experience community, family, or spousal pressure to breastfeed and are sometimes concerned about maintaining the confidentiality of their HIV status; further, formula-feeding logistics are more difficult than those for breastfeeding, particularly in resource-poor areas [14].

Numerous simulations [35,36] have been conducted to prevent MTCT. However, most of them explored the effect of only a single intervention. For example, some studies evaluated the cost - effectiveness of antenatal HIV testing but the remedial measures for untested or testing late HIV-infected mothers were not included [37–40]. Neil Soderlund et al. simulated the cost-effectiveness of four feeding strategies and three antiretroviral interventions but the interventions were considered separately [40]. In practice, however, interventions should not be implemented individually and several interventions can be implemented simultaneously or consecutively. Based on the important changes in South Africa [24] and the South African Antiretroviral Treatment Guideline 2013 recommendations [26], we explored different strategy combinations rather than a single intervention according to the South African HIV-infected mothers' varying status and different designs of feeding patterns. We simulated the different status(prompt treatment, remedial treatments or neither) of HIV infected mothers based on the characters of South African pregnant women in Kesho Bora study and others[16,30,41,42], and we aimed to assess the cost-effectiveness of the feeding patterns of HIV-exposed infants (exclusive breastfeeding or replacement feeding) in light of the mothers' status.

Materials and Methods

Model framework

We developed a decision analytic model using the TreeAge Pro 2011 software package (TreeAge Software, Inc, Williamstown, MA) [45] to compare the cost-effectiveness of two different HIV strategy combinations given only to HIV positive mothers: (1) HIV positive pregnant mothers were tested and treated promptly at any time during pregnancy. They knew their HIV status after antenatal HIV testing in time and received an ARV intervention or standard ART recommended by WHO on the basis of eligibility (Promptly treated cohort). (2) Pregnant mothers did not get tested or treated until after delivery. They presented late in labor without having a diagnosis of their HIV status and thus missed the window of opportunity for prompt interventions. A course of fixed dose combination (FDC) and other treatments were offered as a remedy (Remedy cohort). The first strategy was the gold standard, whereas the second one was remedial when the first wasn't available. The non-responders were assigned as untreated in the two cohorts, and replacement feeding or exclusive breastfeeding was assigned in the two strategies. We evaluated interventions against a 'no intervention' scenario (the mothers'

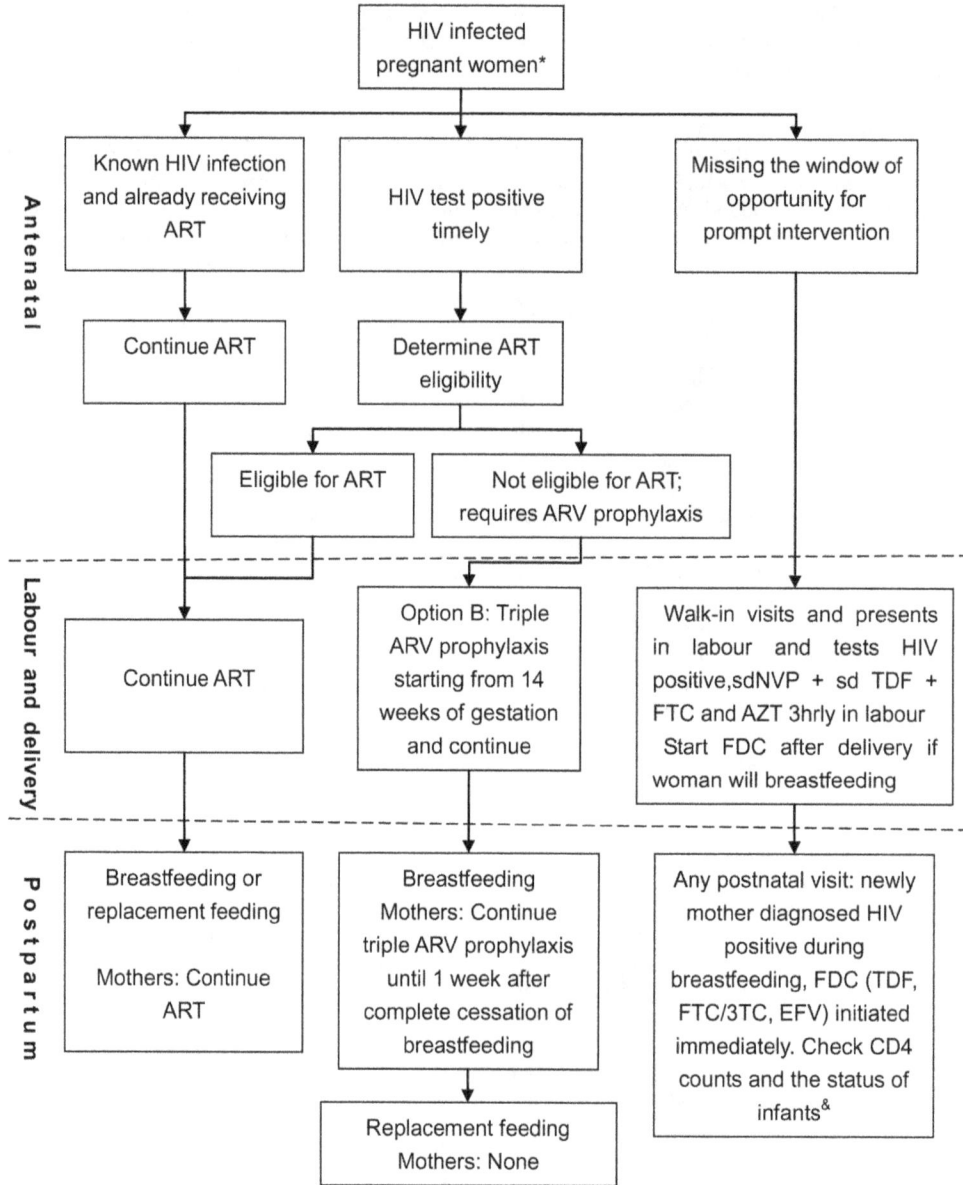

Figure 1. Decision analytic model schematic. & Irrespective of mode of feeding patterns, infants accepted NVP promptly and daily for 6 weeks. ART, antiretroviral therapy; ARV, antiretroviral prophylaxis; sdNVP, single dose nevirapine; sdTDF, single dose Tenofovir; FTC,emtricitabine; AZT, Zidovudine; FDC, fixed dose combination,(TDF, FTC/3TC, EFV); 3TC,Lamivudine; EFV, Efavirenz.

HIV status unidentified and no use of any antiretroviral drugs). The model structures are showed in Figure 1 and Figure 2.

We presented key model outcomes, including the number of infant HIV cases averted, the number of infant life years (LY) saved, the cost per infant HIV case averted, and the cost per LY [40,45] saved from the interventions.

Intervention and settings

The decision analytic model was created to simulate 3–6 cohorts. We used the Monte Carlo simulation method to simulate 10,000 HIV-infected pregnant women from South Africa (average age is 27 years old) in each cohort [16]. The distribution of the

pregnant mothers' age, the CD4 counts and other parameters were all based on the characters of South African pregnant women in Kesho Bora study and others [16,30,41,42]. We simulated the severity and progression of the maternal HIV disease, infants' HIV infections and the time that mothers' highly active antiretroviral therapy (HAART) treatments started based on mothers' CD4 counts during pregnancy. The median CD4 cell count was assumed to be 360×10^6 cells/mm^3. The square root of CD4 count is assumed to be normally distributed within a 95th percentile range of 43 to 984 cells/mm^3 [37]. We assumed that HIV-infected, pregnant women who have CD4 cell counts less than 350 cells/mm^3 received HAART during pregnancy, as the WHO

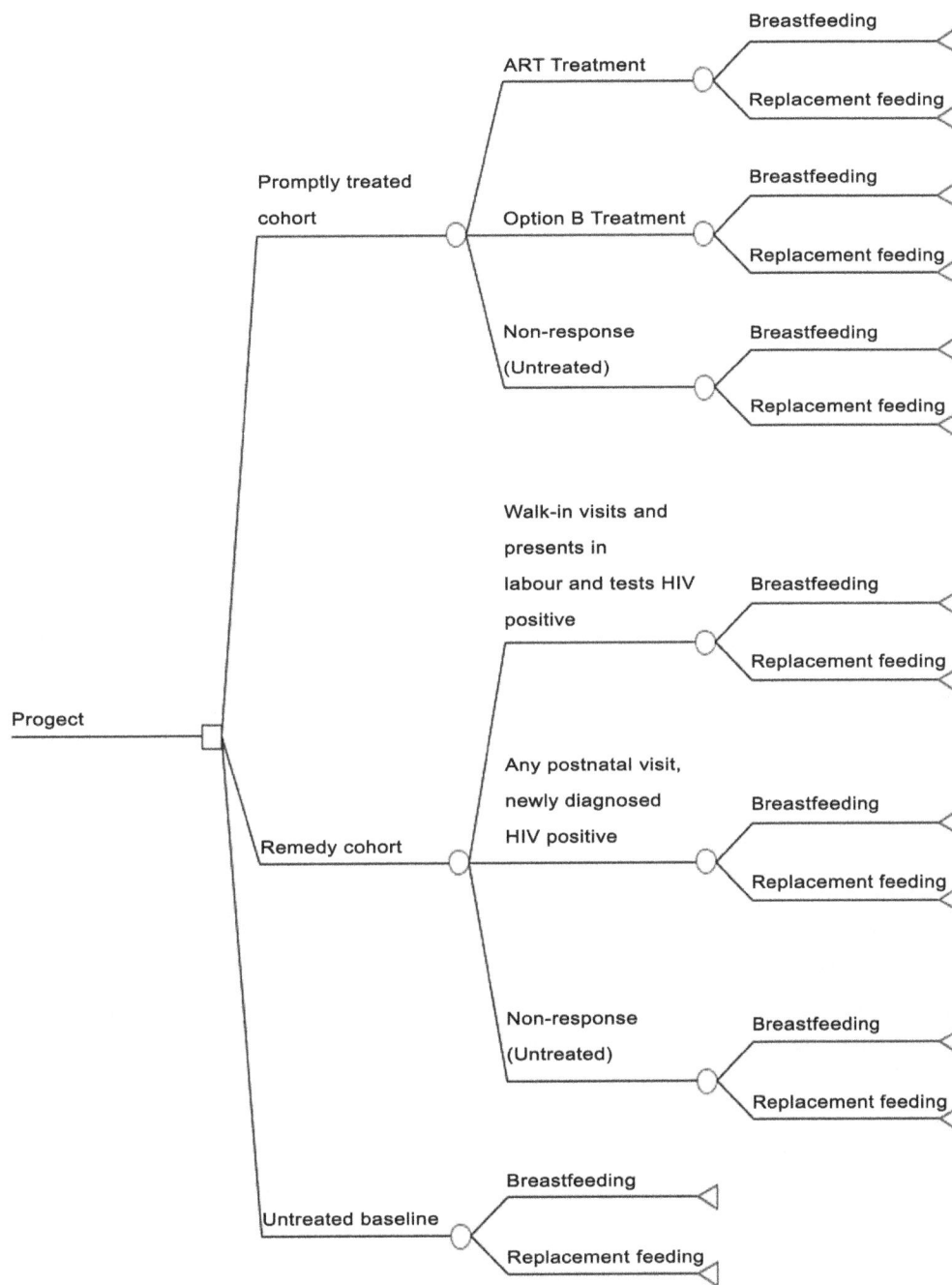

Figure 2. Structure of decision analytic model. ART, antiretroviral therapy.

recently recommended [14]. The intervention approaches assumed that maternal antepartum daily ART continued during pregnancy, delivery, and thereafter. For women who were not eligible for ART, the model used implementation of triple antiretroviral prophylaxis (Zidovudine (AZT) + Lamivudine (3TC) + lopinavir (LPV)) [14], as did the Kesho Bora study conducted in South Africa [16]. Triple ARV prophylaxis started as early as 14 weeks of gestation and continued until delivery; if breastfeeding was applied, it continued until cessation of breastfeeding at 6 months postpartum. All the infants received daily nevirapine (NVP) from birth until age 6 weeks, regardless of the mode of infant feeding.

For HIV-infected mothers who missed the window of opportunity for prompt intervention, some of them were unable to realize their HIV infectious status, which resulted in walk-in labour visits and delayed HIV testing; single-dose nevirapine (sdNVP) + single dose Tenofovir (sdTDF) + emtricitabine (FTC) + Zidovudine (AZT) were then offered at the onset of labor as a remedy, and NVP was also given to their newborn babies daily for 6 weeks [26]. A course of fixed dose combination (FDC) was started after delivery if the woman was assigned to breastfeeding. For others who were diagnosed HIV-positive during breastfeeding at any postnatal visit, FDC (TDF, FTC/3TC, Efavirenz (EFV)) was initiated immediately, and the mothers' CD4 counts and their infants' HIV status were checked. All the interventions mentioned above were in line with recommendations by the South African Antiretroviral Treatment Guideline 2013 [26]. We identified these detailed interventions to ensure the accuracy of the intervention cost and effect.

We also assumed a standard testing strategy consisting of a serum enzyme-linked immunosorbent assay followed by confirmatory Western blotting. We presumed infants complied with exclusive breastfeeding from ages of about 6 weeks to 6 months if their mothers intended to breastfeed, as the WHO recommended [44].

Probabilities

The probabilities and ranges used in the model were derived from published studies of large, population-randomized, controlled trials and published, updated meta-analyses [11,12,15,16,41,43]. We obtained estimates for the model's parameters from South African data when available. Otherwise, we used data from international literatures in an attempt to use estimates from other resource-limited countries. A function to convert annual probability into 18-month probability was used, as follows:

$$P_{18months} = 1 - e^{\ln(1-P_{year}) \times 1.5} [45]$$

The base rates of MTCT were estimated from a randomized controlled trial conducted in Kenya and South Africa by the Kesho Bora study group [16]. In a group of those eligible for ART, the average HIV-positive rate in infants who were breastfed for 18 months was 7.5% (compared with 0.75% in the replacement-feeding group). A range of 3.5%–14.76% was included in the sensitivity analyses, taking the impact of CD4 counts into account. In the group of mothers whose CD4 counts were ≥350 cells/mm^3 and who were assigned to breastfeeding, the converted 18-month infection rate was 6.97% (95% confidence interval (CI) 3.58%–13.62%). The sensitivity analysis includes a lower transmission rate of 1%, derived from an 18-month follow-up study of HIV–infected mothers whose CD4 counts were ≥500 cells/mm^3 in the Kesho Bora study [16,41]. The risk of MTCT was 2% with the use of antiretroviral medicines and avoidance of breastfeeding [43]. 19.5% of exclusively breastfed infants were infected with HIV by 6 months, a figure derived from a intervention cohort study of 1132 HIV positive pregnant women [30]. We used the vertical MTCT rate of HIV infection during postpartum of 15.81% (95% CI 10.7%–21.02%) and 29.03% (95% CI 22.98%–35.26%) without interventions to prevent transmission when the mother was assigned to breastfeeding or replacement feeding, respectively [13,78].

On average, 59% (95% CI 53%–64%) of pregnant women living with HIV were estimated to be eligible for ART on the basis of those with CD4 counts <350 cells/mm^3 receiving lifelong ART [1]. The 83% and 67% South African coverage rates of ART among adults and children (aged 0–14 years), respectively, were assumptions made on the basis of the WHO's Global Update on HIV Treatment 2013 Report [1]. The latest data from 23 countries indicated that the average retention rates for people on ART decrease over time (from about 86% at 12 months to 82% at 24 months) [1]. We assigned 40% and 15.4% as the percentage of women who were selected to exclusive breastfeeding and replacement feeding respectively [30]. Since data to measure precisely the efficacy of remedial intervention in labor and that of FDC during postpartum care are not available, we estimated the

variable efficacy of the remedial intervention in labor as 62.75% (95% CI 40.76%–84.74%), derived from data of the Petra study [46,47]. We rounded the efficacy of FDC to 47.91% (95% CI 43.57%–51.92%), this figure came from a research of 2,127 electronic medical records between July 1999 to June 2006. The hazard ratio (HR) of FDC was 0.92 [48]. In addition, we assumed that the converted 18-month mortality in exclusive breastfeeding infants was 18.9% versus 15.4% in infants given replacement feeds [49], and calculated the adjusted mortality rate which represents the unrelated HIV infection mortality by deducting the under-five mortality rate (42.15/1000 in 2013) [50]. The input probabilities for our decision tree are displayed in Table 1.

Cost estimates

The input cost estimates for our decision tree are presented in Table 2. Cost and utility estimates were also derived from published literatures when necessary. All cost was expressed in 2012 US dollars and South African prices. The total cost included the cost of ART and ARV treatments, the cost of visiting, counseling and testing and the cost of breastfeeding and formula milk [58]. We calculated the cost of mothers from the moment when treatments begin until 1 week after cessation of breastfeeding and the cost during the first 18 months of life for the HIV-exposed infants. The cost-effectiveness was calculated relative to the control group as (IC+NC−HC)/(LS*LE−LL*LE) [40]; where IC = intervention costs, NC = health care costs because of additional morbidity in formula fed children not infected with HIV, HC = costs of HIV related care avoided by preventing infections, LS = lives saved by prevention of HIV infection, LL = lives lost because of formula feeding in children not infected with HIV, and LE = life expectancy. Cost estimates for antiretroviral drugs were based on the Clinton Health Access Initiative (CHAI)'s ceiling price list [51]. The average of the two most common first-line regimens (zidovudine/lamivudine/nevirapine or tenofovir/lamivudine/efavirenz, $146.50/year) were used as the cost of triple ARV during pregnancy [42]. The cost of HAART during pregnancy and lactation were estimated as $76.82 and $50.65, respectively [53,79]. We estimated the baseline cost of a single rapid HIV testing as $2.36 and $6.30, when the testing was negative or positive, respectively [53]. In case of a positive testing, additional confirmatory testing was needed. The cost of CD4 testing was estimated as $5.43 per unit [43,52]. Cost ware discounted by 3% per year [45].

Estimation of life years saved

We focused our analysis on the effectiveness for HIV-exposed infants and estimated the effect using the life years saved. To estimate the number of LY saved induced by the intervention, life expectancy in South Africa at birth was estimated from a review of available demographic data [24], and the base-case calculation used a life expectancy of 60 years. For a child with perinatal transmission of HIV who goes on HAART for life, we estimated a life expectancy approximately two-thirds that of a child without HIV [53,54]. The model used a disease progression scenario in which 25%, 80%, and 100% of children progress to AIDS at 12, 60, and 120 months, respectively. Children were assumed to live for an average of 12 months after progression to AIDS [55,56].

We used the same weights for all infants, irrespective of age. When children were aged less than 5 years, irrespective of their CD4 counts, we assumed they were eligible to start ART. Children aged greater than 5 years were monitored for ART by CD4 testing each year [26]. The parameters are presented in Table 1.

Table 1. References and input probabilities for the decision analytic model.

Reference	Probability Variable	Details	Circumstances	Value	Range
[16]	positive rate of HIV in 18 months	Breastfeeding	ART	7.50%	(3.50%–14.76%)
[16][32]			ARV	6.97%	(1.00%–13.62%)
[13][11]			None treatment	29.03%	(22.98%–35.26%)
[43]		Replacement feeding	ART	0.75%	(0.75%–1.50%)
[43]			ARV	2.00%	-
[13] [78]			None treatment	15.81%	(10.70%–21.02%)
[30]	Efficacy	Using sdNVP + sdTDF + FTC and AZT 3hrly	In labour as a remedy	62.75%	(40.76%–84.74%)
[48]		Initiating FDC immediately	Breastfeeding during postpartum care	47.91%	(43.57%–51.92%)
[2]	Rate of coverage	ART	Among pregnant women	83.00%	(79.00%–87.00%)
		ART	Among infected infants	67.00%	(60.00%–75.00%)
[2]		HIV testing and counseling	Among pregnant women	95.00%	(90.00%–98.00%)
Assumed, [16][27][30]		Exclusive breast feeding	In HIV infected women	40.00%	(8.00%–44.68%)
[30]		Replacement feeding	In HIV infected women	15.4%	-
[2]	Rates of average retention	ART	In 12 months	86.00%	-
			In 24 months	82.00%	-
[13]	Estimated rate of transmission	Breast milk		19.50%	(6.50%–24.90%)
[2]	Average rate of being eligible for ART	Based on CD4<350	Mothers living with HIV	59.00%	(53.00%–64.00%)
Assumed [60],	Proportion of HIV	Infected women among the unidentified	Presented in labor	18.52%	(5.00%–50.00%)
			Diagnosed at postnatal visit	22.22%	(5.00%–50.00%)
[24]	Life experience(year)	Child	Without HIV	60	-
[53] [54]			With prenatal HIV on HAART	40	-
[55]			With prenatal HIV if no no antiretroviral	10	-
[42] [43]			With AIDS	1	-
[50]		Under-five mortality rate		42.15‰	
[49]	Motility rate of infants in 18 months	Breastfeed		18.9%	-
[49]		Replacement feeding		15.4%	-

ART, antiretroviral therapy; ARV, antiretroviral prophylaxis; sdNVP, single dose nevirapine; sdTDF, single dose Tenofovir; FTC, emtricitabine; AZT, Zidovudine; FDC, (TDF, FTC/3TC, EFV); 3TC,Lamivudine; EFV, Efavirenz; HAART, highly active antiretroviral therapy.

Sensitivity and uncertainty analyses

In the sensitivity analyses, the uncertain assumptions about the input cost and behavioral impacts of interventions were varied. An aggregate model was developed using the highest and lowest values and the best fitting parameter. The model's epidemiological values were point estimates and 95% CI for parameters based on published study results. We conducted additional univariate sensitivity analyses with values of cost estimate from one-third to 3 times of their baseline estimates. We also tested the sensitivity of the rankings to variation of the assumptions regarding key parameters.

Results

Three theoretical cohorts(the promptly treated cohort, the remedy cohort and the no intervention control cohort) were applied in our analytic model, all of which were based on estimates of 40% breast feeding coverage and 15.4% replacement feeding rate during postpartum. It is found that the incremental cost per infant HIV case averted were $2063.05 and $3579.66 for the promptly treated cohort and remedy cohort, respectively. Tables 3 reported on the incremental cost-effectiveness ratios (ICER) for interventions, which were listed in the descending order of the infant HIV cases averted. Figure 3 showed an expansion path graphically, with the slope of the line joining any two points indicating the ICER for the more costly option [57]. The remedy strategy did not particularly cost-effective. Compared with the 'no intervention' scenario which leaded to 1127 infected infants, 698 (61.93%) and 110 (9.76%) of pediatric HIV cases were averted in the promptly treated cohort and remedy cohort respectively, with incremental cost-effectiveness of $68.51 and $118.33 per LY, respectively (Figure 3.A).

Because all the HIV-exposed mothers among the two cohorts were designed to have different feeding patterns, we also

Table 2. References and input cost estimates for the decision analytic model.

Reference	Composition of cost	Items	Value($)(year = 2012)
[43][52]	Testing cost	CD4 testing	5.43
[53]		ELISA testing	2.10
[53]		Positive rapid HIV testing	2.36
[53]		ELISA testing and Weston blotting	6.30
[53][79]	HAART cost	HAART in pregnancy	76.82
[53][79]		HAART during lactation	50.65
[2]		ART (first-line regimens)	186.00
[43]	ARV cost	Triple ARV in pregnancy(first-line regimens)	146.50
[51]		sdNVP+sdTDF+FTC and AZT in labor per unit	0.44
[51][43]		FDC(TDF+FTC/3TC+EFV) per year	159.00
[58]	Counseling and Health care cost	Cost of behavior counseling	3.74
[58]	Feeding cost	Breastfeeding (6 month)	153.98
[58]		Formula feeding (6 month)	310.82

ELISA, enzyme-linked immunosorbent assay; HAART, highly active antiretroviral therapy; ART, antiretroviral prophylaxis; ARV, antiretroviral prophylaxis; sdNVP, single dose nevirapine; sdTDF, single dose Tenofovir; FTC, emtricitabine; AZT, Zidovudine; FDC, (TDF, FTC/3TC, EFV); 3TC,Lamivudine; EFV, Efavirenz.

conducted a subgroup analysis according to the feeding patterns, using the untreated cohort (Untreated mothers who were assigned to breastfeeding) for comparison. Compared with the untreated cohort, assigning promptly treated cohort to the replacement feeding strategy was the more cost-effective ($134.88 per infant LY saved), followed by the promptly treated cohort being assigned to breastfeeding ($193.26 infant LY saved), as showed in Figure 3.B. With or without the antenatal testing and treatments, breastfeeding was less cost-effective than replacement feeding strategies.

Sensitivity Analysis

Since the actual values can vary in different settings, both one-way and multivariate sensitivity analyses were conducted to examine the factors that account for the variation in the cost per LY saved. The promptly treated cohort retained a cost-effectiveness ratio lower than $120 per LY in all one-variable sensitivity analyses. When we varied our uncertain assumptions regarding the input parameters, the ranking of interventions remained stable.

If the treatment efficacy of FDC ranged from 25% to 75%, the cost per LY would range $76.5–$223.8 in the remedy cohort. Although the ranking of interventions remained stable under these assumptions, the treatment efficacy of FDC in postnatal intervention significantly influenced the results.

When we decreased the rate of breastfeeding coverage in HIV-infected women from 100% to 5%, the incremental cost-effective per LY increased from $39.02 to $52.95 and from $67.97 to $406.94 in the prompt treated cohort and remedy cohort, respectively. Breastfeeding had a stronger influence on the remedy cohort than the promptly treated cohort. When the rate of breastfeeding coverage in HIV-infected women was reduced by 5% each time, about 57 and 19 infants might be avoided in the promptly treated cohort and remedy cohort, respectively.

Variation in the proportion of newly HIV-infected women presenting in labor and at postnatal visits also substantially affected the result of the remedy cohort. The proportion of HIV-infected women presenting in labor was set to vary by up to 3 times of the point estimate which could entail a ratio as high as 32% of the point estimate ($157 per LY) in the remedy cohort. Similarly, when the proportion of HIV-infected women treated during the

postnatal visits increased from the base-case value of 22% to 80%, the cost per LY increased from $59.20 to $95.15 per LY in the remedy cohort. In conclusion, without consideration of willingness to pay, remedial treatments both in labor and at postnatal visits were worthwhile.

Discussion

In this study, we developed a decision analytic model for prevention of mother-to-child HIV transmission and applied it to discuss the cost-effectiveness of antenatal HIV testing and treatments recommended by WHO versus the interventions used as a remedy in labor and the postpartum period after missing the window of opportunity for prompt intervention.

Early knowledge of HIV status may enable women to make more appropriate decisions with regard to their own health and that of their unborn children [59]. Our study reveals that antenatal testing and prompt treatment will prevent more than half of pediatric HIV cases. Knowledge of the mother's infection status can save an additional 5.9 pediatric LY [37]. There was a correlation coefficient of .66 between the period of confirmed HIV status and receipt of ARV, which illustrated that later confirmation of HIV-infected status led to less possibility of receiving ARV among mothers; this conclusion was derived from an analysis of 108 HIV-infected mothers in China [60]. One research in Hong Kong is also in support of this point of view [61].

Attempts to compare the cost and benefits for testing late and untested HIV-infected women have been previously undertaken [37–39]. However, these analyses failed to account for receipt of remedies in labor and during the postnatal visits among untested HIV-infected women. The guideline in South Africa recommends all pregnant women who need triple therapy and breastfeeding to receive a FDC compatible regimen as a remedy [26], and FDC has been rolled out in South Africa since 2013 [62]. We found that those remedial treatments would avert 9.76% of pediatric HIV cases compared with lack of treatment.

Furthermore, since the differences between the promptly treated cohort and remedy cohort are obvious, our focus was to study the impacts of different feeding patterns and breastfeeding coverage between the two cohorts.

A.

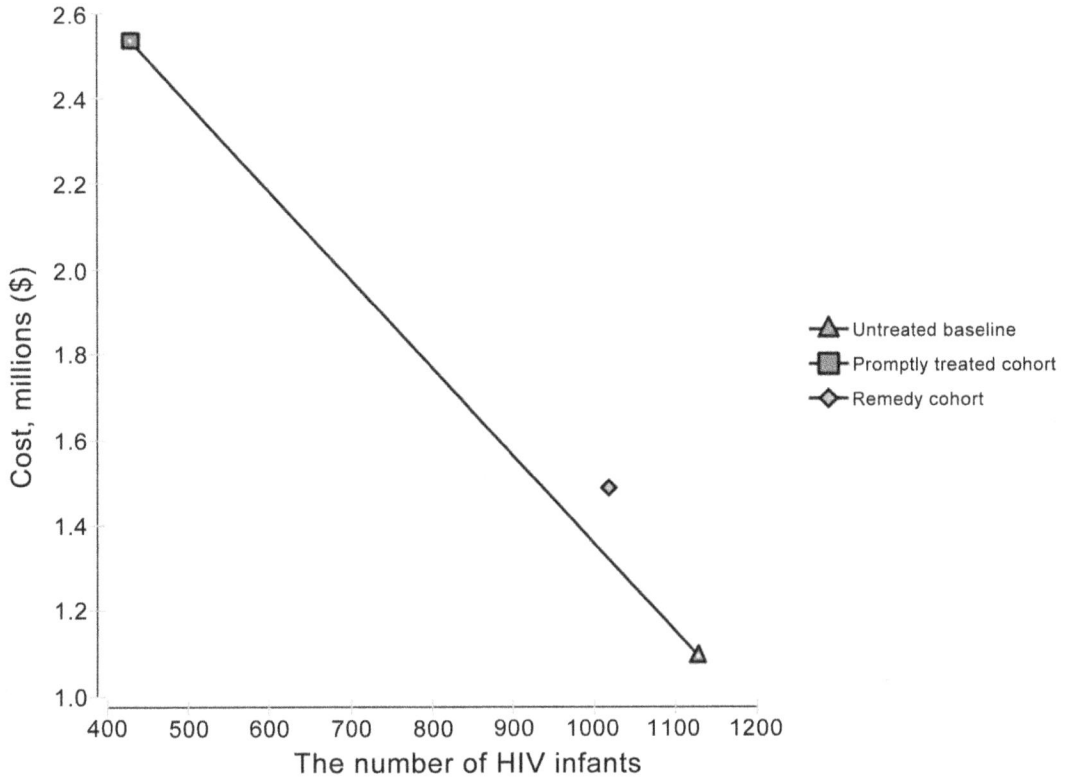

B.

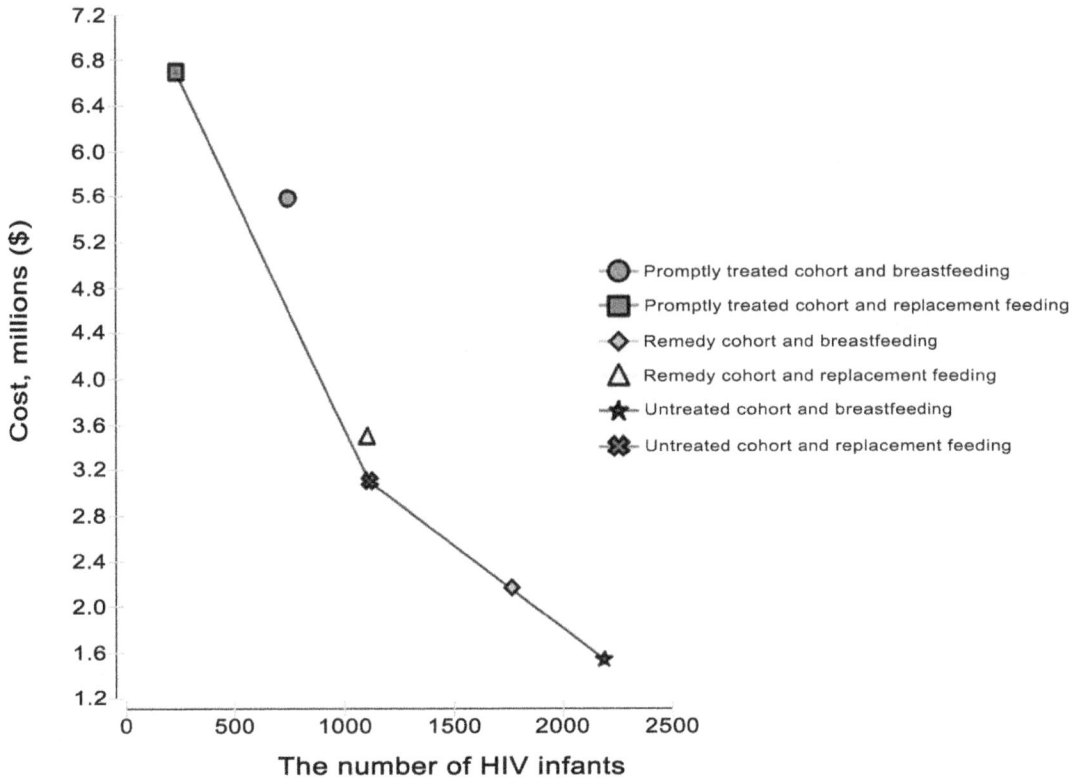

Figure 3. The cost-effectiveness frontier of different strategy combinations. The cost-effectiveness frontier (solid line) includes strategies that maybe cost-effective if the incremental cost-effectiveness ratio is less than the accepted threshold. Strategies that are not on the frontier are dominated, meaning that they are not efficient use of resources. In figure 3.A, irrespective of the feeding patterns, remedial cohort is less cost-effective. In figure 3.B, mothers' prompt treatment and replacement feeding cohort is the most cost-effective intervention, followed by the promptly treated cohort being assigned to breastfeeding.

Our model is in good agreement with other studies [12,35,60] and demonstrates that formula feeding results in a substantial decrease in HIV transmission risk and is cost-effectiveness, but formula is sometimes unaffordable for most HIV infected women because of the resource-limited settings[14,40]. As our results show, although breastfeeding strategy is less cost-effective, we can't ignore the impact of willingness to pay. In sub-Saharan Africa, more deaths would be caused than saved by formula feeding [40]. Breast milk contains nutrients, agents and antibodies that protect the infant from the risk of childhood diseases such as diarrhoea. Without being breastfed, an infant runs the risk of becoming seriously ill with diseases other than HIV. Where treatment for them is limited or inaccessible, an infant's health can be compromised. Similarly, unsafe and unreliable replacement feeding when clean water and resources are unavailable can also be a danger to an infant's health [64]. Breastfeeding is therefore highly widespread in low- and middle-income countries.

One influential factor for MTCT is the coverage of exclusive breastfeeding. Coovadia et al. confirmed that exclusive breastfeeding from about ages of 6 weeks to 6 months carried an HIV transmission risk of about 4% in South Africa [63]. In our study, each time the rate of breastfeeding coverage in HIV-infected women reduced 5%, there were about 59 and 19 infants whose infections were prevented in the promptly treated cohort and remedy cohorts, respectively. In addition, severity of maternal HIV condition influences the breastfeeding coverage and infants' HIV status. Eighteen-month follow-up of an observational cohort in the Kesho Bora study [41] showed that mothers in less severe disease were more willing to breastfeed their children than mothers in serious condition. Maybe they felt too weak to breastfeed and they were more concerned about HIV transmission or ARV toxicity for their breastfed children. Other researches showed that mothers who chose to replacement feed were more likely to have CD4 counts less than 200 cells/mm^3 than those who chose exclusively breastfeeding. [30]This opinion was also supported in a South African study [65]. A reference showed a significant correlation between associated mothers'CD4 counts and infants' HIV status. they found that if the concentration of CD4 counts$\geq$350 cells/mm^3, the HR of infants infected HIV was 0.59 [80]. Delicio found that if the CD4 cell counts lower than 350 cells/mm^3, it would increase the risk of MTCT more than 12 times. [81]What's more, there was no relationship between gestational age and CD4 counts [82].

Early initiation of ART is important for achievement of an undetectable viral load well before delivery. Thus, women should be encouraged to plan pregnancies and attend antenatal care sufficiently early to diagnose HIV infection, assess the HIV stage, and initiate ART or antiretroviral prophylaxis promptly [16]. The latest WHO guidelines stated that lifelong ARV treatment should be provided for all pregnant women and breastfeeding women with HIV, known as Option B Plus [66]. Countries that do not have the resources to provide lifelong ARV should offer the mother ARV for her own health when she finishes breastfeeding, known as Option B. If the mother is not eligible, she may stop taking ARV one full week after cessation of breastfeeding in low- and middle-income countries. In the 22 priority countries of the Global Plan, there are more than half of them implementing the OPTION B regimen policy for preventing the mother-to-child transmission of HIV among pregnant women living with HIV in 2013 [2]. For example, in South Africa, OPTION B is the main regimen policy because of limited resources [2]. Although providing antiretroviral treatment until complete cessation of breastfeeding (Option B) has numerous advantages and has been preferable in our model, and despite the fact that South Africa recently announce a switch to Option B [63], the switch to Option B will present further challenges, such as operational issues, the cost of increasing the number of women on ART, adherence to lifelong ART, emergence of ARV resistance, and long-term side effects to the fetuses, infants, and mothers [67].

Several limitations of this study deserve mention. First, similar to any cost-effectiveness analysis [53,68,69], our study is limited in its inability to model perfectly the complexities of clinical medicine and accurately estimate probabilities and cost. Problems include the lack of empirical data on the effects of FDC [70–72] during postnatal intervention. We have used counseling cost but the cost of home visits, Non-Governmental Organization and community involvement was not included in our model. Further, the sensitivity and specificity of each HIV test were not incorporated into the decision tree.

Second, our model does not reflect the practices of elective cesarean section (ECS). ECS before labor has been introduced as an intervention for the PMTCT of HIV and significantly lowers the risk of mother-to-child transmission of HIV infection [73].However, most of the studies of ECS among HIV infected women were conducted exclusively in North America and Europe [74]. In developing countries, such as South Africa, the risks and benefits associated with ECS are seldom explored [74]. The European Mode of Delivery Collaboration Organization had found that the role of mode of delivery in the management of HIV infected women should be assessed in light of risks as well as benefits and the risk/benefits ratio depended upon the underlying rate of MTCT [74].

The ECS rate is lower in South Africa than that of some developed countries, such as 50.7% in France [75]. A multi-country study in Sub-Saharan Africa showed 1276 women underwent ECS, giving a frequency of 6.2% (range 4.1–16.8%) [74]. Further confirmation was also given by another two studies in South Africa, which showed that only 13.24% and 10.92% of HIV-infected mothers underwent ECS, respectively [16,30,32]. The low rates indicate that ECS may have not served as ubiquitous practices in South Africa. Thus, the effectiveness of ECS in South Africa is also unable to be evaluated due to inadequate parameters in our model.

Third, mixed feeding during the first several months of life which is not included in our model is a influencing factor of HIV transmission [76]. Mixed feeding infants are nearly 11 times (HR 10.87) more likely to acquire infection than the exclusively breastfed children [30]. However, some women in resource-limited settings are malnourished and their breast milk is not sufficient for their infants [77]. As a result, it is difficult to bring the exclusive breastfeeding into force in South Africa [40].

Table 3. Results and Outcomes of each cohorts of 10,000 HIV infected pregnant women.

Status	Feeding patterns	Incremental cost US($)	Infant HIV cases averted		Life years saved		Incremental cost-effectiveness
			Total	Incremental cost (per, $)	Total	Incremental cost(per, $)	
Baseline (no intervention)	-	-	-	-	-	-	-
Promptly treated cohort	-	2063.05	698	1439391.2	21009.8	68.51	Undominated[s]
Remedy cohort	-	3579.66	110	391806.75	3311	118.33	Extended dominated[&]
Untreated cohort	Breastfeed	-	-	-	-	-	-
Untreated cohort	Replacement feed	1461.19	1073	1568400	32297.3	48.56	Undominated
Promptly treated cohort	Replacement feed	4059.88	883	3584863.5	26578.3	134.88	Undominated
Remedy cohort	Breastfeed	1508.69	421	635167.86	12672.1	50.12	Extended dominated
Promptly treated cohort	Breastfeed	5826.72	360	2094217.3	10836	193.26	Extended dominated
Remedy cohort	Replacement feed	3796.63	11	383788.86	331.1	1159.13	Extended dominated

[&]: extended dominated, means exclude any interventions that have a higher ICER than more effective interventions.
[s]: undominated, strategies on the cost-effectiveness frontier, meaning that they are more cost-effective.

In addition, establishment of an intervention to reduce vertical transmission of HIV may have important secondary benefits [55], such as prevention of horizontal transmission, vigilant follow-up infant care to prevent opportunistic infections and etc [71]. These benefits have not been quantified in developing countries and hence are not included in the model.

It should be also noted that in this study, interventions for mothers and exposed infants were only evaluated from the moment when the treatment of the mother began until the end of first 18 months of life for the HIV-exposed infants, although the effectiveness associated with these interventions has been estimated for HIV-exposed infants. Meanwhile, the assumption that infants complied with exclusive breastfeeding from ages of 6 weeks to 6 months if their mothers intended to breastfeed may overestimate the results of exclusive breastfeeding. So we draw our conclusion carefully and do not extend the results throughout the whole period of breast milk exposure. The effectiveness of long-term interventions is unknown.

Another limitation in our study is that we extrapolated most assumptions from a limited number of relatively small-scale studies; thus, precise and reliable estimates of the effectiveness of large-scale prevention programs are needed.

Finally, our estimates of new HIV infections do not take into account dynamic spread at the population level or differences at risk populations, and many factors can cause variability in both the cost and effects of interventions.

Despite all these limitations, our model truly reflected the progress of MTCT. We assigned the HIV-infected pregnant women in South Africa as our target population and once pregnant, individuals were assigned different strategies (promptly treated or not). The CD4 counts were also taken into account as to reflect the severity of the HIV disease. Most of the confirmed interventions were included in our model in light of mothers' HIV-status and the corresponding diseases progress, such as the ART treatment, the Triple ARV prophylaxis and the feeding patterns. In addition, we took remedial preventions and the impacts of different feeding patterns into account. Our study should assist the governments of developing countries, such as South Africa, on strategic decision making regarding the health resource allocation.

Conclusions

In summary, our study demonstrates the cost-effectiveness of antenatal HIV testing and treatments, remedy treatments, and their combinations with different feeding patterns. Antenatal HIV testing and standard prompt treatments constitute a cost-effective strategy even in a resource-limited setting like South Africa. Compared with the promptly treated cohort, remedy during labor or the postnatal period is less cost-effective. Although we should pay more attention to the impact of willingness to pay and the advantages of breastfeeding in resource-limited setting can not be ignored, we still suggest choosing replacement feeding as far as possible. Hopefully, these data will enlighten public health policy decisions in South Africa regarding the implementation of remedial treatments and replacement feeding interventions.

Acknowledgments

The authors gratefully acknowledge X.J. and J. C. for assistance in model development, analyses, and manuscript preparation. Thank the teachers of Department of Epidemiology of School of Public Health of Tianjin Medical University for instruction and copyediting. We are also indebted to the Journal Prep Services Company and RLipkin (City University of New York, New York, USA) and He H.N. for their contributions.

Author Contributions

Conceived and designed the experiments: WY CL. Analyzed the data: WY CL. Wrote the paper: WY CL XF. Designed and revised the figures and tables in the manuscript: XL GZ. Data collection of this study: XF LF. Provided full discussion and revision: ZC JM.

References

1. World Health Organization (2013) Global update on HIV treatment 2013: results, impact and opportunities. Available:http://www.who.int/hiv/pub/progressreports/update2013/en/index.html. Accessed 21 August 2013.
2. World Health Organization (2012) Global report: UNAIDS Report on the global AIDS epidemic. Available:http://www.unaids.org/en/media/unaids/contentassets/documents/epidemiology/2012/gr2012/20121120_UNAIDS_Global_Report_2012_en.pdf. Accessed 15 August 2013.
3. Low A, Gavriilidis G, Larke N, Lajoie M-R, Drouin O, et al. (2013) Impact of antiretroviral on the incidence of opportunistic infections in resource-limited settings: a systematic review and meta-analysis. Available:http://www.who.int/hiv/events/2013/IAS_poster_ARVopport.pdf?ua = 1. Accessed 15 May 2013.
4. Diaz T, Chu SY, Conti L, Nahlen BL, Whyte B, et al. (1994) Health insurance coverage among persons with AIDS: Results from a multistate surveillance project. Am J Public Health 84: 1015–1018.
5. Bassett IV, Regan S, Chetty S, Giddy J, Uhler LM, et al. (2010) Who starts ART in Durban, South Africa? Not everyone who should. AIDS 24 Suppl 1: S37–S44.
6. Sabharwal CJ, Sepkowitz K, Mehta R, Shepard C, Bodach S, et al. (2011) Impact of accelerated progression to AIDS on public health monitoring of late HIV diagnosis. AIDS Patient Care STDS 25: 143–151.
7. Weis KE, Liese AD, Hussey J, Gibson JJ, Duffus WA (2010) Associations of rural residence with timing of HIV diagnosis and stage of disease at diagnosis, South Carolina 2001–2005. J Rural Health 26: 105–112.
8. Ziegler JB, Cooper DA, Johnson RO, Gold J (1985) Postnatal transmission of AIDS-associated retrovirus from mother to infant. Lancet 1: 896–898.
9. Read JS (2000) Preventing mother to child transmission of HIV: the role of caesarean section. Sex Transm Infect 76: 231–232.
10. Read JS (2003) Human milk, breastfeeding and transmission of human immunodeficiency virus type 1 in the United States. American Academy of Pediatrics Committee on Pediatric AIDS. Pediatrics 112: 1196–1205.
11. Horvath T, Madi BC, Iuppa IM, Kennedy GE, Rutherford G, et al. (2009) Interventions for preventing late postnatal mother-to-child transmission of HIV. Cochrane Database Syst Rev CD006734.
12. Nduati R, John G, Mbori-Ngacha D, Richardson B, Overbaugh J, et al. (2000) Effect of breastfeeding and formula feeding on transmission of HIV-1: a randomized clinical trial. JAMA 283: 1167–1174.
13. World Health Organization (2000) Effect of breastfeeding on infant and child mortality due to infectious diseases in less developed countries: a pooled analysis. WHO Collaborative Study Team on the Role of Breastfeeding on the Prevention of Infant Mortality. Lancet 355: 451–455.
14. Bositis CM, Gashongore I, Patel DM (2010) Updates to the World Health Organization's Recommendations for the Use of Antiretroviral Drugs for Treating Pregnant Women and Preventing HIV Infection in Infants. Med J Zambia 37: 111–117.
15. World Health Organization (2006) The role of the health sector in strengthening systems to support children's healthy development in communities affected by HIV/AIDS. Available: http://whqlibdoc.who.int/publications/2007/9789241595964_eng.pdf. Accessed 23 August 2013.
16. de Vincenzi I (2011) Triple antiretroviral compared with zidovudine and single-dose nevirapine prophylaxis during pregnancy and breastfeeding for prevention of mother-to-child transmission of HIV-1 (Kesho Bora study): a randomised controlled trial. Lancet Infect Dis 11: 171–180.
17. Gaillard P, Fowler MG, Dabis F, Coovadia H, Van Der Horst C, et al. (2004) Use of antiretroviral drugs to prevent HIV-1 transmission through breast-feeding: from animal studies to randomized clinical trials. J Acquir Immune Defic Syndr 35: 178–187.
18. Chasela CS, Hudgens MG, Jamieson DJ, Kayira D, Hosseinipour MC, et al. (2010) Maternal or infant antiretroviral drugs to reduce HIV-1 transmission. N Engl J Med 362: 2271–2281.
19. Shapiro RL, Hughes MD, Ogwu A, Kitch D, Lockman S, et al. (2010) Antiretroviral regimens in pregnancy and breast-feeding in Botswana. N Engl J Med 362: 2282–2294.
20. Kramer MS, Chalmers B, Hodnett ED, Sevkovskaya Z, Dzikovich I, et al. (2001) Promotion of Breastfeeding Intervention Trial (PROBIT): a randomized trial in the Republic of Belarus. JAMA 285: 413–420.
21. Wikipedia (15 May 2013) HIV/AIDS in South Africa. Available:http://en.wikipedia.org/wiki/HIV_in_South_Africa. Accessed 04 March 2014.
22. The South African Department of Health (2008) Report on the national hiv and syphilis prevalence survey south africa. Available: http://www.doh.gov.za/docs/antenatal-f.html. Accessed 12 March 2013.
23. The Joint United Nations Programme on HIV and AIDS (2008) 2008 Report On the Global AIDS Epidemic. Available:http://www.amarc.org/documents/manuals/JC1510_2008GlobalReport_en.pdf. Accessed 04 March 2013.
24. Mayosi BM, Lawn JE, van Niekerk A, Bradshaw D, Abdool Karim SS, et al. (2012) Health in South Africa: changes and challenges since 2009. Lancet 380: 2029–2043.
25. Health Department of Republic of South Africa (2010) Annual Report 2010–2011. Available: http://www.doh.gov.za/docs/reports/annual/2011/annual_report2010-11.pdf. Accessed 01 Nov 2013.
26. Health Department of Republic of South Africa (2012) South African antiretroviral treatment guideline2013. Available:http://www.doh.gov.za/docs/policy/2013/ART_Treatment_Guidelines_Final_25March2013.pdf. Accessed 30 August 2013.
27. World Health Organization (2012) Countdown to 2015 maternal,newborn&child surval: building a future for women and children. Available:http://www.countdown2015mnch.org/documents/2012report/2012-complete-no-profiles.pdf. Accessed 09 August 2013.
28. The Joint United Nations Programme on HIV and AIDS (2012) Global Report: UNAIDS Report on the Global AIDS Epidemic 2012. Available:http://www.unaids.org/en/media/unaids/contentassets/documents/epidemiology/2012/gr2012/20121120_UNAIDS_Global_Report_2012_with_annexes_en.pdf. Accessed 11 August 2013.
29. The Joint United Nations Programme on HIV and AIDS (2012) World AIDS Day Report-Results. Available:http://www.unaids.org/en/media/unaids/contentassets/documents/epidemiology/2012/gr2012/jc2434_worldaidsday_results_en.pdf. Accessed 11 August 2013.
30. Coovadia HM, Rollins NC, Bland RM, Little K, Coutsoudis A, et al. (2007) Mother-to-child transmission of HIV-1 infection during exclusive breastfeeding in the first 6 months of life: an intervention cohort study. Lancet 369: 1107–16.
31. Kuhn L, Sinkala M, Kankasa C, Semrau K, Kasonde P, et al. (2007) High Uptake of Exclusive Breastfeeding and Reduced Early Post-Natal HIV Transmission. PLoS ONE 2(12): e1363.
32. Bland RM, Little KE, Coovadia HM, Coutsoudis A, Rollins NC, et al. (2008) Intervention to promote exclusive breast-feeding for the first 6 months of life in a high HIV prevalence area. AIDS 22(7) 883–891.
33. The Joint United Nations Programme on HIV and AIDS (2009) Overview of breastfeeding patterns, Available:http://www.childinfo.org/breastfeeding_overview.html. Accessed 13 May 2013.
34. Leshabari SC, Koniz-Booher P, Åstrøm AN, de Paoli MM, Moland KM (2006) Translating global recommendations on HIV and infant feeding to the local context: the development of culturally sensitive counselling tools in the Kilimanjaro Region, Tanzania. Implementation Science 1:(22).
35. Nagelkerke NJ, Jha P, de Vlas SJ, Korenromp EL, Moses S, et al. (2002) Modelling HIV/AIDS epidemics in Botswana and India: impact of interventions to prevent transmission. Bull World Health Organ 80: 89–96.
36. Grundmann N, Iliff P, Stringer J, Wilfert C (2011) Presumptive diagnosis of severe HIV infection to determine the need for antiretroviral therapy in children less than 18 months of age. Bull World Health Organ 89: 513–520.
37. Gibb DM, Ades AE, Gupta R, Sculpher MJ (1999) Costs and benefits to the mother of antenatal HIV testing: estimates from simulation modelling. AIDS 13: 1569–1576.
38. Mauskopf JA, Paul JE, Wichman DS, White AD, Tilson HH (1996) Economic impact of treatment of HIV-positive pregnant women and their newborns with zidovudine. Implications for HIV screening. JAMA 276: 132–138.
39. Ecker JL (1996) The cost-effectiveness of human immunodeficiency virus screening in pregnancy. Am J Obstet Gynecol 174: 716–721.
40. Soderlund N, Zwi K, Kinghorn A, Gray G (1999) Prevention of vertical transmission of HIV: analysis of cost-effectiveness of options available in South Africa. BMJ 318: 1650–1656.
41. Kesho Bora Study Group (2010) Eighteen-month follow-up of HIV-1-infected mothers and their children enrolled in the Kesho Bora study observational cohorts. J Acquir Immune Defic Syndr 54: 533–541.
42. Estill J, Egger M, Blaser N, Vizcaya LS, Garone D, et al. (2013) Cost-effectiveness of point-of-care viral load monitoring of antiretroviral therapy in resource-limited settings: mathematical modelling study. AIDS 27: 1483–1492.
43. Sturt AS, Dokubo EK, Sint TT (2010) Antiretroviral therapy (ART) for treating HIV infection in ART-eligible pregnant women. Cochrane Database Syst Rev: CD008440.
44. World Health Organization (2006) WHO HIV and Infant Feeding Technical Consultation Held on behalf of the Inter-agency Task Team (IATT) on Prevention of HIV Infections in Pregnant Women, Mothers and their Infants. Available: http://www.who.int/maternal_child_adolescent/documents/pdfs/who_hiv_infant_feeding_technical_consultation.pdf. Accessed 13 May 2013.
45. TreeAge Software Inc (2011) TreeAge Pro 2011 User's Manual. Available: http://installers.treeagesoftware.com/treeagepro/TP2012/TreeAgePro-2012-Manual.pdf. Accessed 21 June 2013.
46. Siegfried N, van der Merwe L, Brocklehurst P, Sint TT (2011) Antiretroviral for reducing the risk of mother-to-child transmission of HIV infection. Cochrane Database Syst Rev: CD003510.
47. The Petra Team (2002) Efficacy of three short-course regimens of zidovudine and lamivudine in preventing early and late transmission of HIV-1 from mother

to child in Tanzania, South Africa, and Uganda (Petra study): a randomised, double-blind, placebo-controlled trial. Lancet.359: 1178–1186.

48. Mosen DM, Horberg M, Roblin D, Gullion CM, Meenan R, et al. (2010) effect of once-daily FDC treatment era on initiation of cART. Dovepress.2: 19–26.

49. Mbori-Ngacha D, Nduati R, John G, Reilly M, Richardson B, et al. (2001) Morbidity and Mortality in Breastfed and Formula-Fed Infants of HIV-1–Infected Women A Randomized Clinical Trial. JAMA. 286(19): 2413–2420.

50. Index mundi (2014) World Facebook, South Africa Infant mortality rate. Available: http://www.indexmundi.com/south_africa/infant_mortality_rate.html. Accessed 20 April 2014.

51. Waning B, Kaplan W, King AC, Lawrence DA, Leufkens HG, et al. (2009) Global strategies to reduce the price of antiretroviral medicines: evidence from transactional databases. Bull World Health Organ 87: 520–528.

52. Kahn JG, Marseille E, Moore D, Bunnell R, Were W, et al. (2011) CD4 cell count and viral load monitoring in patients undergoing antiretroviral therapy in Uganda: cost-effectiveness study. BMJ 343: d6884.

53. Kim LH, Cohan DL, Sparks TN, Pilliod RA, Arinaitwe E, et al. (2013) The cost-effectiveness of repeat HIV testing during pregnancy in a resource-limited setting. J Acquir Immune Defic Syndr 63: 195–200.

54. Antiretroviral Therapy Cohort Collaboration (2008) Life expectancy of individuals on combination antiretroviral therapy in high-income countries: a collaborative analysis of 14 cohort studies. Lancet 372: 293–299.

55. Marseille E, Kahn JG, Mmiro F, Guay L, Musoke P, et al. (1999) Cost-effectiveness of single-dose nevirapine regimen for mothers and babies to decrease vertical HIV-1 transmission in sub-Saharan Africa. Lancet 354: 803–809.

56. Chin J (1991) The epidemiology and projected mortality of AIDS. Available: http://www.popline.org/node/317283. Accessed 20 April 2013.

57. McClamroch K, Behets F, Van Damme K, Rabenja LN, Myers E (2007) Cost-effectiveness of treatment strategies for cervical infection among women at high risk in Madagascar. Sex Transm Dis 34: 631–637.

58. Creese A, Floyd K, Alban A, Guinness L (2002) Cost-effectiveness of HIV/AIDS interventions in Africa: a systematic review of the evidence. Lancet 359: 1635–1643.

59. Westheimer EF, Urassa W, Msamanga G, Baylin A, Wei R, et al. (2004) Acceptance of HIV testing among pregnant women in Dar-es-Salaam, Tanzania. J Acquir Immune Defic Syndr 37: 1197–1205.

60. Li B, Zhao Q, Zhang X, Wu L, Chen T, et al. (2013) Effectiveness of a prevention of mother-to-child HIV transmission program in Guangdong province from 2007 to 2010. BMC Public Health 13: 591.

61. Lee PM, Wong KH (2007) Universal antenatal human immunodeficiency virus (HIV) testing programme is cost-effective despite a low HIV prevalence in Hong Kong. Hong Kong Med J 13: 199–207.

62. South Africa Government Services (2013) Department of Health starts rolling out fixed-dose combination antiretroviral. Available:http://www.services.gov.za/services/content/news/antiretrovirals/en_ZA. Accessed 08 April 2013.

63. Coovadia HM, Rollins NC, Bland RM, Little K, Coutsoudis A, et al. (2007) Mother-to-child transmission of HIV-1 infection during exclusive breastfeeding in the first 6 months of life: an intervention cohort study. Lancet 369: 1107–1116.

64. Avert (2012) HIV & AIDS in South Africa. Available: http://www.avert.org/hiv-aids-south-africa.htm. Accessed 22 April 2013.

65. World Health Organization (2010) Antiretroviral drugs for treating pregnant women and preventing HIV infections in infants: recommendations for a public health approach 2010 geneva switzerland. Available:http://whqlibdoc.who.int/publications/2010/9789241599818_eng.pdf.Acces -sed 25 August 2013.

66. World Health Organization (2013) Consolidated guidelines on the use of antiretroviral drugs for treating and preventing HIV infection:Recommenda-
tions for a public health approach. Available: http://apps.who.int/iris/bitstream/10665/85321/1/9789241505727_eng.pdf. Accessed 01 August 2013.

67. Moodley P, Parboosing R, Moodley D (2013) Reduction in perinatal HIV infections in KwaZulu-Natal, South Africa, in the era of more effective prevention of mother to child transmission interventions (2004–2012). J Acquir Immune Defic Syndr 63: 410–415.

68. McCabe CJ, Goldie SJ, Fisman DN (2010) The cost-effectiveness of directly observed highly-active antiretroviral therapy in the third trimester in HIV-infected pregnant women. PLoS One 5: e10154.

69. Liu X, Li C, Gong H, Cui Z, Fan L, et al. (2013) An economic evaluation for prevention of diabetes mellitus in a developing country: a modelling study. BMC Public Health 13: 729.

70. Jose R, Anton L, Pozniak, Joel E, Gallant, et al. (2008) Tenofovir Disoproxil Fumarate, Emtricitabine and Efavirenz Compared With Zidovudine/Lamivudine and Efavirenzin Treatment-Naive Patients 144-Week Analysis. J Acquir Immune Defic Syndr 47: 74–78.

71. Janssen N, Ndirangu J, Newell M-L, Bland RM (2010) Successful paediatric HIV treatment in rural primary care in Africa. Arch Dis Child 95: 414–421.

72. Gallant JE, Staszewski S, Pozniak AL, De Jesus E, Suleiman JMAH, et al. (2004) Efficacy and Safety of Tenofovir DF vs Stavudine in Combination Therapy in Antiretroviral-Naïve Patients A 3-Year Randomized Trial. JAMA 292: 191–201.

73. The European Mode of Delivery Collaboration (1999) Elective caesarean-section versus vaginal delivery in prevention of vertical HIV-1 transmission: a randomised clinical trial. Lancet 353: 1035–39.

74. Chu K, Cortier H, Maldonado F, Mashant T, Ford N, et al. (2012) Cesarean Section Rates and Indications in Sub-Saharan Africa:A Multi-Country Study from Medecins sans Frontieres. PLoS One 7(9):e44484.

75. Briand N, Jasseron C, Sibiude J, Azria E, Pollet J, et al. (2013) Cesarean section for HIV-infected women in the combination antiretroviral therapy era, 2000–2010. Am J Obstet Gynecol 209: 335.e1–12.

76. Becquet R, Ekouevi DK, Menan H, Amani-Bosse C, Bequet L, et al.(2008) Early mixed feeding and breastfeeding beyond 6 months increase the risk of postnatal HIV transmission: ANRS 1201/1202 Ditrame Plus, Abidjan, Côted'Ivoire. Preventive Medicine 47: 27–33.

77. International Treatment Preparedness Coalition (2009) Missing the Target: Failing Women, Failing Children:HIV, Vertical Transmission and Women's Health. Available:http://www.hivpolicy.org/Library/HPP001643.pdf. Accessed 29 August 2013.

78. Chatterjee A, Bosch RJ, Hunter DJ, Fataki MR, Msamanga GI, et al. (2007) Maternal disease stage and child undernutrition in relation to mortality among children born to HIV-infected women in Tanzania. J Acquir Immune Defic Syndr 46: 599–606.

79. United Nations Programme on HIV/AIDS (2008) Report on the global AIDS epidemic:Executive summary. Available:http://www.unaids.org/en/media/unaids/contentassets/dataimport/pub/globalreport/2008/jc1511_gr08_executivesummary_en.pdf. Accessed 20 August 2013.

80. Kovalchik SA (2012) Mother's CD4+ Count Moderates the Risk Associated with Higher Parity for Late Postnatal HIV-Free Survival of Breastfed Children: An Individual Patient Data Meta-Analysis of Randomized Controlled Trials. AIDS Behav 16: 79–85.

81. Delicio AM, Milanez H, Amaral E, Morais SS, Lajos GJ, et al. (2011) Mother-to-child transmission of human immunodeficiency virus in aten years period. Reprod Health 8: 35.

82. Temmerman M, Nagelkerke N, Bwayo J, Chomba EN, Ndinya-Achola J, et al. (1995) HIV-1 and immunological changes during pregnancy: a comparison between HIV-1-seropositive and HIV-1-seronegative women in Nairobi, Kenya. AIDS 9: 1057–1060.

8

Oral Microbiota Distinguishes Acute Lymphoblastic Leukemia Pediatric Hosts from Healthy Populations

Yan Wang[1,9], Jing Xue[1,9], Xuedong Zhou[1], Meng You[1], Qin Du[1], Xue Yang[2], Jingzhi He[1], Jing Zou[3], Lei Cheng[1], Mingyun Li[1], Yuqing Li[1], Yiping Zhu[2], Jiyao Li[1], Wenyuan Shi[4], Xin Xu[1]*

1 State Key Laboratory of Oral Diseases, West China Hospital of Stomatology, Sichuan University, Chengdu, China, 2 Department of Pediatric Hematology and Oncology, West China Second University Hospital, Sichuan University, Chengdu, China, 3 Department of Pediatric Dentistry, West China Hospital of Stomatology, Sichuan University, Chengdu, China, 4 UCLA School of Dentistry, Los Angeles, California, United States of America

Abstract

In leukemia, oral manifestations indicate aberrations in oral microbiota. Microbiota structure is determined by both host and environmental factors. In human hosts, how health status shapes the composition of oral microbiota is largely unknown. Taking advantage of advances in high-throughput sequencing, we compared the composition of supragingival plaque microbiota of acute lymphoblastic leukemia (ALL) pediatric patients with healthy controls. The oral microbiota of leukemia patients had lower richness and less diversity compared to healthy controls. Microbial samples clustered into two major groups, one of ALL patients and another of healthy children, with different structure and composition. Abundance changes of certain taxa including the Phylum *Firmicutes*, the Class *Bacilli*, the Order *Lactobacillales*, the Family *Aerococcaceae* and *Carnobacteriaceae*, as well as the Genus *Abiotrophia* and *Granulicatella* were associated with leukemia status. ALL patients demonstrated a structural imbalance of the oral microbiota, characterized by reduced diversity and abundance alterations, possibly involved in systemic infections, indicating the importance of immune status in shaping the structure of oral microbiota.

Editor: Yolanda Sanz, Instutite of Agrochemistry and Food Technology, Spain

Funding: This work was supported by the International S&T Cooperation Program of China (grant number: 2011DFA30940), the National Basic Research Program of China ("973 Pilot Research Program," grant Number: 2011CB512108), the National Science & Technology Pillar Program during the 12th Five-year Plan Period (grant number: 2012BAI07B03), National Natural Science Foundation of China (grant number: 81200782) and Doctoral Fund of Ministry of Education of China (grant number: 20120181120002). The funders had no role in study design, data collection and analysis, decision to publish, or preparation of the manuscript.

Competing Interests: The authors have declared that no competing interests exist.

* Email: nixux1982@hotmail.com

⑨ These authors contributed equally to this work.

Introduction

Leukemia is a cancer of the early blood-forming cells. Acute lymphoblastic leukemia (ALL), a malignant disorder of lymphoid progenitor cells, is the most common type of leukemia among children, accounting for 75% of all childhood leukemia and 25% of all malignancy in childhood [1]. Among some individuals leukemia first manifests in oral cavity [2,3]. Oral manifestations that frequently occur in leukemia patients include gingival bleeding, oral ulceration, gingival enlargement, candidiasis and periodontitis [4,5,6]. Oral microbes are believed to be involved in the occurrence or exacerbation of such complications [7]. Certain oral microbiota have been shown to contribute to septicemia, which might delay antineoplastic treatment, compromise treatment efficiency, or even jeopardize the patients' life [8,9]. Therefore, an adequate treatment of oral lesions could lead to a more favorable resolution of both oral and systemic diseases. At present, limited knowledge is available on the oral microbiota of leukemia patients. Previous studies dependent on a culture-based approach have mainly focused on limited cultivable bacterial species and failed to determine the holistic pattern of oral microbiota in leukemia patients [10,11,12,13]. Furthermore, because most previous studies were primarily focused on the effect of antineoplastic treatment on oral microbes, limited information can be obtained on the oral microbiota *per se* under the diseased condition. To determine the role of oral cavity microbiota to local and systemic complications in ALL patients, it is first necessary to generate a more complete picture of the oral cavity microbiota population that is specific to this disease.

In ALL patients, lymphoid progenitor cells are affected, which can partially impair the immune system of the host [14,15]. It is known that microbiota structure within a host is determined by both host and environmental factors. If any one of these factors is greatly perturbed, a drastic composition shift is expected in the oral microbiota, and disease occurs. In the human host, the role of health status in shaping the composition of oral microbiota is still largely unknown. Characterization of the oral microbiome in ALL patients provides information about oral microbiota-host interactions in immunocompromised individuals, and thus contributes to better management of oral and systemic complications associated with immunodeficiency.

To elucidate how a compromised host immune status leads to a perturbed microbial homeostasis necessitates a thorough comparison of the oral microbial composition of ALL patients and ALL-free population. Remarkable advances in high-throughput sequencing have recently improved practicality in analysis of microbiota from a variety of biological and environmental samples under various conditions. Whereas conventional culture-dependent approaches underestimate microbial composition, new culture-independent molecular techniques are capable of investigating entire bacterial communities and characterizing the biodiversity of oral microbiota. High-throughput sequencing has been widely and successfully applied to the exploration of oral microbial diversity in health [16,17,18] and disease-associated communities from those associated with dental caries [19,20], periradicular lesions [21], atherosclerosis [22], and head-neck tumor undergone radiotherapy [23,24]. However, application of these techniques in investigating the oral microbiome under immunocompromised conditions has so far been limited. In this study, we characterized the biodiversity of supragingival plaque microbiota in pediatric clinic ALL patients using a high-throughput sequencing technique (454 pyrosequencing). The oral microbiota compositional profiles were compared to those of ALL-free healthy subjects.

Methods

Ethics Statement

This study was approved by the Ethics Committee of State Key Laboratory of Oral Diseases, Sichuan University, Chengdu, China, and conducted in compliance with the Declaration of Helsinki. Written informed consent was obtained from the parents or guardians of all subjects before the study.

Study Population

Potential study subjects of the leukemia group were selected from a group of patients who were newly diagnosed with acute lymphoblastic leukemia (ALL) in the Department of Pediatric Hematology and Oncology, West China Second University Hospital, Sichuan University. All subjects received no previous antineoplastic treatment. Demographic information was obtained and oral examination was performed. A gender-, age-, and caries status matched healthy counterpart for each leukemia child was recruited from Department of Pediatric Dentistry, West China Hospital of Stomatology, Sichuan University. The detailed eligible

criteria are presented in Table 1. Detailed clinical data of each subject is in Table S1.

Sample Collection and Oral Examination

For each of the 26 subjects, microbial samples were collected at the same time of day, approximately 2 hours after breakfast, using the method mentioned in the Manual of Procedures for Human Microbiome Project (http://hmpdacc.org/tools_protocols/tools_protocols.php) with minor modifications. Briefly, the sampling sites, the teeth in upper right and lower left quadrants or upper left and lower right quadrants, were isolated with cotton rolls and dried before sampling. A sterile Gracey curette was used to collect a pooled supragingival plaque sample from the mesial surfaces of each of these teeth in turn. The collected plaque samples were released from the curette by agitation in 700 µl of TE buffer (10 mM Tris-Cl [pH 7.5] and 1 mM EDTA). The microbial samples were immediately transported on ice to the laboratory and stored at −80°C until further DNA extraction and pyrosequencing analysis.

Oral conditions of each subject, including dentition status, number of teeth, plaque index, caries status, and presence or absence of gingivitis/periodontitis, were recorded after sampling. The presence of caries was further confirmed by periapical radiographs. Plaque-Check+pH kit (GC Corporation, Japan) was used for testing plaque fermentation based on a colourimetric readout of the pH of supragingival plaque corresponding to each sampling site [25].

DNA Extraction

Bacteria were pelleted from dental plaque samples by centrifugation (Thermo Electron Corporation, Boston, MA, USA) at full speed (more than 10,000×g) for 10 min. Bacterial DNA was extracted using QIAamp DNA Micro Kit (QIAGEN, Hilden, Germany) according to the manufacturer's instructions with minor modification. Briefly, 30 µl lysozome solution (50 mg/ml) was added to the mixture at the first step to increase the yield of bacterial DNA from Gram-positive bacteria by hydrolyzing the peptidoglycan cell wall. The amount of DNA extracted per sample was determined using Quant-iT PicoGreen dsDNA Assay Kit

Table 1. Admission criteria.

ALL patients group

Inclusion criteria	Exclusion criteria
(1) Newly diagnosed with acute lymphoblastic leukemia based on bone marrow samples	(1) Previous antineoplastic treatment
(2) No more than eighteen years old	(2) Receiving antibiotics within 3 months before the study
(3) Free of other systemic diseases (including systemic infection)	(3) Local antimicrobial treatment within 2 weeks
(4) Written informed consent	

Healthy control group

Inclusion criteria	Exclusion criteria
(1) Age, socioeconomic and caries status comparable with ALL patients	(1) Systemic or local disorders that cause oral mucosal lesions such as lichen planus
(2) Free of systemic diseases	(2) Periodontal pockets equal to or greater than 4 mm
(3) Written informed consent	(3) Acute oral infection such as dental abscess at enrollment
	(4) Evidence of oral candidiasis
	(5) Receiving antibiotics within 3 months before the study
	(6) Local antimicrobial treatment within 2 weeks

ALL patients: acute lymphoblastic leukemia patients.

(Invitrogen, Carlsbad, USA). Size and integrity of DNA were checked by 1% (w/v) agarose gel electrophoresis in 0.05‰ (v/v) GoldView. The extracted DNA was then stored at $-20°C$ before further analyses.

Pyrosequencing and Data Analysis

The 16S rRNA hypervariable V1–V3 region was amplified using polymerase chain reaction (PCR) with the forward primer 8F (59-AGAGTTTGATCCTGGCTCAG-39) and reverse primer 533R (59-TTACCGCGGCTGCTGGCAC-39) [18]. Unique 10-bp barcodes were incorporated into the reverse primers so that sequences of different samples can be differentiated. Each 25 µl PCR reaction consisted of 1 µl of forward primer (10 µmol/l), 1 µl of barcoded reverse primer (10 µmol/l), 0.5 µl of dNTP mix (10 mmol/l), 2.5 µl of FastStart 10× buffer with 18 mmol/l of $MgCl_2$, 0.25 µl of FastStart HiFi Polymerase (5 U/µl), 1 µl of genomic DNA, and 18.75 µl of water. FastStart HiFi Polymerase, FastStart 10× buffer with $MgCl_2$ and dNTP mix were included in the FastStart High Fidelity PCR System, dNTP Pack (Roche Applied Science). The PCR amplification was performed using the following program: 3 minutes of initial denaturation at 94°C, followed by 25 cycles of denaturation (94°C for 15 seconds), annealing (56°C for 30 seconds) and extension (72°C for 30 seconds) with a final extension of 5 minutes at 72°C. To obtain sufficient PCR products for pyrosequencing, the amplicons of three replicates were pooled. After PCR, amplicons were gel purified using MinElute Gel Extraction Kit (QIAGEN), and then quantified with Quant-iT PicoGreen dsDNA Assay Kit (Invitrogen).The PCR products were combined in equimolar ratios to create a DNA pool used for pyrosequencing. Pyrosequencing was performed according to standard Roche 454 GS-FLX protocols [26].

To optimize raw sequences, the sequence analyzing programs Seqcln (http://sourceforge.net/projects/seqclean/) and MOTHUR (version 1.30.0; http://www.mothur.org) were applied to the data. The primer sequences and 10-bp barcode were removed. The sequences were checked and low quality sequences (quality score <25) were discarded. Sequences that contained ambiguous bases, incorrect primer sequence, or identified to be shorter than 200 bp, or homologous sequences longer than six nucleotides were also removed. UCHIME (http://drive5.com/uchime) was used to detect potentially chimeric artifacts. Sequences were clustered to operational taxonomical units (OTU) using CD-HIT-EST at 97% similarity level. RDP Naïve Bayesian Classifier was applied to perform read level taxonomic assignments with an 80% bootstrap score [27]. Qualified sequences were submitted to the SILVA database (SILVA 111; http://www.arbsilva.de) for taxonomic alignment. Community richness (ACE, Chao1) and diversity indices (Simpson diversity index) were determined by the MOTHUR program at 97% similarity level. The statistical significance of these indices was determined by SPSS 19.0 (SPSS Inc, Chicago, IL, USA) with nonparametric Mann-Whitney U test for independent samples. The heatmap profile was generated by the R program (http://www.r-project.org/). For phylogeny-based cluster comparisons, principal coordinate analysis (PCoA) plots were generated with the distance matrix calculated using the weighted UniFrac algorithm. The composition of the microbial communities present in the samples from the ALL patients (n = 13) and control (n = 12) groups were analyzed using unweighted and weighted UniFrac analysis [28,29] and Parsimony p-tests [30]. Metastats was used to compare the relative abundance of each taxon at different taxonomic levels between ALL patients and healthy children [31], with the p value threshold set at 0.05 and the q value threshold at 0.5 [32].

Sequence Deposition

Sequences were deposited in the NCBI sequence read archive (http://www.ncbi.nlm.nih.gov/Traces/sra/) under accession number SRP034724.

Results

Richness and Diversity of Oral Microbiota in ALL patients and Healthy Children

In total, 356000 qualified sequence reads were obtained and used for analysis, with an average of 13692 sequence reads for each sample. One healthy subject sample (H04) had low sequence counts making the depth of pyrosequencing not comparable to other samples. Thus to avoid potential bias caused by uneven sequence depth, this sample was not subjected to further bioinformatics analyses, leaving 13 ALL patients and 12 healthy control subjects samples for downstream data analyses.

The species-level operational taxonomic units (OTUs) and richness and diversity estimators were generated for each sample (Table S2). Clustering the unique sequences into OTUs at a 0.03 dissimilarity level formed 2280 OTUs per microbiome on average. Richness and diversity estimation of 16S rRNA gene libraries at 97% similarity was calculated and compared between two groups (Table 2). Comparison of species-level OTUs between ALL patients and healthy children revealed that the ALL patients group exhibited lower richness ($p = 0.004$). Furthermore, community richness estimators (Chao 1 and ACE) also revealed a statistically significant lower estimate of richness for ALL patients compared with healthy children. ALL patients showed less diversity compared with healthy subjects as demonstrated by comparing the Simpson Index between the oral microbiota of the two groups ($p = 0.019$).

Structural Comparisons of Oral Microbiota between ALL Patients and Healthy Subjects

No statistically significant difference regarding the demographic information and oral health conditions was observed between the ALL group and the healthy control ($p>0.05$), albeit the ALL patients have a higher incidence of periodontitis compared with the healthy subjects (Table 3). We compared the oral microbial communities present within each of the 13 ALL patients and 12 control subjects using three different types of cluster analysis: OTU-based, taxonomy-based (at the order level) and phylogeny-based cluster analyses. The dendrogram from the OTU-composition presented two clusters, with one cluster composed of leukemia oral samples and the other mainly comprised of healthy control samples (Figure 1). Moreover, the supragingival plaque samples from the ALL patients and healthy controls could be divided into two subsets based on microbiota composition and microbe abundance at the order level. This taxonomy-based clustering at the order level was better associated with the health or disease status (ALL-affected vs. ALL-free) of subjects as shown in Figure S1. Principal coordinate analysis (PCoA) based on the weighted UniFrac metric was also performed. Although 5 subjects from ALL patients group clustered with the healthy controls, a segregation trend for ALL patients and healthy subjects was observed, especially by principal coordinate P1 (Figure 2). To further validate the statistical significance of the aforementioned sample clustering, we performed three different types of pair-wise comparisons, including parsimony test, Unifrac unweighted and Unifrac weighted analyses. A single NJ phylogenetic tree containing all 16S rRNA sequences from the samples from the 13 ALL patients and 12 control subjects (identical to that used for the PCoA analysis) was used as the input for all three methods. All

Table 2. Comparison of richness and diversity estimates of 16S rRNA gene libraries at 97% similarity between the acute lymphoblastic leukemia patients and healthy subjects.

Variables	ALL patients (n = 13)	Healthy control (n = 12)	p value*
OTUs	1778±874	2824±647	0.004
Chao 1[a]	4738.27±2049.02	7215.11±1505.13	0.003
ACE[b]	8305.50±3336.40	12455.82±2400.76	0.004
Simpson[c]	0.0393±0.0246	0.0168±0.0082	0.019

Applicable values are means±SD. ALL patients: acute lymphoblastic leukemia patients.
[a,b]Richness estimators (Chao 1 and ACE) were calculated using MOTHUR.
[c]A higher number indicates less diversity.
*Independent sample nonparametric Mann-Whitney U test was used.

three statistical approaches showed significant difference (parsimony test, $p = 0.006$; Unifrac unweighted, $p = 0.005$; Unifrac weighted, $p < 0.001$), indicating that the oral microbial structure of the ALL-affected population is distinct from that of the healthy controls.

Taxonomy-Based Comparisons of Oral Microbiota between the Two Host Populations

Comparisons of oral microbiota between ALL patients and healthy subjects at each of taxonomical levels of phylum, class, order, family and genus were performed based on Metastats analysis. From the phylum level down to the Genus level, there were no 'leukemia-specific' or 'healthy-specific' taxa unique to either leukemia or healthy hosts. However, 'leukemia-associated' taxa (present in healthy and leukemia populations but differentially distributed) were detected, which were either 'leukemia-enriched' or 'leukemia-depleted' for certain microbe classes (Figure 3; Table S3). A total of 12 phyla were identified in oral microbiota of ALL patients and healthy children in our dataset, which were dominated by six major phyla, including *Proteobacteria*, *Firmicutes*, *Fusobacteria*, *Actinobacteria*, *Bacterioidetes* and candidate division TM7 (Figure S2). Particularly, notable differences in abundance

between ALL patients and healthy subjects were found for the two phyla, i.e. *Firmicutes* ($p = 0.001$) and *Fusobacteria* ($p = 0.003$). *Firmicutes* was more abundant while *Fusobacteria* was less abundant in ALL patients compared to healthy children (Figure 3). Of all genera detected from oral cavity samples, *Abiotrophia* ($p = 0.001$), *Comamonas* ($p = 0.001$), *Granulicatella* ($p = 0.002$), *Leptotrichia* ($p = 0.001$) and *Veillonella* ($p = 0.001$) were significantly different between ALL patients and healthy subjects. Leukemia-enriched genera included *Abiotrophia*, *Granulicatella* and *Veillonella*, while *Comamonas* and *Leptotrichia* constituted leukemia-depleted genera (Figure 3).

Taking taxonomic lineages into account, two lineages were found to be more abundant in the ALL patients compared to the healthy children from the phylum down to the genus level (Table S3). The two leukemia-enriched taxonomic lineages included *Firmicutes* ($p = 0.001$) at Phylum, *Bacilli* ($p = 0.001$) at Class, *Lactobacillales* ($p = 0.001$) at Order, *Aerococcaceae* ($p = 0.001$) at Family and *Abiotrophia* ($p = 0.012$) at genus, as well as *Firmicutes* ($p = 0.001$) at Phylum, *Bacilli* ($p = 0.001$) at Class, *Lactobacillales* ($p = 0.001$) at Order, *Carnobacteriaceae* ($p = 0.002$) at Family and *Granullicatella* ($p = 0.007$) at Genus. Moreover, one leukemia-depleted lineage was found, consisting of *Fusobacteria* ($p = 0.003$) at Phylum, *Fusobacteria* ($p = 0.001$) at Class, *Fusobacteriales* ($p = 0.001$) at Order

Table 3. Demographic and oral health information of acute lymphoblastic leukemia and healthy subjects.

Variables	Characteristics	ALL patients (n = 13)	Healthy control (n = 12)	p value
Age (years)	Mean ± SD	6.69±3.82	7.00±3.05	0.806[a]
Dentition stage	Primary	6	5	0.975[b]
	Mixed	5	5	
	Permanent	2	2	
Sex	Male	8	8	1.000[c]
	Female	5	4	
Caries status	dmfs/DMFS	3.46±3.26	3.00±3.36	0.600[a]
Periodontal condition	Healthy	7	10	0.202[c]
	Gingivitis	6	2	
	Periodontitis	0	0	
Plaque index	Silness-Löe Index	1.41±0.41	1.48±0.70	0.743[a]
Plaque pH	Mean ± SD	5.75±0.28	5.85±0.23	0.350[a]

ALL patients: acute lymphoblastic leukemia patients. dmfs/DMFS: decayed-missing-filled surfaces index in primary and permanent teeth, respectively.
[a]Independent sample nonparametric Mann-Whitney U test was used.
[b]Pearson Chi-Square test was used.
[c]Fisher's Exact test was used.

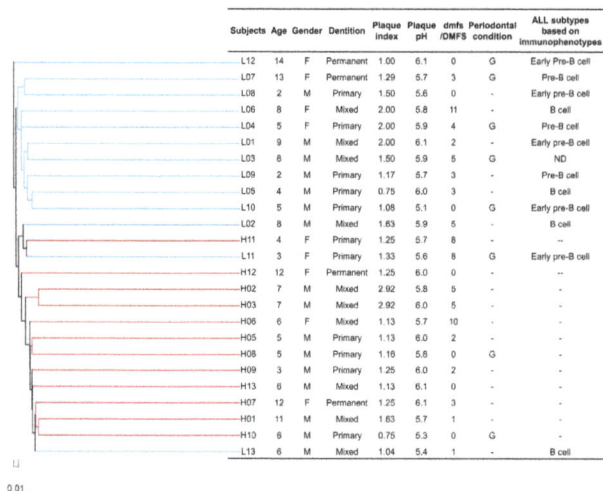

Subjects	Age	Gender	Dentition	Plaque index	Plaque pH	dmfs /DMFS	Periodontal condition	ALL subtypes based on immunophenotypes
L12	14	F	Permanent	1.00	6.1	0	G	Early Pre-B cell
L07	13	F	Permanent	1.29	5.7	3	G	Pre-B cell
L08	2	M	Primary	1.50	5.6	0	-	Early pre-B cell
L06	8	F	Mixed	2.00	5.8	11	-	B cell
L04	5	F	Primary	2.00	5.9	4	G	Pre-B cell
L01	9	M	Mixed	2.00	6.1	2	-	Early pre-B cell
L03	8	M	Mixed	1.50	5.9	5	G	ND
L09	3	M	Primary	1.17	5.7	3	-	Pre-B cell
L05	4	M	Primary	0.75	6.0	3	-	B cell
L10	5	M	Primary	1.08	5.1	0	G	Early pre-B cell
L02	8	M	Mixed	1.63	5.9	5	-	B cell
H11	4	F	Primary	1.25	5.7	8	-	--
L11	3	F	Primary	1.33	5.6	8	G	Early pre-B cell
H12	12	F	Permanent	1.25	6.0	0	-	--
H02	7	M	Mixed	2.92	5.8	5	-	-
H03	7	M	Mixed	2.92	6.0	5	-	-
H06	6	F	Mixed	1.13	5.7	10	-	-
H05	5	M	Primary	1.13	6.0	2	-	-
H08	5	M	Primary	1.16	5.8	0	G	-
H09	3	M	Primary	1.25	6.0	2	-	-
H13	6	M	Mixed	1.13	6.1	0	-	-
H07	12	F	Permanent	1.25	6.1	3	-	-
H01	11	M	Mixed	1.63	5.7	1	-	-
H10	6	M	Primary	0.75	5.3	0	G	-
L13	6	M	Mixed	1.04	5.4	1	-	B cell

0.01

Figure 1. Dendrogram of OTU composition obtained from acute lymphoblastic leukemia-affected children and healthy controls. The dendrogram (left section) indicates the similarity of the microbial communities of supragingival dental plaque between subjects according to their OTU composition, as determined using the Jaccard index (MOTHUR). A summary of patients' clinical information is presented in the right section. H, healthy children. L, acute lymphoblastic leukemia-affected children. dmfs/DMFS, decayed-missing-filled surfaces index in primary and permanent teeth, respectively. G, gingivitis. ND, no data obtained.

and *Fusobacteriaceae* ($p = 0.002$) at Family, but not *Fusobacterium* ($p = 0.009$; q>0.5) at Genus.

Discussion

This study compared the oral microbial composition of acute lymphoblastic leukemia (ALL) and healthy hosts, contributing to a better understanding of the oral microbial profiles in immuno-compromised patients. While there have been several reports investigating oral microbiota in leukemia patients [10,11,12,13,33], most of these studies relied on traditional culturing methods and were focused on only a few kinds of common bacteria, failing to characterize the overall pattern of oral microbiota in leukemia patients. In addition, most of these cross-sectional investigations were focused on the effect of antineoplastic treatment on oral microbiota, and limited information can be obtained regarding the oral microbiota under ALL-associated immunocompromised conditions. These limitations have severely confounded efforts to pinpoint leukemia-associated oral microbiota in patients.

Since gingivitis/periodontitis are common oral pathologies experienced by leukemia patients [4,6], it is critical to distinguish whether a detected microbial change is driven by the global immune status or by the unavoidable existing periodontal pathology. We believe that compared to subgingival and salivary microbiota, which alter under periodontal pathologies [34,35], the supragingival microbiota is less affected by gingivitis/periodontitis, but more by the host immune status given that the caries status is normalized. Therefore, in the present study, we sampled pooled supragingival plaque in carefully controlled ALL and healthy populations, and analyzed its microbial composition via 16S-based 454 pyrosequencing. Oral health conditions, except for periodontal conditions, were well balanced between the ALL patients and healthy groups, further validating the use of supragingival plaque

as a representative microbiota to delineate the influence of the immune status on oral microbiome.

The holistic pattern of leukemia pediatric patients was presented and compared with that of healthy controls, revealing key characteristics of oral microbiota associated with childhood ALL. ALL patients had lower richness and less diversity of oral microbiota compared with healthy subjects. Similar results were reported by Sixou et al, in which the microbial composition of supragingival plaque from the leukemia patients, analyzed by traditional culture methods, were found to be less complex than that of healthy controls [10]. However, Cargill et al. found that the complexity of oral microbiota was not statistically different between leukemia patients and healthy controls until initiation of antineoplastic treatment [33]. This inconsistency might be attributed to techniques used to profile the oral microbiota. Previous studies, mainly using culture methods, based their results on a few selected cultivable bacteria, neglecting characteristics of other bacteria in oral cavity of leukemia patients. At the time of sampling, oral bacteria might have already undergone selection after the disease manifested, with some bacteria inhibited and others thriving, resulting in divergent conclusions from different studies which focused on a few types of bacteria. By using 454 pyrosequencing, a holistic pattern of oral microbiome was presented and bacteria with low abundance and under the detection limit of culture methods could be investigated [36]. A decrease in intestinal microbial diversity was found in pediatric patients with acute myeloid leukemia [37]. The decrease of richness and diversity observed in the current study points to dysbiosis of oral microbiota in ALL patients. In addition to richness and diversity, we report altered structure and composition of oral microbiota in ALL patients. Altered structure and composition of oral microbiota in ALL patients were related to health status of investigated subjects. This was revealed in the separation pattern of samples based on cluster analyses, which were consistent with the presence/absence of leukemia. Since age, dentition stage, plaque pH, plaque index and caries status (dmfs/DMFS) were comparable between ALL patients and healthy children, microbial differences observed in supragingival plaque are likely directly caused by leukemia itself.

It is well-known that the host and microbiota have a dynamic interaction, which is closely associated with health [38]. The host immune system is believed to play an important role in shaping human microbiota [39]. A study on the bacterial and fungal microbiota of the stomach fluid indicated that immune status plays a major role in shaping the gastric fluid microbiota in terms of both diversity and composition [40]. Important effectors of innate immunity, α-defensins that are a kind of secreted antibacterial protein produced by epithelial cells, can affect the composition of intestinal microbial communities [41,42]. Immune-driven dysbiosis in the intestine has been found in mice deficient for the transcription factor T-bet, which is associated with both the innate and the adaptive immune system [2]. Here we showed the importance of the immune system in shaping the oral microbial structure. This is not surprising, because like the small and large intestine, the lamina propria of oral mucosa typically has organized and diffuse lymphoid tissues [43]. In ALL patients, the disorder of lymphoid progenitor cells, the major part of the body's immune system, can lead to impairment of the host immunity [14,15]. The malignant proliferation of lymphocytes in bone marrow infiltrates into the peripheral lymphoid tissues including the lymphoid tissue of oral mucosa, leading to impairment of oral immunity [7,44]. Furthermore, the salivary defense system which contains various antimicrobial components such as secreted immunoglobulin A (SIgA), α-amylase and

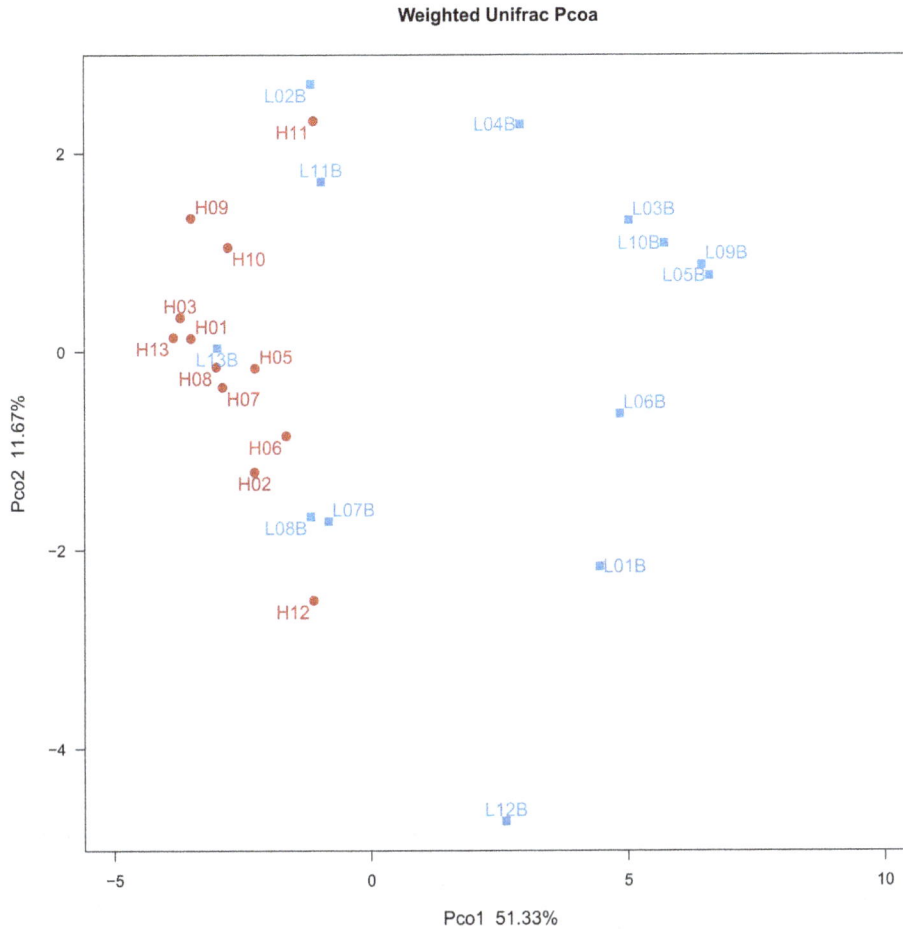

Figure 2. Weighted Unifrac PCoA analysis. The first two principal coordinates (PCo1 and PCo2) from the principal coordinate analysis of weighted UniFrac are plotted for each sample. The variance explained by the PCos is indicated in parentheses on the axes. H, healthy children. L, acute lymphoblastic leukemia-affected children.

lysozyme, has been reported to be significantly impaired in leukemia [45]. However, the exact mechanisms involved in the interaction between the oral immune system and microbiota need further research.

Our investigations of oral microbiota in ALL patients also provided the opportunity for identifying potential microbiota associated with systemic infections in leukemia patients. The present data suggest two taxonomical lineages (*Firmicutes/Bacilli/Lactobacillales/Carnobacteriaceae/Granulicatella*, and *Firmicutes/Bacilli/Lactobacillales/Aerococcaceae/Abiotrophia*) that are much more abundant in the supragingival plaque of ALL patients than healthy controls from the phylum down to the genus level; this indicates that favorable conditions existed for their development in the oral cavity of ALL patients. This could be responsible for an increased risk of bacteremia in leukemia patients. *Granulicatella* and *Abiotrophia*, formerly known as nutritionally variant streptococcus (NVS), have been commonly implicated in endocarditis and bacteraemia, and also in several other infections such as central nervous system infections, otitis media, cholangitis and arthritis [46,47]. A high mortality rate for endocarditis by NVS has been reported [48,49]. Previous studies found that oral bacteria are responsible for 25% to 50% of systemic infections in neutropenic patients [50]. An increase in abundance of opportunistic pathogens might be an important factor to the increased risk of systemic infections in leukemia patients. Altered health status in

ALL patients predisposes the host to developing oral infection by favoring pathogenic bacteria thriving in the oral niche. Prevention of oral microbiota dysbiosis might be a promising measure for decreasing mortality in patients with ALL. It should be noted that the 16S rRNA gene assay has its own limitation, i.e. the detection of 16S rRNA sequences does not imply that live bacteria are present. Therefore, either combination of 16S rRNA gene assay with traditional culture-based approach, or further cohort studies are needed to elucidate the exact relationship between oral microbial disequilibrium and risk of systemic infection in ALL-affected patient.

Conclusion

In summary, by comparing the oral microbial composition of ALL patients and healthy subjects, we have identified a structural imbalance of the oral microbiota, characterized by reduced diversity of microbiota and abundance alterations of certain bacteria, possibly involved in systemic infections, indicating the important role immune status plays in shaping the structure of oral microbiota. Although more works still need to be done, the dysbiosis of oral microbiota identified in this study provides insight into the host-microbe interactions related to the infectious complications of this susceptible population.

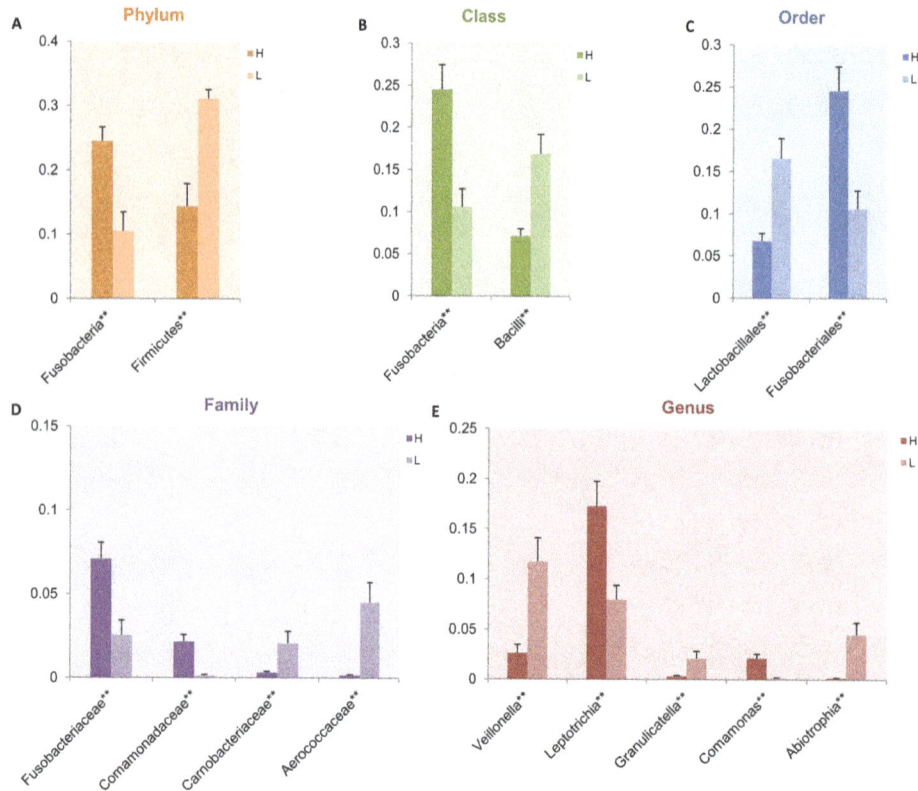

Figure 3. Differential relative abundance of bacterial taxonomy profiles of acute lymphoblastic leukemia and healthy subjects based on Metastats analysis. Comparisons were performed at each of the taxonomical levels of Phylum (A), Class (B), Order (C), Family (D) and Genus (E). Means of the relative abundance for each taxon at each taxonomical level between the healthy and acute lymphoblastic leukemia host-populations are compared, with a p value threshold set at 0.05 (*$p<0.05$; **$p<0.01$) and a q value threshold at 0.5. The discriminating taxa ($p<0.05$ and $q<0.5$) with relative abundance >1% for at least one group at each level are shown. H, healthy children. L, acute lymphoblastic leukemia-affected children.

Supporting Information

Figure S1 Heatmap analysis of the orders detected among all subjects based on microbiota composition and abundance. The colour of each column represents relative abundance of the corresponding order according to the scale at the bottom of the plot. Subject metadata are shown using checkerboard plots based on the following color codes: ALL subjects (black) or healthy children (white); <6 years old (white), 6–12 years (gray) or older than 12 years (black); male (black) or female (white); primary (white), mixed (gray) or permanent (black) dentition; plaque index: <1.00 (white), 1.00–2.00 (gray) or >2.00 (black); plaque pH: <5.4 (white), 5.4–5.7 (gray) or >5.7 (black); dmfs/DMFS: 0–3 (white), 4–7 (gray) or 8–11 (black); gingivitis presence (gray) or absence (white). See figure 1 and table S1 for additional details. H, healthy children. L, acute lymphoblastic leukemia affected children.

Figure S2 Relative abundance of oral microbiota compositions at the phylum level. Comparison of all samples from ALL patients and healthy subjects showed major phyla comprised of *Proteobacteria*, *Firmicutes*, *Fusobacteria*, *Actinobacteria*, *Bacterioidetes* and candidate division TM7. H, healthy children, L, acute lymphoblastic leukemia-affected children.

Table S1 Overview of subject clinical information.

Table S2 The number of OTUs and species richness and diversity estimates in each supragingival plaque microbiome.

Table S3 Differential relative abundance of bacterial taxonomy profiles of acute lymphoblastic leukemia (ALL) patients and healthy (H) subjects based on Metastats analysis.

Acknowledgments

The authors wish to thank Shanghai Majorbio Bio-Pharm Technology Co.,Ltd for the assistance in data analysis.

Author Contributions

Conceived and designed the experiments: XX XDZ JZ LC MYL YQL YPZ JYL WYS. Performed the experiments: YW JX QD XY JZH. Analyzed the data: YW JX MY XX. Contributed reagents/materials/analysis tools: YW JX MY. Wrote the paper: YW XX JX XDZ MY. Agree with manuscript results and conclusions: YW JX XDZ MY QD XY JZH JZ LC MYL YQL YPZ JYL WYS XX.

References

1. Pui CH, Robison LL, Look AT (2008) Acute lymphoblastic leukaemia. Lancet 371: 1030–1043.
2. Garrett WS, Lord GM, Punit S, Lugo-Villarino G, Mazmanian SK, et al. (2007) Communicable ulcerative colitis induced by T-bet deficiency in the innate immune system. Cell 131: 33–45.
3. Barrett AP (1986) Leukemic cell infiltration of the gingivae. J Periodontol 57: 579–581.
4. Hou GL, Huang JS, Tsai CC (1997) Analysis of oral manifestations of leukemia: a retrospective study. Oral Dis 3: 31–38.
5. Meyer U, Kleinheinz J, Handschel J, Kruse-Losler B, Weingart D, et al. (2000) Oral findings in three different groups of immunocompromised patients. J Oral Pathol Med 29: 153–158.
6. Javed F, Utreja A, Bello Correa FO, Al-Askar M, Hudieb M, et al. (2012) Oral health status in children with acute lymphoblastic leukemia. Crit Rev Oncol Hematol 83: 303–309.
7. Paunica SC, Dumitriu A, Mogos M, Georgescu O, Mogos I (2009) The evaluation of the periodontium in patients with leukemia using thermographic imaging. Hematology 14: 341–346.
8. Khan SA, Wingard JR (2001) Infection and mucosal injury in cancer treatment. JNCI Monographs 2001: 31–36.
9. Greenberg MS, Cohen SG, McKitrick JC, Cassileth PA (1982) The oral flora as a source of septicemia in patients with acute leukemia. Oral Surg Oral Med Oral Pathol 53: 32–36.
10. Sixou JL, De Medeiros-Batista O, Gandemer V, Bonnaure-Mallet M (1998) The effect of chemotherapy on the supragingival plaque of pediatric cancer patients. Oral Oncol 34: 476–483.
11. Wahlin YB, Granstrom S, Persson S, Sjostrom M (1991) Multivariate study of enterobacteria and Pseudomonas in saliva of patients with acute leukemia. Oral Surg Oral Med Oral Pathol 72: 300–308.
12. O'Sullivan EA, Duggal MS, Bailey CC, Curzon ME, Hart P (1993) Changes in the oral microflora during cytotoxic chemotherapy in children being treated for acute leukemia. Oral Surg Oral Med Oral Pathol 76: 161–168.
13. Galili D, Donitza A, Garfunkel A, Sela MN (1992) Gram-negative enteric bacteria in the oral cavity of leukemia patients. Oral Surg Oral Med Oral Pathol 74: 459–462.
14. Kitchingman GR, Rovigatti U, Mauer AM, Melvin S, Murphy SB, et al. (1985) Rearrangement of immunoglobulin heavy chain genes in T cell acute lymphoblastic leukemia. Blood 65: 725–729.
15. Zhang XL, Komada Y, Chipeta J, Li QS, Inaba H, et al. (2000) Intracellular cytokine profile of T cells from children with acute lymphoblastic leukemia. Cancer Immunol Immunother 49: 165–172.
16. Li K, Bihan M, Methe BA (2013) Analyses of the stability and core taxonomic memberships of the human microbiome. PLoS One 8: e63139.
17. Zaura E, Keijser BJ, Huse SM, Crielaard W (2009) Defining the healthy "core microbiome" of oral microbial communities. BMC Microbiol 9: 259.
18. Lazarevic V, Whiteson K, Hernandez D, Francois P, Schrenzel J (2010) Study of inter- and intra-individual variations in the salivary microbiota. BMC Genomics 11: 523.
19. Ling Z, Kong J, Jia P, Wei C, Wang Y, et al. (2010) Analysis of oral microbiota in children with dental caries by PCR-DGGE and barcoded pyrosequencing. Microb Ecol 60: 677–690.
20. Yang F, Zeng X, Ning K, Liu KL, Lo CC, et al. (2012) Saliva microbiomes distinguish caries-active from healthy human populations. ISME J 6: 1–10.
21. Saber MH, Schwarzberg K, Alonaizan FA, Kelley ST, Sedghizadeh PP, et al. (2012) Bacterial flora of dental periradicular lesions analyzed by the 454-pyrosequencing technology. J Endod 38: 1484–1488.
22. Koren O, Spor A, Felin J, Fak F, Stombaugh J, et al. (2011) Human oral, gut, and plaque microbiota in patients with atherosclerosis. Proc Natl Acad Sci U S A 108 Suppl 1: 4592–4598.
23. Hu YJ, Shao ZY, Wang Q, Jiang YT, Ma R, et al. (2013) Exploring the dynamic core microbiome of plaque microbiota during head-and-neck radiotherapy using pyrosequencing. PLoS One 8: e56343.
24. Hu YJ, Wang Q, Jiang YT, Ma R, Xia WW, et al. (2013) Characterization of oral bacterial diversity of irradiated patients by high-throughput sequencing. Int J Oral Sci 5: 21–25.
25. Hague A, Baechle M (2008) Advanced caries in a patient with a history of bariatric surgery. J Dent Hyg 82: 22.
26. Margulies M, Egholm M, Altman WE, Attiya S, Bader JS, et al. (2005) Genome sequencing in microfabricated high-density picolitre reactors. Nature 437: 376–380.
27. Wang Q, Garrity GM, Tiedje JM, Cole JR (2007) Naive Bayesian classifier for rapid assignment of rRNA sequences into the new bacterial taxonomy. Appl Environ Microbiol 73: 5261–5267.
28. Lozupone C, Knight R (2005) UniFrac: a new phylogenetic method for comparing microbial communities. Appl Environ Microbiol 71: 8228–8235.
29. Lozupone C, Hamady M, Knight R (2006) UniFrac–an online tool for comparing microbial community diversity in a phylogenetic context. BMC bioinformatics 7: 371.
30. Schloss PD, Handelsman J (2006) Introducing TreeClimber, a test to compare microbial community structures. Appl Environ Microbiol 72: 2379–2384.
31. White JR, Nagarajan N, Pop M (2009) Statistical methods for detecting differentially abundant features in clinical metagenomic samples. PLoS Comput Biol 5: e1000352.
32. Krych L, Hansen CH, Hansen AK, van den Berg FW, Nielsen DS (2013) Quantitatively different, yet qualitatively alike: a meta-analysis of the mouse core gut microbiome with a view towards the human gut microbiome. PLoS One 8: e62578.
33. Lucas VS, Beighton D, Roberts GJ, Challacombe SJ (1997) Changes in the oral streptococcal flora of children undergoing allogeneic bone marrow transplantation. J Infect 35: 135–141.
34. Belstrøm D, Fiehn NE, Nielsen CH, Kirkby N, Twetman S, et al. (2014) Differences in bacterial saliva profile between periodontitis patients and a control cohort. J Clin Periodontol 41: 104–112.
35. Colombo APV, Boches SK, Cotton SL, Goodson JM, Kent R, et al. (2009) Comparisons of subgingival microbial profiles of refractory periodontitis, severe periodontitis, and periodontal health using the human oral microbe identification microarray. J Periodontol 80: 1421–1432.
36. Mardis ER (2008) Next-generation DNA sequencing methods. Annu Rev Genomics Hum Genet 9: 387–402.
37. van Vliet MJ, Tissing WJ, Dun CA, Meessen NE, Kamps WA, et al. (2009) Chemotherapy treatment in pediatric patients with acute myeloid leukemia receiving antimicrobial prophylaxis leads to a relative increase of colonization with potentially pathogenic bacteria in the gut. Clin Infect Dis 49: 262–270.
38. Dethlefsen L, McFall-Ngai M, Relman DA (2007) An ecological and evolutionary perspective on human–microbe mutualism and disease. Nature 449: 811–818.
39. Hooper LV, Littman DR, Macpherson AJ (2012) Interactions between the microbiota and the immune system. Science 336: 1268–1273.
40. von Rosenvinge EC, Song Y, White JR, Maddox C, Blanchard T, et al. (2013) Immune status, antibiotic medication and pH are associated with changes in the stomach fluid microbiota. ISME J 7: 1354–1366.
41. Salzman NH, Ghosh D, Huttner KM, Paterson Y, Bevins CL (2003) Protection against enteric salmonellosis in transgenic mice expressing a human intestinal defensin. Nature 422: 522–526.
42. Salzman NH, Hung K, Haribhai D, Chu H, Karlsson-Sjoberg J, et al. (2010) Enteric defensins are essential regulators of intestinal microbial ecology. Nat Immunol 11: 76–83.
43. Tlaskalová-Hogenová H, Štěpánková R, Hudcovic T, Tučková L, Cukrowska B, et al. (2004) Commensal bacteria (normal microflora), mucosal immunity and chronic inflammatory and autoimmune diseases. Immunol Lett 93: 97–108.
44. Tjwa E, Mattijssen V (2008) Images in clinical medicine. Gingival hypertrophy and leukemia. N Engl J Med 359: e21.
45. Hegde AM, Joshi S, Rai K, Shetty S (2011) Evaluation of oral hygiene status, salivary characteristics and dental caries experience in acute lymphoblastic leukemic (ALL) children. J Clin Pediatr Dent 35: 319–323.
46. Phulpin-Weibel A, Gaspar N, Emirian A, Chachaty E, Valteau-Couanet D, et al. (2013) Intravascular catheter-related bloodstream infection caused by Abiotrophia defectiva in a neutropenic child. J Med Microbiol 62: 789–791.
47. Senn L, Entenza JM, Greub G, Jaton K, Wenger A, et al. (2006) Bloodstream and endovascular infections due to Abiotrophia defectiva and Granulicatella species. BMC Infect Dis 6: 9.
48. Cargill JS, Scott KS, Gascoyne-Binzi D, Sandoe JA (2012) Granulicatella infection: diagnosis and management. J Med Microbiol 61: 755–761.
49. Liao CH, Teng LJ, Hsueh PR, Chen YC, Huang LM, et al. (2004) Nutritionally variant streptococcal infections at a University Hospital in Taiwan: disease emergence and high prevalence of beta-lactam and macrolide resistance. Clin Infect Dis 38: 452–455.
50. Khan SA, Wingard JR (2001) Infection and mucosal injury in cancer treatment. J Natl Cancer Inst Monogr: 31–36.

9

Reducing Deaths from Severe Pneumonia in Children in Malawi by Improving Delivery of Pneumonia Case Management

Penelope M. Enarson[1,2]*, Robert P. Gie[3], Charles C. Mwansambo[4], Ellubey R. Maganga[5], Carl J. Lombard[6], Donald A. Enarson[1,2], Stephen M. Graham[1,7]

1 Child Lung Health Division, International Union Against Tuberculosis and Lung Disease, Paris, France, 2 Desmond Tutu TB Centre, Department of Paediatrics and Child Health, Faculty of Medicine and Health Sciences, Stellenbosch University, Tygerberg, South Africa, 3 Department of Paediatrics and Child Health, Faculty of Medicine and Health Sciences, University of Stellenbosch, Tygerberg, South Africa, 4 Ministry of Health, Lilongwe, Malawi, 5 UNICEF Malawi, Lilongwe, Malawi, 6 Biostatistics Unit, South Africa Medical Research Council (MRC), Cape Town, South Africa, 7 Centre for International Child Health, University of Melbourne Department of Paediatrics and Murdoch Children's Research Institute, Royal Children's Hospital, Melbourne, Australia

Abstract

Objective: To evaluate the pneumonia specific case fatality rate over time following the implementation of a Child Lung Health Programme (CLHP) within the existing government health services in Malawi to improve delivery of pneumonia case management.

Methods: A prospective, nationwide public health intervention was studied to evaluate the impact on pneumonia specific case fatality rate (CFR) in infants and young children (0 to 59 months of age) following the implementation of the CLHP. The implementation was step-wise from October 1st 2000 until 31st December 2005 within paediatric inpatient wards in 24 of 25 district hospitals in Malawi. Data analysis compared recorded outcomes in the first three months of the intervention (the control period) to the period after that, looking at trend over time and variation by calendar month, age group, severity of disease and region of the country. The analysis was repeated standardizing the follow-up period by using only the first 15 months after implementation at each district hospital.

Findings: Following implementation, 47,228 children were admitted to hospital for severe/very severe pneumonia with an overall CFR of 9•8%. In both analyses, the highest CFR was in the children 2 to 11 months, and those with very severe pneumonia. The majority (64%) of cases, 2–59 months, had severe pneumonia. In this group there was a significant effect of the intervention Odds Ratio (OR) 0•70 (95%CI: 0•50–0•98); p = 0•036), while in the same age group children treated for very severe pneumonia there was no interventional benefit (OR 0•97 (95%CI: 0•72–1•30); p = 0•8). No benefit was observed for neonates (OR 0•83 (95%CI: 0•56–1•22); p = 0•335).

Conclusions: The nationwide implementation of the CLHP significantly reduced CFR in Malawian infants and children (2–59 months) treated for severe pneumonia. Reasons for the lack of benefit for neonates, infants and children with very severe pneumonia requires further research.

Editor: Rashida A. Ferrand, London School of Hygiene and Tropical Medicine, United Kingdom

Funding: The CLHP was primarly funded by the MoH of Malawi, who contributed 69% of the running costs comprising facilities and human resources that are part of the existing health system. The Bill and Melinda Gates Foundation funded the remaining 31% of the costs, 21% of which was investment and 79% operating costs. The Bill & Melinda Gates Foundation grant ID#: 413 http://www.gatesfoundation.org/Pages/home.aspx). The external funders had no role in study design, data collection and analysis, decision to publish, or preparation of the manuscript.

Competing Interests: The authors have declared that no competing interests exist.

* Email: penarson@theunion.org

Introduction

Pneumonia is the most frequent cause of death in children less than five years of age [1]. In sub-Saharan Africa, child pneumonia deaths account for an estimated 18% of under-five mortality of which three per cent occur in the neonatal period [1]. The incidence of pneumonia and the case-fatality rate are highest among infants and decline with increasing age [2].

In 1984, the World Health Organization (WHO) introduced standardized case-management (SCM) of pneumonia [3] that became an important part of integrated child health programmes and WHO recommended approaches in clinical care [4]. Pneumonia-related deaths declined following the introduction of community-based SCM [5]. Hospitalized cases represent the more severe spectrum of disease and are more likely to die. The effectiveness of hospital-based SCM on pneumonia-related mortality has not been reported and there are no studies of the effectiveness of nation-wide, hospital-based programmes within existing health services.

The International Union Against Tuberculosis and Lung Disease (The Union) developed the Child Lung Health Programme (CLHP) for SCM of pneumonia in hospitalized children based on its model for tuberculosis services. The Union model for tuberculosis was adopted by the WHO in 1993 as the basis of its global strategy for control of tuberculosis (the DOTS strategy) [6] which the World Bank assessed as among the most cost-effective health interventions in low-income countries [7]. The model includes accurate accounting for services, materials, and training and permits management of supplies to ensure no disruption of essential therapies. The Ministry of Health (MoH), Government of Malawi, requested assistance from The Union to improve the management and outcome of pneumonia in Malawian children. The Union assisted the Ministry of Health to adapt and implement the CLHP within the country's existing health services to ensure sustainability. The model and its implementation have been previously described [8].

The aim of this study was to assess the benefits of this strategy by measuring the trend over time in the case fatality rate (CFR) in neonates, infants and young children (one week to 59 months of age) hospitalized with severe or very severe pneumonia.

Methods

Ethics Statement

The CLHP was routine patient management and data from it was routinely collected. The data used for the study was aggregated data from Monthly Recording Forms - no individual identification appeared on these reports. Permission to use the data was received from the Ministry of Health, Republic of Malawi. Approval to analyze the data was obtained from the Union's Ethical Advisory Group (EAG: 05/10) and the Human Research Ethics Committee (N10/09/285), Faculty of Medicine and Health Sciences, Stellenbosch University.

Intervention Setting

The public health service delivery system in 2000 was district-based with 22 out of 24 districts having one government hospital with satellite health centres. The Government District Health Officer (DHO) was charged with the oversight of services in all government facilities, and co-ordination and supervision of all health providers and programmes in the district. There were three central hospitals (at Blantyre, Lilongwe and Zomba) which were tertiary referral hospitals, but which also acted as district hospitals for their 'host' District.

The DHO reported directly to the central level since the introduction of health sector reform measures removed regional level management in all but the tuberculosis and EPI Programmes. The district health team had a managerial and co-ordinating role, and provided technical support and supervision.

The Ministry of Health (MOH) was entirely financed by the government and external donors. The latter provided most of the development expenditure and financed a large percentage of the recurrent costs of preventive and promotive services [9]. Free medical care in government-run facilities was the policy throughout the country.

Many districts also had a private system, the Christian Health Association of Malawi (CHAM) Hospital within their boundaries. CHAM facilities were independent, owned and run by their respective churches. However, the MOH provided CHAM facilities with staff salaries and subsidised hospitalisation costs (0.75 Malawian Kwacha per day). These facilities were also allowed to operate cost recovery from patients who could afford it.

In 2000 Malawi was the 9th poorest country with a Gross National Product per capita of US$ 170 leading to chronic underfunding of health care services - total public expenditure was 9.0% [9] and only increased to 9.3% by 2005 [10]. This resulted in an on-going chronic shortage of basic health services mainly due to shortage of trained personnel, lack of skills among health professionals to manage severe and very severe pneumonia and lack of essential drugs (especially antibiotics) and supplies (such as oxygen) throughout the country [11].

The main clinical staff was paramedical Clinical Officers and Medical Assistants, supported by State Registered Nurses, State Registered Enrolled Nurses and Midwives. There was an acute shortage of all health personnel with a 39.0% vacancy rate [11]. The MOH employee/ratio to population were as follows: Doctors 1:113,953, Registered Nurses 1:25,857 [11]. Each of the 22 district hospitals had on average a total of 32 health personnel to manage all services within the facility. The distribution was as follows: Medical doctor 1 or none, Clinical Officers 5, Medical Assistants 4 (only worked in the outpatient department), Registered Nurses 5 and Enrolled Nurses/Midwives 17 [11]. The attrition rate of health workers due to death from HIV/AIDS at this time was as high as 41% and also a major cause of absenteeism [12].

In Malawi the ratios of doctors and nurses to population remained lower than those of its neighbouring Sub-Saharan African countries. A comparison of information available from 2004 showed lower ratios for Malawi compared with Tanzania and Zambia/ [13]: for doctors, 1.1 compared with 3.0 and 6.9; for nurses, 25.5 compared with 36.6 and 113. The WHO Standard Doctor/Population Ratio is 10:100,000.

The intervention was carried out in the public health system in Malawi as described above. The CLHP was introduced into 24 of 25 district hospitals in Malawi. Two of these also functioned as a regional referral hospital located in a predominantly urban population while another urban-based regional referral hospital (Malawi's largest hospital based in Blantyre and also the College of Medicine's major teaching hospital) did not participate as it was better staffed and resourced. These were all non-fee paying services. Children with severe or very severe pneumonia may present at any health facility in a district but for inpatient care are referred to the dedicated paediatric wards at the district hospital according to national standards of care.

Situational analysis

A situational analysis prior to the intervention in 2000, found that acute respiratory infection (ARI) was the second leading cause of morbidity in Malawian children below 5 years [14]. Pneumonia or lower respiratory tract infection was the most common diagnosis in hospitalized Malawian children accounting for one-quarter of paediatric admissions. Case-fatality rate for pneumonia prior to the intervention varied between 10% and 26% [15]. Problems identified included inadequate training, insufficient supplies of antibiotics, lack of adequate oxygen therapy, and lack of information to assist in planning services and procurement of essential items [15].

Background child health indicators

In the years just prior to the intervention, Malawi reported a high under-5 mortality of 189 per 1,000 live births for the period 1996–2000.[8] Known risk factors for frequency and severity of child pneumonia such as low birth weight (20% of live births), malnutrition (48% of children with moderate or severe stunting) and HIV infection (91,000 children living with HIV in 2006) were all highly prevalent in Malawi at the time of the intervention [16]. Immunization coverage over the intervention period was reported as relatively high - >90% for BCG and DPT3, and >80% for measles (>80%) - and there were no outbreaks of measles reported. Haemophilus influenzae type b (Hib) conjugate vaccine was introduced in 2002 with high coverage (93%) reported for 2006 [16]. Pneumococcal conjugate vaccine (PCV) was not introduced until 2011 i.e. after the implementation of the CLHP was completed.

National antenatal HIV prevalence in 2001 was estimated to be 17.1% in people 15–24 years of age [17] of age with a prevalence of up to 30% in urban settings [18,19]. HIV prevalence among pregnant women at sentinel sites was 19.5%, 19.8% and 16.9% in 2001, 2003 and 2005. The rate of mother to child transmission in 2001 was 26.9% [20]. The estimated percentage of HIV+ pregnant women who received a full package of care to prevent mother-to-child transmission (MTCT) of HIV in 2004 was only 2.3%.

The majority of HIV-infected infants died before five years of age with pneumonia the most frequent cause of death [21]. The use of cotrimoxazole preventive therapy (CPT) for HIV-exposed infants and HIV-infected children, and the use of anti-retroviral therapy (ART) for HIV-infected children were not routinely available at the time of the intervention. Malawi received funding in 2004 from the Global Fund to Fight AIDS, Tuberculosis and Malaria to start to scale-up ART services but for children this was confined to the 3 government referral hospitals and 2 district hospitals supported by Doctors Without Borders [22].

Intervention Design

The intervention was implemented in a stepped wedge design (non-randomized). Planning commenced on the 1st March 2000 and the first five district hospitals were included on the 1st October 2000. Five to eight additional district hospitals were included annually in a step-wise fashion until all hospitals had been included by July 2003. Data collection ended on the 31st December 2005. The sequence of hospital recruitment was chosen by the Ministry of Health according to service needs, logistical and financial reasons (Figure 1 and 2). The data recorded during the intervention were subsequently collected and analyzed for the present study from July 2011 to December 2012.

A pragmatic evaluation design was planned and was used to analyze the data, beginning with the introduction of a standardized information system that was introduced to ensure that the data generated by the health system were of good quality. Data on pneumonia admissions and outcomes were collected prospectively as part of routine care.

It was planned to use data that was collected during a pre-intervention period as the control group. The patient information forms were introduced into districts on an average of 4 months prior to implementation of the programme. Twelve districts were included and a total of 624 forms (an average 52 forms per district) were collected for analysis. A total of 373 children were admitted with a diagnosis of severe or very severe pneumonia but, of these, 123 records did not include either a diagnosis or known outcome. The remaining 250 forms contained insufficient data to ascertain if a correct diagnosis had been made.

No other reliable pre-intervention data were available. Therefore, for study purposes, it was only possible to use data collected in the first three months following implementation of the CLHP as the 'control' period. These data were of similar quality as that collected during the rest of the study.

Intervention

The CLHP was based on the Union model [23] for delivering health services adapted to standard case management of the child with cough and difficult breathing [24]. The introduction of the CLHP included a substantial programme of work which included establishing an information system, quality assurance mechanisms, training, regular supervision and assurance of provision of antibiotics and oxygen to address all the various problems identified in Table 1.

The essential elements of the CLHP were:

- Political commitment by the Government of Malawi to implement SCM strategies countrywide into the existing secondary health care system. This commitment implied:

  o a structure for delivering the services

  o no discrimination against patients in the delivery of services to promote access.

  o sufficient financial resources for control of lung disease and other childhood illnesses

- Diagnoses and treatment based upon SCM (Table 2) with a system of quality control.
- Training of all paediatric clinical staff in SCM
- Logistics to purchase standardized drugs and to distribute them to ensure uninterrupted supplies at the management level of the District Health Office
- Recording and reporting clinical outcomes of severe and very severe pneumonia
- Supervision and evaluation of the services

Health care workers from the 24 district hospitals that provide inpatient/outpatient care for children were selected for training by each hospital administration as each of the hospitals were recruited for implementation. All paediatric clinical staff was trained as on average this meant only 3–5 nurses and one to two clinical staff per hospital. Therefor it was decided to increase this number to at least 10 and over the intervention period, a total of 312 health care workers (representing approximately 30% of all health care workers in district hospitals) to ensure more staff had received training. This included Clinical Officers (41%), State Registered Nurses (20%), Enrolled Nurses (30%), Medical Assistants (8%), other (1%). As described above there was a chronic shortage of staff and a high attrition rate in those previously trained at the recruited hospitals which meant that the new staff for these hospitals was included in the next training course. To also address this issue ongoing in-service training was provided by senior nurses and clinicians on the paediatric ward using training materials produced by the CLHP.

The training in diagnosis and treatment of children with pneumonia according to WHO SCM guidelines [24,25] comprised an initial five day course during which theoretical and practical training occurred with a one day follow-up training one month later. Training objectives related to skills in standard case management, knowledge of child lung disease and management and planning. These included:

- General assessment of the child or young infant
- Directed history/examination, assessment and classification of a child with cough or difficult breathing

  o assess clinical signs (e.g., respiratory rate, chest indrawing, wheeze)

  o identify any danger signs indicating urgent care is needed

  o assess clinical signs to determine whether pneumonia is present and if so, its severity

Control and intervention periods of 5 implementing groups

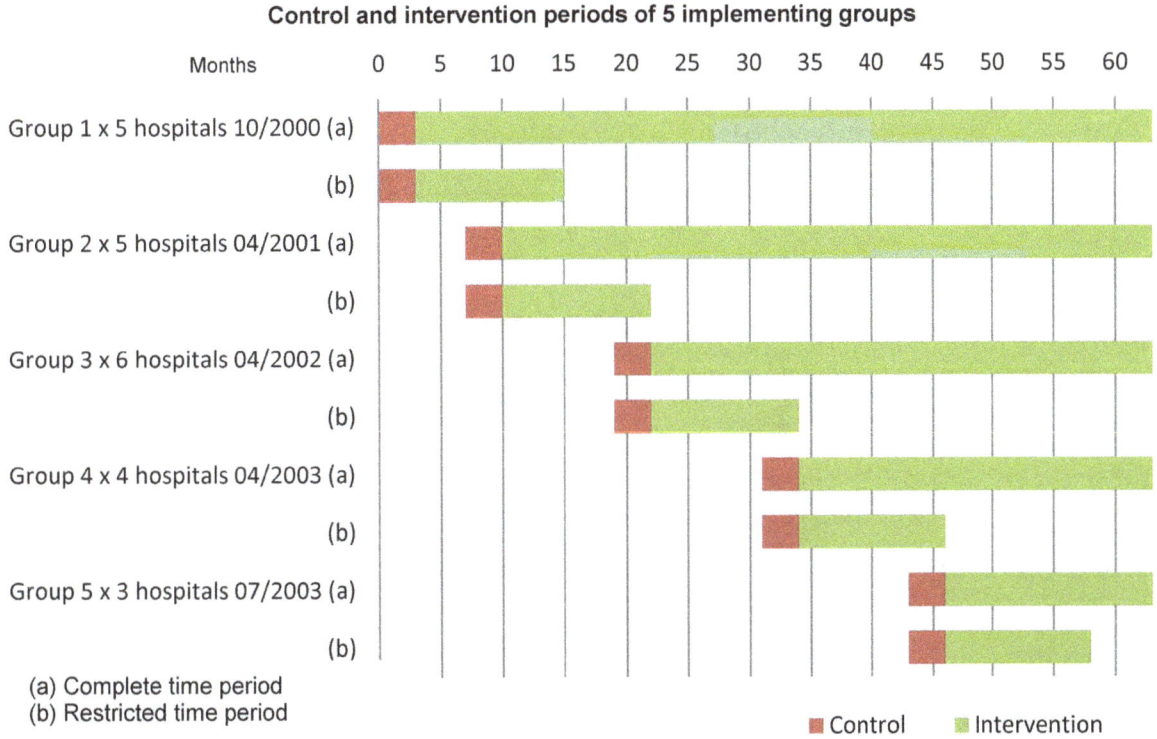

Figure 1. Control and intervention periods for 5 implementing groups for complete and restricted time periods.

Trend in numbers of children admitted to hospital with pneumonia in Malawi, 2000-2005, by group of intake and time since beginning of intervention.

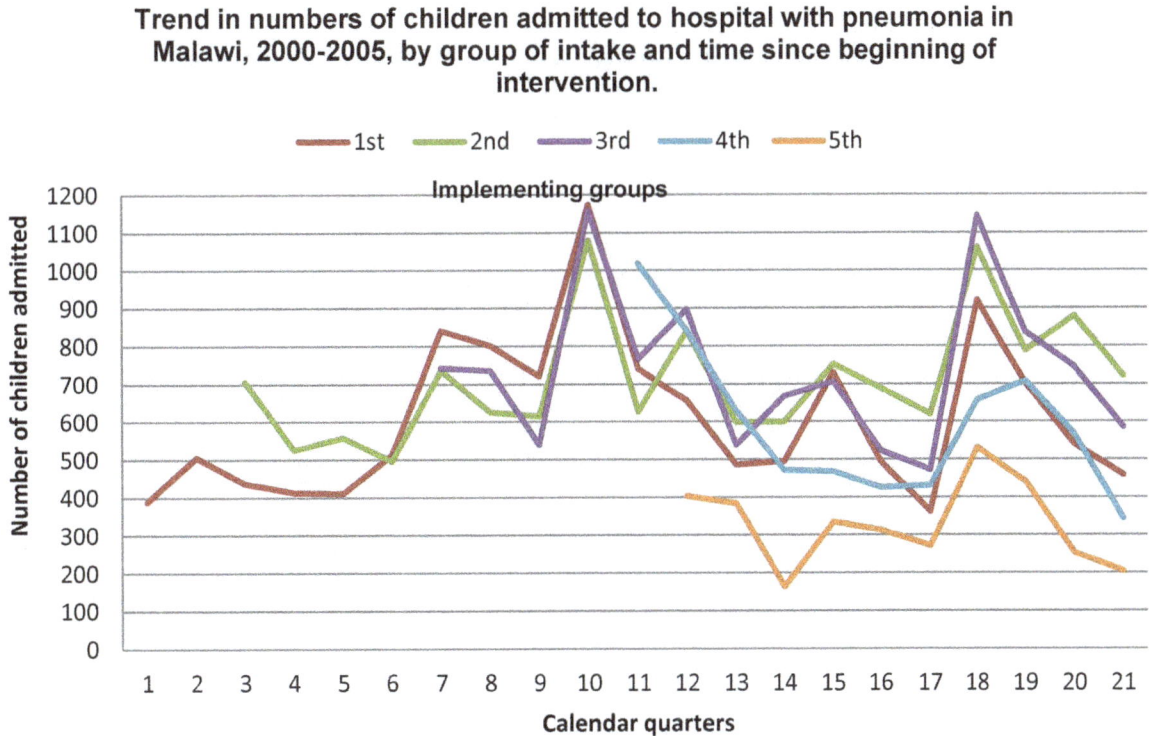

Figure 2. Trend in numbers of children admitted to hospital with pneumonia in Malawi, 2000–2005, by group of intake and time since beginning of intervention.

Table 1. Summary of the situational analysis carried out prior to the implementation of the child lung health programme (CLHP), intended interventions, output indicators and outputs achieved following the CLHP intervention.

Situation Analysis findings	intervention activity	Output indicator	achieved through intervention
No hospital was implementing standard case management guidelines	All children presenting with signs of pneumonia will be managed following the CLHP technical guidelines	Children diagnosed and treated correctly as per standard categories and treatment regimens	Technical guidelines adhered to in >90% of children presenting with respiratory symptoms
Less than 10% of health workers trained in SCM of pneumonia	Health care workers from all district hospitals trained in standard case management of pneumonia	Number of health workers trained in SCM	More than 300 health care workers trained (The target exceeded by 25%
Frequent interruption of supply of antibiotics required for SCM regimens	A material management system introduced at all levels calculated on number of cases. Antibiotic reserve stock supplied	Regular uninterrupted supply of antibiotics at central, regional and district levels	No stock outs of antibiotics experienced at all levels.
No regular supply of oxygen available on paediatric wards	One designated oxygen concentrator be provided for each paediatric ward implementing CLHP	All infants <2 months admitted with severe/very severe pneumonia, all children 2–59 months admitted with very severe pneumonia or a RR≥70 received oxygen therapy	All hospitals provided with an oxygen concentrator and personnel trained at central and district level in use and maintenance.
No regular reporting system in place	Each district hospital CLHP Coordinator to fill Monthly Reports on cases and treatment outcomes and submit to central level management unit	Monthly reports on Cases of Pneumonia and on Treatment Results	99.4% achievement as of December 2005 i.e. of 2274 reports expected 2260 were received
No regular standardized supervisory/support visits being carried out by Central Level Unit	Implementation of regular standardized supervisory/support visits to implementing hospitals by Central Level Unit	Regular standardized supervisory/ support visits to implementing hospitals carried out by Central Level Unit	Standardized supervision tool developed and implemented. Monthly visits carried out for 6 months then quarterly
No evaluation of ARI control activities regularly carried out	A report on external evaluation/ technical support visits to the CLHP sent to the MOH every 6 months	Evaluation reports	Eight external evaluation/technical support visits plus 1 independent external review visit to the CLHP carried out and a report on each visit sent to MOH.

o   identify other conditions and comorbidities (fever, anaemia, malnutrition, tuberculosis, malaria, asthma, HIV-related lung disease) that can be treated

o   Identify differential diagnosis

• Prescribe appropriate treatment
• Supportive care
• Monitor child's progress
• Counselling and discharge planning
• Complete Recording Form

In addition the District Hospital Programme Coordinator was taught how to complete monthly reports and maintain adequate supply of drugs and supplies.

The training was followed by regular supervision visits to the hospitals six weeks after the training, with monthly visits for the first six months then regular three-monthly visits. On initiation of the CLHP the amount of antibiotics required for each district hospital was calculated, including one-month consumption needs plus one-month buffer stock. One year buffer stock was held at the central medical store. During supervision visits stock was checked to prevent stock-outs of antibiotics during the intervention.

Oxygen was available in a minority of district hospitals prior to the initiation of the CLHP. The CLHP acquired and installed oxygen concentrators in each district hospital paediatric ward [26].

Patients and standard case-management

All children aged up to 59 months hospitalized with a clinical diagnosis of severe or very severe pneumonia were included. They were classified at the time of admission as severe or very severe pneumonia according to WHO recommendations. Neonates, less than two months of age, with severe and very severe pneumonia were combined in a single category. The CLHP was implemented within existing services, using treatment for pneumonia as recommended by the MoH protocols consistent with WHO guidelines [25]. Table 2 outlines the standard case management of children with pneumonia as recommended by the World Health Organization and used within the CLHP for training purposes and to guide patient care. These treatment protocols have since been updated in 2005 and 2013 [27].

Data Collection

Demographic and clinical information was transcribed to the Hospital Inpatient Pneumonia Register, aggregated monthly and sent to a data management centre where they were entered into an EXCEL spread-sheet. The aggregated data included the following variables used in the analysis: Number of cases by age groups - <2 months, 2–11 months and 12–59 months; number of males and females; number of cases by severity – non-severe, severe and very severe and number of cases by outcome (died). There was no individual patient clinical data recorded on the monthly reports. Errors were followed up and corrected. At each supervision visit, a random sample of recording forms was checked for accuracy and

Table 2. WHO standard case management of pneumonia defined by age groups and severity of disease.

Diagnosis	Standard Case Management	
	Presenting signs and symptoms	Recommended treatment regimens
Child 2–59 months		
Severe pneumonia	Respiratory rate: ≥50 aged 2–11 months	**Penicillin** 50 000 units/kg IM/IV Q6h for 3 days if
	≥40 aged 12–59 months	improved then oral **amoxicillin** 25 mg/kg three times
	Lower chest wall in-drawing	daily for total of 5 to 8 days
	Respiratory rate:	
	≥50 aged 2–11 months	
Very severe	≥40 aged 12–59 months	**Chloramphenicol** 25 mg/kg IM/IV 8 hourly for 5
pneumonia	Lower chest wall in-drawing	days if improved then three times daily for total
	Cyanosis	of 10 days antibiotic treatment
	Unable to drink	
	Reduced level of consciousness	Oxygen therapy
	Severe respiratory distress	
Infant <2 months		
	Respiratory rate: ≥60	**Gentamicin** 7.5 mg/kg once daily for 8 days
	Severe lower chest wall in-	**Penicillin** 50 000 units/kg Q6h IM/IV for three days if
Severe/Very severe	drawing	improved then oral **amoxicillin** 25 mg/kg three time
pneumonia	Unable to breast-feed	daily for a total of 8 days antibiotic treatment
	Grunting	
	Apneic spells	Oxygen therapy
Co-morbid conditions		
Pneumonia in severely malnourished child	Signs and symptoms for severe/very severe pneumonia as above PLUS signs and symptoms for any of the following	**Cotrimoxazole** prophylaxis on admission if not acutely ill
	Marasmus	Treatment for severe or very severe pneumonia as
	Kwashiorkor	above PLUS **Gentamicin** (7.5 mg/kg IM/IV) once daily for 7 days
	<60 Weight for Height	If the child fails to improve within 48 hours, add **Chloramphenicol** (25 mg/kg IM/IV 8-hourly) for 5 days
	2–6-month-old child with central	
	cyanosis	
	Hyper-expanded chest	**Continue first-line antibiotic** (such as
	Fast breathing	**Chloramphenicol**) as mixed infection with
Known/suspected	Chest X-ray changes, but chest	bacteria occurs
PcP	clear on auscultation	
	Enlarged liver, spleen, lymph	**Oral Cotrimoxazole**: 120 mg three times daily if less
	nodes	than 5 kg; 240 mg three times daily if 5 kg or more for
	HIV test positive in mother or	21 days
	child	

consistency. (See Text S1 for supplementary material for recording and reporting).

Statistical Analysis

Statistical analysis was that used for a cluster-randomized trial with a stepped wedge design. Five groups of hospitals were included with different starting points. The hospitals within each group started simultaneously so providing contemporaneous data. Monthly reports formed the units of analysis. The first three months after implementation in each cohort, was taken as the 'control' period for purposes of comparison, and each of the months following that, the intervention period. The analysis used two approaches: 1) analysis using the entire follow-up of 63 months (unrestricted) and 2) analysis of first 15 months follow-up (restricted) at each district hospital. The latter was used to limit the influence of the underlying trend in improvement of outcome occurring over time.

The primary outcome was the proportion of children who died while in hospital (case fatality rate). In addition to an implementation indicator link to intervention month, other variables included: 1) Year of the implementation; 2) Age group: <2 months, 2–11 months and 12–59 months; 3) Severity category at diagnosis: In children 2–59 months there were two categories severe and very severe which were recorded separately; 4) Region of the country: North, Central and South and 5) Season defined by month of year.

The time factor used in the analysis was month. Data within each facility were reported by this time period broken down by the covariates used in the analysis. It was then possible to recreate the individual records from the monthly report since the information reported the number of children who survived and died by unique covariate pattern. Hospitals were the clusters. All monthly records compiled at the districts were included in the analysis depending on the analysis restriction applied as outlined above.

Due to the pragmatic nature of the intervention and the stepwise implementation of the intervention it was decided to test the intervention effect in a fully adjusted model. Thus all covariates that were available from the monthly reports were included in the analysis. Interactions with the intervention were also considered. Calendar trend was extracted from the timing of the report as well as the region of the hospital.

A logistic regression model was used to estimate odds ratios and their standard errors for all the interactions of the covariates with the intervention. Of the interactions investigated only those with significant interaction between severity and intervention were retained. The clustering of children within districts was taken into account using a robust cluster variance approach. Taking only the basic design into account an overall crude intervention effect was estimated in a separate model with CLHP implementation as the only dependent variable.

As implementation began at varying times, the length of follow-up for different groups of hospitals varied, with those beginning the implementation having the longest follow-up. Therefore, the analysis was repeated (restricted analysis) using only the first 15 months follow-up at each district hospital in order to standardize the length of the intervention in the various hospitals (Figure 1). The restricted analysis became part of the model strategy to ensure contemporaneous time periods were not dominated by the intervention periods at the end of the intervention for those hospitals which started the implementation earliest. This approach was considered more objective as it limited the influence of the underlying trend in improvement of outcome that might have occurred over time in those hospitals with the longest implementation period.

Results

Table 1 summarizes the results of the situation analysis undertaken prior to commencing implementation within the district hospitals and gives an outline of the elements of the intervention introduced by the CLHP, the output indicators used to monitor progress and the operational achievements during the course of the program. Adherence to guidelines improved from zero to over 90% among children presenting for care. Training of staff increased from less than ten per cent to over the target set for training all staff engaged in the care of small children. While interruption of essential supplies was frequent prior to the introduction of the program, it never occurred again after the program was introduced. All hospitals received the facility of oxygen supply during the implementation of the program. The poor case records and lack of routine reporting at the outset (preventing the use of any data on patient care prior to implementing the program) had been corrected with almost all

(99.4%) reports being submitted by the end of the intervention period.

A total of 48 285 children were recorded in the intervention of which 1057 (2•2%) cases were admitted for non-severe pneumonia and were excluded from further analysis resulting in 47 228 cases of severe and very severe pneumonia being analysed. Of the 2274 monthly report forms generated during this period, 2260 (99•4%) were received for analysis. Figure 1 indicates the routine data that were used for analysis within the intervention. It is clear that the follow-up periods varied according to the point of introduction of the program. The follow-up period was standardized within the restricted analysis by truncating the analysis at the same point of follow-up for each of the groups of hospitals.

Hospitals reported a mean number of children treated for severe or very severe pneumonia of 1968 (range: 807 to 4458). Figure 2 indicates the trend in numbers of children with severe and very severe pneumonia admitted to hospital over the course of the intervention, by the hospital group of intake. The hospital intake per calendar quarter showed no significant change over the period of the intervention. The trend was similar for the proportion by age group (Figure 3) with no important change over the intervention period. There was some change in the distribution by severity grade among the children admitted to hospital (Figure 4), with a decline in the proportion of children aged two to 59 months with very severe pneumonia and a concomitant rise in the proportions classified as severe in this age group. The trend in proportions of young children (aged less than two months) showed no change over the period.

Table 3 shows the distribution of numbers of children admitted to hospital by calendar year, by age group and by classification of severity, for the entire period of follow-up and for the restricted period of follow-up. It also indicates the number and proportion of the children who died during the course of treatment. Overall, 4,605 children (9.8%) died compared with 1,600 (11.3%) when considering the more restricted period. Case fatality rate was highest for children with very severe pneumonia and was higher for younger as compared with older children. There was a steady decline in case fatality rate by calendar year overall and, to a lesser extent within the restricted period of follow-up. Deaths were equally likely to occur within the first 24 hours of hospitalization as compared with later in the course of treatment in the whole group (Table 4). The exception was the youngest age group in which a higher proportion of deaths occurred in the earlier time period. This was even more apparent for cases within the restricted period of follow-up.

Table 5 shows the results of statistical analysis of likelihood of death, overall and for the restricted period of follow-up. Deaths were not associated with the region of the country with results not significantly different for the north, central and southern regions. There was a significant variation by calendar month with fewer deaths occurring in the middle quarters of the year. Deaths were much more likely to occur in younger children.

Multivariate analysis of the trend in deaths over the intervention period, adjusted for age, severity, calendar month and region, showed a significant decline over the calendar years of the intervention in the overall intervention group. In comparison, although there was a decline in the likelihood of death over the intervention period, the decline was not statistically significant in the group with the restricted period of follow-up. The significant reduction in likelihood of death overall was restricted to the group of older children with severe pneumonia; there was no difference at all among the older children with very severe pneumonia or for the group of younger children. These results remained significant in the analysis of the restricted period of follow-up.

Trend , by age group, of children admitted to hospital with pneumonia in Malawi, 2000-2005.

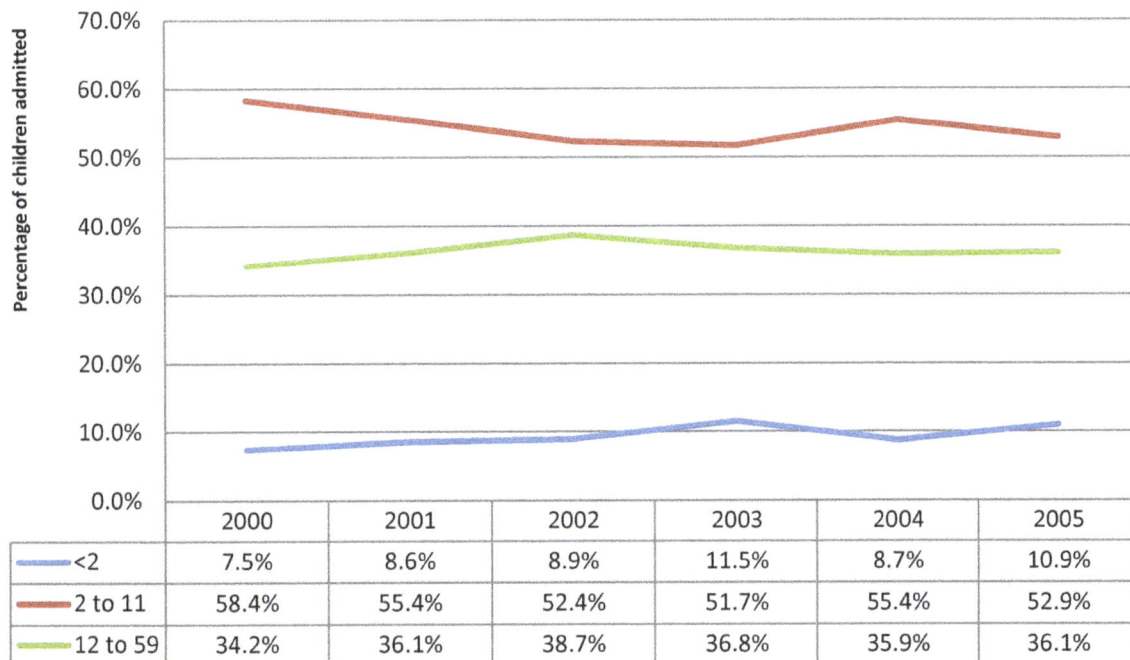

	2000	2001	2002	2003	2004	2005
<2	7.5%	8.6%	8.9%	11.5%	8.7%	10.9%
2 to 11	58.4%	55.4%	52.4%	51.7%	55.4%	52.9%
12 to 59	34.2%	36.1%	38.7%	36.8%	35.9%	36.1%

Figure 3. Trend by age group of children admitted to hospital with pneumonia in Malawi, 2000–2005.

Trend , by severity category, of children admitted to hospital with pneumonia in Malawi, 2000-2005.

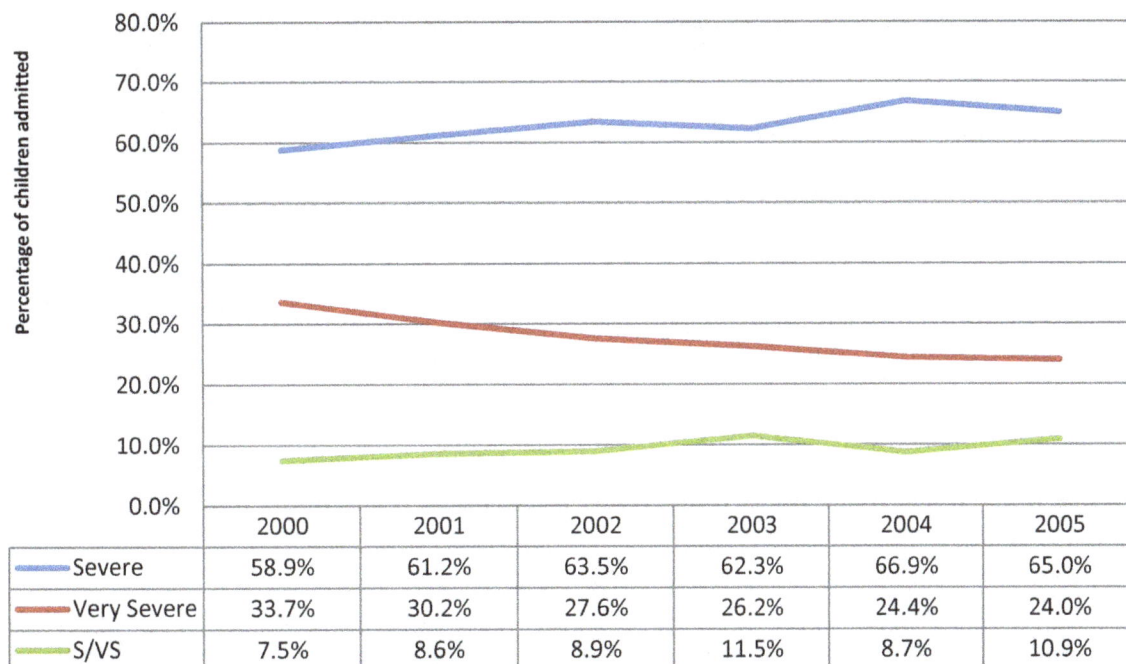

	2000	2001	2002	2003	2004	2005
Severe	58.9%	61.2%	63.5%	62.3%	66.9%	65.0%
Very Severe	33.7%	30.2%	27.6%	26.2%	24.4%	24.0%
S/VS	7.5%	8.6%	8.9%	11.5%	8.7%	10.9%

Figure 4. Trend by severity category of children admitted to hospital with pneumonia in Malawi, 2000–2005.

Table 3. Numbers of children (0–59 months) treated for pneumonia by age, severity and case-fatality rate by year in district hospitals in Malawi, 2000–2005 for the restricted and unrestricted time periods.

Year	RESTRICTED n = 14 162			UNRESTRICTED n = 47 228		
	All	Died	CFR	All	Died	CFR
	Cases	No	%	cases		%
2000	389	73	18·8	389	73	18·8
2001	3558	473	13·3	3558	473	13·3
2002	3249	368	11·3	7364	771	10·5
2003	5216	560	10·7	12849	1225	9·5
2004	1750	126	7·2	9986	938	9·4
2005	-	-	-	13082	1125	8·6
Total	14162	1600	11·3	47228	4605	9·8
	RESTRICTED n = 14 162			UNRESTRICTED n = 47 228		
	All	Died	CFR	All	Died	CFR
	Cases	No.	%	Cases	No.	%
Age group (months)*						
<2	1386	156	11·3	4773	492	10·3
2–11	7640	1023	13·4	25153	2998	11·9
12–59	5136	421	8·2	17302	1115	6·4
Severity grade (aged 2–59 months)**						
severe	8727	509	5·8	30267	1445	4·8
very severe	4049	935	23·1	12188	2668	21·9

* % of total number in age categories.
** infants <2 months were not categorized or analyzed by separate degree of severity.

In an effort to estimate an overall crude intervention effect, a logistic regression analyses without covariates taking only the basic design into account was estimated in a separate model with CLHP implementation as the only dependent variable. This showed that in the restricted analysis the overall effect of the CLHP did not significantly decrease CFR for children admitted to hospital for pneumonia (OR = 0•82; 95%CI 0•63–1•06; p = 0•14) However in contrast to the unrestricted analysis showed there was a significant overall effect of the intervention in decreasing the CFR for all degrees of severity and age groups (OR = 0•79; 95% CI 0•64–0•99; p-value = 0•040).

Discussion

The trend in case fatality rates in infants and young children (1 week to 59 months of age) hospitalized and treated for severe and very severe pneumonia was evaluated over the course of the implementation of a nationwide programme to deliver standardized case management for childhood pneumonia. We were able to demonstrate the significant decline in CFR overall was no longer significant when the period of follow-up was standardized in the restricted analysis, there remained a significant decrease in CFR in children, aged 2–59 months, treated for severe pneumonia. Similarly the CFR for neonates admitted for severe/very severe pneumonia remained unchanged. An important strength of this intervention was the nation-wide implementation of the program, the prevention of antibiotics stock outs and the comprehensive and complete set of data collected over the duration of the intervention.

The high overall CFR of around 10% is within the range of that reported from nine district hospitals in Kenya but higher than the overall CFR of 6% in the study [28]. The higher case-fatality rate associated with young age and very severe pneumonia is expected and consistent with other studies [3,29–31]. The lack of intervention effect in infants and children younger than 59 months suffering from very severe pneumonia is disappointing but the CFR is similar to other studies from the African region even when the studies have been conducted in central hospitals that have better resources than district hospitals [29,31].

The introduction of the CLHP included a substantial programme of work which included establishing an information system, quality assurance mechanisms, training, regular supervision and provision of antibiotics and oxygen to address all the various problems identified in Table 1 simultaneously. Interventions that may have contributed to improved outcomes were the continuous provision of antibiotics and oxygen. Due to the planning and supervision of CLHP no shortages of antibiotics at any stage were experienced. Oxygen concentrators were acquired and installed in all district hospitals during the course of the CLHP implementation, as previously described [26]. Few district hospitals had oxygen available at the beginning of the implementation. Oxygen therapy was delivered via nasal prongs and was indicated on the basis of clinical indicators as oximetry was not available. Clinical indicators are known to be inaccurate in detecting all cases of hypoxaemia and so the use of oximetry along with supplemental oxygen could potentially have further improved outcomes [32]. The outcome of the intervention might have been influenced by the attrition of health care workers trained in the

Table 4. Deaths before and after 24 hours of commencement of treatment by age and severity of pneumonia for the restricted and unrestricted pre and post intervention time periods.

UNRESTRICTED N = 47 228					
Characteristic	Deaths	Died<24	%	Died>24	%
Age (months)					
<2	492	298	60.6	194	39.4
2–11	2998	1378	46.0	1620	54.0
12–59	1115	559	50.1	556	49.9
Total	4605	2235	48.5	2370	51.5
Severity grade					
(2–59 months)*					
severe	1445	586	40.5	859	59.5
very severe	2668	1351	50.6	1317	49.4
RESTRICTED N = 14 162					
Characteristic	Deaths	Died<24	%	Died>24	%
Age (months)					
<2	156	103	66.0	53	34.0
2–11	1023	489	47.8	534	52.2
12–59	421	227	53.9	194	46.1
Total	1600	819	51.2	781	48.8
Severity grade					
(2–59 months)*					
severe	509	209	41.1	300	58.9
very severe	935	507	54.2	428	45.8

*Infants <2 months were not categorized or analyzed by separate degree of severity.

SCM of pneumonia. To minimize this effect an additional 30% more health care workers were trained.

It was not possible to determine the factors contributing to a poor outcome. There are a number of reasons that might explain a lack of benefit as seen in this analysis, especially for neonatal and very severe pneumonia in infants. First, neonates with pneumonia and infants with very severe pneumonia who are critically ill on presentation to the health services are high-risk groups for a poor outcome and often die within the first 24 hours after admission. The main impact of improved case management is likely to reduce deaths after 24 hours by clinical improvement in those that are not so critically ill at presentation, such as those with severe pneumonia.

In the HIV endemic setting, antibiotics and oxygen may not be effective against all causes of pneumonia. *Pneumocystis* pneumonia (PcP) which was common at the time of this intervention and usually fatal in Malawian infants presenting with very severe pneumonia would not have responded to first line antibiotics [30,31]. The impact of HIV is highlighted by studies carried out in urban hospitals in South Africa showing that HIV is associated with treatment failure and poor outcomes [29]. While health workers were trained to recognise and treat PcP and other HIV-related lung disease this almost certainly did not occur as almost all participants' HIV status was recorded as unknown. Although improved HIV/AIDS services in the country would be expected to also improve outcome of treatment of children with pneumonia, the improvement in such services has not been demonstrated and therefore could not have been sufficient to explain the effect we demonstrated. Similarly, the inclusion of the 13-valent PCV into

the Malawi EPI schedule since November 2011 is likely to further reduce the incidence and CFR of pneumonia in young children irrespective of HIV status [33,34].

The intervention did show a beneficial effect in infants and children with severe pneumonia but this may have been lessened by co-morbidities or clinical overlap with pathogens that would not be responsive to standard first-line therapy, such as *Mycobacterium tuberculosis*, malaria or non-typhoidal *Salmonella*. Malawi is endemic for tuberculosis (TB), and studies from the Africa region have shown that TB is common and sometimes fatal in infants and young children with acute severe pneumonia [29–31,35]. TB is likely to be under-recognised as a potential cause of acute severe pneumonia as health workers are trained to consider TB as a chronic disease associated with persistent rather than acute symptoms.

Severe malaria is common and seasonal in Malawi and can present with clinical features similar to pneumonia [36], especially severe malarial anaemia where fast breathing and chest in-drawing are common features [37]. Invasive salmonellosis is commonly associated with malarial anaemia, often presents with clinical features of pneumonia and is commonly fatal [38]. First-line antibiotics currently used for severe pneumonia in Malawi are not effective against sepsis due to non-typhoidal *Salmonella* [39]. It is notable that CFR was highest early in the rainy season and this is a peak time of year for severe malarial anaemia and invasive salmonellosis. Malnutrition is another important co-morbidity with a similar seasonal effect that could also increase the risk of poor outcome from pneumonia [40,41]. Childhood malnutrition is

Table 5. Odds ratios from logistic regression models for mortality on the covariates including intervention period for the restricted and unrestricted analyses.

Factor	Level	Restricted period				Unrestricted period			
		Odds ratio	95% CI Lower	Upper	P value*	Odds ratio	95% CI Lower	Upper	P value*
Year	2000	1			0·36	1			<0·001
	2001	0·925	0·64	1·33		0·98	0·74	1·28	
	2002	0·798	0·48	1·32		0·79	0·54	1·15	
	2003	0·704	0·42	1·18		0·72	0·51	1·00	
	2004	0·533	0·24	1·18		0·75	0·52	1·06	
	2005	N/A				0·69	0·5	0·95	
Month	January	1			<0·001	1			<0·001
	February	0·78	0·60	1·02		0·72	0·60	0·88	
	March	0·53	0·35	0·80		0·61	0·49	0·76	
	April	0·75	0·55	1·02		0·77	0·63	0·93	
	May	0·69	0·51	0·94		0·72	0·57	0·92	
	June	0·65	0·50	0·85		0·81	0·68	0·96	
	July	0·72	0·56	0·92		0·77	0·63	0·95	
	August	0·77	0·52	1·14		0·74	0·60	0·91	
	September	0·69	0·51	0·93		0·81	0·68	0·97	
	October	0·85	0·66	1·10		0·95	0·76	1·17	
	November	0·92	0·68	1·26		1·00	0·81	1·22	
	December	0·86	0·64	1·15		0·99	0·83	1·20	
Region	South	1			0·63	1			0·87
	Central	0·86	0·57	1·31		0·98	0·74	1·30	
	North	1·00	0·72	1·37		0·94	0·73	1·23	
Age	2–59 months	1			<0·001	1			<0·001
	2–11 months	1·72	1·41	2·09		1·86	1·69	2·05	
Intervention by age and severity									
2–59 months					0·0305				0·0052
Severe	pre	1				1			
	post	0·70	0·50	0·98	0·04	0·63	0·47	0·84	0·002
Very severe	pre	1				1			
	post	0·97	0·72	1·30	0·80	0·94	0·73	1·21	0·57
<2 months**	pre	1				1			
	post	0·83	0·56	1·22	0·34	0·80	0·57	1·14	0·20

* p-value for factor.
** infants <2 months were not categorized or analyzed by separate degree of severity.

very common in Malawi with high rates of stunting and wasting [42,43].

An important limitation is that the analysis is based on routinely collected aggregate data in the district hospitals after training had been undertaken. By using the first three months of data collected after training as the baseline for comparison due to the poor quality of available data prior to the intervention is likely to have underestimated the impact of the intervention. This underestimation is supported by the high CFR (10–26%) observed during the situational analysis prior to the implementation of the CLHP [15]. The trend of improved outcomes following the first three months of intervention is noteworthy as it suggests sustained improvements in care due to this CLHP approach, rather than a temporary improvement only following training as might have been expected.

In 2005, based on the programme's success the MoH included the CLHP (within inpatient services) in the Essential Health Package funded through the Sector Wide Approach. It would have been beneficial and informative to have undertaken a formal costing but this was not possible at the time. The CLHP has been sustained beyond the cycle of external funding due to the programme's success. The CLHP has now been maintained for 8 years since the end of external project funding and is currently being expanded to 16 nongovernment hospitals. All components of the programme were still functioning well.

Improvements in child survival are being noted in many settings but consistently child pneumonia-related mortality and neonatal mortality are two of the major challenges that need to be addressed in order to reach Millennium Development Goal targets and beyond [1]. This comprehensive prospective study of the intervention to improve case-management in district hospitals in Malawi has highlighted the on-going challenges in these high mortality groups.

Supporting Information

Text S1 Supplementary material for recording and reporting.

Acknowledgments

We wish to thank the Malawi MoH for its request to The Union to assist with the implementation of the CLH Programme and its continued support throughout the scale-up process and beyond the funding cycle. Partial funding was provided by the Bill and Melinda Gates Foundation. We wish to express our appreciation to all members of the training teams for donating their time so readily. We particularly wish to thank the Community Health Science Unit ARI/CLHP Management Team who were involved in running, monitoring and evaluating the ongoing programme; the District Health Officers for their continued support and the CLHP Coordinators whose work made it all possible.

Author Contributions

Conceived and designed the experiments: PME RPG DAE. Performed the experiments: PME RPG CCM ERM SMG DAE. Analyzed the data: PME CJL RPG DAE. Contributed reagents/materials/analysis tools: PME RPG ERM CJL DAE. Wrote the paper: PME RPG CCM ERM SMG DAE CJL.

References

1. Liu L, Johnson HL, Cousens S, Perin J, Scott S, et al. (2012) Global, regional, and national causes of child mortality: an updated systematic analysis for 2010 with time trends since 2000. Lancet 379: 2151–2161.
2. Reed C, Madhi SA, Klugman KP, Kuwanda L, Ortiz JR, et al. (2012) Development of the respiratory index of severity in children (RISC) score among young children with respiratory infections in South Africa. PLoS ONE 7: e27793. doi:10.1371/journal.pone.0027793.
3. Shann F, Hart K, Thomas D (1984) Acute lower respiratory tract infections in children: possible criteria for selection of patients for antibiotic therapy and hospital admission. Bull World Health Organ 62: 749–753.
4. WHO (2005) Hospital care for children: guidelines for the management of common illnesses with limited resources. World Health Organization, Geneva.
5. Theodoratou E, Al-Jilaihawi S, Woodward F, Ferguson J, Jhass A, et al. (2010) The effect of case management on childhood pneumonia mortality in developing countries. Intô Jô Epidem 39: i155–i171.
6. Bukhman G, Kidder A (2008) Cardiovascular disease and global health equity: Lessons from tuberculosis control then and now. Amô Jô Public Health; 98: 44–54.
7. World Bank (1993) World Development Report 1993: Investing in health. World Bank, Oxford University Press, Oxford.
8. Enarson PM, Gie R, Enarson DA, Mwansambo C (2009) Development and implementation of a national programme for the management of severe and very severe pneumonia in children in Malawi. PLoS Med 6: e1000137. doi:10.1371/journal.pmed.1000137.
9. Government of Malawi (1999) Malawi Fourth National Health Plan, 1999–2004: Health sector human resources plan. Ministry of Health and Population, Lilongwe.
10. Government of Malawi (2005) Integrated household survey 2004–2005. National Statistical Office of Malawi, Zomba.
11. Government of Malawi (1999) Malawi Fourth National Health Plan, 1999–2004: Health sector human resources plan. Ministry of Health and Population, Lilongwe.
12. Gonani A, Makuti M, Macheso A, Shongwe S, Kinoti S, et al. (2005) The impact of HIV/AIDS on the health workforce in Malawi. Ministry of Health, Malawi.
13. O'Neil M, Jarrah Z, Nkosi L, Collins D, Perry C, et al. (2010) Evaluation of Malawi's Emergency Human Resources Program. Management Sciences for Health and DFID. Cambridge, Massachussets.
14. Government of Malawi (2001) Malawi demographic and health survey 2000. National Statistical Office and ORC Macro, Zomba.
15. Enarson P, Campbell H, Nolan C, Pio A (2000) Integrated child lung health project Malawi situation analysis report. International Union Against Tuberculosis and Lung Disease, Paris.
16. United Nations Children's Fund (2007) The State of the World's Children 2007 Report. UNICEF, New York.
17. National AIDS Control Commission, Malawi (2001) Estimating National HIV Prevalence in Malawi from Sentinel Surveillance Data, The National AIDS Control Programme & The POLICY Project, Lilongwe.
18. Graham SM, Coulter JBS, Gilks CF (2001) Pulmonary disease in HIV-infected African children. Intô Jô Tuberc Lung Dis 5: 12–23.
19. Rogerson SR, Gladstone M, Callaghan M, Erhart L, Rogerson SJ, et al. (2004) HIV infection among paediatric in-patients in Blantyre, Malawi. Transô Rô Soc Trop Med Hyg 98: 544–555.
20. UNICEF (2002) Sentinel Surveillance Report, National AIDS Control Commission, 2001 Programme data for PMTCT programmes, UNICEF, New York.
21. Enarson PM, Gie RP, Enarson DA, Mwansambo C, Graham SM (2010) The impact of HIV on standard case management for the inpatient treatment of childhood pneumonia in high HIV prevalence countries. Expert Rev Resp Med 4: 211–220.
22. Ellis J, Molyneux EM (2007) Experience of anti-retroviral treatment for HIV-infected children in Malawi: the 1st 12 months. AnnTrop Paediatr 27: 261–267.
23. Enarson DA (1995) The International Union Against Tuberculosis and Lung Disease Model National Tuberculosis Programmes. Tuber Lung Dis 76: 95–99.
24. Enarson PM, Enarson DA, Gie RP (2005) Management of the child with cough or difficult breathing, A Guide for Low Income Countries. 2nd ed. The International Union Against Tuberculosis and Lung Disease, Paris.
25. WHO/UNICEF(2000) Management of the child with a serious infection or severe malnutrition: Guidelines for care at the first-referral level in developing countries. World Health Organisation, Geneva, WHO/FCH/CAH/001.
26. Enarson P, La Vincente S, Gie RP, Maganga ER, Chokani C (2008) Implementation of an oxygen concentrator system in district hospital paediatric wards throughout Malawi: Lessons from the field. Bull World Health Organ 86: 344–348.
27. WHO (2013). Pocket book of hospital care for children: guidelines for the management of common childhood illnesses – Second edition. World Health Organization, Geneva.
28. Ayieko P, Okiro EA, Edwards T, Nyamai R, English M (2012) Variations in mortality in children admitted with pneumonia to Kenyan hospitals. PLoS ONE 7: e47622. doi:10.1371/journal.pone.0047622.
29. McNally LM, Jeena PM, Gajee K, Thula SA, Sturm AW, et al. (2007) Effect of age, polymicrobial disease, and maternal HIV status on treatment response and

cause of severe pneumonia in South African children: a prospective descriptive study. Lancet 369: 1440–1451.

30. Graham SM, Mankhambo L, Phiri A, Kaunda S, Chikaonda T, et al. (2011) Impact of human immunodeficiency virus infection on the etiology and outcome of severe pneumonia in Malawian children. Pediatr Infect Disô J 30: 33–38.

31. Graham SM, Mtitimila EI, Kamanga HS, Walsh AL, Hart CA, Molyneux ME (2000) The clinical presentation and outcome of *Pneumocystis carinii* pneumonia in Malawian children. Lancet 355: 369–373.

32. Duke T, Wandi F, Jonathan M, Matai S, Kaupa M, et al. (2008) Improved oxygen systems for childhood pneumonia: a multihospital effectiveness study in Papua New Guinea. Lancet 372: 1328–1333.

33. O'Brien KL, Wolfson LJ, Watt JP, Henkle E, Deloria-Knoll M, et al. (2009) Burden of disease caused by *Streptococcus pneumonia* in children younger than 5 years: global estimates. Lancet 374: 893–902.

34. Everett DB, Cornick J, Denis B, Chewapreecha C, Croucher N, et al. (2012) Genetic characterisation of Malawian pneumococci prior to the roll-out of the PCV13 vaccine using a high-throughput whole genome sequencing approach. PLoS One. 7: e44250.

35. Nantongo JM, Wobudeya E, Mupere E, Joloba M, Ssengooba W, et al. (2013) High incidence of pulmonary tuberculosis in children admitted with severe pneumonia in Uganda. BMC Pediatr; 13: 16.

36. Roca-Feltrer A, Kwizombe CJ, Sanjoaquin MA, Sesay SS, Faragher B, et al. (2012) Lack of decline in childhood malaria, Malawi, 2001–2010. Emerg Infect Dis 18: 272–278.

37. Bronzan RN, Taylor TE, Mwenechanya J, Tembo M, Kayira K, et al. (2007) Bacteremia in Malawian children with severe malaria: prevalence, etiology, HIV co-infection and outcome. Jô Infect Dis 195; 895–904.

38. Graham SM, English M (2009) Nontyphoidal salmonellae: a management challenge for children with community acquired invasive disease in tropical African countries. Lancet 372: 267–269.

39. Gordon M, Graham SM, Walsh AL, Wilson L, Phiri A, et al. (2008) Epidemics of invasive *Salmonella enteritidis* serovar Enteritidis and S.Typhimurium infections among adults and children, associated with multidrug resistance in Malawi. Clin Infect Dis 46: 963–969.

40. Chisti MJ, Terbruegge M, La Vincente S, Graham SM, Duke T (2009) Pneumonia in severely malnourished children in developing countries – mortality risk, aetiology and validity of WHO clinical signs: a systematic review. Trop Med Int Health 14: 1173–1189.

41. Rice AL, Sacco L, Hyder A, Black RE (2000) Malnutrition as an underlying cause of childhood deaths associated with infectious diseases in developing countries. Bull World Health Organ 78: 1207–1221.

42. Government of Malawi (2011) Malawi demographic and health survey 2010. National Statistical Office and ICF Macro, Zomba.

43. UNICEF (2012) The State of the World's Children 2012 Report. United Nations Children's Fund, New York.

10

Scaling-Up Access to Family Planning May Improve Linear Growth and Child Development in Low and Middle Income Countries

Günther Fink[1]*, Christopher R. Sudfeld[1], Goodarz Danaei[1], Majid Ezzati[2], Wafaie W. Fawzi[1]

1 Harvard School of Public Health, Boston, Massachusetts, United States of America, 2 MRC-PHE Centre for Environment and Health, Departments of Epidemiology and Biostatistics, Imperial College London, London, United Kingdom

Abstract

Background: A large literature has indicated a robust association between birth spacing and child survival, but evidence on the association of birth timing with physical growth in low and middle income countries (LMICs) remains limited.

Methods and Results: Data from 153 cross-sectional Demographic and Health Surveys (DHS) across 61 LMICs conducted between 1990 and 2011 were combined to assess the association of birth timing with child stunting (height-for-age z-score <-2). A total of 623,789 children of birth order 1–5 contributed to the maternal age analysis, while the birth spacing dataset consisted of 584,226 children of birth order 2 and higher. Compared to 27–34 year old mothers, maternal age under 18 years was associated with a relative stunting risk of 1.35 (95% CI: 1.29–1.40) for firstborn children, whereas the relative risk was 1.24 (95% CI: 1.19–1.29) for mothers aged 18–19 years. The association of young maternal age with stunting was significantly greater for urban residents and those in the top 50% of household wealth. Birth intervals less than 12 months and 12–23 months had relative risks for stunting of 1.09 (95% CI: 1.06–1.12) and 1.06 (95% CI: 1.05–1.06) as compared to a 24–35 month inter-pregnancy interval, respectively. The strength of both teenage pregnancy and short birth interval associations showed substantial variation across WHO region. We estimate that 8.6% (6.9–10.3%) of stunted cases in the South Asian DHS sample would have been averted by jointly eliminating teen pregnancies and birth intervals less than 24 months, while only 3.6% (1.5–5.7%) of stunting cases would have prevented in the Middle East and North Africa sample.

Conclusions: Postponing the age of first birth and increasing inter-pregnancy intervals has the potential to significantly reduce the prevalence of stunting and improve child development in LMICs.

Editor: Nyovani Janet Madise, University of Southampton, United Kingdom

Funding: This project was supported by Grand Challenges Canada through the Saving Brains Project. The funders had no role in study design, data collection and analysis, decision to publish, or preparation of the manuscript.

Competing Interests: The authors have declared that no competing interests exist.

* Email: gfink@hsph.harvard.edu.

Introduction

Approximately 16 million teenagers (under 20 years of age) give birth each year worldwide, of which more than 90% reside in low and middle income countries (LMICs) [1]. Childbirth at an early age and short birth spacing have been shown to be associated with increased risk of birth complications [2], child mortality [3–5], and physical growth restrictions [4,6–10]. Studies primarily conducted in high income settings have also found young maternal age to be associated with poor cognitive and behavioral outcomes for children [11,12].

Approximately one-third of children under age 5 in LMICs, or about 314 million children, are currently affected by linear growth restriction or stunting [13]. Stunting has long been recognized as a principal risk factor for child morbidity and mortality, but more recent work has also shown consistent associations with cognitive

deficits and underachievement in school [14,15] and lower adult earnings [14,16,17].

While previous studies have documented associations between birth timing and child physical growth [4,18,19], relatively little is known about the relative magnitude of these associations across socioeconomic and cultural settings. Given the complex biological, social, and behavioral mechanisms underlying birth timing [20–22], there variations across regions as well as within countries are potentially large [23]. In this study, we use the most comprehensive global dataset with birth timing available to date in order to update risk estimates of young maternal age and short birth spacing with child linear growth, examine differences in the associations across geographic and socioeconomic strata, and quantify the potential impact of eliminating high risk birth timing on the prevalence of child stunting in LMICs.

Methods

Data Sources

The dataset utilized for this study was pooled from 153 cross-sectional Demographic and Health Surveys (DHS) conducted 1990 to 2011 in 61 low and middle income countries. DHS are nationally representative surveys of households that collect a wide-range of data with emphasis on maternal and child health indicators. The 61 DHS countries (shown in Table S1 and Figure S4 in File S1) included in this dataset cover 83% of the total population residing low-income countries and 48% of the population of middle-income countries as classified by the World Bank in 2010 [24].

Study Population

In total 768,504 children aged 6–59 months were included in the 153 DHS which included child anthropometric measurements. A total of 17,962 children (1.1%) were excluded due to implausible height-for-age z-scores (HAZ) (< -6SD or >6SD), and an additional 138 children (0.1%) were excluded due to missing covariate information. The maternal age analysis was restricted to 623,789 children of birth order 1–5 due to the implausibility of having more than five children during the teenage years, while the birth interval dataset included all 584,226 children of birth order 2 and higher.

Exposures, Covariates, and Outcomes

Maternal age and birth spacing was assessed by self-report of the mother. Given that exact dates of conception are not available within the DHS dataset, we follow the previous literature [18,19] in defining birth spacing as the number of months between the birth month for the child under observation and the birth month of the preceding birth. Covariates were selected based on a literature review and included: birth order, child age, child sex, multiple gestation, location of delivery, breastfeeding for the first six months of life, urban/rural residence, maternal education, mother's partner vital status, maternal partner education, household wealth quintile, and year of the DHS. Descriptive statistics for all covariates in both the maternal age and birth spacing dataset are presented in Table S2 in File S1. Household wealth quintiles were calculated by creating a wealth score based on ownership of materials and household characteristics based on principal component analysis as recommended by Filmer and Pritchett [25]. HAZ was computed from the crude child height and age data employing the Anthro Software package which utilizes the WHO Child Growth Standard [26]. Stunting was defined as a HAZ more than 2 standard deviations below the reference mean [27].

Analysis

Log-poisson models were used to estimate relative risks for stunting employing the methodology of Zou [28]. Restricted cubic splines were first used to assess potential non-linear relationship of continuous maternal age and birth spacing with child stunting [29,30]. To test for non-linearity, the likelihood ratio test was used to compare the model with only the linear term to the model with the linear and the cubic spline terms. We utilized the shape of the spline analysis with commonly used cut-offs to present a categorical analysis of maternal age (<18, 18–20, 20–26, 27–34, 35+ years) and birth spacing (<12, 12–23, 24–35, 36+ months). We also present a continuous analysis of birth spacing, since the spline analysis indicated a linear relationship.

A priori we decided to present stratified categorical analyses by sex, urban/rural residence, household wealth (poorest 50% vs.

wealthiest 50%), and WHO World Bank region to assess heterogeneity in estimates. Potential modification of the maternal age association by birth order (firstborn versus birth order 2–5), birth spacing by birth order (birth order 2–5 versus 5+), and birth spacing by maternal age were also assessed. The Wald test for risk-ratio homogeneity was used to assess the statistical significance of the interaction. If significant effect modification was detected, stratified analyses were presented. As robustness check, multivariate linear regression models analyzing HAZ as a continuous outcome are also presented in the Tables S3 and S4 in File S1. All multivariate analyses included a fixed effect for each survey and the multivariate birth interval analysis also included categorical adjustment for maternal age. P-values for trend in categorical analyses were calculated by treating the median value of each maternal age or birth interval category as a continuous variable. P-values were two-sided with clustered robust standard errors to allow for local residual correlation as a result of the complex survey design utilized in DHS [31]. All regression analyses were conducted using STATA version 12 [32].

We then calculated the partial population-attributable risk percentage (PAR%) for teenage pregnancy and birth spacing <24 months by World Bank region for the DHS sample [33]. Partial PAR%s were calculated to estimate the percent of stunting cases that would not have occurred in the DHS sample if a hypothetical family planning intervention eliminated teen pregnancy and short birth intervals, but other risk factors for stunting did not change as a result of the intervention. We considered a hypothetical intervention which led all teenage pregnancies to occur at a maternal age of 20–26 years and all birth intervals <24 months to occur at 24–36 months. All region specific prevalences and effect sizes for other risk factors for stunting included in the multivariate model were assumed to remain constant in calculation of partial PAR%.

Ethics Statement

De-identified secondary data was obtained through the Measure DHS website. The project involved no human subjects research.

Results

Sample Characteristics

The mean age at first birth across the 153 DHS was 20.4 years with 19% of all births occurring to teenage mothers (<20 years at birth). The DHS with the highest percentage of teenage pregnancies was Bangladesh with 34.8% in 2004, while the lowest was Rwanda in 2005 (6.8%). The median birth spacing interval for the sample was 33 months, with 21.7% of all births occurring less than 24 months from the preceding birth. The DHS with the highest percentage of births with an inter-pregnancy birth interval of less than 24 months was Jordan in 1990 (48.0%), while the lowest was Zimbabwe in 2010 (7.4%).

The covariate distribution among the total sample of children 6–59 months is summarized in Table S2 in File S1. Briefly, 49.4% of children were female, the mean child age was 30 months, 24.0% were firstborn children, 27.4% were of birth order 5 or higher, and the majority of children resided in rural areas (61.4%). As for mothers, 91.4% were married or living with a partner and 37.5% never attended any schooling. In terms of temporal coverage, 6.8% of children in the sample were born in the 1980s, 42.3% in the 1990s, and 50.9% in the 2000s.

Maternal Age

There were 184,278 firstborn and 439,511 children of birth order 2–5 that contributed to the analysis of maternal age. The association of maternal age with stunting was significantly modified by birth order and as a result stratified analyses are presented (p-value for interaction: <0.001). The crude stunting prevalence for firstborn children was >50% for mothers reporting to be under 13 years of age and gradually declined to roughly 20% for mothers 27 years and older (Figure S5 in File S1). A multivariate restricted cubic spline analysis of continuous maternal age and stunting among firstborn children determined a significantly non-linear relationship (p-value for non-linear relationship: <0.001) which is presented in Figure 1. The estimated adjusted risk ratio for stunting declined gradually from a peak of 1.5 at age 13 years to the reference maternal age of 27 years (RR: 1.0). There was no indication of increased risk of stunting for maternal ages greater than 27 years, but statistical power was lacking due to low prevalence of first births among mothers in their thirties in LMICs. A similar relationship was found in a multivariate continuous analysis of maternal age and stunting among children of birth order 2–5, but the slope in risk of stunting was flatter for maternal ages less than the 27 year reference with maternal age less than 13 years carrying the greatest relative risk of 1.3 (not presented).

Table 1 shows the results of a multivariate categorical analysis of maternal age. The adjusted relative risk of stunting among firstborn children was 1.35 (95% CI: (1.30–1.40), 1.24 (95% CI: 1.19–1.29) and 1.15 (95% CI: 1.11–1.20) for maternal age groups <18, 18–19, and 20–26 years as compared to the reference group of mothers aged 27–34 years, respectively (p-value for trend: < 0.001). Additional adjustment for birth spacing (a potential mediator) did not appear to reduce the strength of the association.

Among children of birth order 2–5, there was also a significant association of maternal age with stunting, but the magnitude of the association was weaker (p-value for trend: <0.001) (Table 1). The adjusted relative risk of stunting among children birth order 2–5 was 1.20 (95% CI: (1.18–1.22), 1.14 (95% CI: 1.12–1.15) and 1.08 (95% CI: 1.06–1.09) for maternal age groups <18, 18–19, and 20–26 as compared to the 27–34 years reference, respectively. Secondary analysis of HAZ as a continuous outcome showed a similarly muted relationship of maternal age with stunting for children of birth order 2–5 as compared to firstborns (Table S3 in File S1).

In Table 1 stratified results of multivariate categorical models by child sex, urban/rural residence, household wealth, and World Bank region are also presented for firstborn children. There was no significant difference in the strength of association by sex (p-value for interaction: 0.136), but a significantly stronger association of maternal age with stunting was observed for children in urban areas as compared to rural (p-value for interaction: 0.016) and for households in the top 50% of household wealth as compared to bottom 50% (p-value for interaction: <0.001). The association of maternal age with stunting also significantly varied by WHO region (p-value <0.001). At the regional level, the strongest association between maternal age at first birth and stunting among firstborn children was found in the Latin America and Caribbean region, whereas the weakest was for the Middle East and North Africa region (MENA).

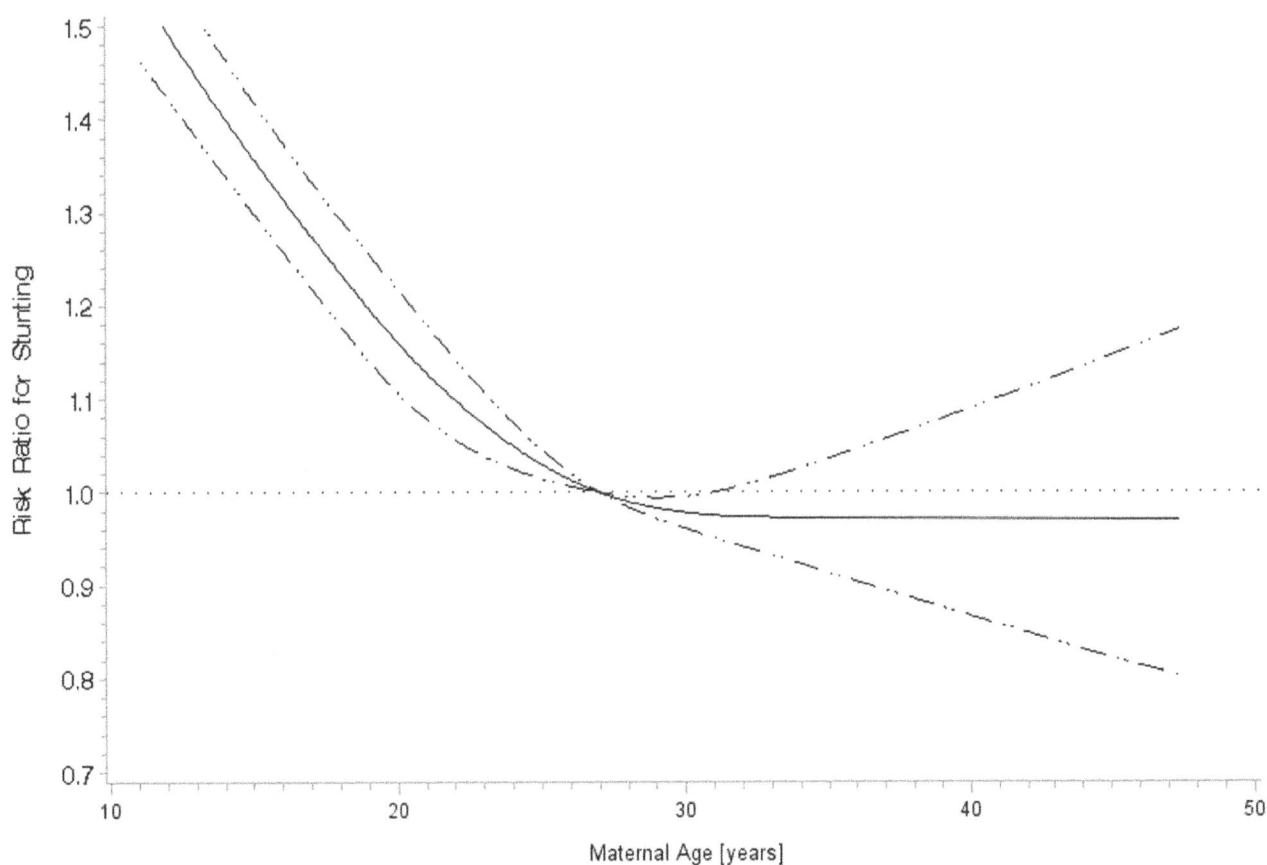

Figure 1. **Non-linear adjusted[a] relationship of maternal age with stunting for firstborn children[b].** [a]Adjusted for same factors as Table 1 Caption. [b] 27 years is the reference group (p-value for non-linear relationship: <0.001).

Table 1. Association of maternal age with stunting for children aged 6–59 months by birth order, sex, household wealth, and World Bank region.

Subgroup	n	% Stunted	Adjusted[a] Relative Risk of Stunting by Maternal Age (95% CI)					p-value for trend	p-value for interaction
			<18 years	18–19 years	20–26 years	27–34 years	35+ years		
Firstborn	184,278	35.0	1.38 (1.33–1.43)	1.27 (1.22–1.31)	1.16 (1.12–1.20)	1.0 [Ref.]	0.99 (0.91–1.09)	<0.001	<0.001
Birth order 2–5[b]	439,511	40.6	1.23 (1.21–1.26)	1.16 (1.14–1.17)	1.10 (1.09–1.11)	1.0 [Ref.]	0.92 (0.90–0.93)	<0.001	
Among Firstborn Children									
Males	93,171	36.8	1.35 (1.29–1.42)	1.24 (1.18–1.30)	1.14 (1.08–1.19)	1.0 [Ref.]	0.96 (0.85–1.09)	<0.001	0.136
Females	91,107	33.1	1.40 (1.33–1.48)	1.30 (1.23–1.37)	1.18 (1.12–1.25)	1.0 [Ref.]	1.03 (0.90–1.18)	<0.001	
Urban	78,907	24.1	1.58 (1.49–1.68)	1.38 (1.30–1.47)	1.22 (1.15–1.29)	1.0 [Ref.]	0.91 (0.78–1.07)	<0.001	0.016
Rural	105,371	43.1	1.26 (1.21–1.32)	1.18 (1.13–1.23)	1.09 (1.05–1.14)	1.0 [Ref.]	1.05 (0.94–1.17)	<0.001	
Poorest 50%	93,976	40.1	1.21 (1.15–1.26)	1.11 (1.06–1.17)	1.06 (1.01–1.11)	1.0 [Ref.]	1.02 (0.91–1.14)	<0.001	<0.001
Wealthiest 50%	90,302	29.6	1.56 (1.48–1.65)	1.42 (1.34–1.50)	1.25 (1.18–1.32)	1.0 [Ref.]	0.94 (0.81–1.09)	<0.001	
East Asia	3,782	46.3	1.23 (1.05–1.43)	1.17 (1.01–1.37)	1.11 (0.96–1.28)	1.0 [Ref.]	0.98 (0.73–1.31)	0.001	<0.001
Europe and Central Asia	6,264	18.0	1.53 (1.19–1.96)	1.38 (1.09–1.73)	1.13 (0.91–1.40)	1.0 [Ref.]	1.29 (0.84–1.98)	0.002	
Latin America and Caribbean	43,971	20.1	1.63 (1.48–1.79)	1.43 (1.30–1.57)	1.21 (1.10–1.33)	1.0 [Ref.]	0.91 (0.74–1.14)	<0.001	
Middle East and North Africa	18,465	23.7	1.09 (0.97–1.22)	1.11 (1.00–1.24)	1.07 (0.97–1.18)	1.0 [Ref.]	0.87 (0.66–1.15)	0.025	
South Asia	38,929	44.3	1.36 (1.27–1.46)	1.30 (1.21–1.39)	1.17 (1.09–1.25)	1.0 [Ref.]	0.97 (0.79–1.18)	<0.001	
Sub-Saharan Africa	72,867	42.6	1.33 (1.26–1.41)	1.22 (1.15–1.29)	1.14 (1.08–1.21)	1.0 [Ref.]	1.12 (0.97–1.29)	<0.001	

[a]Adjusted for child age in months, child sex, multiple birth, location of delivery, breastfeeding in first six months, rural residence, maternal education category, paternal education category, household wealth quintile, five-year period of birth, and survey fixed effects. Standard errors are clustered at the survey-cluster level to adjust for complex survey design used in the DHS data.
[b]Also adjusted for birth order.

Birth Spacing

The sample size for birth spacing analyses was 584,226 children of birth order 2 or higher. Crude stunting prevalence was the highest for birth intervals less than 12 months (>40%) and gradually declined with increased birth interval length up to 60 months (5 years) (Figure S6 in File S1). Figure 2 shows the results of a multivariate restricted cubic spline analysis of birth spacing and stunting, which found a significantly linear relationship (p-value for linear relationship: <0.001). Similar to the crude data, the adjusted relative risk of stunting appeared to continuously decrease with increasing birth intervals and there was no indication of a plateau of the association.

In Table 2 results of multivariate categorical (<12, 12–23, 24–35, and ≥ 36months) and linear analyses of birth spacing are presented. The categorical analyses determined the relative risk of stunting for birth intervals <12 months and12–23 months were 1.09 (95% CI 1.06–1.12) and 1.06 (95% CI 1.05–1.06) as compared the reference of group 24–35 months, respectively. A birth interval of ≥36 months was associated with significantly decreased risk of stunting as compared to the 24–35 month reference group (RR: 0.91; 95% CI: 0.90–0.91) (p-value for trend: <0.001). In a multivariate linear analysis, each additional 6 months in the inter-pregnancy interval was associated with a 2.1% reduction in the relative risk of stunting (RR: 0.979; 95% CI: 0.977–0.979; p<0.001). Secondary analysis of HAZ score continuously found a similar relationship (Table S4 in File S1).

Stratified results of multivariate categorical models for birth spacing by birth order, sex, urban/rural residence, household wealth, and World Bank region are also presented in Table 2. There was no significant difference in the strength of the association of birth spacing with stunting by birth order, child sex, or household wealth (all p-value for interaction >0.05). Nevertheless, there was significant heterogeneity in the association by WHO region (p-value for interaction <0.001).

Estimated Population-Level Impact

Due to substantial variation in both the estimated relative risk and the prevalence of teenage pregnancy, the estimated population impact of eliminating teenage pregnancies in the DHS sample varied widely by WHO region. As Table 3 shows, in the South Asian DHS sample an estimated 6.9% (6.2–7.6%) of stunting cases could have been averted by eliminating teenage pregnancies, while the same is true for only 0.8% of stunting cases (0–1.6%) in the MENA region. The percentage of stunting cases attributed to birth intervals <24 months was relatively similar across region. The highest PAR% estimate for short birth intervals was observed for the MENA region (3.0%; 95% CI: 1.7–4.2%), while the lowest was determined for Latin America and the Caribbean (1.2%; 95% CI: 0.2–2.1%). We also estimate that by eliminating both teenage pregnancy and birth intervals <24 months, 8.6% (6.9–10.3%) of stunting cases could have been averted in the South Asian DHS sample, while only 3.6% (95% CI: 1.5–5.7) would have been prevented in the MENA region sample.

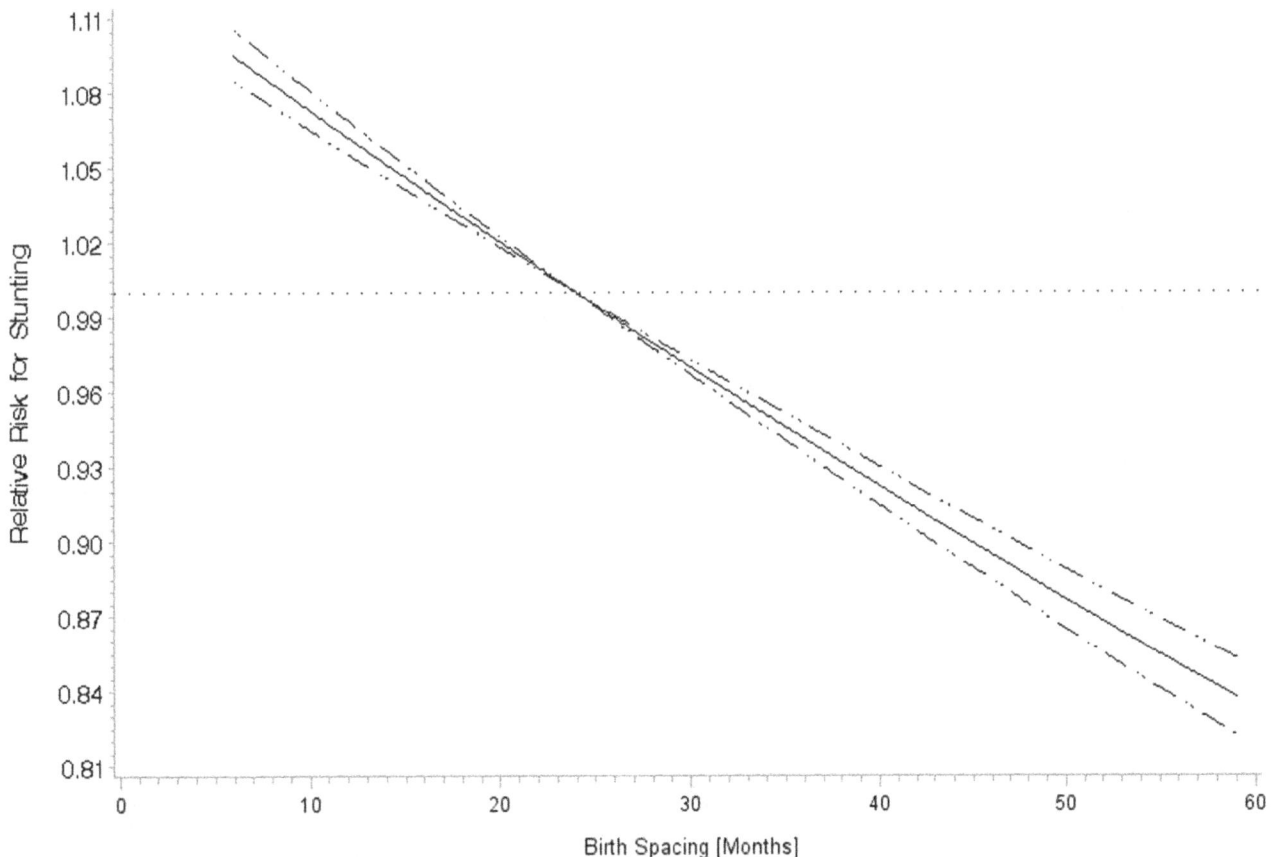

Figure 2. Linear adjusted[a] relationship of birth spacing with stunting[b] among children of birth order 2-5. [a] Adjusted for same factors as Table 1 Caption. [b] 24 months is the reference group (p-value for linear relationship: <0.001).

Table 2. Association of birth interval with stunting for children aged 6–59 months by birth order, sex, household wealth, and World Bank region.

Sub Group	n	% Stunted	Adjusted[a] Relative Risk of Stunting by Birth Interval (95% CI)				p-value for trend	p-value for interaction
			<12 months	12–23 months	24–35 months	>36 months		
Birth order 2–5	439,511	40.6	1.11 (1.07–1.14)	1.06 (1.05–1.07)	1.0 [Ref.]	0.89 (0.89–0.90)	<0.001	0.280
Birth order 6+	144,715	47.8	1.05 (1.00–1.10)	1.05 (1.03–1.06)	1.0 [Ref.]	0.90 (0.89–0.92)	<0.001	
Among birth order 2–5								
Males	222,566	42.1	1.13 (1.08–1.18)	1.07 (1.05–1.08)	1.0 [Ref.]	0.91 (0.90–0.92)	<0.001	0.100
Females	216,945	39.0	1.08 (1.03–1.12)	1.06 (1.04–1.07)	1.0 [Ref.]	0.88 (0.87–0.89)	<0.001	
Urban	155,356	28.9	1.20 (1.13–1.27)	1.08 (1.06–1.11)	1.0 [Ref.]	0.86 (0.85–0.88)	<0.001	0.506
Rural	284,155	47.0	1.07 (1.03–1.10)	1.05 (1.04–1.06)	1.0 [Ref.]	0.91 (0.90–0.92)	<0.001	
Poorest 50%	247,845	45.1	1.06 (1.03–1.11)	1.05 (1.04–1.06)	1.0 [Ref.]	0.91 (0.90–0.92)	<0.001	0.063
Top 50%	191,666	34.8	1.17 (1.11–1.23)	1.08 (1.06–1.09)	1.0 [Ref.]	0.88 (0.87–0.89)	<0.001	
East Asia	9,796	52.2	1.15 (0.95–1.39)	1.03 (0.98–1.08)	1.0 [Ref.]	0.90 (0.86–0.94)	<0.001	<0.001
Europe and Central Asia	9,936	43.7	1.35 (1.07–1.71)	1.07 (0.99–1.17)	1.0 [Ref.]	0.86 (0.79–0.94)	<0.001	
Latin America and Caribbean	88,086	28.6	1.21 (1.12–1.31)	1.06 (1.03–1.08)	1.0 [Ref.]	0.77 (0.75–0.79)	<0.001	
Middle East and North Africa	45,101	26.5	1.22 (1.10–1.36)	1.12 (1.08–1.16)	1.0 [Ref.]	0.91 (0.87–0.94)	<0.001	
South Asia	80,059	52.5	1.09 (1.03–1.14)	1.05 (1.03–1.06)	1.0 [Ref.]	0.91 (0.90–0.93)	<0.001	
Sub-Saharan Africa	206,533	44.4	1.04 (0.99–1.09)	1.06 (1.04–1.07)	1.0 [Ref.]	0.92 (0.91–0.93)	<0.001	

[a]Adjusted for maternal age, birth order, child age in months, child sex, multiple birth, location of delivery, breastfeeding in first six months, rural residence, maternal education category, paternal education category, household wealth quintiles, five-year period of birth, and survey fixed effects. Standard errors are clustered at the survey-cluster level to adjust for complex survey design used in the DHS data.

Table 3. Estimated percent reduction in stunted children by eliminating teenage pregnancy and birth intervals <24 months* by World Bank region within DHS sample.

	% of births occurring to teenage mothers	% of births occurring <24 months birth spacing	Partial PAR% Teenage pregnancy	Partial PAR% <24 months birth spacing	Partial PAR% Teenage Pregnancy and <24 months birth spacing
East Asia and Pacific	10.6	18.4	2.3 (1.0–3.5)	2.2 (−0.2–4.6)	4.3 (0.6–7.9)
Europe and Central Asia	16.4	18.5	5.3 (3.9–6.7)	1.8 (−1.7–5.3)	6.6 (1.4–11.8)
Latin America and the Caribbean	21.5	17.8	5.2 (4.7–5.8)	1.2 (0.2–2.1)	5.6 (4.0–7.1)
Middle East and North Africa	11.9	21.9	0.8 (0–1.6)	3.0 (1.7–4.2)	3.6 (1.5–5.7)
South Asia	23.8	16.3	6.9 (6.2–7.6)	2.3 (1.5–3.2)	8.6 (6.9–10.3)
Sub-Saharan Africa	18.3	14.6	3.8 (3.4–4.3)	2.0 (1.6–2.4)	5.4 (4.5–6.2)

PAR%= Population attributable risk % or the % of stunting cases that can be attributed to the risk factor(s) of interest.
* Assuming all teenage pregnancies would occur at a maternal age of 20–26 years and all birth intervals <24 months would occur at 24–36 month intervals. Regional specific also used in calculation of partial PAR%.

Discussion

The individual and population level analyses of birth timing presented in this work have yielded several key findings. Foremost, young maternal age at first birth is a substantial risk factor for child stunting, while the association of short birth intervals with restricted linear growth appears to be weak. In terms of the shape of these relationships, the risk of stunting was highest for maternal ages under 18 years with declines in risk up to 27 years. As for birth spacing, the highest risk of stunting was observed for birth intervals of less than 12 months with gradual linear decreases in risk for longer birth intervals.

In the DHS sample stunting rates are substantially lower for firstborn children as compared to children of higher birth order, while the reverse is true for infant mortality [4]. In the British context, firstborn children were shown to be smaller at birth but then exhibited rapid catch-up growth and reached greater heights as compared to higher birth order children by 12 months of age [34]. A similar growth catch-up mechanism may partially explain the low prevalence of stunting for firstborn children in LMICs. Most studies from developing countries have found the association of maternal age with child mortality to be weak [4,35], whereas the relative risk of child mortality appears to sharply increase for birth intervals of less than 18 months [18,19]. Our results suggest the opposite is true for linear growth, that there is a relatively small increase in the risk of stunting associated with short birth intervals, while the risk of stunting is substantial for children born to teenage mothers. As a result, the mechanisms underlying the observed relationships of birth timing with mortality and physical growth are likely to be different. It is possible the biological factors which lead to a generally strong association of short birth intervals with early infant mortality and reduced birth size are not as significant contributors to childhood stunting due to the potential for growth catch-up [34,36,37]. This is in contrast to the social, economic, and behavioral consequences of young maternal age which may persist as key drivers of physical growth throughout childhood.

Our results also suggest remarkable heterogeneity in the strength of the maternal age and stunting association across socioeconomic groups and by urban/rural residence. Even though we hypothesized a priori there would be significant heterogeneity in the association of birth timing with stunting, the finding that young maternal age at first birth is relatively more harmful in urban and in wealthier households as compared to rural and poorer households was not anticipated. This finding is partially driven by the use of relative risk measures in our primary analysis, as the significantly lower prevalence of stunting in urban and wealthy households may result in the same absolute increase in the probability of stunting yielding a larger observed relative risk. Nevertheless, the heterogeneous relationship remained when analyzing HAZ continuously (Tables S3 and S4 in File S1). One potential mechanism for the observed effect modification is that income differentials between older and younger mothers are more pronounced in urban and wealthier strata and the relatively simple asset score used by DHS does not completely capture these differences. An alternative explanation is that in rural areas and among poorer households stunting may be primarily the result of inadequate food availability and variety [38], micronutrient deficiency [39], or poor sanitation [40] while having a young mother may not be as important of a factor for children facing significant nutritional and environmental adversity. The relatively higher impact in urban strata may also reflect the relatively high risk faced by young mothers in urban slum neighborhoods, which we cannot directly identify in the DHS data, and which may appear relatively wealthy in asset-based indices. Independent of the mechanisms driving this heterogeneity, it seems likely that the relative importance of young maternal age as a population-level risk factor for stunting will increase over the coming years as LMICs become increasingly urbanized and also develop economically [41].

The associations of maternal age and birth spacing with child stunting also varied substantially across WHO region, which may reflect differences in wealth and urbanization along with other regional factors like social support and family structure, prevalence of childhood infections, and food security.

Overall, our results suggest that the combined burden of teenage motherhood and short birth intervals is largest for the South Asian region, where we estimate that close to 9% of stunting cases could be averted with improved birth spacing, followed by Europe and Central Asia (6.6%), Latin America and the Caribbean (5.6%), Sub-Saharan Africa (5.4%), East Asia and Pacific (4.3%) and MENA (3.6%). The larger impact in the first three regions is primarily the result of their high prevalence of teenage motherhood, which is relatively rare in the East Asia and MENA regions. In terms of birth spacing, largest improvements seem possible for the MENA region, where more than one in five children are born within less than 24 months of the preceding birth.

A primary concern in the interpretation of DHS analyses is the cross-sectional nature of the data. While reverse causality concerns are often salient in cross-sectional studies, the potential for reverse causation should be minimal in this analysis due to the known temporal ordering of events. Nevertheless, residual or unmeasured confounding is possible. Residual confounding by socioeconomic status may be of particular importance because household asset ownership may not completely capture relative economic standing, especially for households in urban slum areas. More generally, birth timing decisions are the result of a complex set of individual, social, and other contextual factors, whose omission could potentially bias the results presented, so that the estimated associations may not necessarily reflect the true causal effect of interest.

The results presented in this study suggest that young maternal age and short birth intervals are risk factors for restricted linear growth, which implies that lowering adolescent fertility and increasing birth intervals has the potential to substantially reduce the number of stunted children, particularly for the South Asian region. Even though birth timing is the result of a complex combination of biological, social, and behavioral factors [3,5,18,20,22,23,35,42,43], large reductions in adolescent fertility [44] and short birth intervals [21] through increased availability and use of contraceptives seems possible. More than 900 million women are estimated to still face unmet needs for contraception globally [45], and the potential improvements in child physical growth shown in this paper provide further evidence in support of expansion of family planning services.

Supporting Information

File S1 Contains the following files: Table S1: Survey List. Table S2. Covariate distribution for Maternal Age (n = 623,789) and Birth Interval (n = 584,226) Datasets. Table S3. Association of Maternal Age with HAZ for Children Aged 6-36. Table S4. Association of Birth Spacing with HAZ for Children Aged 6-36. Figure S4: Geographical Coverage of 61 Sample Countries. Figure S5. Crude stunting prevalence for first born children by maternal age. Figure S6. Crude stunting prevalence for first born children by birth interval.

Author Contributions

Conceived and designed the experiments: GF CS ME WF. Performed the experiments: GF CS GD. Analyzed the data: GF CS. Contributed reagents/materials/analysis tools: GF CS GD. Contributed to the writing of the manuscript: GF CS GD ME WF.

References

1. WHO (2011) WHO guidelines on preventing early pregnancy and poor reproductive health outcomes among adolescents in developing countries. Geneva: WHO.
2. Mayor S (2004) Pregnancy and childbirth are leading causes of death in teenage girls in developing countries. BMJ 328: 1152.
3. Alam N (2000) Teenage motherhood and infant mortality in Bangladesh: maternal age-dependent effect of parity one. J Biosoc Sci 32: 229–236.
4. Finlay JE, Ozaltin E, Canning D (2011) The association of maternal age with infant mortality, child anthropometric failure, diarrhoea and anaemia for first births: evidence from 55 low- and middle-income countries. BMJ Open 1: e000226.
5. Raj A, Saggurti N, Winter M, Labonte A, Decker MR, et al. (2010) The effect of maternal child marriage on morbidity and mortality of children under 5 in India: cross sectional study of a nationally representative sample. BMJ 340: b4258.
6. Gupta N, Kiran U, Bhal K (2008) Teenage pregnancies: obstetric characteristics and outcome. Eur J Obstet Gynecol Reprod Biol 137: 165–171.
7. Guimaraes AM, Bettiol H, Souza LD, Gurgel RQ, Almeida ML, et al. (2013) Is adolescent pregnancy a risk factor for low birth weight? Rev Saude Publica 47: 11–19.
8. Zabin LS, Kiragu K (1998) The health consequences of adolescent sexual and fertility behavior in sub-Saharan Africa. Stud Fam Plann 29: 210–232.
9. Senderowitz J, Paxman JM (1985) Adolescent fertility: worldwide concerns. Popul Bull 40: 1–51.
10. Chen XK, Wen SW, Fleming N, Demissie K, Rhoads GG, et al. (2007) Teenage pregnancy and adverse birth outcomes: a large population based retrospective cohort study. Int J Epidemiol 36: 368–373.
11. Shaw M, Lawlor DA, Najman JM (2006) Teenage children of teenage mothers: psychological, behavioural and health outcomes from an Australian prospective longitudinal study. Soc Sci Med 62: 2526–2539.
12. Coyne CA, Langstrom N, Lichtenstein P, D'Onofrio BM (2013) The association between teenage motherhood and poor offspring outcomes: a national cohort study across 30 years. Twin Res Hum Genet 16: 679–689.
13. Stevens GA, Finucane MM, Paciorek CJ, Flaxman SR, White RA, et al. (2012) Trends in mild, moderate, and severe stunting and underweight, and progress towards MDG 1 in 141 developing countries: a systematic analysis of population representative data. Lancet 380: 824–834.
14. Grantham-McGregor S, Cheung YB, Cueto S, Glewwe P, Richter L, et al. (2007) Developmental potential in the first 5 years for children in developing countries. Lancet 369: 60–70.
15. Kar BR, Rao SL, Chandramouli BA (2008) Cognitive development in children with chronic protein energy malnutrition. Behav Brain Funct 4: 31.
16. Heckman J, Stixrud J, Urzua S (2006) The effects of cognitive and noncognitive abilities on labor market outcomes and social behavior. Journal of Labor Economics 24: 411–482.
17. Heckman JJ (2007) The Economics, Technology, and Neuroscience of Human Capability Formation. Proceedings of the National Academy of Sciences 104: 13250–13255.
18. Rutstein SO (2005) Effects of preceding birth intervals on neonatal, infant and under-five years mortality and nutritional status in developing countries: evidence from the demographic and health surveys. Int J Gynaecol Obstet 89 Suppl 1: S7–24.
19. Rutstein SO (2008) Further evidence of the effects of preceding birth intervals on neonatal, infant, and under-five-years mortality and nutritional status in developing countries: Evidence from the demographic health surveys. DHS Working Paper 41.
20. Adhikari R (2003) Early marriage and childbearing: risks and consequences. In: Bott S, Jejeebhoy S, Shah I, Puriet C, editors. Towards adulthood: exploring the sexual and reproductive health of adolescents in South Asia: World Health Organization:. pp. 62–66.
21. Alvergne A, Lawson DW, Clarke PM, Gurmu E, Mace R (2013) Fertility, parental investment, and the early adoption of modern contraception in rural Ethiopia. Am J Hum Biol 25: 107–115.
22. Reynolds HW, Wong EL, Tucker H (2006) Adolescents' use of maternal and child health services in developing countries. Int Fam Plan Perspect 32: 6–16.
23. Conde-Agudelo A, Rosas-Bermudez A, Castano F, Norton MH (2012) Effects of birth spacing on maternal, perinatal, infant, and child health: a systematic review of causal mechanisms. Stud Fam Plann 43: 93–114.
24. World Bank (2012) World Development Indicators Online database.
25. Filmer D, Pritchett LH (2001) Estimating wealth effects without expenditure data - or tears: An application to educational enrollments in states of India. Demography 38: 115–132.
26. WHO (2006) Anthro Software for assessing growth and development of the world's children. Geneva: WHO.
27. WHO Multicentre Growth Reference Study Group (2006) WHO Child Growth Standards: Length/height-for-age, weight-for-age, weight-for-length, weight-for-height and body mass index-for-age: Methods and development. Geneva: World Health Organization.
28. Zou G (2004) A Modified Poisson Regression Approach to Prospective Studies with Binary Data. American Journal of Epidemiology 159: 702–706.
29. Durrleman S, Simon R (1989) Flexible regression models with cubic splines. Stat Med 8: 551–561.
30. Govindarajulu US, Spiegelman D, Thurston SW, Ganguli B, Eisen EA (2007) Comparing smoothing techniques in Cox models for exposure-response relationships. Stat Med 26: 3735–3752.
31. ICF International (2012) Demographic and Health Survey - Sampling and Household Listing Manual In: MEASURE DHS, editor. Calverton, Maryland USA.
32. StataCorp (2011) Stata Statistical Software: Release 12. College Station, TX: StataCorp LP.
33. Spiegelman D, Hertzmark E, Wand HC (2007) Point and interval estimates of partial population attributable risks in cohort studies: examples and software. Cancer Causes Control 18: 571–579.
34. Ong KK, Preece MA, Emmett PM, Ahmed ML, Dunger DB (2002) Size at birth and early childhood growth in relation to maternal smoking, parity and infant breast-feeding: longitudinal birth cohort study and analysis. Pediatr Res 52: 863–867.

35. Scally G (2002) Too much too young? Teenage pregnancy is a public health, not a clinical, problem. Int J Epidemiol 31: 554–555.

36. Prentice AM, Ward KA, Goldberg GR, Jarjou LM, Moore SE, et al. (2013) Critical windows for nutritional interventions against stunting. Am J Clin Nutr 97: 911–918.

37. Wells JCK, Hallal PC, Reichert FF, Dumith SC, Menezes AM, et al. (2011) Associations of Birth Order With Early Growth and Adolescent Height, Body Composition, and Blood Pressure: Prospective Birth Cohort From Brazil. American Journal of Epidemiology 174: 1028–1035.

38. UNICEF (1990) Strategy for improved nutrition of children and women in developing countries. New York, NY: UNICEF.

39. Caulfield LE, Richard SA, Rivera JA, Musgrove P, Black RE (2006) Stunting, Wasting, and Micronutrient Deficiency Disorders. In: Jamison D, Breman J, Measham A, editors. Disease Control Priorities in Developing Countries. Washington (DC): World Bank.

40. Fink G, Günther I, Hill K (2011) The effect of water and sanitation on child health: evidence from the demographic and health surveys 1986–2007. Int J Epidemiol 40: 1196–1204.

41. Bloom DE, Canning D, Fink G, Khanna T, Salyer P (2010) Urban Settlement: Data, Measures, and Trends. In: Beall J, Huha-Khasnobis B, Kanbur R, editors. Urbanization and Development: Multidisciplinary Perspectives: Oxford University Press.

42. King JC (2003) The risk of maternal nutritional depletion and poor outcomes increases in early or closely spaced pregnancies. J Nutr 133: 1732S–1736S.

43. Stewart CP, Katz J, Khatry SK, LeClerq SC, Shrestha SR, et al. (2007) Preterm delivery but not intrauterine growth retardation is associated with young maternal age among primiparae in rural Nepal. Matern Child Nutr 3: 174–185.

44. Yen S, Martin S (2013) Contraception for adolescents. Pediatr Ann 42: 21–25.

45. Alkema L, Kantorova V, Menozzi C, Biddlecom A (2013) National, regional, and global rates and trends in contraceptive prevalence and unmet need for family planning between 1990 and 2015: a systematic and comprehensive analysis. Lancet 381: 1642–1652.

11

Outcome for Children with Metastatic Solid Tumors over the Last Four Decades

Stephanie M. Perkins[1], Eric T. Shinohara[2], Todd DeWees[1], Haydar Frangoul[3]*

1 Department of Radiation Oncology, Washington University School of Medicine, Saint Louis, Missouri, United States of America, **2** Department of Radiation Oncology, Vanderbilt University School of Medicine, Nashville, Tennessee, United States of America, **3** Department of Pediatrics, Vanderbilt University School of Medicine, Nashville, Tennessee, United States of America

Abstract

Background: Outcomes for pediatric solid tumors have significantly improved over the last 30 years. However, much of this improvement is due to improved outcome for patients with localized disease. Here we evaluate overall survival (OS) for pediatric patients with metastatic disease over the last 40 years.

Procedure: The United States Surveillance, Epidemiology, and End Results (SEER) database was used to conduct this study. Patients diagnosed between 0 and 18 years of age with metastatic Ewings sarcoma, neuroblastoma, osteosarcoma, rhabdomyosarcoma or Wilms tumor were included in the analysis.

Results: 3,009 patients diagnosed between 1973–2010 met inclusion criteria for analysis. OS at 10 years for patients diagnosed between 1973–1979, 1980–1989, 1990–1999 and 2000–2010 was 28.3%, 37.2%, 44.7% and 49.3%, respectively (p<0.001). For patients diagnosed between 2000–2010, 10-year OS for patients with Ewing sarcoma, neuroblastoma, osteosarcoma, rhabdomyosarcoma and Wilms tumor was 30.6%, 54.4%, 29.3%, 27.5%, and 76.6%, respectively, as compared to 13.8%, 25.1%, 13.6%, 17.9% and 57.1%, respectively, for patients diagnosed between 1973–1979. OS for neuroblastoma significantly increased with each decade. For patients with osteosarcoma and Ewing sarcoma, there was no improvement in OS over the last two decades. There was no improvement in outcome for patients with rhabdomyosarcoma or Wilms tumor over the last 30 years.

Conclusions: OS for pediatric patients with metastatic solid tumors has significantly improved since the 1970s. However, outcome has changed little for some malignancies in the last 20–30 years. These data underscore the importance of continued collaboration and studies to improve outcome for these patients.

Editor: David Loeb, Johns Hopkins University, United States of America

Funding: The authors have no support or funding to report.

Competing Interests: The authors have declared that no competing interests exist.

* E-mail: Haydar.frangoul@vanderbilt.edu

Introduction

With advances in medical therapy, survival for pediatric solid tumors has significantly improved over the past 30 years. This improvement has been achieved through improvements in efficacy and reductions in toxicity of multi-modal therapy that includes chemotherapy, surgery and/or radiation therapy. While patients with localized disease have experienced the largest improvement in outcome, improvement in survival for patients with metastatic disease has been more limited [1–6].

The approach to treating pediatric patients with metastatic disease is unique from that of adults in that treatment is often approached with curative intent with the use of intensive therapy. Through pediatric cooperative groups in both the United States and abroad, numerous clinical trials including phase III randomized trials, have been completed or are currently being conducted. These studies not only allow for the inclusion of patients with metastatic disease but, in many cases, are also specifically designed for this subset of patients [7–12].

There has clearly been an effort to improve outcome for pediatric patients with metastatic disease. Using National Cancer Institute's Surveillance, Epidemiology, and End Results (SEER) registry, we evaluated outcome for patients less than 19 years of age diagnosed with metastatic Ewing sarcoma, neuroblastoma, osteosarcoma, rhabdomyosarcoma and Wilms tumor between 1973–2010.

Materials and Methods

The United States Surveillance, Epidemiology, and End Results (SEER) database was used to conduct this study [13]. This research was determined to be exempt from IRB oversight by the IRB at Washington University School of Medicine. SEER*Stat version 8.1.2 (Surveillance Research Program, National Cancer Institute, Bethesda, MD, USA) was used to compile data from the SEER public-use database. Patients diagnosed between 1973–2010 provided by 18 registries were identified. Patients between 0 and 18 years of age diagnosed with metastatic disease from the following malignancies were included in the study: Ewing sarcoma, neuroblastoma, osteosarcoma, rhabdomyosarcoma and Wilms tumor. The following International Classification for Childhood Cancer site recode extended ICD-0-3 histology codes were included: 8900–8902, 8910, 8912, 8920, 8921, 8960, 9180–9183, 9186, 9192, 9193, 9260 and 9500. Patients with a prior diagnosis of cancer were excluded from analysis. Patient demographic information including age, race, gender, year of diagnosis, follow-up time, vital status at last follow-up and cause of death were collected. Overall survival (OS) was evaluated using the Kaplan-Meier method. Hazard ratios (HRs) for risk of mortality were calculated comparing patients by decade of diagnosis using the Cox proportional hazards model. Statistical analysis was performed using SAS version 9.2 (Cary, NC).

Results

A total of 10,938 pediatric patients with Ewing sarcoma, neuroblastoma, osteosarcoma, rhabdomyosarcoma, and Wilms tumor were identified. Of these patients, 3,009 patients had metastatic disease at diagnosis and met inclusion criteria for analysis. Patient demographic information is presented in Table 1. Overall, 27.5% of patients were found to have metastatic disease at diagnosis. The percentage of patients presenting with metastatic disease did not significantly change over time ranging from 26% in the 1970s to 27% in the 2000s. The rate of metastatic disease was 22.3% for Ewing sarcoma, 49.1% for neuroblastoma, 22.5% for rhabdomyosarcoma, 13.1% for osteosarcoma and 20.4% for Wilms tumor. However, the number of children with metastatic disease included in the SEER registry increased with each decade. This is a reflection of the increasing number of SEER registry sites. In the 1970's there were 9 SEER registry sites and by the end of this study period, there were 18 SEER registry sites.

Median follow-up of all patients was 2.3 years (range 0–37.8 years). OS over time for each tumor type is presented in

Figure 1. HRs for risk of mortality OS for each tumor type over time are presented in Table 2. For patients with Ewing sarcoma, 10-year OS for patients diagnosed between 2000–2010 was 30.6% as compared to 13.8% for patients diagnosed between 1973–1979. Patients diagnosed between 1980–1989 experienced worse OS compared to patients diagnosed between 2000–2010 (HR = 1.48, 95% CI 1.01–2.17); however, there was no significant difference in OS for patients diagnosed in the 1990's versus 2000–2010 (HR = 0.94, 95% CI 0.65–1.37).

For patients with neuroblastoma, OS significantly increased during each decade (Figure 1). When compared to patients diagnosed between 2000–2010, HRs for risk of mortality were significantly worse for each previous decade (Table 2). OS at 10 years for patients diagnosed between 1973–1979, 1980–1989, 1990–1999 and 2000–2010 were 25.1%, 32.9%, 43.5% and 54.4%, respectively (p<0.001). For neuroblastoma patients greater than or equal to 2 years old at diagnosis there is also steady significant improvement in outcome over time. In the 1970s and 1980s, 10-year OS for these older children was 2.0% and 10.9%, respectively. By the 1990s, 10-year OS increased to 26.8% and for patients diagnosed after 1999 10-year OS was 38.9%. Patients diagnosed prior the age of two years diagnosed between 1973–1979, 1980–1989, 1990–1999 and 2000–2010 experienced 10-year overall-survival of 42.9%, 52.7%, 59.1%, and 71.5%, respectively (p<0.001). For patients two years of age or older, OS between 1973–1979, 1980–1989, 1990–1999 and 2000–2010 was 2.0%,10.9%, 26.8%, and 38.9%, respectively (p<0.001). HRs for risk of mortality for neuroblastoma patients stratified by age less than 2 years of age are presented in Table 2.

OS at 10 years for osteosarcoma patients with metastatic disease diagnosed between 1973–1979, 1980–1989, 1990–1999 and 2000–2010 were 13.6%, 5.1%, 23.9% and 29.3%, respectively. Patients diagnosed between 2000–2010 experience improved survival over patients diagnosed in the 1970s and 1980s; however,

Table 1. Patient Information.

	All Patients N(%)	Ewing Sarcoma	Neuroblastoma	Osteosarcoma	habdomyosarcoma	Wilms Tumor
Patients N (%)	3009	289 (9.6)	1478 (49.1)	266 (8.8)	441 (14.7)	535 (17.8)
Mean Age in Years at Diagnosis (range)	5.6 (0–18)	12.7 (0–18)	2.4 (0–18)	13.3 (2–18)	9.0 (0–18)	4.1 (0–17)
Gender						
Male	1681 (55.9)	171 (59.2)	839 (56.8)	169 (63.5)	257 (58.3)	245 (45.8)
Female	1328 (44.1)	118 (40.8)	639 (43.2)	97 (36.5)	184 (41.7)	290 (54.2)
Race						
White	2359 (78.4)	263 (91.0)	1137 (76.9)	199 (74.8)	335 (76.0)	425 (79.4)
Black	297 (13.2)	6 (2.1)	186 (12.6)	43 (16.2)	76 (17.2)	86 (16.1)
Other	234 (7.8)	20 (6.9)	140 (9.5)	23 (8.6)	29 (6.6)	22 (4.1)
Unknown	19 (0.6)	0	15 (1.0)	1 (0.4)	1 (0.2)	2 (0.4)
Year of Diagnosis						
1973–1979	248 (8.2)	32 (11.1)	117 (7.9)	22 (8.3)	28 (6.3)	49 (9.2)
1980–1989	458 (15.2)	47 (16.3)	215 (14.5)	39 (14.7)	64 (14.5)	93 (17.4)
1990–1999	653 (21.7)	61 (21.1)	319 (21.6)	71 (26.7)	86 (19.5)	116 (21.7)
2000–2010	1650 (54.8)	149 (51.6)	827 (56.0)	134 (50.4)	263 (59.6)	277 (51.8)

Abbreviations: N = number.

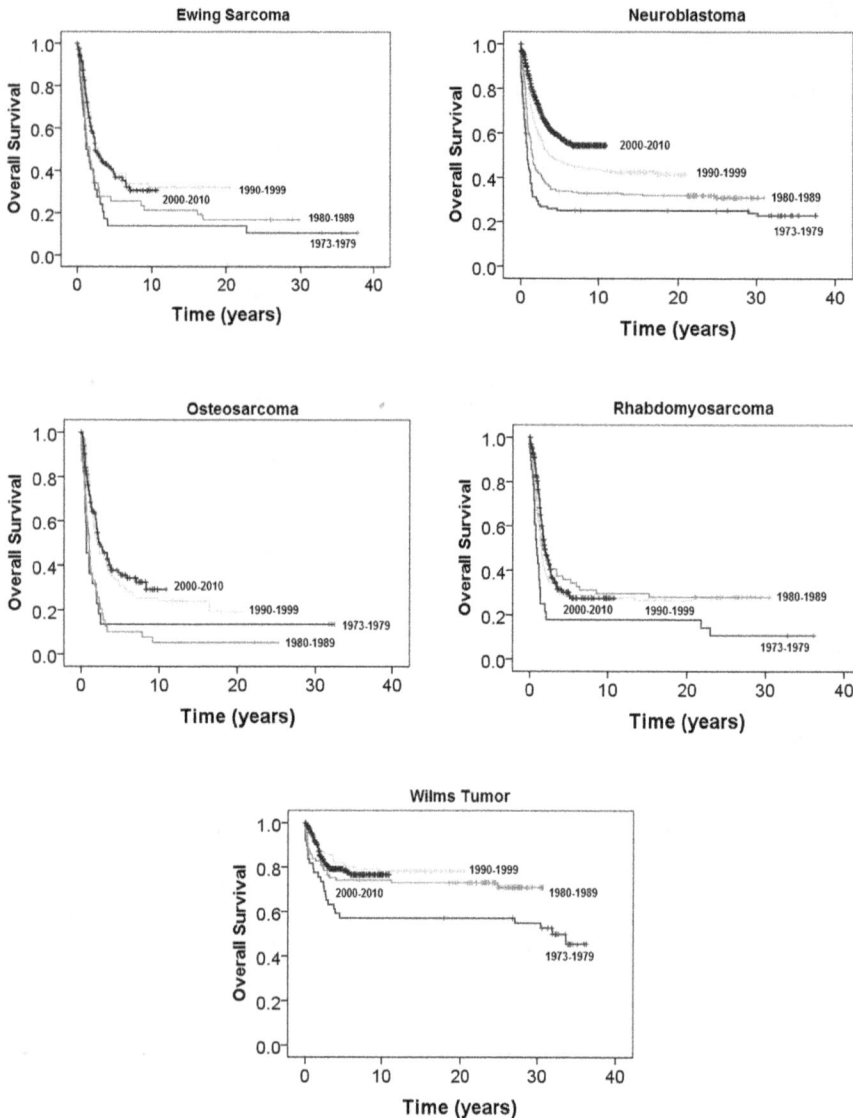

Figure 1. Overall survival based on tumor type.

there has been no significant improvement in outcome compared to patients treated in the 1990s.

For patients with metastatic rhabdomyosarcoma, 10-year OS for the past 30 years was nearly identical. OS at 10 years for patients diagnosed between 1980–1989, 1990–1999 and 2000–2010 was 29.7%, 29.1% and 27.5%, respectively. However, patients diagnosed between 2000–2010 did experience a significant increase in survival as compared to patients diagnosed between 1973–1979 (HR = 2.01, 95% CI 1.31–3.08). For patients with embryonal rhabdomyosarcoma (n = 192), OS at 10 years for patients diagnosed between 1973–1979, 1980–1989, 1990–1999, 2000–2010 was 27.8%, 37.2%, 35.0% and 40.5%, respectively. There were few patients with known alveolar histology diagnosed prior to 2000 (n = 46). For patients diagnosed between 2000–2010 with alveolar histology, 10-year OS was 19.5%.

Wilms tumor patients with metastatic disease diagnosed between 1973–1979, 1980–1989, 1990–1999 and 2000–2010 experienced 10-year OS of 57.1%, 74.2%, 78.3%, and 76.6%, respectively. Patients diagnosed between 1973–1979 experienced

an increased risk of mortality compared to patients diagnosed between 2000–2010 (HR = 2.11, 95% CI 1.28–3.50). However, there has been no significant increase in survival since that time.

Discussion

Our study shows that despite improvements in survival in children with metastatic diseases over the past four decades the outcome in some disease continues to be poor. This is especially true for patients with bone and soft tissue sarcoma. Rhabdomyosarcoma is the most common soft tissue sarcoma and a quarter of the patients present with metastatic disease [5]. The Intergroup Rhabdomyosarcoma Study Group (IRSG) was formed in 1972 to systematically study the therapy and biology of children with rhabdomyosarcoma. The first study by the group was IRS-I (1972–1978) that evaluated the addition of doxorubicin to vincristine, dactinomycin, and cyclophosphamide (VAC) plus radiation [14]. The OS of those patients was 20%. The IRS-II study conducted 1978–1984 evaluated the use of repetitive cycles of VAC compared to alternating cycles of VAC and vincristine,

Table 2. Hazard Ratio of overall survival for each tumor type based on decade of diagnosis.

	10-year Overall Survival (%)	Hazard Ratio of Overall Survival (95% CI)	P value
Ewing Sarcoma			
2000–2010	30.6	1.0	
1990–1999	32.2	0.94 (0.65–1.37)	0.75
1980–1989	21.3	1.48 (1.01–2.17)	0.046
1973–1979	13.8	1.84 (1.20–2.83)	0.005
Neuroblastoma			
All Patients			
2000–2010	54.4	1.0	
1990–1999	43.5	1.45 (1.20–1.74)	<0.0001
1980–1989	32.9	2.15 (1.76–2.63)	<0.0001
1973–1979	25.1	3.08 (2.43–3.92)	<0.0001
<2 years old			
2000–2010	71.5	1.0	
1990–1999	59.1	1.50 (1.10–2.05)	0.010
1980–1989	52.7	2.00 (1.44–2.79)	<0.0001
1973–1979	42.9	2.76 (1.89–4.01)	<0.0001
≥2 years old			
2000–2010	38.9	1.0	
1990–1999	26.8	1.41 (1.20–1.91)	0.0005
1980–1989	10.9	3.00 (2.34–3.86)	<0.0001
1973–1979	2.0	6.5 (4.73–9.00)	<0.0001
Osteosarcoma			
2000–2010	29.3	1.0	
1990–1999	23.9	1.11 (0.78–1.56)	0.57
1980–1989	5.1	2.31 (1.56–3.42)	<0.0001
1973–1979	13.6	2.14 (1.29–3.55)	0.003
Rhabdomyosarcoma			
2000–2010	27.5	1.0	
1990–1999	29.1	1.15 (0.86–1.54)	0.36
1980–1989	29.7	1.00 (0.72–1.40)	0.99
1973–1979	17.9	2.01 (1.31–3.08)	0.001
Wilms Tumor			
2000–2010	76.6	1.0	
1990–1999	78.3	0.91 (0.56–1.46)	0.91
1980–1989	74.2	1.22 (0.76–1.97)	0.40
1973–1979	57.1	2.11 (1.28–3.50)	0.003

Abbreviation: CI, Confidence Interval; NR, not yet reached.

doxorubicin, and cyclophosphamide [15]. Although the complete remission rate for those patients was 53% the OS was 26%. The IRS-III study, conducted between 1984–1991, examined the addition of cisplatin and etoposide to the previous regimens used in IRS-II, but failed to improve the survival of patients with group IV disease with 5-year OS of 27% [16]. Between 1991–1997, IRS-IV study evaluated the addition of ifosfamide and etoposide to VAC and the result also showed no significant improvement in the 3-year event free survival (25%) and 3-year OS (39%) of patients with group IV disease compared to prior studies [17]. Our findings in this study reflect the lack of improvement of outcome of those patients since 1980. The improvement observed in our study

between the 1970s to 1980s likely reflects the introduction of IRS therapy in the 1970s.

Ewing sarcoma represents the second most common soft tissue sarcoma and the second most common primary bone sarcoma in children. Although the use of chemotherapy has significantly improved the outcome of patients with localized disease from an OS of <20% to 70–80%, it has not been as effective in patients with metastatic disease [3]. In the 1960s, patients were treated with single agent chemotherapy with dismal survival. In the 1970s, combination chemotherapy was used primarily consisting of VAC [18]. A large intergroup study was conducted from 1973 to 1978 that randomized patients to VAC with or without doxorubicin [19]. Patients with localized disease randomized to VAC plus doxorubicin had significantly improved survival compared to those receiving VAC alone. In a landmark study conducted between 1988–1992, patients were randomly assigned to receive 49 weeks of standard chemotherapy with doxorubicin, vincristine, cyclophosphamide, and dactinomycin or experimental therapy with these four drugs alternating with courses of ifosfamide and etoposide [20]. Although patients with localized disease had significantly improved survival with the addition of ifosfamide those with metastatic disease had no benefit with an OS of 22%. Although the survival of children with localized disease is 73% [21], the 10-year OS for children diagnosed after 1999 with metastatic disease in our study remains low at 30.6% with very limited improvement in survival since the 1980s and 1990s.

Osteosarcoma is the most common primary bone tumor in children and 15% to 20% of patients present with metastatic disease. The treatment prior to the 1970s consisted mainly of surgery with single agent chemotherapy [2]. Meyers et al reported on a study conducted from 1975 to 1984 using multi-agent neoadjuvant chemotherapy followed by surgery in children with metastatic disease but only 11% of the patients survived [22]. The survival improved in the 1990s to 29% with the addition of cisplatin to the chemotherapy regimen [10]. These results are consistent with our observation with survival improving from 10% in the 1980s to the 31% in the 1990s; however, no significant improvement has been made since the 1990s.

Although the improvement in patients with soft tissue sarcoma has been stagnant for the past two to three decades there has been consistent improvement in the survival in patients with metastatic neuroblastoma. We observed a significant increase in survival in every decade since the 1970s. This improvement is likely related to the intensification of multi-agent chemotherapy and radiation therapy for these patients [4]. In the 1990s, the introduction of autologous stem cell transplant (ASCT) and 13-cis-retinoic acid therapy improved the survival of high risk neuroblastoma patients [23]. In the past 10 years, survival was further improved with using immune therapy with Anti-GD2 therapy following ASCT [24]. Our data shows significant improvement in survival of patients who are older than 2 years of age at diagnosis as well as those who are less than 2 years. The survival of those who are less than 2 years of age is 71.5% while the survival of older patients, which generally have more biologically aggressive disease, remains low at 38.9%.

Wilms tumor is the most common renal tumor in children. Combination chemotherapy with vincristine and actinomycin D was used as early as the late 1950s and early 1960s [25]. The National Wilms Tumor Study (NTWS) group was established in 1968 to systematically study therapies for patients with Wilms tumor. The third NTWS (1979–1986) evaluated the addition of

doxorubicin to the two drug regimen and resulted in an improved survival of 80% for patients with stage IV favorable histology disease [26]. The outcome for children with stage IV disease with diffuse anaplasia has remained poor with an OS of 33% in the most recent NTWS-5 study [27]. In our analysis the OS of children with stage IV disease has not improved since 1980s.

It is important to discuss the strengths and weaknesses of these data. The SEER database offers the unique ability assess outcome for large numbers of patients with these rare diagnoses who were treated throughout the United States over the last 40 years. Limitations to these data are that the SEER database does not provide details on the use of radiotherapy nor does it provide any information regarding the chemotherapy employed in the treatment of these children. Additionally, the SEER database provides limited biological information. While we are able to differentiate embryonal versus alveolar histology for many rhabdomyosarcoma patients, other biological information such as N-MYC amplification for neuroblastoma patients or anaplastic histology for Wilms tumor patients were either unavailable or available for very few patients. Another possible limitation to the data is the issue of stage migration in more modernly treated patients. However, we noticed no significant increase in the percentage of patients diagnosed with metastatic disease in any of the tumor types over the decades in this study. Our study is a comprehensive and provocative analysis of the outcome of children with advanced solid tumors over four decades.

The improvement in outcome for childhood cancer patients is a testament to the collaborative approach in pediatric oncology which extends nationally and internationally. However, with the exception of neuroblastoma, little improvement has been made in the last 20–30 years for children with metastatic solid tumors. These results reinforce the importance of continued collaborative efforts evaluating targeted therapy and further research to understand the underlying biology of these diseases.

Key Message

Outcome for children with metastatic solid tumors has significantly improved since the 1970's. However, with the exception of neuroblastoma, there has been little improvement in other solid tumors in the last 20–30 years.

Author Contributions

Conceived and designed the experiments: SP HF. Performed the experiments: SP. Analyzed the data: SP HF ES TD. Contributed reagents/materials/analysis tools: SP ES TD HF. Contributed to the writing of the manuscript: SP HF ES TD.

References

1. Kalapurakal JA, Dome JS, Perlman EJ, Malogolowkin M, Haase GM, et al. (2004) Management of Wilms' tumour: current practice and future goals. Lancet Oncol 5: 37–46.
2. Jaffe N (2009) Osteosarcoma: review of the past, impact on the future. The American experience. Cancer Treat Res 152: 239–262.
3. Balamuth NJ, Womer RB (2010) Ewing's sarcoma. Lancet Oncol 11: 184–192.
4. Park JR, Bagatell R, London WB, Maris JM, Cohn SL, et al. (2013) Children's Oncology Group's 2013 blueprint for research: neuroblastoma. Pediatr Blood Cancer 60: 985–993.
5. Malempati S, Hawkins DS (2012) Rhabdomyosarcoma: review of the Children's Oncology Group (COG) Soft-Tissue Sarcoma Committee experience and rationale for current COG studies. Pediatr Blood Cancer 59: 5–10.
6. Smith MA, Seibel NL, Altekruse SF, Ries LA, Melbert DL, et al. (2010) Outcomes for children and adolescents with cancer: challenges for the twenty-first century. J Clin Oncol 28: 2625–2634.
7. Ladenstein R, Potschger U, Le Deley MC, Whelan J, Paulussen M, et al. (2010) Primary disseminated multifocal Ewing sarcoma: results of the Euro-EWING 99 trial. J Clin Oncol 28: 3284–3291.

8. Carli M, Colombatti R, Oberlin O, Bisogno G, Treuner J, et al. (2004) European intergroup studies (MMT4-89 and MMT4-91) on childhood metastatic rhabdomyosarcoma: final results and analysis of prognostic factors. J Clin Oncol 22: 4787–4794.
9. Seibel NL, Krailo M, Chen Z, Healey J, Breitfeld PP, et al. (2007) Upfront window trial of topotecan in previously untreated children and adolescents with poor prognosis metastatic osteosarcoma: children's Cancer Group (CCG) 7943. Cancer 109: 1646–1653.
10. Kager L, Zoubek A, Potschger U, Kastner U, Flege S, et al. (2003) Primary metastatic osteosarcoma: presentation and outcome of patients treated on neoadjuvant Cooperative Osteosarcoma Study Group protocols. J Clin Oncol 21: 2011–2018.
11. Green DM, Breslow NE, Evans I, Moksness J, D'Angio GJ (1996) Treatment of children with stage IV favorable histology Wilms tumor: a report from the National Wilms Tumor Study Group. Med Pediatr Oncol 26: 147–152.
12. Matthay KK, Reynolds CP, Seeger RC, Shimada H, Adkins ES, et al. (2009) Long-term results for children with high-risk neuroblastoma treated on a

randomized trial of myeloablative therapy followed by 13-cis-retinoic acid: a children's oncology group study. J Clin Oncol 27: 1007–1013.

13. Surveillance E, and End Results (SEER) Program (www.seer.cancer.gov) SEER*Stat Database: Incidence – SEER 18 Regs Research Data + Hurricane Katrina Impacted Louisiana Cases, Nov 2012 Sub (1973–2010 varying) – Linked To County Attributes – Total U.S., 1969–2011 Counties, National Cancer Institute, DCCPS (released April 2013, based on the November 2012 submission): Surveillance Research Program, Surveillance Systems Branch.

14. Maurer HM, Beltangady M, Gehan EA, Crist W, Hammond D, et al. (1988) The Intergroup Rhabdomyosarcoma Study-I. A final report. Cancer 61: 209–220.

15. Maurer HM, Gehan EA, Beltangady M, Crist W, Dickman PS, et al. (1993) The Intergroup Rhabdomyosarcoma Study-II. Cancer 71: 1904–1922.

16. Crist W, Gehan EA, Ragab AH, Dickman PS, Donaldson SS, et al. (1995) The Third Intergroup Rhabdomyosarcoma Study. J Clin Oncol 13: 610–630.

17. Breneman JC, Lyden E, Pappo AS, Link MP, Anderson JR, et al. (2003) Prognostic factors and clinical outcomes in children and adolescents with metastatic rhabdomyosarcoma – a report from the Intergroup Rhabdomyosarcoma Study IV. J Clin Oncol 21: 78–84.

18. Jaffe N, Paed D, Traggis D, Salian S, Cassady JR (1976) Improved outlook for Ewing's sarcoma with combination chemotherapy (vincristine, actinomycin D and cyclophosphamide) and radiation therapy. Cancer 38: 1925–1930.

19. Nesbit ME Jr., Gehan EA, Burgert EO Jr., Vietti TJ, Cangir A, et al. (1990) Multimodal therapy for the management of primary, nonmetastatic Ewing's sarcoma of bone: a long-term follow-up of the First Intergroup study. J Clin Oncol 8: 1664–1674.

20. Grier HE, Krailo MD, Tarbell NJ, Link MP, Fryer CJ, et al. (2003) Addition of ifosfamide and etoposide to standard chemotherapy for Ewing's sarcoma and primitive neuroectodermal tumor of bone. N Engl J Med 348: 694–701.

21. Womer RB, West DC, Krailo MD, Dickman PS, Pawel BR, et al. (2012) Randomized controlled trial of interval-compressed chemotherapy for the treatment of localized Ewing sarcoma: a report from the Children's Oncology Group. J Clin Oncol 30: 4148–4154.

22. Meyers PA, Heller G, Healey JH, Huvos A, Applewhite A, et al. (1993) Osteogenic sarcoma with clinically detectable metastasis at initial presentation. J Clin Oncol 11: 449–453.

23. Matthay KK, Villablanca JG, Seeger RC, Stram DO, Harris RE, et al. (1999) Treatment of high-risk neuroblastoma with intensive chemotherapy, radiotherapy, autologous bone marrow transplantation, and 13-cis-retinoic acid. Children's Cancer Group. N Engl J Med 341: 1165–1173.

24. Yu AL, Gilman AL, Ozkaynak MF, London WB, Kreissman SG, et al. (2010) Anti-GD2 antibody with GM-CSF, interleukin-2, and isotretinoin for neuroblastoma. N Engl J Med 363: 1324–1334.

25. Green DM (2013) The evolution of treatment for Wilms tumor. J Pediatr Surg 48: 14–19.

26. Breslow NE, Churchill G, Nesmith B, Thomas PR, Beckwith JB, et al. (1986) Clinicopathologic features and prognosis for Wilms' tumor patients with metastases at diagnosis. Cancer 58: 2501–2511.

27. Dome JS, Cotton CA, Perlman EJ, Breslow NE, Kalapurakal JA, et al. (2006) Treatment of anaplastic histology Wilms' tumor: results from the fifth National Wilms' Tumor Study. J Clin Oncol 24: 2352–2358.

12

Braving Difficult Choices Alone: Children's and Adolescents' Medical Decision Making

Azzurra Ruggeri[1]*, **Michaela Gummerum**[2], **Yaniv Hanoch**[2]

1 Max Planck Institute for Human Development, Berlin, Germany, **2** University of Plymouth, Plymouth, England

Abstract

Objective: What role should minors play in making medical decisions? The authors examined children's and adolescents' desire to be involved in serious medical decisions and the emotional consequences associated with them.

Methods: Sixty-three children and 76 adolescents were presented with a cover story about a difficult medical choice. Participants were tested in one of four conditions: (1) own informed choice; (2) informed parents' choice to amputate; (3) informed parents' choice to continue a treatment; and (4) uninformed parents' choice to amputate. In a questionnaire, participants were asked about their choices, preference for autonomy, confidence, and emotional reactions when faced with a difficult hypothetical medical choice.

Results: Children and adolescents made different choices and participants, especially adolescents, preferred to make the difficult choice themselves, rather than having a parent make it. Children expressed fewer negative emotions than adolescents. Providing information about the alternatives did not affect participants' responses.

Conclusions: Minors, especially adolescents, want to be responsible for their own medical decisions, even when the choice is a difficult one. For the adolescents, results suggest that the decision to be made, instead of the agent making the decision, is the main element influencing their emotional responses and decision confidence. For children, results suggest that they might be less able than adolescents to project how they would feel. The results, overall, draw attention to the need to further investigate how we can better involve minors in the medical decision-making process.

Editor: Amanda Bruce, University of Missouri-Kansas City, United States of America

Funding: The authors have no support or funding to report.

Competing Interests: The authors have declared that no competing interests exist.

* Email: ruggeri@mpib-berlin.mpg.de

Introduction

As part of an attempt to increase children's participation in decision making, Articles 12 and 13 of the United Nations Convention on the Rights of the Child specify that minors have the right to express themselves freely, be heard on all matters affecting them, and have their views taken seriously [1]. In recent years, there has been a shift from a paternalistic medical model, where physicians and parents hold an authoritative role in determining a child's treatment, to one advocating minors' involvement in their medical treatment [2]. Simultaneously, the US Supreme Court has come to recognize that minors who show maturity and competence deserve a voice in determining their medical treatment and even allows minors, in cases such as abortion, treatments for substance abuse and sexually transmitted diseases, and contraception, to receive treatment without parental consent or notification [3]. According to the Article 6 of the Convention for the Protection of Human Rights and Dignity of the Human Being with regard to the Application of Biology and Medicine: Convention on Human Rights and Biomedicine, ratified in Italy in 2001, "the opinion of the minor shall be taken into consideration as an increasingly determining factor in proportion to his or her age and degree of maturity." Yet, a number of important questions remain open. Do children and

adolescents welcome this change, wishing to be actively involved and taking responsibility for medical decisions regardless of the severity of the decision? Can they anticipate their emotional reactions to these choices?

Research on shared medical decision making among minors has so far focused on legal and ethical issues (e.g.,[4]), cognitive competency (e.g., [5]), and providing recommendations for determining children's level of involvement [2]. Although these are important issues, researchers have neglected to examine minors' views and feelings about this decision-making process. To the best of our knowledge, this is the first study to investigate (a) children's and adolescents' desire for autonomy, (b) their confidence that the right decision was made, and (c) their emotional reactions when faced with what Botti, Orfali, and Iyengar [6] called "tragic" medical choices.

What did Botti et al. mean by tragic choices? Imagine facing the following scenario: A premature baby's life is sustained by a ventilator, and after 3 weeks of treatment the baby's condition has not improved. The attending physician informs you (the parent) that you have a choice between continuing the treatment (with 40% probability of death or a crippling neurological condition if the baby survives) or withdrawing the treatment (resulting in the baby's death). Moreover, envision that you can make the decision yourself or have the physician assume responsibility for the decision [6]. Thus, according to Botti et al., tragic choices are ones that are difficult or distressing to make and have no clear positive outcome for the decision maker.

In three studies, Botti et al. [6] examined adults' desire for autonomy and their emotional reactions to this and other hypothetical dilemmas. They showed that adults for whom the doctor made the decision reported significantly fewer negative emotions than adults who made the choice themselves. They proposed that ascribing personal causation to an event intensifies negative emotions associated with a difficult choice. Consequently, it is possible that "individuals are likely to be better off if those choices are either physically or psychologically removed from them [6]. Two additional findings from Botti et al. study are of interest. First, not informing participants about treatment options and their outcomes eliminated the emotional advantages associated with transferring the choice to another agent. Second, despite feeling worse after the decision, choosers were reluctant to give up their autonomy.

Whether children and adolescents behave and react similarly when making difficult choices is an open and important question. If medical professionals are to include minors in the medical decision-making process, there may be times when they have to present minors with difficult choices (e.g., treatment options for diabetes, see [7]). In this study, we first manipulated who made the decision: the minor or the minor's parents; second, we manipulated which option was chosen by parents; and, finally, we manipulated whether information was given about all the possible treatment options. This allowed us to examine which of these factors (agent making the choice, choice taken, information provided) affect children's and adolescents' decision confidence and emotional reactions in difficult choice situations and, ultimately, whether minors prefer to make a difficult choice themselves, despite being able to anticipate the negative emotional consequences associated with this choice. Given the paucity of data on the topic, our investigation could have clinical implications for physicians (and possibly parents) who must decide whether to include minors in the medical decision-making process.

There is good evidence that adolescents in particular are increasingly interested in making decisions independent of adults [8], [9]. Compared to children, adolescents regard more issues as a matter of personal choice, have a stronger desire to be independent, and are more likely to question authority figures' decisions [10]. Hence, we expected that when faced with difficult medical decisions, adolescents (compared to children) would show a stronger preference for making autonomous decisions (Hypothesis 1).

According to Botti et al. [6], being responsible of a decision intensifies negative emotions associated with a difficult choice. Thus, despite children's and adolescents' willingness to make a decision autonomously, we would expect participants to experience a less negative emotional response when the difficult choice was made by their parents (Hypothesis 2). Indeed, even though adolescents want to be autonomous decision-makers, they are still seeking advice from a person they consider more competent and knowledgeable than themselves [11]. This is particularly true when decisions involve physical harm or moral and social-conventional transgressions [12]. Adolescents acknowledge that authority-based decision procedures can be more suitable in some environments where adults might have more competence and better knowledge (e.g., in school;[13], [14]).

Similarly, the confidence that the best decision was made might depend on either the agent (minor or parent) making the decision or the decision option chosen. We therefore explored two

alternative—but not mutually exclusive—hypotheses: (a) If the agent making the decision is the most important element, we expected that participants, and especially adolescents, would show higher decision confidence when they made the decision themselves than when the parents made the decision, independent of the decision option chosen by the parents; (b) if the decision option chosen influences decision confidence, participants should be equally confident that the right decision was made when one particular option was chosen, independent of who (they themselves or the parents) made the decision (Hypotheses 3a and 3b respectively).

We also investigated *which* decision children and adolescents take, and explored whether and how the decision taken affected desire for autonomy, emotional response and decision confidence.

Finally, we hypothesized that minors would be sensitive to the information provided to make a decision (Hypothesis 4). That is, the negative emotional response and the confidence that the best decision was made would be worse if no information about the treatment options and outcomes were provided (see [6]).

Methods

Participants

Sixty-three 4th-grade children, aged 8 to 11 years (29 female, $M_{age} = 9.6$ years, SD = 0.6), and 76 high school students, aged 15 to 17 years (43 female, $M_{age} = 16.5$ years, SD = 0.7), were recruited from two schools in Livorno, Italy. Participants were all white, and none of them suffered a chronic medical or psychiatric condition that could have constrained or influenced a correct and neutral understanding of the instructions.

The experimental procedures were approved by the ethics committee of the Max Planck Institute for Human Development, and all the parents of the children involved, as well as the teachers and the schools' Institutional Review Board, were informed and consented (in written form) to let the children participate prior to data collection. Participants were asked to give their assent to participate, and were free to leave the classroom and withdraw from the experiment at any time.

Design and procedure

All participants received a piece of paper with an introduction to a scenario, common to all conditions, and a description of the specific condition to which they were assigned (see below). All participants of one age group assigned to the same condition were tested together. The experimenter read the scenario aloud. Participants were asked to imagine they had had an accident 1 week before: They had been hit by a car while walking home from school. As a result of the accident, they had a broken leg and were suffering from a severe infection. After the first 10 days of treatment they did not get any better.

Participants were randomly assigned to one of four conditions: 1) own informed choice; 2) informed parents' choice to amputate; 3) informed parents' choice to continue the treatment; and 4) uninformed parents' choice to amputate. The number of participants in each condition for each age group is presented in Table 1. In the informed Conditions 1, 2, and 3, the doctor presented to the participants and their parents two alternatives: Continue the treatment or amputate the leg. If they continued with the treatment, there were 4 chances out of 10 that the infection would dangerously spread, and 6 chances out of 10 that the doctors would save the leg. Even if the doctors saved the leg, it would be seriously damaged and would hurt a lot, and the participant would not be able to run again. These survival odds were the same as in the Botti et al. [6] study but presented in a

Table 1. Means and Standard Deviations for Participants' Preference for the Condition They Were Assigned to[a], Choice Made in Condition 1, Willingness to Have Been Assigned to the Other Type of Choice Condition[a,b], Emotional Response[c], and Decision Confidence[a].

	Children		Adolescents		Total	
	M	SD	M	SD	M	SD
Condition 1: Own informed choice (amputate)						
Prefer my choice condition	5.9	3.4	7.0	1.4	6.1	3.0
Prefer the other type of choice condition	3.3	2.8	2.5	2.1	3.1	2.6
Emotional response	4.2	1.8	4.8	1.4	4.3	1.7
Decision confidence	6.4	3.6	6.0	0.0	6.3	3.2
Condition 1: Own informed choice (not amputate)						
Prefer my choice condition	8.3	1.2	7.0	2.0	7.2	1.9
Prefer the other type of choice condition	2.7	2.9	1.9	1.2	2.0	1.5
Emotional response	4.7	1.0	6.3	1.5	6.0	1.5
Decision confidence	8.7	0.6	7.3	1.9	7.5	1.8
Condition 2: Informed parents' choice (amputate)						
Prefer my choice condition	3.4	1.8	2.1	1.7	2.5	1.8
Prefer the other type of choice condition	6.4	2.8	7.9	1.3	7.4	2
Emotional response	6.6	1.3	7.9	0.6	7.5	1.0
Decision confidence	2.2	1.8	4.8	2.0	3.9	2.3
Condition 3: Informed parents' choice (not amputate)						
Prefer my choice condition	3.6	2.8	3.0	2.4	3.3	2.6
Prefer the other type of choice condition	5.0	3.5	7.6	1.7	6.1	3.2
Emotional response	4.6	2.1	5.6	1.7	5.0	2.0
Decision confidence	6.2	3.1	7.1	1.8	6.6	2.7
Condition 4: Uninformed parents' choice (amputate)						
Prefer my choice condition	3.3	3.2	2.5	1.9	2.8	2.4
Prefer the other type of choice condition	6.5	3.3	7.6	1.6	7.3	2.3
Emotional response	6.0	1.3	7.5	0.9	7.0	1.3
Decision confidence	3.3	2.6	4.7	2.5	4.3	2.6

[a]On a scale from 1, *not at all*, to 9, *extremely*.
[b]For participants who made their own choice (Condition 1), switching to parents' choice (Condition 2, 3 and 4) and vice versa.
[c]Average of five negative emotions (nervous, upset, unhappy, concerned, guilty), each reported on a scale from 1, *not at all*, to 9, *extremely*.

frequency format to make them easier for children to understand [15].

In Condition 1 (own informed choice), participants were asked to decide whether to amputate their leg. In Condition 2 (informed parents' choice), participants' parents made the decision to amputate the leg. In Condition 3 (informed parents' opposite choice), participants' parents made the decision not to amputate but to continue the treatment. In Condition 4 (uninformed parents' choice), the doctor did not mention the option to continue the treatment nor the outcome probabilities associated with the two alternatives, and the decision to amputate the leg was made by the parents.

After hearing the scenario, each group completed a questionnaire, almost identical to the one administrated by Botti et al. [6]. Only participants in Condition 1 (own informed choice) were asked for their decision on whether to amputate the leg and their reasons for their choice. Participants in all conditions were asked to indicate to what extent each of five negative emotions (nervous, upset, unhappy, concerned, guilty) described how they felt about the treatment decision on a scale from 1, *not at all*, to 9, *extremely*. (We left out one of the emotional states from the original

questionnaire, "distressed," as in Italian the two words for "distressed" and "concerned" are hard to tell apart). Next, participants had to indicate how confident they were that the best decision had been made on a scale from 1, *not at all*, to 9, *extremely*. The final two questions measured participants' preference for decision autonomy. Participants in Condition 1 (own informed choice) were asked how much they liked having to make the decision and how much they would have preferred that their parents made the decision for them. Participants in Conditions 2, 3, and 4 (informed parents' choice, informed parents' opposite choice, uninformed parents' choice) were asked how much they liked not having to make the decision and how much they would rather have made the choice themselves. The response scale for both questions ranged from 1 (*not at all*) to 9 (*extremely*).

A similar scenario and questionnaire was piloted with 128 participants from six classes and two different schools in Livorno, Italy: 63 children aged 9–10 years ($M_{age} = 9.5$ years, $SD = 0.6$), and 65 young students aged 14–16 years ($M_{age} = 15.0$ years, $SD = 0.8$). The pilot was followed by a spontaneous discussion in class, aimed at testing participants' understanding of the scenario, of the consequences of the actions presented in the scenario, and of the questions included in the questionnaire.

Results

Choice taken

Eighty-seven percent of the adolescents chose not to amputate, whereas only 27% of the children chose not to amputate, $\chi^2(1,27) = 10.1$, $p = 0.001$. 36% of the children (25% of which had chosen to amputate) and 41% of the adolescents (86% of which had chosen not to amputate) did not provide a reason for their choices. Most of the participants who provided a reason for their choices referred only to the anticipated outcomes of their choice. All participants who chose to amputate said that they would rather avoid suffering. Participants who decided not to amputate argued that they did not want to give up hope of once again being able to run, walk or do sport. Only few adolescents (N = 5) mentioned in their comments the information about the alternative outcomes presented in the scenario: "Even though the chances are low, they are there"

Preference for autonomy

A univariate analysis of variance (ANOVA) indicated a main effect of condition on how much participants liked being assigned to the condition they were in, $F(3,137) = 16.2$, $p<0.001$, $\eta^2 = 0.3$. A Bonferroni post hoc analysis confirmed that participants in Condition 1 (own informed choice) preferred to make the decision themselves more than participants in Conditions 2, 3, and 4 (parents' choice) preferred not to make the decision ($p<0.001$, Table 1). Post-hoc analyses (with Bonferroni correction) did not reveal any difference between Conditions 2, 3 and 4. Also, we found no differences between age groups or interaction effects.

An ANOVA with the choice made in Condition 1 as independent variable, confirmed that preference for autonomy was also not influenced by the choice made by participants in Condition 1, $p = .329$, nor by the age group, $p = .933$. The analysis did not reveal any interaction effect.

An ANOVA on how much participants wanted to change from their assigned condition to another condition indicated a main effect of condition, $F(3,137) = 20.6$, $p<0.001$, $\eta^2 = 0.30$. Bonferroni post hoc analyses showed that participants assigned to Conditions 2, 3, and 4, where parents made the choice, were significantly more likely to want to change their condition than those in Condition 1 (own informed choice; $p<0.001$, Table 1). No significant differences emerged between conditions 2, 3 and 4 (all $ps>0.05$).

The analysis also showed a main effect of age, $F(1,137) = 4.9$, $p = 0.029$, $\eta^2 = 0.04$: Children, overall, were less likely to desire to change condition than adolescents. Moreover, we found an Age × Condition interaction, $F(3,137) = 3.37$, $p = 0.020$, $\eta^2 = 0.07$. Children in Condition 1 (own informed choice) were more willing to leave the decision to their parents than the adolescents in Condition 1, whereas adolescents in Conditions 2, 3, and 4 (where parents made the choice) were more interested than the children in being transferred to Condition 1. All post hoc analyses revealed no difference between Conditions 2, 3, and 4 ($p>0.1$): Providing information about the alternatives to parents as decision makers did not affect the preference for autonomy for either age group.

An ANOVA with the choice made in Condition 1 as independent variable, confirmed that willingness to change to a more autonomous condition was also not influenced by the choice made by participants in Condition 1, $p = .557$, nor by the age group, $p = .456$. The analysis did not reveal any interaction effect.

Emotional response

We collapsed the participants' emotion ratings (nervous, upset, unhappy, concerned, guilty; Overall $\alpha = 0.77$; Children $\alpha = 0.68$; Adolescents $\alpha = 0.77$) into one negative emotion score and conducted an ANOVA with condition and age as the independent variables. This analysis revealed the two main effects of condition, $F(3,137) = 14.2$, $p<0.001$, $\eta^2 = 0.25$, and age, $F(3,137) = 23.1$, $p< 0.001$, $\eta^2 = 0.15$. As can be seen in Table 1, participants in Conditions 1 and 3 expressed significantly fewer negative emotions than participants in the other two conditions. All post hoc analyses revealed significant differences ($p<0.001$) between Condition 1 or 3 and Condition 2 or 4, whereas the emotional responses did not differ between Conditions 1 and 3 ($p = 0.789$) or between Conditions 2 and 4 ($p = 0.731$). Overall children reported fewer negative emotions than adolescents (see Table 1).

Decision confidence

Regarding the participants' confidence that the best decision had been made, we found the two significant main effects of condition, $F(3,137) = 14.5$, $p<0.001$, $\eta^2 = 0.25$, and age, $F(3,137) = 7.2$, $p = 0.0008$, $\eta^2 = 0.05$. As displayed in Table 1, participants in Conditions 1 and 3 exhibited significantly higher confidence that the choice made was the best one compared to participants in Conditions 2 and 4. A Bonferroni post hoc analysis showed significant differences ($p<0.001$) between Condition 1 or 3 and Condition 2 or 4, and no differences between Conditions 1 and 3 ($p = 0.805$) or between Conditions 2 and 4 ($p = 0.956$). Children's confidence was overall lower than that of adolescents (see Table 1).

Preference for autonomy or treatment choice?

The above analyses indicate children's and adolescents' emotional responses and decision confidence was affected by which choice condition they were assigned to (own choice, parents' choice), but also by the treatment choice (amputation, no amputation, including participants in Condition 1). We conducted two sets of hierarchical linear regression analyses to assess the influence of these two components (choice condition and treatment choice) on the dependent variables emotional response and decision confidence while controlling for (potential) age differences. Step 1 of the hierarchical linear regression analysis contained the independent variables choice condition (own vs. parents' choice), treatment choice (no amputation vs. amputation) and age group (children vs. adolescents). Step 2 additionally contained the interactions of Choice Condition × Age Group and Treatment Choice × Age Group.

As shown in Table 2, both age group and treatment choice significantly predicted emotional response, $F(3, 135) = 20.91$, $p< .001$. Adolescents reported more negative emotional responses than children. Participants who decided to amputate reported significantly more negative emotional responses. Choice condition did not significantly predict emotional response. Regression model 2, which included the variables choice condition, treatment choice, and age group as well as the interaction terms of Choice Condition × Age group and Treatment Choice × Age Group did not lead to a significant change in R^2 compared to regression model 1, $\Delta R^2 = .02$, $\Delta F(2, 133) = 2.01$, $p = .14$ (Table 2). Therefore, the marginally significant interaction of Choice Condition × Age group was not further investigated.

Table 3 shows the results of the regression analyses for the dependent variable decision confidence. Regression model 1 revealed that both choice condition and treatment choice, but not age group, significantly predicted decision confidence, $F(3, 134) = 13.13$, $p<.001$. Participants who made their own choice

Table 2. Results of Hierarchical Regression Analysis Predicting Emotional Response.

	Emotional response	
Independent variables	β	ΔR^2, ΔF, df, p
Step 1		.32, 20.91, 3, .001
Choice condition	.13	
Treatment choice	.34**	
Age group	.41**	
Step 2		.02, 2.01, 2, .14
Choice condition	.14	
Treatment choice	.38**	
Age group	.96*	
Choice condition × Age group	−.69†	
Treatment choice × Age group	.12	

†p<.10 * p<.05, ** p<.01.

were more confident about their decision. Furthermore, those who chose not to amputate showed higher decision confidence. Regression model 2, which additionally contained the interaction variables of Choice Condition × Age group and Treatment Choice × Age led to a significant change in R^2 compared to regression model 1, $\Delta R^2 = .04$, $\Delta F(2, 132) = 3.66$, $p = .03$. Table 3 shows that participants who made their own choice, those who chose not to amputate, and adolescents showed higher decision confidence. The interaction of Choice Condition × Age Group additionally predicted decision confidence. Subsequent regression analyses of the effect of choice condition on decision confidence within each age group showed that while participants in both age groups felt more confident in the own choice than parents' choice conditions, this difference was significant for adolescents, â = −.25, $t(73) = 2.21$, $p = .03$, but not for children, â = .23, $t(61) = 1.82$, $p = .10$ (see Figure 1).

Discussion

The United Nations Convention on the Rights of the Child, the US Supreme Court, and, most importantly, the medical establishment, at least in the United States, have all come to recognize the importance of giving minors a say in making medical decisions. So far, researchers have tended to focus on the relationship between minors' cognitive abilities and decision competence [5], [2], [4]. With few exceptions (see[16]), what has been missing is insight into whether children and adolescents want to be involved in the process of making decisions about their medical treatment even when those decisions are difficult and might be emotionally taxing for them.

Our data clearly indicate that children and adolescents want to be involved in the decision process, even when the outcome involves serious negative consequences. Participants preferred making the decision themselves rather than having an authority figure (a parent) decide for them. Desire for autonomy was independent of the decision made by parents (i.e., amputate in

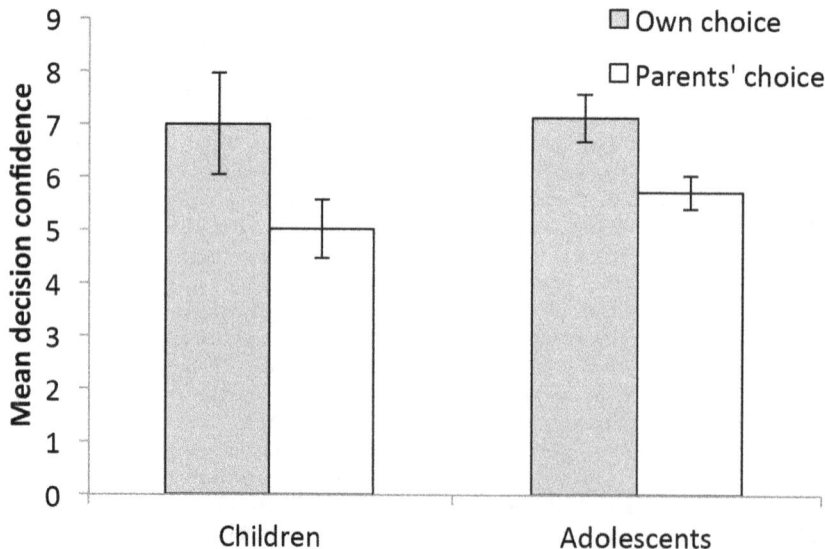

Figure 1. Mean decision confidence as a function of choice condition and age group. Error bars display standard errors.

Table 3. Results of Hierarchical Regression Analysis Predicting Decision Confidence.

Independent variables	Decision Confidence	
	β	ΔR^2, ΔF, df, p
Step 1		.23, 13.13, 3, .001
Choice condition	−.20*	
Treatment choice	−.40**	
Age group	.14	
Step 2		.04, 3.65, 2, .03
Choice condition	−.25**	
Treatment choice	−.48**	
Age group	.97*	
Choice condition × Age group	−.92*	
Treatment choice × Age group	.27	

* $p<.05$, ** $p<.01$.

Condition 2 vs. not amputate in Condition 3) and of the decision made by participants in Condition 1 (i.e., whether to amputate or not). As hypothesized (Hypothesis 1), this willingness to make autonomous decisions and not to let parents make the choice was stronger for adolescents than children. Our findings, thus, are nicely aligned with results of previous developmental research showing adolescents' greater desire for autonomous decision making in more everyday contexts with less difficult outcomes (e.g.,[9], [10]). Adolescents might feel that they are grown up and as such deserve to be independent and are entitled to decide about their own medical treatment.

In Condition 1, most of the adolescents (87%) chose not to amputate, whereas only 27% of the children chose not to amputate. This was an unexpected result. Children consistently reported to be worried about feeling pain for their entire life if they do not amputate. This was the only other alternative to amputation mentioned by the doctor in the given scenario. Because the doctor is an expert adult, it is not too surprising that children believed that the given alternatives were the only two available and decided to avoid the possibility of future pain and amputate. They might even have perceived that the doctor was indirectly suggesting that it would have been better to amputate, because he presented the other alternative as very unattractive. Indeed, two children explicitly mentioned that "this is what the doctor would do". Adolescents, in contrast, reported that they "did not want to give up" and to "believe there was still hope of saving the leg without necessarily having to suffer in the future", even though this possibility was not mentioned by the doctor in the scenario.

This result might relate to adolescents' well-documented illusion of invincibility [17]. Invincibility is a typical phase of social and cognitive development of adolescence that peaks in early adolescence and is dominated by egocentric thinking, a side effect of the teen's search for identity. Teens believe that they are the focus of everyone's attention and are constantly being evaluated by others. This belief further engenders feelings of uniqueness, as teens perceive their feelings and experiences as exceptional and not subject to the laws governing others' lives, and promote the illusion of being special and invulnerable to the consequences of dangerous or risky behavior [18], [19]. Such illusion and feeling of uniqueness might help explaining why adolescents, ignoring the

options given by the doctor, thought there was still a chance for them to save their legs without having to suffer pain forever.

We know that adolescents are very accurate and predictive when they make probability judgments for a number of significant life events, except for judging the probability of dying prematurely [20], [21]. What about children's and adolescents' ability to forecast their emotional reactions to difficult choices? Even though there has been a growing interest in adults' ability to forecast their emotional responses to various health decisions and conditions [22], [23], to our knowledge, this line of investigation has not been applied to minors (see [24]). Botti et al. [6] proposed that personal responsibility was associated with greater negative emotional responses (Hypothesis 2). However, we found that participants in Condition 1 (own informed choice) reported similar negative emotions to those of participants in Condition 3 (informed parents' choice to continue treatment), and lower negative emotional responses than participants in Conditions 2 and 4 (informed parents' choice to amputate; uninformed parents' choice to amputate). In this sense, it is evident that the choice condition alone is not enough to predict participants' emotional responses, but the decision outcome (amputate vs. not amputate) has to be considered as well. Indeed, participants reported lower negative emotional responses when the decision choice was "no amputation". Future research might systematically vary the seriousness of the decision outcome and investigate its effect on emotional responses.

Treatment choice (amputate vs. not amputate) also affected decision confidence, and our results support both Hypotheses 3a and 3b: Participants reported higher confidence that the right decision has been made when they themselves (versus the parents) made the decision. Furthermore, those who chose not to amputate expressed higher decision confidence.

Moreover, children's decision confidence was overall lower than that of adolescents, and they also reported fewer negative emotions than adolescents. A possible interpretation of these results is that children are less able than adolescents to project how they would feel, that is, to form a counterfactual scenario of how it would feel to have lost a leg or live with pain (see[25], [26]).

In contrast to Botti et al.'s findings [6], we also found that not providing information about the alternatives at stake (in Condition 4 compared to Condition 2) did not affect participants' responses (see Hypothesis 4). These results might be due to children's and adolescents' inability to conceptualize and utilize the information provided. This result reinforces the need to design health and risk communications in a transparent and easy-to-understand way for patients of all ages [27]–[29].

Our study is not without limitations. First, our sample is one of convenience and the study was conducted at school rather than in a clinic or in a hospital. Second, the scenarios presented to children were hypothetical by nature and only focused on a single health related problem. It is unclear whether our results are robust enough to generalize to other health issues such as diabetes or cancer. While future studies should examine clinical samples, our novel results, nonetheless, highlight the need to further explore children's and adolescents' desire to be actively involved in their health decision making.

In conclusion, our results suggest that age and cognitive competence are not the only factors that should be taken into account when considering whether minors *deserve* a voice in medical decision making. Children and adolescents want to be involved in medical decisions, even when the choice is a difficult one. A future direction would be to investigate how medical decisions are and should be *negotiated* within families, for example, to minimize the negative emotional impact the choice and the choice outcomes have on all family members. This line of research would tap not only into the literature on shared decision making about health [30]–[32], but also into the more recent studies reporting systematic differences between the treatment choice one recommends for another person vs. makes for oneself (see [23], [33]). How can we better involve minors and their families in the process of making medical decisions?

Acknowledgments

Thanks to Claudia Mazzeranghi and Marianna Sgherri for collecting the data, and to the teachers of the participating schools for their support. Thanks to Nicolai Bodemer and Anita Todd for their useful comments and feedbacks.

Author Contributions

Conceived and designed the experiments: AR MG YH. Performed the experiments: AR. Analyzed the data: AR MG. Wrote the paper: AR MG YH.

References

1. Lansdown G (2005) The evolving capacities of the child. UNICEF.
2. McCabe MA (1996) Involving children and adolescents in medical decision making: Developmental and clinical considerations. J Pediatr Psychol 21: 505–516. doi:10.1093/jpepsy/21.4.505
3. Hickey K (2007) Minors' rights in medical decision making. JONA's Healthcare Law, Ethics, and Regulation 9: 100–104.
4. Wadlington W (1994) Medical decision making for and by children: Tensions between parent, state, and child. University of Illinois Law Review 2: 311–336.
5. Kuther TL (2003) Medical decision-making and minors: Issues of consent and assent. Adolescence 38: 343–358.
6. Botti S, Orfali K, Iyengar SS (2009) Tragic choices: Autonomy and emotional responses to medical decisions. J Consum Res 36: 337–352. doi:10.1086/598969
7. Danne T, Lange K, Kordonouri O (2007) New developments in the treatment of type 1 diabetes in children. Arch Dis Child 92: 1015–1019. doi:10.1136/adc.2006.094904
8. Steinberg LD (2010) Adolescence: New York: McGraw-Hill.
9. Zimmer-Gembeck MJ, Collins WA (2003) Autonomy development during adolescence. In Adams GR & Berzonsky MD, editors. Blackwell handbook of adolescence, 175–204. Malden, MA: Blackwell.
10. Smetana JG, Asquith P (1994) Adolescents' and parents' conceptions of parental authority and personal autonomy. Child Dev 65: 1147–1162. doi:10.1111/j.1467-8624.1994.tb00809.x
11. Lewis CC (1981) How adolescents approach decisions: Changes over grades seven to twelve and policy implications. Chid Dev 52: 538–544. doi:10.1111/j.1467-8624.1981.tb03078.x
12. Laupa M (1995) Children's reasoning about authority in home and school contexts. Soc Dev 4: 1–16. doi:10.1111/j.1467-9507.1995.tb00047.x
13. Helwig CC, Arnold ML, Tan D, Boyd D (2003) Chinese adolescents' reasoning about democratic and authority-based decision making in peer, family, and school contexts. Child Dev 74: 783–800. doi:10.1111/1467-8624.00568
14. Helwig CC, Kim S (1999) Children's evaluations of decision-making procedures in peer, family, and school contexts. Child Dev 70: 502–512. doi:10.1111/1467-8624.00036
15. Zhu L, Gigerenzer G (2006) Children can solve Bayesian problems: The role of representation in mental computation. Cognition 98: 287–308. doi:10.1016/j.cognition.2004.12.003
16. Lyon ME, McCabe MA, Patel KM, D'Angelo LJ (2004) What do adolescents want? An exploratory study regarding end-of-life decision-making. J Adolescent Health: official publication of the Society for Adolescent Medicine 35: 529.e1–6. doi:10.1016/j.jadohealth.2004.02.009
17. Elkind D (1970) Children and adolescents: Interpretive essays on Jean Piaget. New York: Oxford University Press.
18. Donovan RJ, Henley N, Jalleh G, Slater C (1995) Road safety advertising: An empirical study and literature review. Canberra, Australia: Donovan Research Federal Office of Road Safety.
19. Henley N, Donovan RJ (2003) Young people's response to death threat appeals: Do they really feel immortal? Health Educ Res 18: 1–14.
20. de Bruin WB, Parker AM, Fischhoff B (2007) Can adolescents predict significant life events? J Adolescent Health 41: 208–210.
21. Fischhoff B, Bruine de Bruin W, Parker AM, Millstein SG, Halpern-Felsher BL (2010) Adolescents' Perceived Risk of Dying. J Adolescent Health 46: 265–269. doi:10.1016/j.jadohealth.2009.06.026
22. Halpern J, Arnold RM (2008) Affective forecasting: An unrecognized challenge in making serious health decisions. J Gen Intern Med 23: 1708–1712. doi:10.1007/s11606-008-0719-5
23. Ubel PA, Loewenstein G, Schwarz N, Smith D (2005) Misimagining the unimaginable: The disability paradox and health care decision making. Health Psychol 24:(Suppl), S57–S62. doi:10.1037/0278-6133.24.4.S57
24. Albert D, Steinberg L (2011) Judgment and decision making in adolescence. J Res Adolescence 21: 211–224. doi:10.1111/j.1532-7795.2010.00724.x
25. Guttentag R, Ferrell J (2004) Reality compared with its alternatives: Age differences in judgments of regret and relief. Dev Psychol 40: 764–775. doi:10.1037/0012-1649.40.5.764
26. Guttentag R, Ferrell J (2008) Children's understanding of anticipatory regret and disappointment. Cognition Emotion 22: 815–832. doi:10.1080/02699930701541542
27. Gigerenzer G (2011) Better doctors, better patients, better decisions: Envisioning health care 2020. Cambridge, MA: MIT Press.
28. Gigerenzer G, Gaissmaier W, Kurz-Milcke E, Schwartz LM, Woloshin S (2007) Helping doctors and patients make sense of health statistics. Psychol Sci Publ Interest 8: 53–96. doi:10.1111/j.1539-6053.2008.00033.x
29. Bodemer N, Gaissmaier W (2012) Risk communication in health. In S. . Roeser, R. . Hillerbrand, P. . Sandin, & M. . Peterson, editors. Handbook of risk theory. 621–660. Dordrecht, the Netherlands: Springer Netherlands.
30. Edwards A, Elwyn G (2009) Shared decision-making in health care: Achieving evidence-based patient choice. Oxford, England: Oxford University Press.
31. Feufel MA, Bodemer N (2012) Finding the right tool to improve health decisions: Nudging, social marketing, empowerment? Manuscript submitted for publication.
32. McNutt RA (2004) Shared medical decision making: Problems, process, progress. JAMA-J Am Med Assoc 292: 2516–2518. doi:10.1001/jama.292.20.2516
33. Zikmund-Fisher BJ, Sarr B, Fagerlin A, Ubel PA (2006) A matter of perspective: choosing for others differs from choosing for yourself in making treatment decisions. J Gen Intern Med 21: 618–22. doi:10.1111/j.1525-1497.2006.00410.x

13

Depression and Health Related Quality of Life in Adolescent Survivors of a Traumatic Brain Injury

Ashley Di Battista[1,2,3]*, **Celia Godfrey**[3], **Cheryl Soo**[3], **Cathy Catroppa**[1,3,5], **Vicki Anderson**[1,3,4,5]

1 School of Behavioural Science, University of Melbourne, Melbourne, Australia, 2 Department of Psychology, The Hospital for Sick Children, Toronto, Ontario, Canada, 3 Clinical Sciences, Murdoch Children's Research Institute, Royal Children's Hospital, Melbourne, Australia, 4 Psychology, Royal Children's Hospital, Melbourne, Australia, 5 Department of Paediatrics, University of Melbourne, Melbourne, Australia

Abstract

Traumatic brain injury is (TBI) a leading cause of morbidity and mortality in youth. Adult survivors of a severe pediatric TBI are vulnerable to global impairments, including greater employment difficulties, poor quality of life (HRQoL) and increased risk of mental health problems. When estimating the health related quality of life in adolescents, the presence of anxiety and depression and the quality of social relationships are important considerations, because adolescents are entrenched in social development during this phase of maturation. The influence of anxiety, depression and loneliness on health related quality of life in adolescent survivors of TBI has not been documented. This pilot study aimed to identify and measure the relationship between anxiety, depression and loneliness and perceived health related quality of life in adolescent survivors of a TBI. Method: mixed method/cohort pilot study (11 adolescents, mild to severe TBI; 9 parents), using self-report and proxy-report measures of anxiety, depression, health related quality of life, loneliness and clinical psychiatric interviews (adolescent only). Results: Self-reported depression was significantly correlated with self-reported HRQoL (rs [11] = −0.88, $p<0.001$). Age at injury was significantly correlated with self-reported HRQoL (rs [11] = −0.68, $p = 0.02$). Self-reported depression predicted self-reported HRQoL ($R^2 = 0.79$, F [1,10] = 33.48, $p<0.001$), but age at injury did not ($R^2 = 0.19$, F [1,10] = 2.09, $p = 0.18$). Conclusions: Our results suggest that depression is a predictor of health related quality of life in youth post-TBI. The possibility of using targeted assessment and therapy for depression post-TBI to improve health related quality of life should be explored.

Editor: Amanda Bruce, University of Missouri-Kansas City, United States of America

Funding: Funding provided by Victorian Government Operational Infrastructure Scheme, Victorian Neurotrauma Initiative – fellowship to CS, Australian National Health & Medical Research Council – fellowships to VA and CC and Canadian Institutes of Health Research – Doctoral Research Award to AD. This research was supported in part by grants from the Canadian Institutes of Health Research (CIHR) Doctoral Research Award (DRA), Canada – awarded to ADB, and the Victorian Government Operations Infrastructure Funding, Australia. The funders had no role in study design, data collection and analysis, decision to publish, or preparation of the manuscript.

Competing Interests: The authors have declared that no competing interests exist.

* Email: ashley.dibattista@sickkids.ca

Introduction

Traumatic brain injury (TBI) is a leading cause of morbidity and mortality in children and adolescents in first world nations [1]. In recent years there has been a move towards assessing sequelae of TBI beyond cognitive domains, including quality of life (HRQoL) and mood disorders, such as ADHD, depression and anxiety post-injury [2]. Research from our team investigating adult survivors of pediatric TBI has reported that survivors of severe TBI are particularly vulnerable to global functional impairments, including poorer school performance, greater employment difficulties, poor HRQoL and increased risk of mental health problems [3]. However, the majority of research into pediatric and adolescent TBI outcomes in the psychosocial domain focuses on parent or clinician proxy assessment. The appropriateness of proxy reporting for internalizing conditions, such as quality of life (QoL), depression and anxiety has been criticized for many years in the broader psychology literature

[4,5], yet parental proxy reporting remains the most often used method of assessment for these states in the pediatric TBI field [6].

Epidemiology: Anxiety, Depression and HRQoL

Anxiety disorders are the most commonly diagnosed mental disorders in childhood and adolescence [7]. There is a high point prevalence of depression in otherwise healthy adolescents, with estimates as high as 6% [8]. In addition, there is a strong co morbidity between depression and anxiety, with reported co morbidity as high as 90% in those with an already diagnosed anxiety disorder experiencing a concurrent depressive episode [9].

The recent systematic review of HRQoL in pediatric survivors of a TBI [6] highlighted that all of the data available on pediatric HRQoL post-TBI are dependent on proxy reporting (clinician or physician), and adhere to the HRQoL paradigm, most frequently employing the Pediatric Quality of Life Inventory (PedsQL 4.0; [10]). Our systematic review [6] also found that good outcomes were contingent on milder injuries, proxy reporting and early assessment whereas poor outcomes occurred in the context of more severe injuries and later assessment (≤6 months vs. ≥1 year post-trauma, respectively). Recent work from our group has identified that the relationship between parental report and self-report in adolescent HRQoL ratings is poor and caution needs to be taken when interpreting HRQoL data derived from solely parent proxy sources [11].

Current Research in Adolescent Anxiety, Depression and HRQoL

The small body of literature on affective symptomatology and disorders following pediatric TBI has begun to describe elevated levels of anxiety and depression following brain injury in both children and adolescents [12–16]. These data, however, are plagued by methodological constraints, most notably the use of parent-proxy observers to rate anxiety and depression symptoms [4,5]. The few studies that have used diagnostic interview or self-report scales suggest a link between TBI, anxiety and depression [2,14–17]. Recent data [2] have also identified the development of novel definite or subclinical anxiety disorders in children during the first six months after a TBI, but no information is available on later time points (e.g. beyond the relatively acute post-injury period of 6 months), or for older adolescents. The limited data are consistent with adult TBI literature which shows linkages between brain injury and the development of new onset disorders or persistence and worsening of pre-existing anxious or depressive conditions [18,19].

Methodological Constraints – Concordance between Self-Report and Parent Proxies on Measures of Anxiety, Depression and HRQoL

The concordance between self-report and proxy-reporting of anxiety and depressive symptomatology reflects similar findings to those reported in the HRQoL literature. A meta-analysis of 119 studies by Acenbach, McConaughy and Howell [20] assessed the consistency between ratings of behavioral and emotional problems from various proxies, including parents, teachers, mental health workers, observers and peers and their child/adolescent counterpart. Overall correlations were higher for younger children with proxy reporting, but decreased with adolescents. The authors suggested that, given the overall modest correlations between proxies and children and adolescents, the process of using proxy reports are ineffective and promoted use of multiple sources to achieve the best possible ratings [20]. Kazdin, Esveldt-Dawson, Unis & Rancurello [21] have also reported little or no relationship between mother or father proxy reports and that of their children on measures of depression.

Social Relationships in Adolescence – Impact on Anxiety, Depression and HRQoL

When estimating HRQoL and internalizing behaviours in adolescents, the quality of social relationships and friendships is an important consideration because adolescence is a period of intense and rapid social development. Adolescents are particularly sensitive to social comparison and concerns regarding their status among peers [22,23]. Depression, anxiety and low self-esteem have been associated with peer difficulties during childhood and adolescence [24,25]. Anxiety in children and adolescence has been linked to peer rejection [26]. The impact of loneliness on the adolescent post-TBI may be even more problematic when young people experience social withdrawal due to cognitive difficulties (e.g. remedial classes), social interaction problems (e.g. behavioural sequelae post-trauma) or functional impairments that limit interaction with others at school and leisure (e.g. motor co-ordination problems, speech impairment, etc). The compounding effects of cognitive, behavioural and social difficulties in adolescents post TBI [26,27] make this group especially vulnerable to anxiety and depression and predictors of these affective conditions warrant investigation.

The aim of this study was to explore the role of anxiety, depression and loneliness and their association with perceived HRQoL in adolescent survivors of a TBI. The concordance between parent proxy and adolescent self-report on measures of anxiety, depression and HRQOL was also explored.

We hypothesized that: 1.Self-reported anxiety and or depression would be related to poorer self-reported HRQoL; 2. that loneliness would be associated with greater depression and anxiety, as well as poorer HRQoL ratings from adolescents; 3.there would be poor concordance between all proxy and self-report measurements on the self-reported and parent proxy reported anxiety, depression and QoL measures.

Methods

Ethics Statement

The study was approved by the Royal Children's Hospital (RCH) Human Research Ethics Committee on 11 January, 2011. HREC 30198 A, Quality of life in adolescents following traumatic brain injury: the impact of anxiety and depression. Date of original approval: 11 January 2011. Duration: 36 months. Date of approval expiry: 11 January 2014. Please note that this application was recommended for Chairman's approval (expedited review). All Chair approvals are ratified at the subsequent Human Research Ethics Committee (HREC) meeting. In the interim, the HREC require the approved materials to be used, as listed on the attached Approval Certificate. The Royal Children's Hospital Human Research Ethics Committee (RCH HREC) is constituted in according to the National Health and Medical Research Council's 'National Statement on Ethical Conduct in Human Research (2007). The committee operates in accordance with these guidelines and is registered with the NHMRC.

All participants were required to provide written consent to participate in the study, in the form of a signed consent letter (parents and/or legal guardians) and assent forms for adolescents. All participants in this study provided written informed consent from parents or guardians on behalf of the minors/children enrolled in this study.

Procedure

Potential participants were identified via: 1. clinical audits of admission to the Emergency Department; 2. private referrals; 3. participants previously enrolled in other studies who agreed to future contact about upcoming studies conducted at RCH.

Assessments were conducted at the RCH in outpatient clinics, in a private room. Parents were asked to complete parent versions of questionnaires while they were waiting for the young people to complete the assessment. For older participants who did not attend with a parent (e.g. 18 years and older) questionnaires were supplied to the adolescent to give to their parent. Completion of parental questionnaires was not mandatory for participants aged 18 and over. For those families who agreed but could not attend RCH for the assessment (n = 1), questionnaire packages were mailed to the home, along with consent forms to sign and return (with a postage paid return envelope provided). Rural participants who could not attend RCH (n = 1) were also offered the opportunity to conduct the clinical interview (K-SADS, SCID; see measures section) over the telephone.

Participants

A total of 581 patients were identified via two clinical audits and private referrals (see Figure 1). Correcting for duplicate and non-TBI entries, a total of 153 were deemed eligible to contact, based on the inclusion criteria. In accordance with ethics approval and associated Australian privacy laws, a tracing letter and follow up phone call were provided to all 153 families. Two families were excluded due to difficulties with English language identified via phone call. A total of 106 potential participants could not be contacted (e.g. outdated phone number, outdated address). Of the remaining 47 eligible families, 27 families declined participation. No reasons were provided. Twenty families consented to participate. Of these, 7 did not attend. Two participants were fully assessed but later excluded from analyses, due to etiological and methodological issues. One participant was excluded after assessment due to etiology of trauma (acquired brain injury (ABI) via tumor, not TBI; incorrect documentation) and one participant was excluded due to the time since injury, which was double that of the other participants (16 years post trauma) and represented a significant outlier in terms of time since injury. As a result, a total of 11 full cases were analyzed. Nine parents participated in the assessment, rendering a total final sample of n = 20. Attrition analyses revealed no significant differences between participants and non-participants on TBI severity X^2 (1, N = 152) = 1.60, $p = 0.21$, age at injury X^2(4, N = 152) = 2.27, $p = 0.69$ or gender X^2 (1, N = 152) = 0.52, p = 0.47.

Inclusion/Exclusion Criteria

Inclusion criteria were: 1). Aged 10–25 years at time of approach and assessment; 2). Diagnosis of TBI, 3). Medical records sufficient to determine injury severity; 4). No pre-injury history of neurological, developmental, or psychiatric disorder; 5). English speaking; 6.) minimum of one year post TBI. Exclusion criteria were: non-English speaking, non-accidental injury, and pre-injury diagnosis of neurological, developmental, or psychiatric disorder, IQ below 70.

Measures

1. DEMOGRAPHICS AND INJURY CHARACTERIS-TICS. Socioeconomic status, age, gender, IQ, age at injury, injury severity and time since injury were collected. IQ was assessed using the two-subtest form of the Wechsler Abbreviated Scale of Intelligence (WASI; [28]). The two-subtest form yields a full scale IQ (FSIQ). Standardized age appropriate norms were recorded. As a result of inconsistent injury severity data recorded in patient medical files, the TBI severity was classified according to the Mayo Classification System for Traumatic Brain Injuries [29]. The Mayo Classification System [29] was used as it was designed to permit TBI severity classifications of injuries in instances where data relating to the injury, e.g. post-traumatic amnesia duration (PTA), loss of consciousness (LOC) duration, etc., may be missing. The Mayo Classification System maximally uses the available information to classify TBIs into the following categories: (a) Moderate-Severe (Definite) TBI, (b) Mild (Probable) TBI, (c) Symptomatic (Possible) TBI.

2. QUESTIONNAIRES. The questionnaires were completed in order to screen for current, point-prevalence (e.g. most recent seven days) of anxiety and depressive symptomatology. Cut off scores (where available) and total scores were used to identify experiences of both anxiety and depression. Individual adolescents were administered all of the self-report measures plus a clinical interview, using the age-appropriate version. Parent proxies completed the CDI, SCARED and PedsQL parent proxy reports.

i. **ANXIETY:** Participants were administered either the Screen for Anxiety Related Disorders (SCARED [30]; ≤18 years old) or the State-Trait Anxiety Inventory (STAI [31]; 19–25 years)

a. The SCARED was administered to those participants who were ≤18 years old. The SCARED is a 41-item self-report questionnaire assessing five domains of anxiety: Generalized Anxiety Disorder, Separation Anxiety Disorder, Social Anxiety Disorder, Significant School Avoidance and Panic Disorder/Significant Somatic Symptoms. A total score is also provided, where scores ≥25 indicate the presence of an anxiety disorder, and those with scores ≥30 are more specific of a disorder. Cut off scores for the SCARED are supplied for a "Total Anxiety" score as well as five subtest: Panic/somatic, general anxiety, separation anxiety, social phobia and school phobia. Cut off scores are those provided by SCARED developers, who generated cut off values for optimal sensitivity and specificity.

b. The STAI was administered to those participants who were aged 19 years and older. The State-Trait Anxiety Inventory Form Y (STAI) clearly differentiates between the temporary condition of "state anxiety" and the more general and long-standing quality of "trait anxiety." The STAI-assesses feelings of apprehension, tension, nervousness, and worry. Individuals respond to each item on a four-point Likert scale, indicating the frequency with which each strategy is used.

ii. **DEPRESSION**– the Child Depression Inventory (CDI [32]; ≤17 years) or the Centre for Epidemiology Studies Depression Scale (CESD [33] 18–25 years).

a. the Child Depression Inventory (CDI) was administered to those participants aged ≤17 years). The CDI is a 27 item self-report questionnaire assessing feelings and thoughts related to depression in the past 2 weeks. Each item consists of three statements that are ranked on a Likert-type scale from 0–2 for severity. Total scores range from 0–54. There are five subscales to the CDI, including: "Negative mood"; "Interpersonal Problems"; "Ineffectiveness"; "Anhedonia"; "Negative Self-Esteem". Cut-off values of raw scores and t-scores are available for the self-report versions of the CDI, but not for the parental proxy. Raw scores ≥19 (t-score ≥65) endorse a clinically significant level of depression.

b. the Centre for Epidemiologic Studies Depression Inventory (CES-D) was administered to those participants aged >17 years. The scale contains 20 questions, and each item is rated on a scale from 0 to 3 on the basis of "how often you have felt this way during the past week": 0 = rarely or none of the time (less than 1 day), 1 = some or a little of the time (1–2 days), 2 = occasionally or a moderate amount of time (3–4 days), and 4 = most or all of the time (5–7 days). Total severity is calculated by summing all of the scores. Scores range from 0 to 60; higher scores indicate more severe depressive symptoms. A cut-off score of 16 is indicative of "significant" or "mild" depressive symptomatology.

iii. **LONELINESS:** Loneliness was assessed using the Peer network and Dyadic Loneliness Scale (PNDLS [34] for adolescents up to 17 years of age, and The Differential

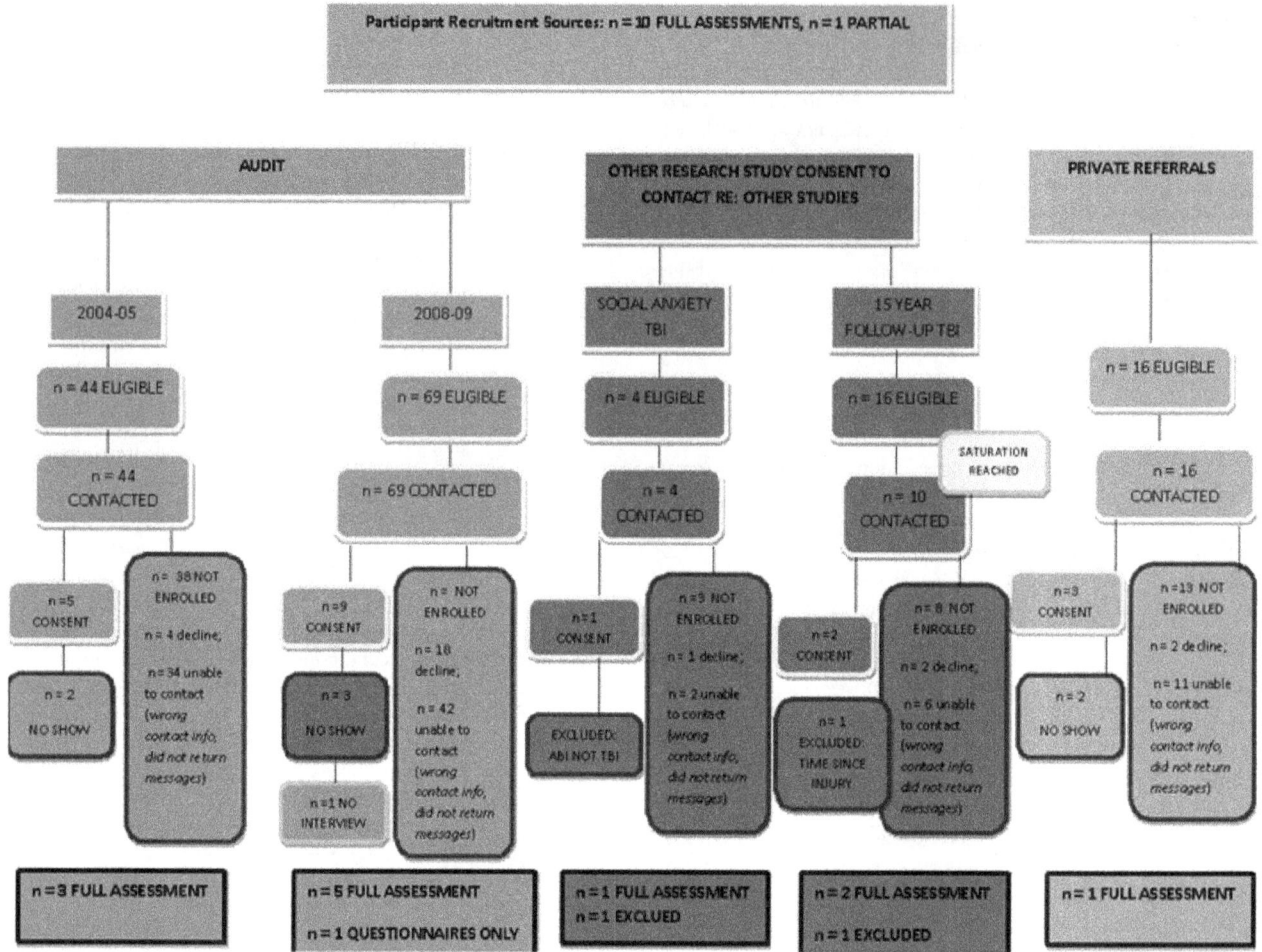

Figure 1. Participant Recruitment and Final Sample Flow Diagram. This figure documents the participant recruitment process, sources, participation and decline rates, accounting for the final sample.

Loneliness Scale for Non-Student Populations [35] were used for those adolescents aged 18 and older.

a. The Peer Network and Dyadic Loneliness Scale (PNDLS) was administered to those adolescents 17 years of age and younger. The PDNLS is a 16 item, four point scale self-report measure. The PNDLS yields two subscale scores, one for peer network loneliness and one for peer dyadic loneliness. Higher scores indicate greater loneliness. Scores are computed for each subscale by summing the child's self-ratings on the eight items comprising the subscale and dividing by eight. Therefore, subscale scores range from 1 (very low loneliness) to 4 (very high loneliness).

b. The Differential Loneliness Scale for Non-Student Populations assesses loneliness in the context of: familial relationships, romantic relationships, friendships, relationships with family and with larger groups. The self-report measure contains 60 true/false questions and was administered to those participants aged 18 and older.

iv. **QUALITY OF LIFE:** Participants (*aged <19 years of* age) and their parents were given the PedsQL 4.0 [10], a self-

report measure to assess current quality of life, or the SF-36 version 2 [36] for participants aged 19–20 years.

a. The PedsQL 4.0 is a 20 item self-report questionnaire that assesses five domains of quality of life: 1.) physical functioning (8 items); 2.) emotional functioning (5 items); 3.) social functioning (5 items); and 4.) school functioning (5 items). Individual scales can be combined to yield 3 summary measures of physical (same as physical functioning scale), psychosocial (emotional, social and school functioning scales) and total health (all 4 scales). Scale scores range from 0 to 100; higher scores connote better quality of life.

b. The SF-36 is a self-report questionnaire that yields 8 scales (and two summary measures), assessing: 1.) physical functioning; 2.) physical role; 3.) bodily pain; 4.) general health; 5.) vitality; 6.) social functioning; 7.) emotional role; and 8.) mental health. The two summary indices separate the physical from the mental component of the health-related HRQoL. In norm-based scoring, each scale was scored to have same average (50) and the same standard deviation (10 points).

v. **DIAGNOSTIC INTERVIEWS:** In addition to self-report measures, clinical interviews were employed to determine lifetime anxiety and or depression. The Kiddie-SADs-Present and Lifetime version (KSADS-PL [37]) was used for those aged 18 and younger and The Structured Clinical Interview for DSM-IV-TR, Research Non-Patient Edition (SCID-R: [38] First, Psitzer, Gibbon, Williams, 1997) was used for participants over the age of 18 years. The original scoring method provided by the developers of the SCID and the KSADS-PL were employed.

a. The Kiddie-Sads-Present and Lifetime version (KSADS-PL) primary diagnoses assessed with the K-SADS-PL include: Major Depression, Dysthymia, Mania, Hypomania, Cyclothymia, Bipolar Disorders, Schizoaffective Disorders, Schizophrenia, Schizophreniform Disorder, Brief Reactive Psychosis, Panic Disorder, Agoraphobia, Separation Anxiety Disorder, Avoidant Disorder of Childhood and Adolescence, Simple Phobia, Social Phobia, Overanxious Disorder, Generalized Anxiety, Obsessive Compulsive Disorder, Attention Deficit Hyperactivity Disorder, Conduct Disorder, Oppositional Defiant Disorder, Enuresis, Encopresis, Anorexia Nervosa, Bulimia, Transient Tic Disorder, Tourette's Disorder, Chronic Motor or Vocal Tic Disorder, Alcohol Abuse, Substance Abuse, Post-Traumatic Stress Disorder, and Adjustment Disorders. Only the modules pertaining to Mood Disorder (Depression and Suicidality) and Anxiety (Panic Disorder, Agoraphobia, Separation Anxiety Disorder, Avoidant Disorder of Childhood and Adolescence, Simple Phobia, Social Phobia, Overanxious Disorder, Generalized Anxiety, Obsessive Compulsive Disorder) were used in the assessment.

b. The Structured Clinical Interview for DSM-IV-TR, Research Non-Patient Edition (SCID-R) is for use in studies in which the subjects are not identified as psychiatric patients (e.g., community surveys, family studies, research in primary care). The diagnostic modules of the SCID-I/NP are the same as those of the SCID-I/P (W/PSYCHOTIC SCREEN); the only difference in the two versions is in the Overview section. In the SCID-I/NP there is no assumption of a chief complaint, and other questions are used to inquire about a history of psychopathology.

Diagnostic interviews were conducted by the lead author, who is a practicing psychologist and holds a Ph.D. in psychology. Participants were coded into de-identified study numbers before interview. The interviewer did not review the details of the case prior to interview, however, the interviewer was not blind to TBI severity or time since injury.

Statistical Analysis

Data acquired were normal, albeit derived from a small sample. Given that the sample size was small non-parametric correlations were used. Correlation analysis of the relationship between self-reported anxiety and or depression on quality of life was conducted using Spearman Rank Correlations. Gender, social economic status, TBI severity, age at injury, time since injury and cognitive functioning were correlated with anxiety, depression, loneliness and HRQoL variables. Concordance between proxy and self reports was conducted via Spearman Rank correlation.

Single factor linear regressions were performed using those independent variables which had strong correlations and effect sizes with the dependant variable (HRQoL) (see Results section). This process of using multiple single independent variable regressions was conducted in order to account for the small sample size (e.g. inefficient power for multiple variable entries) and to determine directionality of relationship versus simple correlations.

As different measures were required for different aged participants, the measures specific to the domain of interest were combined to create grouped variables. In order to ensure that all measures were assigned a value appropriate to a standard metric, all total raw scores were re-coded using the lowest common denominator (LCD). The LCD was calculated and all variables were multiplied by their corresponding value to render each appropriate in the new metric. For example, if measure A was out of 12 and measure B was out of 20 would have resulted in the following calculation: LCD = 60; therefore [(Measure A Total Raw Score * 5)+(Measure B Total Raw Score *3)] = Combined A+ B Measure. The measures were equivalent in terms of domains assessed, thus rendering the measures appropriate to be analyzed together. This process included the following: the SCARED and the STAI were combined to generate a total anxiety measure; the Peds QL was combined with the SF-36, the CDI's (version 1 and 2) and the CESD were combined; the PDNLS and The Differential Loneliness scales were combined.

Frequency of endorsed symptomatology for clinically relevant anxiety and depression (parent proxy and self-reported) are presented in table 1. Parent proxy and self-reported 'good' versus 'poor' quality of life as well as endorsed loneliness rates are also presented in table 1. Life-time history of depression and anxiety are also reported. Life-time history of depression and anxiety are the subject of another companion paper, and so are reported briefly here.

Results

Participant characteristics and injury details for n = 11 participants included in the final analyses are presented in Table 2. Information on TBIs in the group varied, with inconsistent information available across subjects (e.g. missing information on Glasgow Coma Score at scene, no documentation regarding Post-Traumatic Amnesia, etc). Using the Mayo Classification System for Traumatic Brain Injuries, the majority (63.6%) were moderate-severe definite. There were 6 moderate-severe (definite), 3 mild (probable) TBI and 2 symptomatic (possible) TBI in the final analysis. The average age at injury was 12.48 (3.06) years [range: 4.33–16 years]. The average age at assessment was 17.09 (1.81) years [range: 13.92–19.5 years]. The average time since injury at assessment was 4.62 (2.89) years [range: 1.92–10.75 years].

The majority of the sample (64%) was male. The majority of the sample (54.5%) was enrolled in high school at the time of assessment. Three (27.3%) of the participants were enrolled in university studies, one (9.1%) was enrolled in a apprenticeship course, and one (9.1%) was employed in full-time work. The socioeconomic status of the sample (Australian Bureau of Statistics Socio-Economic Indices for Areas; SEIFA 2006 [39]) ranged from the third decile (e.g. lowest 30% of population) with a relative socio-economic disadvantage decile of 6 to the highest possible status (decile = 10; relative socio-economic disadvantage = 10). One participant fell below the 6th decile. The majority of participants (91%) were at or above the 6th decile, with an average decile of 7.8, The FSIQ was available for nine participants; two did not complete the assessment, one as a result

Table 1. Anxiety, Depression and HRQoL Ratings Stratified by Self-Report and Parental Proxy Report.

Sample	Anxiety Clinically Relevant n, (%)	Depression Clinically Relevant n, (%)	Good Overall HRQoL n, (%)	Poor Overall HRQoL n, (%)	Peer Network Loneliness - Lonely n, (%)	Peer Dyadic Loneliness - Lonely n, (%)	Differential Loneliness - Lonely n, (%)
Self-Report, Current Screen	3, (27.2%)	2, (18.2%)	7, (67%)	4, (36.4%)	1, (9.1%)	4, (36.4%)	0, (0%)
Parent Proxy	1, (11.1%)	1, (11.1%)	7 (78.8%)	2, (22.2%)	N/A	N/A	N/A

of completing questionnaire packages and returning them via mail (rural participant) and the other was unable to complete the assessment in the time available. Of the nine participants assessed, the average FSIQ was 104 (15.3), range: 83.3–133.0.

Two of the participants did not have corresponding parental data; all analyses correlating parent and proxy data are based on the n = 9 full data sets.

Lifetime presence of clinically significant anxiety and or depression was assessed in 10 participants (one declined interview). Lifetime anxiety was present in 2 participants, (aged 15 years and 12 years, 3 months respectively at the time of injury). Lifetime depression was present in one participant. The one participant who endorsed previous lifetime depression also experienced co-morbid anxiety. Table 1 outlines the lifetime anxiety and depression reported, via interview, as well as the endorsed self-reported and parent proxy reported anxiety and depression data.

None of the parental proxy and self-report measures were correlated: HRQoL (rs [9] = −0.27, p = 0.49); anxiety (rs [9] = 0.65, p = 0.06); depression (rs = 0.07, p = 0.86).

Self-reported depression was significantly correlated with self-reported HRQoL (rs [11] = −0.88, p<0.001). Loneliness was significantly correlated with anxiety (rs [11] = 0.72, p = 0.01) but not depression (rs [11] = −0.43, p = 0.19) or HRQoL (rs [11] = 0.37, p = 0.27). Self-reported anxiety was not correlated with self-reported HRQoL (rs [11] = −0.02, p = 0.95). FSIQ was not correlated with any of the outcome variables: QoL (rs [9] = −0.49, p = 0.19), depression (rs [9] = −0.63, p = 0.07), anxiety (rs [9] = −0.10, p = 0.81) or loneliness (rs [9] = −0.0, p = 0.99).

Age at injury was significantly correlated with self-reported HRQoL (rs [11] = −0.68, p = 0.02). Age at testing was significantly correlated with self-reported anxiety (rs [11] = −0.66, p = 0.03). Injury severity was not correlated with any of the self-reported outcome variables: anxiety (rs [11] = 0.44, p = 0.18), depression (rs [11] = 0.29, p = 0.39), HRQoL (rs [11] = −0.33, p = 0.32), loneliness (rs [11] = 0.39, p = 0.24), or parent-proxy reported outcome variables: anxiety (rs [9] = 0.52, p = 0.15), depression (rs [9] = 0.38, p = 0.31), or HRQoL (rs [9] = −0.46, p = 0.91). Table 1 outlines the self-reported and proxy ratings of anxiety, depression and HRQoL.

The regression model with a single predictor (self-reported depression) found that self-reported depression predicted self-reported HRQoL (R^2 = 0.79, F [1,10] = 33.48, p<0.001) (see Figure 2). A separate single predictor regression using age at injury found that age at injury was not a significant predictor of self-reported HRQoL (R^2 = 0.19, F [1,10] = 2.09, p = 0.18).

Discussion

Our results suggest that self-reported current depressive symptoms predict self-reported current HRQoL in adolescent survivors of a TBI. Importantly, the causality of the relationship, that is, does depression predict quality of life, or does quality of life predict depression, remains unclear at this stage. What is apparent is the significant relationship between the two domains, and that their potentially synergistic association. This seems so for young people for whom their TBI has caused limitations in activities that had been a big part of the adolescents' life before the injury. For example, one participant expressed grief about no longer being able to ride his bike, which had been an important part of his pre-injury life. There also seemed to be a relationship between what the adolescent had hoped to do in future and an impact on mood, for example, one adolescent was upset at the loss of opportunity to learn how to drive. He was especially sad because his friends were currently meeting this developmental goal without him. While age

Table 2. Participant Demographics and Injury Characteristics.

GENDER	AGE INJURY, AGE AT ASSESSMENT	TIME SINCE INJURY	CAUSE OF INJURY	TYPE OF INJURY	GCS Scene; GCS Lowest	PTA (days, hours)	LOC	SURGICAL INTERVENTION (YES, NO)	CT (Abnormal, Normal)	NEUROLOGICAL SIGNS (present, absent)	TBI SEVERITY
M	16 y, 17 y 9 m	1 yr 11 mo	MVA (occupant)	Acceleration/deceleration	NA; GCS=4	21 DAYS	NA	NO	ABNORMAL	PRESENT	MSD
F	11 y 9 m, 13 y, 11 M	2 yrs 2 mo	Sports-related head collision with stationary object	Direct Impact, head against object. Skull fracture.	NA; GCS=12	24 HOURS	<1 MIN	YES	ABNORMAL	PRESENT	MSD
M	14 y, 10 m 17 y, 1 m	2 yrs 3 mo	Sports-related head collision with ground	Direct impact, head against object	NA; GCS=13	NA	<1 MIN	NO	NORMAL	PRESENT	MP
M	13 y, 3 m 15 y, 5 m	2 yrs 2 mo	Sports-related head collision with ground	Direct impact, head against object	NA; NA	NA	SHORT DURATION	NO	NORMAL	PRESENT	MP
M	12 yrs, 10 mo 17 y	4 yrs 2 mo	MVA (occupant)	Acceleration/deceleration	NA; GCS=3	NA	NA	YES	ABNORMAL	PRESENT	MSD
*F	15 yrs, 0 mo 18 y, 5 m	3 yrs 5 mo	Violence/assault	Direct impact, blow to the head	NA; NA	NA	NA	NO	NORMAL	PRESENT	SP
M	12 yrs, 3 mo 19 y, 2 m	6 yrs 11 mo	Violence/assault	Direct impact, head against object	NA; NA	NA	NA	NO	NORMAL	PRESENT	SP
M	4 yrs, 4 mo 15 y, 1 m	10 yrs 9 mo	MVA (occupant)	Acceleration/deceleration	NA; GCS=7	NA	NA	YES	ABNORMAL	PRESENT	MSD
F	11 yrs, 3 mo 18 y, 6 m	7 yrs 3 mo	MVA (occupant)	Acceleration/deceleration	NA; NA	NA	SHORT DURATION	NO	ABNORMAL	PRESENT	MSD
F	12 yrs, 9 mo 19 y, 6 m	6 yrs 7 mo	MVA (pedestrian)	Direct impact, head against object	NA; GCS=13	NA	NA	NO	ABNORMAL	PRESENT	MSD
M	13 yrs, 0 mo 16 y	3 yrs, 0 mo	Sports-related head collision with ground	Direct impact, head against object	NA; NA	NA	SHORT DURATION	NO	NORMAL	PRESENT	MP

NA = information was not documented in medical file; Short Duration = written as "short duration" in the medical file, no time/quantifiable duration recorded; TBI severity reported according to Mayo Classification System [29]; SP = symptomatic possible TBI; MP = mild probable TBI; MSD = Moderate-severe definite TBI. *Previous skull fracture as infant (<1 year of age).

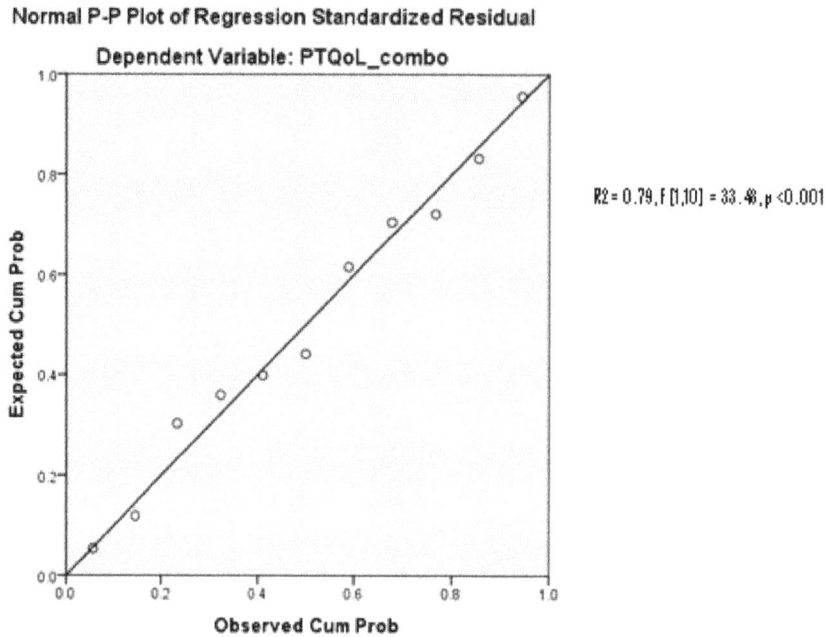

Figure 2. Regression Model, Self-Reported Depression and HRQoL. Cumulative distribution functions (fit between probability distributions) of self-reported depression against self-reported HRQoL. The Probability-Probability (P-P) plot demarks the fit of probability distributions, The data presented are approximately linear, which suggests that the specified theoretical distribution was the correct model (e.g. a good fit between the specific distribution and the observed data).

at injury was correlated with HRQoL, it did not predict HRQoL in our sample. Neither anxiety nor loneliness was associated with HRQoL. As expected, self-report and parent proxy reports were non-concordant.

Hornerman et al. [18] found that at 10 years post-injury, adolescents and young adults experience worse quality of life than healthy controls and those who have undergone organ transplantation when compared on domains of mobility, vision, hearing, eating, speech, mental status, depression, distress and usual activity involvement. When these data are considered against our sample, which were on average 4.6 years post-injury, it could be hypothesized that early identification and treatment of depression could prevent ongoing depression symptoms overtime. Recent adult TBI literature reported an increase in major depressive disorder and generalized anxiety disorder in adults with a severe TBI at 18 months post-injury, which impact on HRQoL [40].

Interestingly we found a relationship between age at injury and self-reported quality of life, where younger age at injury was correlated with a better HRQoL. When a TBI occurs early in childhood, the young person may have little recall of pre-injury life. It is possible that a younger age at injury resulting in a less dramatic life-change for the adolescent, who may have experience life as a continuation post-trauma, versus a change due to the injury. For example, one of the participants stated that he did not know a life pre-injury because he was too young to remember a life prior to the trauma. Severity of injury was not correlated with any of the outcome variables in either parents or self-reports. This result is particularly interesting, given the temptation to assume that mood and quality of life must be impaired as a result of a more significant injury.

While anxiety was not found to be a statistically significant contributor to HRQoL, it was related to both age at testing and loneliness. It is possible that anxiety and loneliness may interact in such a way as to influence the ongoing social development

trajectory of these adolescents. Current findings suggest a sequential nature of depressive co-morbidity, e.g. where the onset of depression follows the onset of most anxiety subtypes [41], suggesting that further examination of possible interaction effects of anxiety and depression in adolescent TBI survivors is warranted.

A systematic review found that children as young as 6 years of age were competent in providing reliable, valid accounts of their health [42], the overreliance on parental proxies in TBI research [6] may be due to concerns regarding individual insight into their TBI and less so attributable to the validity of response due to age. Although this study did not assess insight outright, it may be inferred that insight is intact in the adolescent sample assessed in this study, given up to 36% endorsed depression, anxiety, loneliness and quality of life related deficits. Endorsement of these symptoms requires that the individual is aware of their current level of functioning, at an emotional level. While the question regarding insight into the actual TBI is unknown in this sample, the results suggest that insight into one's own emotional state in a reasonable proportion of the sample is intact. By the same token, the non-significant, inverse relationship between parental proxies and adolescents suggests that the awareness of parents to mood and or quality of life related issues is not objective and may be inaccurate.

Limitations

The sample size for this study was small, therefore generalizations to all adolescents with a TBI cannot be made and our pilot results must be interpreted with caution. While every attempt was made to encourage participation of adolescents within our reach, unfortunately we were unable to satisfy a large sample. Federal privacy legislation and resultant restrictive methods for identify potential participants (clinical audit) limited our sample size which potentially introduces bias into the sample. The sample may be biased towards unusually keen families, or perhaps those who had personal reasons for participation, such as personal benefit or an opportunity to speak about their experiences. Small sample sizes are a common limitation in TBI outcome research; speculation on effective ways to address this problem may be to involve more interaction between research groups and divisions across the hospital setting, to organize a systematic approach of families, who may be overwhelmed with multiple research requests. Importantly, adolescents are entirely within their rights to decline participation in research studies, regardless of whether or not their parents consent. The failure to achieve a large samples size is partially reflected by adolescents' authority to say 'no' to research studies, which overrides parental interest in research. Efforts to ask adolescents why they do and do not wish to participate in research studies may help to provide insights into how to better market research studies to youth. Sample size limitations must also be considered in light of our attrition analyses, which revealed no significant differences between participants and non-participants on TBI severity, age at injury or gender. The attrition analyses suggest that although our pilot sample was small it was representative of the available pool of adolescents who experienced a TBI on key factors (TBI severity, gender and age). Importantly, small sample sizes do not preclude statistical analyses; rather, they require specific statistical analyses appropriate to small samples. The key limitation of using a small sample size is low power to detect large differences between designs or measures [43]. Of note, the results of the current study identified large effects from a small sample, which suggests that the findings are valid for the sample assessed in this study. Future research on larger samples is required to determine if our findings are generalizable to all survivors of adolescent TBI. Importantly, should depression continue to be a strong predictor of HRQoL in this group, routine assessment of depressive symptoms and HRQoL may help to inform targeted, individual-specific rehabilitation strategies aimed at ameliorating depressive symptomatology and improving HRQoL. Re-assessment of the role of anxiety and loneliness may also be relevant, as a large sample size may yield alternate trends to those reported here. Family history of psychiatric diagnoses were beyond the scope of the current study, but future research may wish to examine what role, if any, family history of psychiatric diagnoses play in adolescent experiences following a TBI. The current study did not collect contextual data regarding participants', including family situations, which may have impacted on their psychological well-being.

Future research should also consider alternate definitions of quality of life beyond the HRQoL model, especially considering the importance of emotional states described in this study.

Assessing the subjective-well being of adolescents may be especially well equipped to disentangle the relationships between mood and QoL.

While our sample size is small and results must be interpreted with caution, this pilot study supports a directional relationship between depression and reduced HRQoL in adolescent survivors of a TBI. Age at injury was correlated with HRQoL, but was not a statistically significant predictor of HRQoL in this sample. Neither loneliness nor anxiety was directly correlated with HRQoL, but they were related to each other. Age at injury was related to HRQoL, but was unable to predict it. As expected, parent proxy and self-reports of anxiety, depression and HRQoL were non-concordant.

Anxiety and depression are the most commonly occurring mental health concerns in otherwise healthy youth. Prevalence and incidence data on anxiety and depression in youth often rely on proxy reporting; despite evidence to suggest that proxy reporting is invalid for this purpose. Anxiety and depression are highly co morbid conditions in the general public. TBI has been consistently linked to new onset or worsening of persisting depression and anxiety across the lifespan, spanning childhood to adulthood. Recent research has supported a link between younger age at injury and development of new onset anxiety disorders, with novel depressive disorders co-morbid with these anxious states. Taken together, there is a reasonable suggestion that adolescent survivors of a TBI are at an increased risk for developing or worsening of anxious and or depressive states, given the impact of sequelae following injury that may interfere with their cognitive, psychosocial and interpersonal functioning. The findings from this pilot study support an important predictive role for depressive symptoms on self-reported HRQoL in adolescent survivors of a TBI.

Acknowledgments

People: Stephen Hearps, BPsych, PGDipPsych. Data Analyst. Mr Hearps has provided insight and guidance into statistical analysis for this study, in conversation with Dr. Ashley Di Battista. The corresponding author confirms that she has listed everyone who contributed significantly to the work in the Acknowledgments section.

Author Contributions

Conceived and designed the experiments: ADB. Performed the experiments: ADB. Analyzed the data: ADB. Contributed reagents/materials/analysis tools: ADB CC VA. Wrote the paper: ADB. Edited the manuscript: CG CC VA. Contributed to the study design: CC CS VA CG.

References

1. Langois JA, Rutland-Brown W, Wald MM (2006) The epidemiology and impact of traumatic brain injury: A brief overview J Head Trauma Rehabilitation 21: 375–378.
2. Max JE, Keatley E, Wilde EA, Bigler ED, Levin HS, et al. (2011) Anxiety disorders in children and adolescents in the first six months after traumatic brain injury J Neuropsychiatry 23: 29–39.
3. Anderson VA, Brown S, Newitt H (2010) What contributes to quality of life in adult survivors of childhood traumatic brain injury? J Neurotrauma 27: 1–8.
4. Hodges K (1993) Structured interview for assessing children J Child Psychol Psychiatry 34: 49–68.
5. Fletcher JM, Levin HS, Lachar D, Kusnerik L, Harward H, et al. (1996) Behavioral outcomes after pediatric closed head injury: Relationship with age severity and lesion size J Child Neurology 11: 283–290.
6. Di Battista A, Soo C, Catroppa C, Anderson V (2012) Quality of life in children and adolescents post-TBI: A systematic review and meta-analysis J Neurotrauma 29: 1717–1727.
7. Beesdo K, Knappe S, Pine DS (2009) Anxiety and anxiety disorders in children and adolescents: Developmental issues and implications for DSM-V Psychiatric Clinics of North America 32: 482–524.
8. Eapen V, Crncec R (2012) Strategies and challenges in the management of adolescent depression Current Opinion in Psychiatry 25: 7–13.
9. Ressler KJ, Mayberg HS (2007) Targeting abnormal neural circuits in mood and anxiety disorders: From the laboratory to the clinic Nature Neuroscience 10: 1116–1124.
10. Varni JW, Seid M, Kurtin PS (2001) PedsQL 4 0: reiability and validity of the Pediatric Quality of LIfe Inventory version 4. 0 generic core scales in healthy and patient populations Med Care 39: 800–812.
11. Green L, Godfrey C, Soo C, Anderson V, Catroppa C (2012) Agreement between parent-adolescent ratings on psychosocial outcome and qualtiy of life following childhood traumatic brain injury Developmental Neurorehabilitation 15: 105–113.
12. Barker-Collo S (2007) Depression and anxiety 3 months post stroke: Prevalence and correlates Archives of Clinical Neuropsychology 22: 519–531.
13. McCarthy ML, Mackenzie EJ, Dennis R, Durbin DR, Aitken ME, et al. (2006) Health-related quality of life during the first year after traumatic brain injury Arch Phys Med Rehabil 160: 253–260.

14. Luis CA, Mittenberg WI (2002) Mood and anxiety disorders following pediatric traumatic brain injury: A prospective study Journal of Clinical and Experimental Neuropsychology 24: 270–279.

15. Kirkwood M, Jansuz J,Yeats KW, Taylor HG, Wade SL, et al. (2000) Prevalence and correlates of depressive symptoms following traumatic brain injuries in children Child Neuropsychology 6: 195–208.

16. Max JE, Schachar RJ, Levin H, Ewing-Cobbs L, Chapman SB, et al. (2005) Predictors of attention-deficit/hyperactivigy disorder within 6 months after pediatric traumatic brain injury Journal of the American Academy of Child and Adolescent Psychiatry 44: 1032–1040.

17. Bloom D, Saunders A, Song J, Ewing-Cobbs L, Levin H, Fletcher JM, et al. (1997) Psychiatric disorders following pediatric TBI Journal of the International Neuropsychological Society 5: 127.

18. Hornerman MD, Selassie AW, Lineberry L, Ferguson PL, Labbate LA (2008) Predictors of psychological symptoms 1 year after traumatic brain injury: A population-based epidemiological study Journal of Head Trauma Rehabilitation 23: 74–83.

19. Hibbard MR, Uysal S, Kepler K, Bogandy J, Silver J (1998) Axis I psychopathology in individuals with traumatic brain injury Journal of Head Trauma Rehabilitation 13: 24–39.

20. Achenbach T, McConaughy S, Howell C (1987) Child/adolescent behavioral and emotional problems: implications of cross-informant correlations for situational specificity Psychol Bulletin 101: 213–232.

21. Kazadin AE, Esveldt-Dawson K, Unis AS, Rancurello MS (1983) Child and parent evaluation of depression and aggression in psychiatric inpatient children Journal of the American Academy of Child and Adolescent Psychiatry 22: 157–164.

22. Baumeister R, Leary M (1995) The need to belong: Desire for interpersonal attachments as a fundamental human motivation Psychological Bulletin 117: 497–529.

23. Irons C, Gilbert P (2005) Evolved mechanisms in adolescent anxiety and depression symptom: The role of the attachment and social rank systems Journal of Adolescence 28: 325–341.

24. Hawker DS, Boulton MJ (2000) Twenty years' research on peer victimization and psychosocial maladjustment: A meta-analytic review of cross-sectional studies Journal of Child Psychology and Psychiatry 41: 441–445.

25. Juvonen J, Graham S (2001) Peer harassment in school: The plight of the vulnerable and victimized New York: Guilford.

26. Muscara F, Catroppa C, Anderson V (2008) The impact of injury severity on executive function 7–10 years following pediatric traumatic brain injury Developmental Neuropsychology 5: 623–636.

27. Cattelani R, Lombardi F, Brianti R, Marzzuxxhi A (1998) Traumatic brain injury in childhood: Intellectual behavioural and social outcome into adulthood Brain Injury 12: 283–296.

28. Wechsler D (1999) Wechsler Abbreviated Scale of Intelligence In: Corporation TP editor Harcourt Brace & Company New York NY USA.

29. Malec J, Brown A, Leibson C, Flaada J, Mandrekar J, et al. (2007) The Mayo classification system for traumatic brain injury severity J Neurotrauma 24: 1417–1424.

30. Birmaher B, Khetarpal S, Brent D, Culy M, Balach L, et al. (1997) THe screen for child anxiety related emotional disorders (SCARED): Scale construction and psychometric characteristics J Am Acad Child Adolesc Psychiatry 36: 545–553.

31. Spielberger CD (1989) State-Trait Anxiety Inventory: Bibilgraphy Palo Alto CA: Consulting Psychologists Press.

32. Kovacs M (1992) The Children's Depression Inventory North Tonawanda NY: Multi-Health Systems.

33. Radloff LS (1977) The CES-D Scale: A self-report depression scale for research in the general population Applies Psychological Measurement 1: 385–401.

34. Hoza B, Bukowski WM, Beery S (2000) Assessing peer network and dyadic loneliness Journal of Clinical Child Psychology 29: 1119–1128.

35. Schmidt N, Sermat V (1983) Measuring loneliness in different relationships Journal of Personality and Social Psychology 44: 1038–1047.

36. Ware JE, Kosinski M, Keller SK (1994) SF-36 Physical and mental health summary scales: A user's manual Boston MA: The Health Institue.

37. Kaufman J, Birmaher B, Brent DA, Ryan ND, Rao U (1997) Schedule for affective disorders and schizophrenia for school-age children-present and lifetime version (K-SADS-PL): Initial reliablity and validity data Journal of the American Academy of Child and Adolescent Psychiatry 36: 980–998.

38. First MB, Psitzer RL, Gibbon M, Williams JB (1997) User's guide for Structured Clinical Interview for DSM-IV Axis I Disorders Washington: American Psychiatric Press.

39. Statistics ABo (2008) 2033 0 55 001 Socio-economic Indexes for Areas (SEIFA) 2006 In: Statistics ABo editor Updated 17 July 2013 ed Canberra: Commonwealth of Australia.

40. Diaz A, Schwarzbold M, Thais M, Hohl A, Bertotti M, et al. (2012) Psychiatric disorders and health-related quality of life after severe traumatic brain injury: A prospective study Journal of Neurotrauma 29: 1029–1037.

41. Avenevoli S, Stolar M, Li J, Dierker L, Ries Merikangas K (2001) Comorbidity of depression in children and adolescents: Models and evidence from a prospective high-risk family study Biological Psychiatry 49: 1071–1081.

42. Riley AW (2004) Evidence that school-age children can self-report on their health Ambul Pediatr 4: 371–376.

43. Saro J (2013) Best practices for using statistics on small sample sizes 2013; Available: https://www.measuringusability.com/blog/small-n.php.

14

HIV Drug Resistance Early Warning Indicators in Namibia with Updated World Health Organization Guidance

Anna Jonas[1], Victor Sumbi[2], Samson Mwinga[2], Michael DeKlerk[1], Francina Tjituka[2], Scott Penney[3], Michael R. Jordan[3,4], Tiruneh Desta[5], Alice M. Tang[3], Steven Y. Hong[3,4]*

1 Directorate of Special Programmes, Republic of Namibia Ministry of Health and Social Services, Windhoek, Namibia, 2 Strengthening Pharmaceutical Systems, Management Sciences for Health, Windhoek, Namibia, 3 Department of Public Health and Community Medicine, Tufts University School of Medicine, Boston, Massachusetts, United States of America, 4 Division of Geographic Medicine and Infectious Diseases, Tufts Medical Center, Boston, Massachusetts, United States of America, 5 World Health Organization Namibia, Klein Windhoek, Namibia

Abstract

Background: In response to concerns about the emergence of HIV drug resistance (HIVDR), the World Health Organization (WHO) has developed a comprehensive set of early warning indicators (EWIs) to monitor HIV drug resistance and good programme practice at antiretroviral therapy (ART) sites.

Methods: In 2012, Namibia utilized the updated WHO EWI guidance and abstracted data from adult and pediatric patients from 50 ART sites for the following EWIs: 1. *On-time Pill Pick-up*, 2. *Retention in Care*, 3. *Pharmacy Stock-outs*, 4. *Dispensing Practices*, and 5. *Virological Suppression*.

Results: Data for EWIs one through four were abstracted and validated. *EWI 5 – Virological Suppression* was not included due to poor data entry at many sites. *On-time Pill Pick-up* national estimate was 87.9% (87.2–88.7) of patients picking up pills on time for adults and 90.0% (88.9–90.9) picking up pills on time for pediatrics. *Retention in Care* national estimate was 82% of patients retained on ART after 12 months for adults and 83% for pediatrics. *Pharmacy Stock-outs* national estimate was 99% of months without a stock-out for adults and 97% for pediatrics. *Dispensing Practices* national estimate was 0.01% (0.003–0.064) of patients dispensed mono- or dual-therapy for adults and 0.25% (0.092–0.653) for pediatrics.

Conclusions: The successful 2012 EWI exercise provides Namibia a solid evidence base, which can be used to make national statements about programmatic functioning and possible HIVDR. This evidence base will serve to contextualize results from Namibia's surveys of HIVDR, which involves genotype testing. EWI abstraction has prompted the national program and its counterparts to engage sites in dialogue regarding the need to strengthen adherence and retention of patients on ART. The EWI collection process and EWI results will serve to optimize patient care and support Namibia in making evidence-based recommendations and take action to minimize the emergence of preventable HIVDR.

Editor: Omar Sued, Fundacion Huesped, Argentina

Funding: This work was supported by funding from the Republic of Namibia Ministry of Health and Social Services, National Institutes of Health, NIH L30 AI080268-02 (SYH), NIH 1K23AI097010-01A1 (SYH), NIH K23 AI074423-05 (MRJ), and NIH P30 AI42853-10 (AMT). Travel expenses for this study were supported in part by the Harold Williams Tufts Medical Student Research Fellowship (SP). The funders had no role in study design, data collection and analysis, decision to publish, or preparation of the manuscript.

Competing Interests: The authors have declared that no competing interests exist.

* Email: shong@tuftsmedicalcenter.org

Introduction

Background

In recent years, the rapid scale up of antiretroviral therapy (ART) for treatment of HIV infection in resource-limited countries has been highly successful resulting in 9.7 million people receiving ART in low- middle-income countries as of December 2012 [1]. The public health approach to scaling up ART in resource-limited settings involves the use of standardized and simplified treatment regimens that are consistent with international standards, and appropriate to local circumstances. Because of the high mutation rate and high replication rate of HIV, the chronic nature of HIV

infection and the need for lifelong treatment, the emergence of some drug resistance is inevitable in populations taking ART [2–3].

In response to countries concerns about the emergence of HIV drug resistance (HIVDR), the World Health Organization (WHO) has developed a comprehensive HIVDR surveillance and monitoring strategy based on public health principles. The updated 2012 global HIVDR surveillance and monitoring strategy contains 5 key elements: *1. Monitoring of Early Warning Indicators (EWI) of HIVDR, 2. Surveillance of transmitted drug resistance (TDR) in recently infected populations, 3. Surveillance of HIVDR in populations initiating*

ART, 4. Surveillance of acquired HIVDR in populations on ART, and 5. Surveillance of HIVDR in children <18 months of age [4].

HIVDR Early Warning Indicators

The purpose of routine monitoring of HIVDR EWIs is to assess the extent to which ART sites and programmes are functioning by monitoring factors at individual ART sites known to create situations favourable to the emergence of HIVDR. The monitoring of EWIs provides the context for interpreting the results from surveys of HIVDR. Specifically, EWI results permit the timely identification of ART sites not achieving a globally suggested standard target, which supports tailoring of appropriate interventions that can potentially optimize care and treatment and reduce the risk of population-level HIVDR emergence. Drug resistance will not necessarily result immediately if an indicator shows non-optimal performance; however, achieving the best possible performance as measured by these indicators will help to minimize preventable HIVDR.

In 2012, WHO updated its 2010 EWI guidance by conducting a critical review of the available medical literature and the multiple challenges observed with data collection and reporting. EWI definitions were simplified and harmonized with other monitoring and evaluation frameworks and processes, including those of the Global Aids Response Progress Reporting (GARPR) and the United States President's Emergency Plan for AIDS Relief (PEPFAR) [4]. The number of core indicators was reduced to four: on-time pill pick-up, dispensing practices, drug supply continuity and clinic retention at 12 months. A fifth indicator, viral load suppression at 12 months, was recommended to be monitored only at sites where viral load testing was routinely performed on all patients 12 months after therapy initiation. EWI targets were adjusted to take into account new scientific evidence on optimal programme management and performance.

HIV in Namibia

Namibia is a resource-limited country in sub-Saharan Africa that has been severely affected by the HIV epidemic. In Namibia, there are approximately 200,000 people living with HIV in a population of 2.1 million [5]. Among 15–49 year olds, approximately 18.2% are infected with HIV-1. [unpublished data] The epidemic is predominantly spread via heterosexual contact, and prevalence estimates vary by region with up to 37.7% infected with HIV-1 in the most heavily affected areas in the north. [unpublished data]

ART rollout

ART has been available in Namibia's private sector since 1997 and in the public sector since 2003. At 84%, Namibia has one of the highest ART coverage rates in Sub-Saharan Africa with 107,154 eligible patients on ART as of March 2013. At present, ART is available at all 40 public hospitals and at an additional 111 satellite/outreach service points, as well as 30 Integrated Management of Adolescent and Adult Illness (IMAI) sites. [unpublished data] Of these sites, the national ART program considers 44 to be main ART sites. Main sites dispense ART independently and to patients at IMAI and satellite/outreach sites. (Figure 1)

In the public sector, ART is provided free of charge following a population-based model of care with one primary first-line regimen and three alternate first-line regimens consisting of two nucleoside reverse transcriptase inhibitors (NRTI) combined with a non-nucleoside reverse transcriptase inhibitor (NNRTI). The recommended second-line regimen consists of 2 NRTIs with a ritonavir-boosted protease inhibitor (PI). ART initiation is based

on WHO clinical staging and/or CD4 cell count ≤ 350 cells/mm^3. All public ART sites have access to first- and second-line ART regimens. At all public ART sites, viral load testing is performed six months after ART initiation and targeted viral load testing is performed to confirm clinical or immunological failure beyond six months [6]. With support from Management Sciences for Health (MSH) Namibia, a standardized pharmacy record system, the Electronic Dispensing Tool (EDT), is used to dispense all ART. In the private sector, ART is provided utilizing an individual model of care with ART regimens selected based on results of drug resistance testing. (16% of patients on ART in Namibia)

Early Warning Indicators in Namibia

In 2009, Namibia piloted five EWIs at nine ART sites [7]: 1) *ART prescribing practices*, 2) *Patients lost to follow-up (LTFU) at 12 months*, 3) *Patient retention on first-line ART at 12 months*, 4) *On-time ARV drug pick-up*, and 5) *ARV drug-supply continuity*. Records supported monitoring of three of these five EWIs. Nine of nine (100%) sites met the target of 100% initiated on appropriate first-line regimens. Eight of nine (89%) sites met the target of $\leq 20\%$ LTFU. Six of nine (67%) sites met the target of 0% switched to a second-line regimen. In 2010, Namibia scaled-up these same three EWIs from nine to 33 ART sites [8]. Twenty-two of 33 (67%) sites met the target of 100% initiated on appropriate first-line regimens. Seventeen of 33 (52%) sites met the target of $\leq 20\%$ LTFU. Fifteen of 33 (45%) sites met the target of 0% switched to a second-line regimen. EWI monitoring directly resulted in public health action to optimize the quality of care, specifically the strengthening of ART record systems, engagement of ART sites, and operational research for improved adherence assessment and improved ART patient defaulter tracing.

Methods

Early Warning Indicators selection

Based on discussion with WHO consultants and review of pertinent record-keeping systems, the Namibia HIVDR technical working group (TWG) determined to abstract the following EWIs for abstraction in 2012 with the corresponding WHO-recommended targets summarized in Table 1: *On-time pill pick-up, Retention in care, Pharmacy stock-outs, Dispensing practices,* and *Virological Suppression (Namibia-specific definition due to routine viral load testing done at 6 months in Namibia).*

EWI performance was rated according to WHO recommended scorecards. (Table 1) The scorecards utilize three classifications: red (poor performance, below desired level), amber (fair performance, not yet at desired level), and green (excellent performance, achieving desired level). Also, the scorecards allow for a "grey" classification if a site does not monitor a specific EWI or a "white" classification if an indicator is not reported according to national regulations [4].

EWIs are monitored separately for adult and pediatric populations. Recommended targets are identical for adult and pediatric populations except for the indicator assessing desirable rates of virological suppression.

Ethics statement

Ethical review was not required as this data was public health surveillance data abstracted from existing routinely collected ministry of health medical records. Only anonymized data were abstracted from the medical records for public health surveillance purposes. Names, dates of birth, addresses, and unique patient identifier numbers were not abstracted from records. After discussion with the Tufts Medical Center institutional review

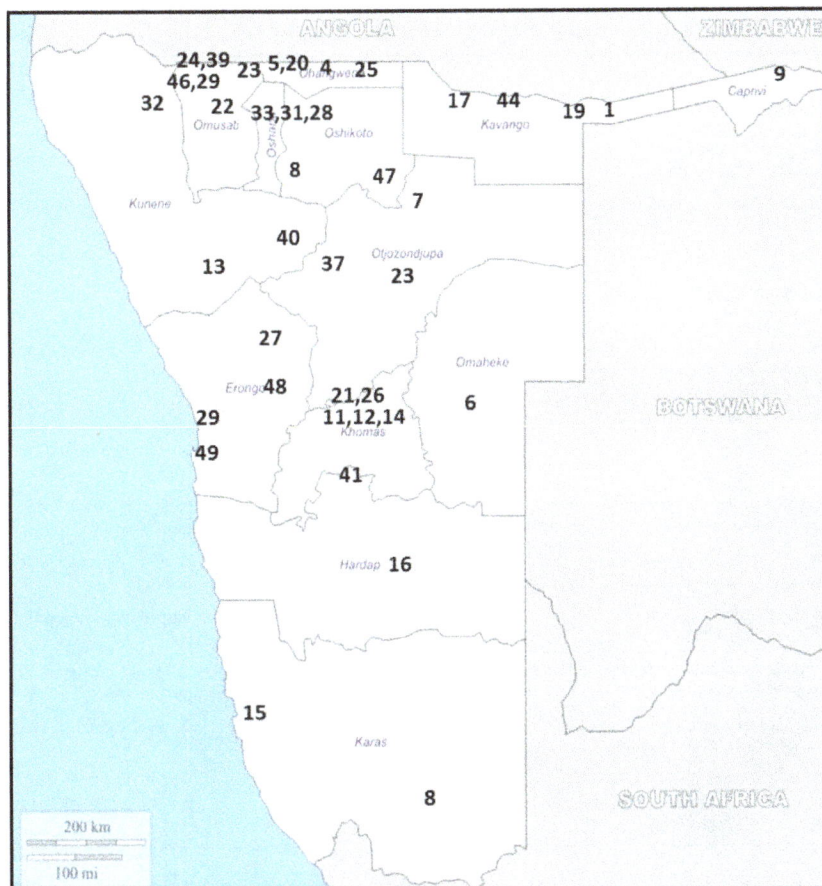

Figure 1. Geographic Location of ART Sites. This figure illustrates the public ART sites located in Namibia. The map is adapted from: http://d-maps.com/carte.php?num_car=4824&lang=en.

board, it was determined that because this was routine public health de-identified data analyzed within the Ministry of Health and Social Services in Namibia, no formal written waiver was necessary. The data used for this study was obtained from and analyzed by the Ministry of Health and Social Services (MoHSS) of Namibia.

Site selection and data abstraction

EWIs are designed to be collected routinely from all sites within a country, or a large number of representative sites. All 44 main ART delivery sites and 6 outreach sites that had disaggregated EDT data were chosen for EWI abstraction in 2012 including sites that participated in EWI abstraction in 2010. Data for ART outreach sites without disaggregated EDT data were included in this year's EWI abstraction exercise within the main ART sites. EWI data abstraction was conducted centrally in August 2012 by a data abstraction team formed by the TWG in collaboration with the WHO and the MoHSS. The team consisted of 4 members trained on the WHO methodology of EWI abstraction. Data for *On-time pill pick-up*, *Retention in care*, and *Dispensing Practices* were downloaded from the national EDT database through automatic queries into MS Excel and calculated according to WHO guidance. Data for *Pharmacy stock-outs* were calculated from monthly ART site reporting. Data for *Virological suppression at 6 months* were downloaded centrally from the national electronic patient medical system (ePMS) database into MS Excel.

Data quality assessment

Data quality assessments were implemented throughout the EWI process. Three elements of data quality were considered in the assessments: data reliability, data completeness, and data consistency [9]. Data reliability, which is an assessment of the quality of the abstraction, was assessed by confirming 10% of the centrally-queried data to the existing data in the EDT. Data completeness was assessed from the centrally-queried data; and sites with a large percentage of data missing were removed from EWI analyses (1 site). Finally, assessment of data consistency was initially performed during the pilot of EWIs [7] and the most optimal source for each variable was determined. EDT data were considered the gold standard for pharmacy pick-up dates and ART regimens dispensed, while ePMS and paper records (Patient Care Booklets) were considered the gold standard for information about patient status such as dates of transfer in and transfer out, dates of death, and dates of stop. Therefore, EDT data for patients who had incomplete pill pick-ups were validated and corrected by comparing records in ePMS and Patient Care Booklets, looking for dates of transfer out, death or ART stop. Centrally-queried EDT data for patients who had inappropriate ART regimens at start or at 12 months were validated and corrected with the site-specific EDT system to ensure accuracy of the queries. Validation with ePMS and paper medical records was performed by the individual ART sites that were trained on EWI methodology at a national EWI conference.

Table 1. Selected 2012 WHO Early Warning Indicator Definitions (Numerator/Denominator) and Targets.

Early Warning Indicator	Definitions (Numerator/Denominator)	Targets[#]
On-time pill pick-up	Numerator: number of patients picking up their ART on time* at first drug pick-up after a defined baseline pick-up date.	Red: <80%
	Denominator: number of patients who picked up drugs on or after the designated EWI sample start date.[§]	Amber: 80–90%
		Green: >90%
Retention in care	Numerator: number of adults or children who are still alive and on ART 12 months after initiating treatment.	Red: <75% retained after 12 months of ART
	Denominator: total number of adults or children who initiated ART who were expected to achieve 12-month outcomes within the reporting period, including those who have died since starting therapy, those who have stopped therapy, and those recorded as lost to follow-up[†] at month 12.[∞]	Amber: 75–85% retained after 12 months of ART
		Green: >85% retained after 12 months of ART
Pharmacy stock-outs	Numerator: number of months in the designated year in which there were no stock-out[‡] days of any (adult or pediatric) ARV drug routinely used at the site.	Red: <100% of a 12-month period with no stock-outs
	Denominator: 12 months.	Green: 100% of a 12-month period with no stock-outs
Dispensing practices	Numerator: number of patients (adults or children) who pick up form the pharmacy, a regimen consisting of one or two ARVs.	Red: >0% dispensing of mono- or dual therapy
	Denominator: number of patients (adults or children) picking up ART on or after the designated EWI sample start date. Sampling continues until the full sample size is reached.	Green: 0% dispensing of mono- or dual therapy
Virological suppression at 6 months^	Numerator: number of patients receiving ART and a viral load at the site after the first 6 months of ART whose viral load is<1000 copies/mL.	Targets to be determined by WHO
	Denominator: consecutive ART starters from 1 January, 2010 until 31 December 2010 and have viral load results after 6-months available (between 5–12 months from ART initiation).	

ART – Antiretroviral therapy.
ARV – Antiretrovirals.
*On-time pill pick-up: Pick up pills no more than two days late on their first pick-up after a baseline pick-up.
[§]EWI sample start date: The date designated as the start of the sampling. The sample start date is fixed by the HIVDR Working Group.
[†]Lost to follow-up: Patients who had not returned to the pharmacy or clinic ≤90 days after the last ART run-out date during the 12-months after the date of ART initiation were classified as LTFU. Stopping therapy without restarting was classified as not LTFU if the patient continued to attend clinic appointments.
[∞]Transfers of care to another site were excluded from the denominator.
[‡]Stock-out: Any occurrence of zero stock of a routinely-used ARV drug at the site at which the patient routinely picks up ARVs.
[#]Adult and pediatric targets are the same. Targets for *Virological Suppression at 6-months* have not been determined by WHO.
^Due to routine data collection of viral load at 6 months, Namibia chose to monitor *Virological suppression at 6 months* instead of the WHO recommendation of 12 months.
Table adapted from WHO HIV Drug Resistance EWI guidance report [4].

Sample size

In order to make the results generalizable to the patient population at the ART site, the sampling strategy was based on calculating a minimum sample size for each indicator at each site, based on the number of eligible patients for each EWI. For *On-time pill pick-up* and *Dispensing practices*, the number of eligible patients at each site to be sampled was the number of patients who were "active" on ART at the time of the sample start date (1 January, 2012). WHO recommends data abstraction on a minimum number of consecutive patients following the sample size criteria below to provide a 95% CI of ±7%. However, data abstraction was oversampled by 20% to account for potential censoring of patients; therefore the true confidence intervals are <±7%. All sites began abstraction from the sample start date, and abstracted data until appropriate sample size for each site was reached; regardless of how many months it took to reach the appropriate sample size. Sample sizes for sites were based on the numbers of patients at each participating ART site meeting the eligibility definition of patients to be represented for each EWI according to WHO guidance [4]. For *Retention in care*, a census of all patients initiating ART in the 12 months of 2010 was taken (consistent with

GARPR/PEPFAR). For *Virological suppression at 6 months*, a census of all patients starting ART in 2010 with 6-month viral load data available was obtained.

Calculation of national estimates

The national estimates for adult and pediatric EWIs were calculated by summing the numerators and denominators for each EWI found in Figures 2 and 3, respectively, to get a cumulative percentage of all ART sites. (Table 2) The national statistics are representative of Namibia's public ART sites because data for all outreach sites not listed in this report were included within the main sites. This means that all patients receiving ART in the public sector in Namibia were included in the sample frame.

The confidence intervals for EWIs 1 and 4 were weighted by number of active patients and proportion of total patients sampled at each ART site. Confidence intervals were calculated separately for adults and pediatrics populations attending the same clinic. *Retention in care* and *Pharmacy stock-out* confidence intervals were not calculated because retention is measured as a census of all patients and stock outs are reports of actual drug shortages.

Site	On-time pill pick-up	Retention in care	Pharmacy stock-outs	Dispensing practices
1.	178/210 (85%)	217/265 (82%)	12/12 (100%)	0/210 (0%)
2.	112/132 (85%)	61/70 (87%)	11/12 (92%)	0/132 (0%)
3.	171/236 (72%)	424/486 (87%)	12/12 (100%)	0/240 (0%)
4.	200/238 (84%)	628/788 (80%)	12/12 (100%)	0/240 (0%)
5.	176/210 (84%)	233/337 (69%)	12/12 (100%)	0/210 (0%)
6.	176/210 (84%)	259/332 (78%)	12/12 (100%)	0/210 (0%)
7.	160/189 (85%)	42/66 (64%)	12/12 (100%)	0/192 (0%)
8.	144/252 (57%)	710/846 (84%)	12/12 (100%)	0/254 (0%)
9.	180/208 (87%)	111/170 (65%)	12/12 (100%)	0/210 (0%)
10.	231/251 (92%)	1222/1517 (81%)	12/12 (100%)	0/252 (0%)
11.	177/185 (96%)	176/217 (81%)	12/12 (100%)	0/186 (0%)
12.	155/160 (97%)	84/105 (80%)	12/12 (100%)	0/161 (0%)
13.	225/252 (89%)	669/806 (83%)	12/12 (100%)	0/251 (0%)
14.	184/210 (88%)	180/209 (86%)	12/12 (100%)	0/210 (0%)
15.	171/190 (90%)	183/231 (79%)	12/12 (100%)	1/191 (<1%)
16.	165/209 (79%)	145/190 (76%)	12/12 (100%)	0/210 (0%)
17.	16/16 (100%)	78/78 (100%)	12/12 (100%)	0/16 (0%)
18.	179/209 (86%)	222/270 (82%)	12/12 (100%)	0/210 (0%)
19.	199/209 (95%)	204/228 (89%)	11/12 (92%)	0/210 (0%)
20.	184/210 (88%)	192/230 (83%)	12/12 (100%)	0/210 (0%)
21.	236/240 (98%)	400/447 (89%)	12/12 (100%)	0/240 (0%)
22.	127/144 (88%)	60/65 (92%)	10/12 (83%)	0/144 (0%)
23.	162/213 (76%)	295/367 (80%)	12/12 (100%)	0/216 (0%)
24.	190/209 (91%)	239/270 (89%)	12/12 (100%)	0/210 (0%)
25.	230/246 (93%)	22/22 (100%)	12/12 (100%)	0/249 (0%)
26.	157/186 (84%)	129/152 (85%)	12/12 (100%)	0/186 (0%)
27.	244/257 (95%)	1146/1333 (86%)	12/12 (100%)	0/258 (0%)
28.	118/186 (63%)	112/113 (99%)	12/12 (100%)	0/186 (0%)
29.	196/209 (94%)	181/189 (96%)	12/12 (100%)	0/210 (0%)
30.	174/210 (83%)	369/398 (93%)	12/12 (100%)	0/210 (0%)
31.	162/192 (84%)	119/160 (74%)	12/12 (100%)	0/192 (0%)
32.	245/258 (95%)	1981/2335 (85%)	12/12 (100%)	0/258 (0%)
33.	222/240 (93%)	552/659 (84%)	12/12 (100%)	0/240 (0%)
34.	-	86/93 (92%)	12/12 (100%)	-
35.	54/60 (90%)	13/18 (72%)	12/12 (100%)	0/59 (0%)
36.	192/216 (89%)	366/438 (84%)	12/12 (100%)	1/216 (<1%)
37.	111/130 (85%)	63/69 (91%)	12/12 (100%)	0/132 (0%)
38.	247/252 (98%)	753/856 (88%)	12/12 (100%)	0/252 (0%)
39.	159/185 (86%)	136/198 (69%)	12/12 (100%)	0/18 (0%)
40.	174/192 (91%)	144/218 (66%)	12/12 (100%)	0/192 (0%)
41.	163/185 (88%)	151/163 (93%)	12/12 (100%)	0/186 (0%)
42.	47/52 (90%)	51/62 (82%)	12/12 (100%)	0/53 (0%)
43.	204/252 (81%)	783/1023 (77%)	12/12 (100%)	0/252 (0%)
44.	207/240 (86%)	404/468 (86%)	12/12 (100%)	0/240 (0%)
45.	182/210 (87%)	211/263 (80%)	12/12 (100%)	0/210 (0%)
46.	185/209 (89%)	260/315 (83%)	12/12 (100%)	0/210 (0%)
47.	153/166 (92%)	105/120 (88%)	11/12 (92%)	0/168 (0%)
48.	222/238 (93%)	573/660(87%)	11/12 (92%)	0/240 (0%)
49.	189/210 (90%)	310/384 (81%)	12/12 (100%)	0/210 (0%)

Figure 2. Adult Site-specific EWI Results. EWI – Early Warning Indicator. Green indicates sites that achieved excellent performance, desired target level. Yellow indicates sites that achieved fair performance, progressing towards desired target level. Red indicates poor performance, below desired target level. Gray indicates that data was not available from that site.

Results

Namibia abstracted data on four EWIs for both adults and pediatrics: *On-time pill pick-up, Retention in care, Pharmacy stock-outs,* and *Dispensing practices.* Data from 28,909 adults and 6,086 pediatric patients were abstracted and analyzed. Site-specific EWI results for adults are presented in Figure 2 and for pediatrics in Figure 3. The national EWI summary for adults and pediatrics is presented in Table 2. Data collected for *Virological suppression at 6*

months was determined to be unreliable due to site-level data entry errors.

On-time pill pick-up

For adults, 42% of sites achieved "excellent" performance (≥ 90%) for *On-time pill pick-up,* 48% of sites had "fair" performance (80–90%), and 10% of sites had "poor" performance (<80%). The rates from all adult sites ranged from 57% to 100%. For pediatrics,

Site	On-time pill pick-up	Retention in care	Pharmacy stock-outs	Dispensing practices
1.	72/89 (81%)	22/27 (81%)	12/12 (100%)	0/90 (0%)
2.	13/16 (81%)	6/6 (100%)	11/12 (92%)	0/16 (0%)
3.	122/166 (73%)	60/73 (82%)	11/12 (92%)	0/168 (0%)
4.	138/185 (75%)	60/81 (74%)	11/12 (92%)	0/186 (0%)
5.	102/120 (85%)	13/22 (59%)	12/12 (100%)	0/120 (0%)
6.	78/89 (88%)	18/25 (72%)	11/12 (92%)	0/89 (0%)
7.	22/24 (92%)	2/2 (100%)	12/12 (100%)	0/24 (0%)
8.	179/186 (96%)	84/112 (75%)	12/12 (100%)	0/186 (0%)
9.	46/58 (79%)	4/8 (50%)	11/12 (92%)	0/58 (0%)
10.	103/120 (86%)	41/56 (73%)	12/12 (100%)	0/120 (0%)
11.	4/6 (67%)	2/3 (67%)	12/12 (100%)	0/6 (0%)
12.	24/25 (96%)	4/5 (80%)	12/12 (100%)	0/25 (0%)
13.	172/185 (93%)	72/83 (87%)	9/12 (75%)	0/186 (0%)
14.	53/60 (88%)	7/7 (100%)	12/12 (100%)	0/60 (0%)
15.	53/62 (85%)	19/23 (83%)	12/12 (100%)	0/62 (0%)
16.	105/119 (88%)	13/15 (87%)	12/12 (100%)	0/120 (0%)
17.	-	7/7 (100%)	12/12 (100%)	-
18.	109/120 (91%)	30/41 (73%)	12/12 (100%)	0/120 (0%)
19.	112/120 (93%)	23/27 (85%)	12/12 (100%)	0/120 (0%)
20.	70/75 (93%)	5/7 (71%)	12/12 (100%)	0/75 (0%)
21.	153/158 (97%)	59/65 (91%)	12/12 (100%)	0/158 (0%)
22.	25/31 (81%)	6/6 (100%)	11/12 (92%)	0/31 (0%)
23.	162/186 (87%)	47/58 (81%)	12/12 (100%)	0/186 (0%)
24.	100/120 (83%)	26/30 (87%)	12/12 (100%)	0/120 (0%)
25.	9/9 (100%)	1/1 (100%)	12/12 (100%)	0/9 (0%)
26.	34/42 (81%)	7/9 (78%)	12/12 (100%)	0/42 (0%)
27.	194/216 (90%)	115/130 (88%)	12/12 (100%)	3/216 (1%)
28.	55/74 (74%)	25/25 (100%)	12/12 (100%)	0/74 (0%)
29.	110/120 (92%)	22/23 (96%)	12/12 (100%)	0/120 (0%)
30.	135/144 (94%)	42/49 (86%)	12/12 (100%)	0/144 (0%)
31.	19/23 (83%)	1/4 (25%)	12/12 (100%)	0/23 (0%)
32.	199/209 (95%)	182/215 (85%)	12/12 (100%)	0/209 (0%)
33.	181/185 (98%)	64/74 (86%)	12/12 (100%)	0/186 (0%)
34.	-	7/7 (100%)	12/12 (100%)	-
35.	8/8 (100%)	1/1 (100%)	12/12 (100%)	0/8 (0%)
36.	109/120 (91%)	15/18 (83%)	10/12 (83%)	1/120 (<1%)
37.	10/11 (91%)	5/5 (100%)	12/12 (100%)	0/11 (0%)
38.	182/191 (95%)	95/107 (89%)	12/12 (100%)	0/192 (0%)
39.	22/27 (81%)	9/14 (64%)	12/12 (100%)	0/27 (0%)
40.	45/48 (94%)	5/5 (100%)	10/12 (83%)	0/47 (0%)
41.	9/12 (75%)	2/2 (100%)	12/12 (100%)	0/12 (0%)
42.	2/3 (67%)	1/1 (100%)	12/12 (100%)	0/3 (0%)
43.	161/174 (93%)	96/121 (79%)	12/12 (100%)	0/174 (0%)
44.	93/108 (86%)	14/16 (88%)	11/12 (92%)	0/113 (0%)
45.	95/120 (79%)	17/19 (89%)	12/12 (100%)	0/120 (0%)
46.	69/72 (96%)	14/17 (82%)	11/12 (92%)	1/72 (1%)
47.	25/27 (93%)	10/10 (100%)	12/12 (100%)	0/27 (0%)
48.	113/120 (94%)	18/25 (72%)	7/12 (58%)	1/120 (<1%)
49.	2/3 (67%)	1/1 (100%)	12/12 (100%)	0/3 (0%)

Figure 3. Pediatric EWI Site-specific Results. EWI – Early Warning Indicator. Green indicates sites that achieved excellent performance, desired target level. Yellow indicates sites that achieved fair performance, progressing towards desired target level. Red indicates poor performance, below desired target level. Gray indicates that data was not available from that site.

49% of the sites achieved "excellent" performance (≥90%), 32% of sites had "fair" performance (80–90%), and 19% of sites had "poor" performance (<80%). The rates from all pediatric sites ranged from 67% to 100%. The national estimate for *On-time pill pick-up* was 87.9% (87.2–88.7) of patients picking up pills on time for adults and 90.0% (88.9–90.9) picking up pills on time for pediatrics.

Retention in care

For adults, 45% of the sites achieved "excellent" performance (≥85%) for *Retention in care*, 41% of sites had "fair" performance (75–85%), and 14% of sites had "poor" performance (<75%). The retention rates from the adult sites ranged from 64% to 100%. For pediatric sites, 57% of sites achieved "excellent" performance (≥ 85%), 21% of sites had "fair" performance (75–85%), and 22% of sites had "poor" performance (<75%). The retention rates at the

Table 2. National EWI Summary Report.

Early Warning Indicator	EWI Target for all sites (time period)	Number adult of sites meeting EWI target (% of sites meeting target)	Number pediatric of sites meeting EWI target (% of sites meeting target) N = X ART sites	National Adult Estimates % (CI)	National Pediatric Estimates % (CI)
On-time pill pick-up	Green: >90%	Green 20/48 (42%)	Green 23/47 (49%)	87.9% (87.2–88.7)*	90.0% (88.9–90.9)*
	Amber: 80–90%	Amber 23/48 (48%)	Amber 15/47 (32%)		
	Red: <80%	Red 5/48 (10%)	Red 9/47 (19%)		
	(1 Jan 2012-)				
Retention in care	Green: >85%	Green 22/49 (45%)	Green 28/49 (57%)	15,957/19,299 (82%)	1,399/1,688 (83%)
	Amber: 75–85%	Amber 20/49 (41%)	Amber 10/49 (21%)		
	Red: <75%	Red 7/49 (14%)	Red 11/49(22%)		
	(1 Jan 2010–31 Dec 2010)				
Pharmacy stock-outs	Green: 100%	Green 44/49 (90%)	Amber 37/49 (76%)	582/588 (99%)	568/588 (97%)
	Red: <100%	Red 5/49 (10%)	Red 12/49 (24%)		
	(1 April 2012–31 Mar 2013)				
Dispensing practices	Green: 0%	Green 46/48 (96%)	Green 42/47 (89%)	0.01% (0.003–0.064)*	0.25% (0.092–0.653)*
	Red: >0%	Red 2/48 (4%)	Red 5/47 (11%)		
	(1 Jan 2012-)				

EWI – Early Warning Indicator.
*National estimates were weighted by the number of active patients and proportion of patients sampled from each ART site.

pediatric sites ranged from 25% to 100%. The national estimate for *Retention in care* is 82% of patients retained on ART after 12 months for adults and 83% for pediatrics.

Pharmacy stock-outs

For adults, 90% of sites achieved "excellent" performance with 100% of months without a pharmacy stock-out and 10% were classified as "poor" performance with <100% of months without a pharmacy stock-out. For pediatrics, 76% of sites achieved "excellent" performance and 24% of sites were classified as "poor" performance. The national estimate for *Pharmacy stock-outs* is 99% of months without a stock-out for adults and 97% for pediatrics.

Dispensing practices

For adult sites, 96% achieved "excellent" performance with 0% of patients dispensed mono- or dual therapy, and 4% were classified as "poor" performance with >0% of patients mono- or dual-therapy. For pediatric sites, 91% of achieved "excellent" performance and 9% were classified as "poor" performance. Only 8 of 14,008 patients were dispensed dual therapy. There was no dispensing of mono-therapy. The national estimates for *ARV dispensing practices* are 0.01% (0.003–0.064) of patients dispensed mono- or dual-therapy for adults and 0.25% (0.092–0.653) for pediatrics.

Virological suppression at 6 months

It was discovered that in many sites, ART clerks were not entering VL data into the ePMS that had the results "target not detected" (undetectable). Therefore, VL suppression data are expected to be underestimates. So the decision was made to report these data as "grey" for "data not available". It was also

discovered that a proportion of VL were being conducted before ART start at some sites.

Discussion

This paper presents the first published HIVDR EWIs using the new 2012 WHO guidance and the first published pediatric EWI data for Namibia. Namibia successfully abstracted data on four WHO recommended EWIs and scaled-up monitoring to 50 ART sites throughout the country from the previous 33 ART sites in 2010: *On-time pill pick-up, Retention in care, Pharmacy stock-outs*, and *Dispensing practices*. The 50 ART sites which include data from main and outreach/satellite sites represent the public ART sites throughout the country. For the first time in Namibia, existing medical and pharmacy records (ePMS, EDT, and Patient care booklets) allowed for accurate monitoring of four EWIs. Also pediatric data were abstracted for the first time. Accurate monitoring of *Virological suppression at 6 months* was not accomplished due to systematic data entry errors at site-level. For the previous EWI exercise in 2010, accurate data abstraction was not possible from existing medical and pharmacy records to report *On-time pill pick-up, Pharmacy stock-outs*, or pediatric EWI data. The 2010 EWI exercise resulted in important modifications to the data abstraction tool to make this EWI data abstraction possible [8].

On-time pill pick-up is an important measure of patient adherence that is associated with LTFU [10], HIVDR [11–13] virological failure [14–17], and increased mortality [18–20]. In Namibia, over 40% of adult and pediatric sites achieved the target of ≥90% *On-time pill pick-up* rates. In previously published EWI data in other African settings, only 15% of the 321 adult sites monitoring *On-time pill pick-up* achieved their target of ≥90% [21]. Similarly, published data from Cameroon revealed 0% of their sites achieving ≥90% on-time pill pick-up rates [22]. However, comparisons are limited because Namibia utilized the new WHO definition of *On-time pill pick-up*. With these data, Namibia plans to design operational research to investigate the sites performing poorly for site-level factors contributing to poor population adherence.

In Namibia, less than half of all adult ART sites achieved the target of ≥85% retention at 12 months with pediatric sites performing only slightly better. According to Fox and Rosen [23], sub-Saharan Africa reported an average of 80.2% retention at 12 months with LTFU being the highest contributing factor to attrition. In Namibia, data suggest a significant proportion of patients are not retained in care due to LTFU or transferring out to other ART clinics without informing their previous clinic. A recent paper in Malawi [24] found that out of 2,183 LTFU patients who were traced and alive, 1,226 (56%) were reported to be still taking ART from the original clinic or another clinic. Out of the 1,226, 293 (24%) patients reported treatment gaps. Therefore, it is possible that the low observed retention rates may be underestimates. Nevertheless, a substantial proportion of these patients may be at high risk for experiencing treatment interruptions and developing HIVDR [25–26]. According to Brinkhof et al [27], patients that are not retained have increased mortality, 40% of LTFU patients, with most of the mortality occurring during the first 6 months of disengagement with care. Namibia's broad range of retention rates between ART sites suggest there may be factors at site-level that are influencing retention. Efforts should be made to investigate reasons for disengagement from care in order to strengthen and standardize existing defaulter tracing mechanisms. Acting upon EWI data, Namibia has initiated operational research to examine reasons for LTFU and factors associated with LTFU. Additionally, an intervention study is planned to investigate the effect of defaulter tracing.

In previous EWI exercises in Namibia, it was not possible to monitor *Pharmacy stock-outs* or drug supply continuity due to inaccurate stock records [7–8]. However, modifications to the stock reporting system resulted in available data abstraction for this important EWI. In 2012, very few adult sites and a small number of pediatric sites had ART stock outs in Namibia. According to Bennett et al, in Africa 63% percent of 537 adult sites achieved the target of 100% of 12 months with no stock-outs in a 2012 aggregate analysis [21]. Additionally, Billong et al [22] reported 45% of 38 adult sites and Sigaloff et al [28] documented 75% of 12 adult sites reaching the WHO target. *Pharmacy stock-outs* is an important EWI to report because it is strongly associated with HIVDR and virological suppression [29]. The reasons for stock-outs in Namibia were poor inventory management practices, storage space constraints, and short-dated ARVs. Based on these data Namibia plans to strengthen supervision by regional pharmacists in order to ensure proper drug forecasting, procurement, and supply distribution. Long-term solutions for lack of storage space at certain ART sites are being investigated. Also, communication between the ART logistics pharmacist and the Central Medical Stores are being strengthened in order to determine appropriate ARV stock levels.

In Namibia, very few sites were found to have inappropriate prescribing of adult or pediatric regimens. In other African countries the reported percent of sites meeting the WHO target were, 74% of 907 sites [21], 90% of 40 sites [22], 88% of 81 sites [30], and 85% of 13 sites [28]. However, comparisons are limited by the change in the WHO definition for inappropriate regimens. Using the updated WHO definition (mono- or dual-therapy), very few ART sites in Namibia did not meet the WHO target for inappropriate dispensing. Furthermore, the small percentage of sites that did not meet the WHO target had <1% of patients dispensed mono or dual therapy. In investigating these cases of

mono- or dual-therapy, most were found to be transfers in from the private sector which were continued on these regimens by the ART clinic staff. Based on these data, Namibia plans to use clinical mentors to investigate patients on inappropriate regimens. In addition, plans are underway to engage the private sector in order to determine prescribing practices.

Due to availability of data, Namibia chose to monitor *Virological suppression at 6 months* instead of the WHO EWI recommendation of monitoring viral load at 12 months [4]. In the data analysis phase, it was discovered that data clerks at many ART sites were not correctly entering in undetectable viral loads into the ePMS. Therefore, the viral load suppression rates are likely gross underestimates. Although this exercise resulted in inaccurate estimates of virological suppression, lessons learned will be used to educate lab data entry clerks on the proper procedures for entering undetectable viral loads so that this important indicator can be accurately monitored in future years.

Since Namibia sampled representatively from all public ART sites in the country, a national estimate of each EWI was calculated. A nationally representative estimate can be used to monitor trends over time and compare the functioning of the ART program with internationally accepted standards. Also, individual ART sites can be compared to the national standard in order to determine sites underperforming and need further investigation. In addition, sites performing above national standards can be investigated for best practices which can then be applied to other ART sites. Comparisons were also made between adult and pediatric ART sites, which did not find any notable difference.

One important limitation of this EWI exercise is the inability to collect reliable data on *Virological suppression at 6 months*. Strengthening of ART data quality, as mentioned above, is an important factor for future monitoring. An additional limitation is these data were not disaggregated into outreach/satellite and IMAI sites for analysis, even though data for these sites were included in the main sites. Moving forward, Namibia plans to disaggregate EWI data into the IMAI and outreach/satellite sites from the main sites so that programmatic functioning can be assessed at every level of care. Also, as decentralisation of ART services continues, data quality will be strengthened at IMAI and outreach sites. Finally, the limitation to engage the private sector in EWI exercises prevents the ability to make broader statements about ART delivery and HIVDR in Namibia. Also, many patients in the public sector transfer in from the private sector and the lack of communication may lead to inaccurate data. Efforts are being made to include the private sector in future EWI exercises.

The successful 2012 EWI exercise built upon two previous rounds of EWIs [7–8] provides Namibia a solid evidence base, which can be used to make national statements about programmatic functioning in the context of HIVDR and related factors. This evidence base will serve to contextualize results from Namibia's surveys of HIVDR, which involve HIV genotype testing. Currently, analysis of data from national surveys of acquired and transmitted HIVDR is ongoing; nationally representative surveillance of pre-treatment and acquired HIVDR is planned.

The EWI abstraction process has mobilized the national ART program and its partners to institute minor adjustments in existing databases, which will facilitate abstraction of WHO recommended EWIs in the future (viral load suppression), and yield a more accurate assessment of overall programmatic functioning. Importantly, three successful rounds of EWI monitoring have highlighted the potential for HIVDR emergence in Namibia due to sites not optimizing adherence and retention of patients. These data have prompted the national program and its counterparts to engage sites in dialogue regarding the need to strengthen adherence and retention of patients on ART. The EWI collection process and EWI results will serve to optimize patient care and support Namibia in making evidence-based recommendations and take action to minimize the emergence of preventable HIVDR.

EWIs in Namibia have been integrated into the routine Monitoring and Evaluation activities of the MoHSS, thereby ensuring sustainability into the future. EWIs are routinely monitored at site level and reported as an ongoing activity with continuous validation along with annual national reporting.

Acknowledgments

The Republic of Namibia Ministry of Health and Social Services, WHO-Namibia, Management Sciences for Health/Systems for Improved Access to Pharmaceuticals and Services funded by USAID, Namibia Institute of Pathology, Tufts University School of Medicine (Christine Wanke, Megan Kassick), and WHO-Geneva.

Author Contributions

Conceived and designed the experiments: AJ VS MRJ TD SYH. Performed the experiments: VS SM MD SP SYH. Analyzed the data: AJ VS FT SP MRJ TD AMT SYH. Wrote the paper: AJ VS SP MRJ AMT SYH.

References

1. UNAIDS (2013) Global Report: UNAIDS report on the global AIDS epidemic 2013. Available at: http://www.unaids.org/en/media/unaids/contentassets/documents/epidemiology/2013/gr2013/UNAIDS_Global_Report_2013_en.pdf. Accessed December 5, 2013.
2. Coffin J (1995) HIV population dynamics in vivo: implications for genetic variation, pathogenesis, and therapy. Science 267(5197): 483–9.
3. Bennett DE, Bertagnolio S, Sutherland D, Gilks CF (2008) The World Health Organization's global strategy for prevention and assessment of HIV drug resistance. Antivir Ther 13(2): 1–13.
4. WHO (2012) Report on assessment of World Health Organization HIV drug resistance early warning indicator advisory panel meeting. Available at: http://apps.who.int/iris/bitstream/10665/75186/1/9789241503945_eng.pdf. Accessed September 26, 2013.
5. Central Intelligence Agency (2009) "Namibia". The World Factbook. Available at: https://www.cia.gov/library/publications/the-world-factbook/geos/wa.html. Accessed September 26, 2013.
6. Republic of Namibia Ministry of Health and Social Services Directorate of Special Programs (2010) National guidelines for antiretroviral therapy. Third edition. July 2010. Available at: http://www.who.int/hiv/pub/guidelines/namibia_art.pdf. Accessed September 26, 2013.
7. Hong SY, Jonas A, Dumeni E, Badi A, Pereko D, et al. (2010) Population-based Monitoring of HIV Drug Resistance in Namibia with Early Warning Indicators. J Acquir Immune Defic Syndr (55): 27–31
8. Jones A, Gweshe J, Siboleka M, DeKlerk M, Gawanab M, et al. (2013) HIV Drug Resistance Early Warning Indicators in Namibia for Public Health Action. PLoS ONE 8(6): e65653.
9. WHO (2010) World Health Organization indicators to monitor HIV drug resistance prevention at antiretroviral treatment sites. Available at: http://www2.paho.org/hq/dmdocuments/2010/hivdr-early-warning-indicators---updated-april-2010.pdf. Accessed September 26, 2013.
10. Toure S, Kouadio B, Seyler C, Traore M, Dakoury-Dogbo N, et al. (2008) Rapid scaling-up of antiretroviral therapy in 10,000 adults in Cote d'Ivoire: 2-year outcomes and determinants. AIDS (22): 873–82.
11. Bangsberg DR, Acosta EP, Gupta R, Guzman D, Riley ED, et al. (2006) Adherence-resistance relationships for protease and non-nucleoside reverse transcriptase inhibitors explained by virological fitness. AIDS (20): 223–31.
12. Sethi AK, Celentano DD, Gange SJ, Moore RD, Gallant JE (2003) Association between adherence to antiretroviral therapy and human immunodeficiency virus drug resistance. Clin Infect Dis (37): 1112–8.
13. Harrigan PR, Hogg RS, Dong WW, Yip B, Wynhoven B, et al. (2005) Predictors of HIV drug- resistance mutations in a large antiretroviral-naive cohort initiating triple antiretroviral therapy. J Infect Dis (191): 339–47.
14. Nachega JB, Hislop M, Dowdy DW, Chaisson RE, Regensberg L, et al. (2007) Adherence to non-nucleoside reverse transcriptase inhibitor-based HIV therapy and virologic outcomes. Ann Intern Med (146–8): 564–573.
15. Martin M, Del Cacho E, Codina C, Tuset M, De Lazzari E, et al. (2008) Relationship between adherence level, type of the antiretroviral regimen, and plasma HIV type 1 RNA viral load: a prospective cohort study. AIDS Res Hum Retroviruses (24): 1263–8.
16. Maggiolo F, Ravasio L, Ripamonti D, Gregis G, Quinzan G, et al. (2005) Similar adherence rates favor different virologic outcomes for patients treated with non- nucleoside analogues or protease inhibitors. Clin Infect Dis (40): 158–63.
17. Paterson DL, Swindells S, Mohr J, Brester M, Vergis EN, et al. (2000) Adherence to protease inhibitor therapy and outcomes in patients with HIV infection. Ann Intern Med (133): 21–30.
18. Lima VD, Harrigan R, Bangsberg DR, Hogg RS, Gross R, et al. (2009) The combined effect of modern highly active antiretroviral therapy regimens and adherence on mortality over time. J Acquir Immune Defic Syndr (50): 529–36.
19. Garcia de Olalla P, Knobel H, Carmona A, Guelar A, Lopez-Colomes JL, et al. (2002) Impact of adherence and highly active antiretroviral therapy on survival in HIV-infected patients. J Acquir Immune Defic Syndr (30): 105–10.
20. Nachega JB, Hislop M, Dowdy DW, Lo M, Regensberg L, et al. (2006) Adherence to highly active antiretroviral therapy assessed by pharmacy claims predicts survival in HIV-infected South African adults. J Acquir Immune Defic Syndr (43): 78–84.
21. Bennett DE, Jordan MR, Bertagnolio S, Hong SY, Ravasi G, et al. (2012) HIV drug resistance early warning indicators in cohorts of individuals starting antiretroviral therapy between 2004 and 2009: World Health Organization global report from 50 countries. Clin Infect Dis (54–4): S280–9.
22. Billong SC, Fokam J, Nkwescheu AS, Kembou E, Milenge P, et al. (2012) Early warning indicators for HIV drug resistance in Cameroon during the year 2010. PLoS One 7(5): e36777.
23. Fox MP, Rosen S (2010) Patient retention in antiretroviral therapy programs up to three years on treatment in sub-Saharan Africa, 2007–2009: systematic review. Trop Med Int Health (15): 1–15.
24. Tweya H, Feldacker C, Estill J, Jahn A, Ng'ambi W, et al. (2013) Are they really lost? "True" status and reasons for treatment discontinuation among HIV infected patients on antiretroviral therapy considered lost to follow up in urban Malawi. PLoS ONE 8(9): e75761.
25. Parienti JJ, Massari V, Descamps D, Vabret A, Bouvet E, et al. (2004) Predictors of virologic failure and resistance in HIV-infected patients treated with nevirapine- or efavirenz-based antiretroviral therapy. Clin Infect Dis (38): 1311–16.
26. Oyugi JH, Byakika-Tusiime J, Ragland K, Laeyendecker O, Mugerwa R, et al. (2007) Treatment interruptions predict resistance in HIV-positive individuals purchasing fixed-dose combination antiretroviral therapy in Kampala, Uganda. AIDS (21): 965–971.
27. Brinkhof MW, Pujades-Rodriguez M, Egger M (2009) Mortality of patients lost to follow-up in antiretroviral treatment pro- grammes in resource-limited settings: systematic review and meta-analysis. PLoS One (4): e5790.
28. Sigaloff KC, Hamers RL, Menke J, Labib M, Siwale M, et al. (2012) Early warning indicators for population-based monitoring of HIV drug resistance in 6 African countries. Clin Infect Dis 54(4): S294–9.
29. Marcellin F, Boyer S, Protopopescu C, Dia A, Ongolo-Zogo P, et al. (2008) Determinants of unplanned antiretroviral treatment interruptions among people living with HIV in Yaoundé, Cameroon (EVAL survey, ANRS 12-116). Trop Med Int Health (13): 1470–78.
30. Dzangare J, Gonese E, Mugurungi O, Shamu T, Apollo T, et al. (2012) Monitoring of early warning indicators for HIV drug resistance in antiretroviral therapy clinics in Zimbabwe. Clin Infect Dis (54): S313–6.

15

Life Course Impact of School-Based Promotion of Healthy Eating and Active Living to Prevent Childhood Obesity

Bach Xuan Tran[1], Arto Ohinmaa[1], Stefan Kuhle[2], Jeffrey A. Johnson[1], Paul J. Veugelers[1]*

1 School of Public Health, University of Alberta, Edmonton, Alberta, Canada, **2** Department of Pediatrics, Obstetrics & Gynecology, Dalhousie University, Halifax, NS, Canada

Abstract

Background: The Alberta Project Promoting active Living and healthy Eating in Schools (APPLE Schools) is a comprehensive school health program that is proven feasible and effective in preventing obesity among school aged children. To support decision making on expanding this program, evidence on its long-term health and economic impacts is particularly critical. In the present study we estimate the life course impact of the APPLE Schools programs in terms of future body weights and avoided health care costs.

Method: We modeled growth rates of body mass index (BMI) using longitudinal data from the National Population Health Survey collected between 1996–2008. These growth rate characteristics were used to project BMI trajectories for students that attended APPLE Schools and for students who attended control schools (141 randomly selected schools) in the Canadian province of Alberta.

Results: Throughout the life course, the prevalence of overweight (including obesity) was 1.2% to 2.8% (1.7 on average) less among students attending APPLE Schools relative to their peers attending control schools. The life course prevalence of obesity was 0.4% to 1.4% (0.8% on average) less among APPLE Schools students. If the APPLE Schools program were to be scaled up, the potential cost savings would be $33 to 82 million per year for the province of Alberta, or $150 to 330 million per year for Canada.

Conclusions: These projected health and economic benefits seem to support broader implementation of school-based health promotion programs.

Editor: Melania Manco, Scientific Directorate, Bambino Hospital, Italy

Funding: The Provincial evaluation was funded through a contract with Alberta Health. The APPLE Schools program was funded through a donation to the School of Public Health at the University of Alberta. The research was funded by an operating grant by the Canadian Institutes for Health Research (FRN: 91061), Heart and Stroke Foundation of Canada and Canadian Population Health Initiative, and through Canadian Institutes for Health Research and Alberta Innovates Health Solutions (AIHS) postdoctoral fellowships to Dr. Bach Tran, and a Canada Research Chair in Population Health, an Alberta Research Chair in Nutrition and Disease Prevention and AIHS Health Scholarship to Dr. Paul J. Veugelers. Dr. J. A. Johnson is a Centennial Professor at the University of Alberta and a Senior Health Scholar with AIHS. All interpretations and opinions in the present study are those of the authors. The funders had no role in study design, data collection and analysis, decision to publish, or preparation of the manuscript.

Competing Interests: The authors have declared that no competing interests exist.

* Email: paul.veugelers@ualberta.ca

Introduction

Obesity affects the health of Canadians and costs the nation approximately $1.27 to 11.08 billion per year in health care [1]. A myriad of psychological and physical consequences hamper obese individuals to function as healthy and productive members of the society. The physical consequences include chronic and fatal diseases such as cardiovascular disease, type 2 diabetes, and various cancers [2,3].

Poor eating habits and sedentary lifestyles are the established risk factors for obesity. Promotion of healthy eating and active living is considered to be most effective when targeting childhood years [4,5]. In the Canadian province of Alberta, we recently demonstrated the feasibility and effectiveness of a school-based program in preventing childhood obesity [6]. This Alberta Project Promoting active Living and healthy Eating in Schools (APPLE Schools) is a comprehensive school health program that started as

a pilot in 2008 in 10 elementary schools. The intervention involved a full-time School Health Facilitator in each school for implementing healthy eating and active living policies, practices and strategies while engaging stakeholders, including parents, staff and the community. School Health Facilitators contributed to the schools' health curriculum, and organized nutrition programs such as cooking clubs and healthy breakfast, lunch and snack programs, after school physical activity programs, walk-to-school days, community gardens, weekend events and circulated newsletters. By 2010 the eating habits and physical activity levels of students attending APPLE Schools had significantly improved whereas the prevalence of obesity had declined relative to their peers attending other Albertan schools [6]. These findings are consistent with other school-based programs internationally that took a comprehensive approach to promoting healthy eating and active living [5,7–9].

It is recognized that health status in early periods of life form the foundation for a healthier life course and that obesity in childhood often persists into adulthood. However, to date little is known about the long-term implications of successful prevention of childhood obesity [10]. Public health decision makers wish to be informed on the long-term health benefits and financial implications of these prevention programs. Guyer et al acknowledged the need for well-designed longitudinal studies to determine the importance of childhood interventions for health outcomes in adulthood, or in other words, to estimate the impact of early interventions on the life-course of the youngsters who had been subjected to these intervention (a life-course approach) [10]. The purpose of this study is to estimate the life course impact of the APPLE Schools program in terms of future body weight status and avoided health care costs.

Materials and Methods

This study has been reviewed and approved by the Health Research Ethics Board of the University of Alberta, Edmonton, Alberta, Canada.

Data source and statistical analysis

We previously published that the prevalence of obesity among grade five students (typically 10 or 11 years of age) attending APPLE Schools reduced 2.2% between 2008 and 2010 as compared to a 2.8% increase in the prevalence of obesity among grade fivers attending other schools [6]. This difference is equivalent to reductions of 0.26 and 0.17 kg/m^2 in body mass index (BMI) per year among girls and boys, respectively, participating in APPLE Schools programs. These intervention benefits were used as the starting points of life course BMI trajectories to estimate the life course impact of the APPLE Schools intervention.

For the purpose of determining longitudinal BMI trajectories throughout the life course, we accessed longitudinal data of persons of all ages who participated in the Canadian National Population Health Surveys (NPHS). The NPHS included longitudinal assessment of 17,276 persons selected from each of the 10 Canadian provinces [11–13]. The data were anonymized and we accessed and analyzed the data at the Research Data Center of the University of Alberta, Edmonton, AB, Canada. The NPHS employed a stratified two-stage sample design based on the Labour Force Survey in all provinces except for the province of Québec, where the another survey, the Enquête Sociale et de Santé, was used. Participants were followed up and interviewed every two years (cycles) using a common set of health questions. Follow up response rates ranged from 92.8% in cycle 2 to 70.7% in cycle 8. Data collection continued when participants were institutionalized in a long-term care facility and included verification of vital status. Data collection at baseline (cycle 1 in 1994/1995) was through in-person interviews, and in subsequent cycles through telephone interviews [11]. To minimize systematic differences in data collection, we excluded cycle 1 from the present analysis. Cycle 2 to 8 provide longitudinal data for 1996 to 2008 that included self-reported heights and weights. We restricted our analyses to observations of individuals in the age range of 11 to 70 years, as 11 is the typical age students reach while in grade five (i.e., the grade level of the assessment of the APPLE Schools program effectiveness). Age 70 was set as the upper labour age in light of assessing potential economic implications. We used standards set by the World Health Organization to classify adult body weight categories; underweight (BMI <18.5), normal weight (BMI ≥

18.5 to <25), overweight (BMI ≥25 to <30), and obesity (BMI ≥ 30).

We applied growth curve models to the longitudinal NPHS data to quantify individual changes in BMI over time. These BMI trajectories were estimated for 5 different age period: 11 to <23, 23 to <35, 35 to <47, 47 to <59, and 59 to 70 years of age. This staggered modeling approach provided flexibility to the full life course BMI trajectory and improved our ability to estimate the models since each NPHS participant was tracked for 14 years over 7 NPHS cycles. The growth curve models describe BMI changes in one age category as a function of the development of BMI in the previous age category. In other words, for each age category, the growth curve model estimates the changes in BMI based on the BMI starting value in that particular age category. For example, we estimated the BMI growth for the age 11 to less than 23 years using the BMI at age 11 years. This would provide a projected BMI at age 22.99 years, which would then be the starting value for the estimation of the BMI growth in the subsequent age category, 23 to less than 34 years, and so on.

The model selection was purposive, and we applied an analytical procedure that had been used in previous studies and shown to be robust in estimating trajectories of BMI of individuals using this data set [14,15]. The models were adjusted for survey sampling weights, sex, body weight status, and calendar year. We further considered interaction terms of sex and age, and of sex and the quadratic form of age [14]. Body weight status (at the beginning of each age category) was considered as a random effect in these models, as were sex as well as intercept and linear slope [14]. The growth curve models were considered to have an unstructured covariance matrix [14]. We computed Bosker/Snijders and Bryk/Raudenbush R-square values for mixed models with two levels.

To project the life course BMI trajectories of grade five students in Alberta, we applied the parameters from the above described growth curve models to overweight and obesity prevalence rates of Alberta [6]. These prevalence rates originated from a population-based survey including 3,398 grade five students from 141 randomly selected schools from across Alberta in 2010 [6]. We then repeated the projection of the life course BMI trajectories adjusting the starting prevalence rates for the reduction in BMI resulting from the APPLE Schools program. The differences between the two models then represent the potential life course impact of the APPLE School program on the projected BMI status.

Projection of health care cost savings by reduction in the prevalence of overweight and obesity was estimated by multiplying the total direct health care cost for obesity by the proportion of overweight and obese cases prevented by the intervention. An updated estimation by Anis et al showed that the annual direct health care cost of overweight and obesity in Canada was $ 6 billion in 2006 [16]. We assumed that this cost remained unchanged overtime and for every overweight and obese case that we prevented, we avoided the costs for health conditions related to obesity.

Results

Table 1 presents the parameter estimates for each of the 5 age-specific growth curve models used to project life course changes in BMI for grade five students in Alberta. Figure 1 presents the projected body weight status for grade five students with normal weight using the parameter estimates of Table 1. Approximately 40% of normal weight youth are estimated to progress to overweight by the time they turn 25 years of age. This percentage will further increase to 60% by the time they turn 35 years of age. Figure 2 depicts the projected body weight status for grade five students who were overweight and shows that 60% will progress to obesity by the time they turn 30 years of age. Very few overweight youth enter adulthood as normal weight (Figure 2). Lastly, figure 3 shows that nearly all obese youth progresses to obese adults.

When applying the grow curves to grade five students attending APPLE Schools, we estimated that for every unit increase in BMI at age 11, 23, 35, 47, and 59, the BMI growth rate over the five corresponding age-specific periods increased by 0.82, 0.890, 0.969, 0.930, and 0.863 kg/m^2 respectively (p<0.05). Comparing the estimates of the growth curves applied to students attending APPLE Schools and attending other Alberta schools, we quantified the benefits of the APPLE Schools program throughout the students' lifetime. This is presented in Figure 4. The lifetime prevalence of overweight (including obesity) was 1.2% to 2.8% (1.7 on average) less among students attending APPLE Schools relative to those attending other Alberta schools. The prevalence of obesity was 0.4% to 1.4% (0.8% on average) less among students attending APPLE Schools students relative to those attending other Alberta schools (Figure 4). We estimated that 2% to 5.5% of overweight cases and 3% to 6.5% of obesity cases could be prevented through the APPLE Schools program (Figure 5).

If this program were to be scaled up to Canada that spends approximately 6 billion dollars for health care for people with excess body weight, the potential cost savings would be 150 to 330

million dollars per year (Figure 6) [16]. Similarly, if this program were to be scaled up to Alberta, it could save 33–82 million dollars for obesity-related health care in Alberta (Figure 6). The avoided health care costs were in average higher at younger ages (Figure 6).

Discussion

We projected of body weight trajectories of youth in Alberta and forecasted that more than two thirds is likely to develop excess body weight at some point in their lives. We further modeled the long-term benefits of the APPLE Schools intervention and forecasted that the prevalence of overweight (including obesity) among students attending APPLE Schools is 2% to 6% less relative to the prevalence among their peers who are attending other schools in Alberta. With a nationwide implementation of the APPLE Schools program, this could result in 150 to 330 million dollars per year in cost savings due to avoided health care services.

We forecasted that more than two thirds of current youth is likely to become overweight or obese at some point in their lives. This seems higher that the forecasts by Kuhle [17] who reported that 45% of youth would have excess body weight by 2006 and 55% by in 2026. Forecasts in the US had revealed that in 2010 the obesity prevalence of sex and racial subgroups ranges from 33 to 55% and that the national prevalence of obesity is expected to increase to 51% by 2030 [18,19].

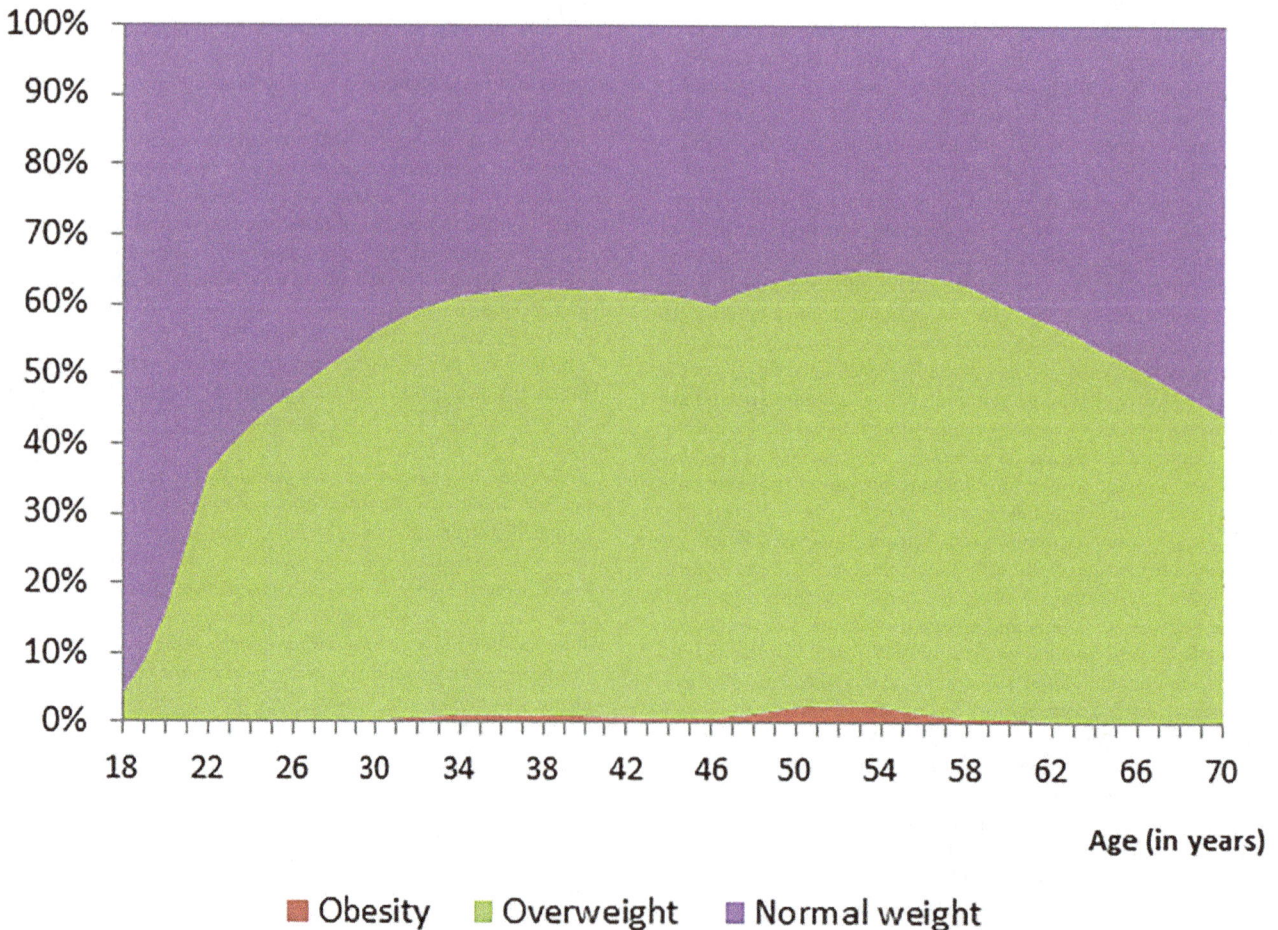

Figure 1. Life course weight status projections of normal weight grade five students.

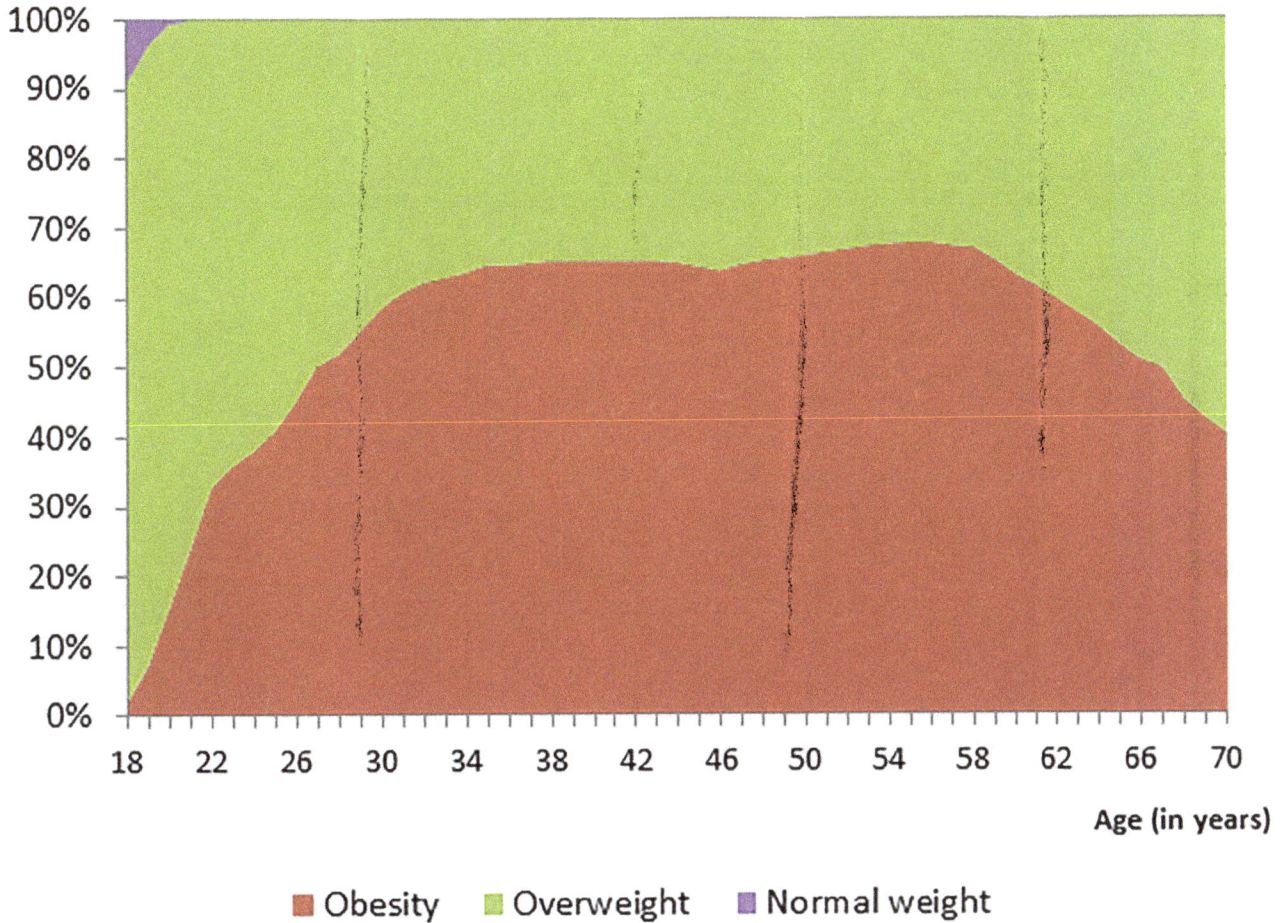

Figure 2. Life course weight status projections of overweight grade five students.

The present study is the first to follow a life course approach for the purpose of quantifying the impact on adulthood obesity of school-based promotion of healthy eating and active living. Our findings are consistent with the existing evidence that interventions at an early age are effective in influencing body weight status later in life and that school-based prevention programs may therefore be cost effective [5,20–26]. In the United States, Wang et al. developed a progression model to project the long-term benefits of a school based intervention and reported a 1% reduction in overweight and obese and $586 million in cost savings [27]. We estimated direct health care costs savings of $150 to 330 million per year in Canada, based on the prevention of 2% to 6% of the projected cases of overweight and obesity. If these estimates hold true, it would seem that small reductions in childhood obesity prevalence translate into large costs savings at the population level, and thus school programs and other initiatives that can further reduce overweight prevalence rates will further contribute to program effectiveness and cost savings.

Body weight in childhood is an established predictor of body weight at a later age [20,28–35]. For example, Magarey et al had tracked the weight status of Finnish children and identified weight status at age 6 as a strong predictor of weight status in adulthood [28], and Starc and Strel tracked 4,833 Slovenian children and found that those who were obese at age 18 years, 40% of males and 48.6% of females had been obese at 7 years [31]. It is for this reason that we had considered early body weight in our growth

curves, and our analyses confirmed the importance of body weight for growth in body weight. However, reduction in the prevalence of excess body weight was not the only benefit reported for APPLE Schools. We had also reported benefits to healthy eating and active living [6], that were achieved throughout a comprehensive approach that improved students' knowledge levels, attitudes, self-efficacy and leadership skills related to making healthy choices. Where knowledge, attitudes and life skills may persist over the life course of APPLE Schools graduates, they may contribute to healthier choices later in life and herewith to more prevention of excess body weight. The health and costs benefits revealed in this study may therefore not have fully captured the potential impacts of the APPLE Schools program, and comprehensive school health programs in general.

A strength of the present study is that it was based on large established national and provincial studies as well as a feasible school-based intervention that will improve the generalizability of the findings. More over, we followed a life course approach to provide insight into the future health benefits and cost implications of interventions. Where students' heights and weights were measured in APPLE Schools and control schools, heights and weights in the longitudinal NPHS were obtained through self-report. Self-report of height and weight is prone to error which we acknowledge as a study limitation. Other study limitations may relate to the use of administrative health care databases for the purpose of estimating avoided health case costs. Furthermore,

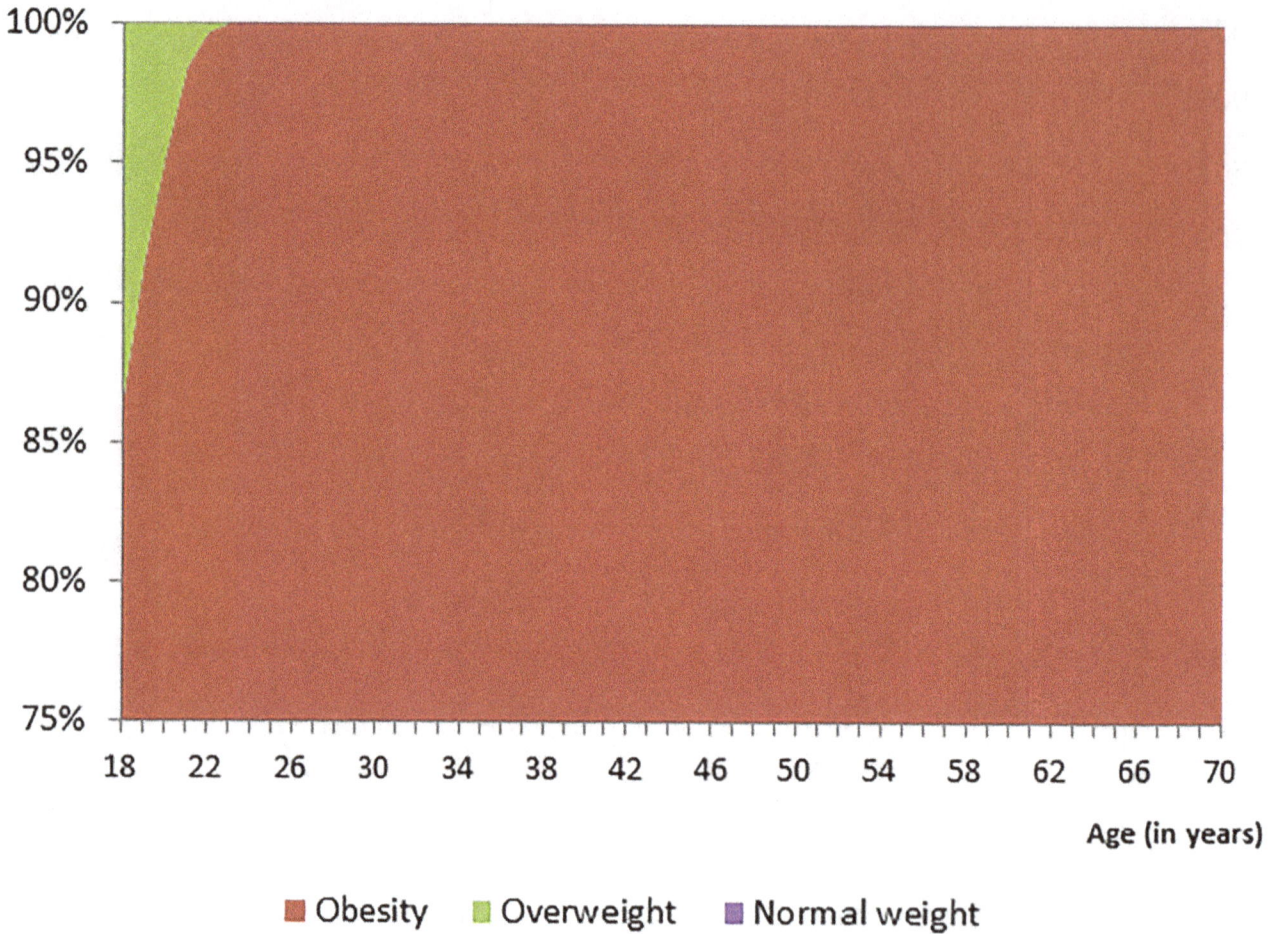

Figure 3. Life course weight status projections of obese grade five students.

Table 1. Growth curve modeling of BMI for five age categories of participants of the Canadian National Population Health Survey.

	Age: 11,<23	Age: 23,<35	Age: 35,<−47	Age: 47,<59	Age: 59,<71
Boy	**7.767**	**15.442**	**29.673**	**2.766**	−0.300
Girl	**4.800**	**13.915**	**11.684**	9.631	−1.674
Boy×Age	**1.285**	**0.571**	−0.201	**0.903**	0.903
Girl×Age	**1.701**	0.569	**0.604**	0.562	0.903
Boy×Age^2	**−0.023**	−0.008	0.003	**−0.008**	−0.008
Girl×Age^2	**−0.040**	−0.008	−0.007	−0.005	−0.007
Year					
1996	reference	reference	reference	reference	reference
1998	−0.134	**0.207**	**0.220**	0.117	0.029
2000	−0.013	**0.358**	**0.589**	**0.380**	**0.328**
2002	0.162	**0.811**	**0.882**	**0.683**	**0.647**
2004	0.367	**0.911**	**0.978**	**0.643**	**0.673**
2006	0.058	**1.002**	**1.232**	**0.868**	**0.923**
2008	0.029	**1.139**	**1.299**	**1.011**	**1.082**
R2 coefficient	0.33	0.12	0.08	0.04	0.02

Note: Figures in bold represent statistically significant estimates (p < 0.05).

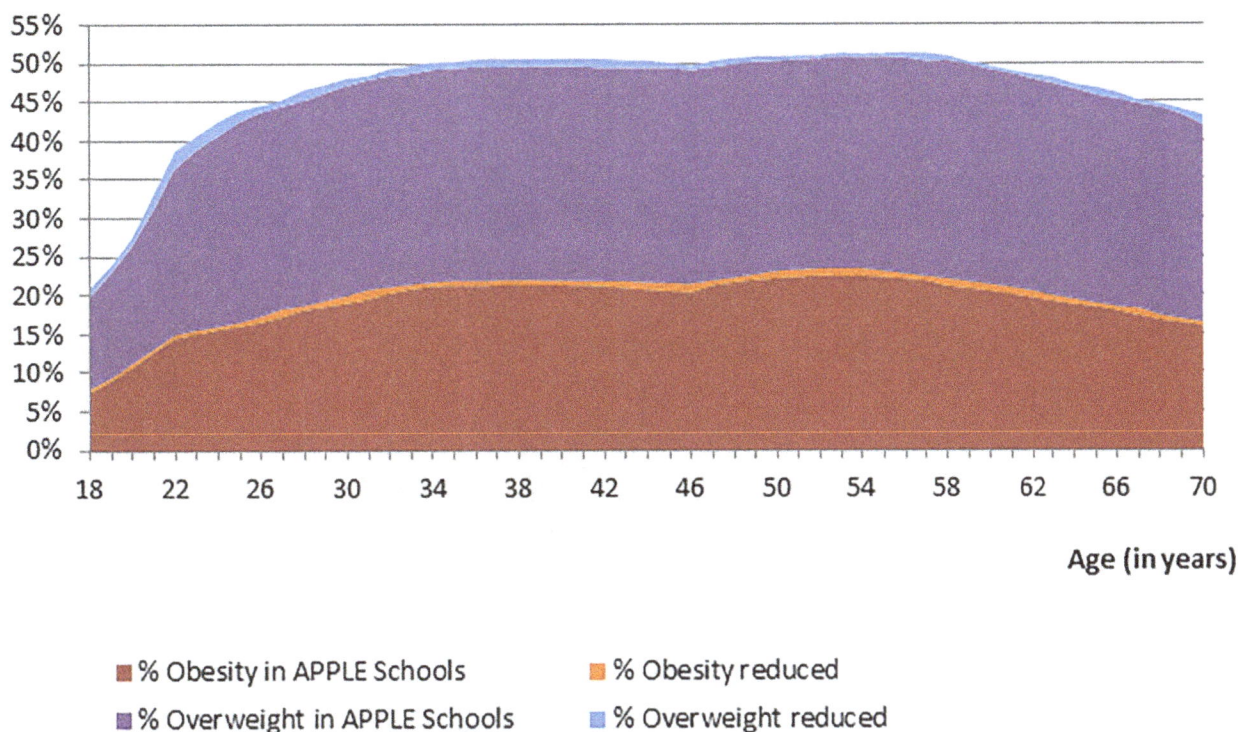

Figure 4. Life course weight status projections for the grade five students attending the APPLE Schools program and those who are not. Figure 4 footnote: Purple represents the percentage of students attending APPLE Schools who are projected to become overweight; Blue represents the percentage students attending other Alberta schools who are projected to become overweight; Red represents the percentage of students attending APPLE Schools who are projected to become obese; Orange represents the percentage students attending other Alberta schools who are projected to become obese.

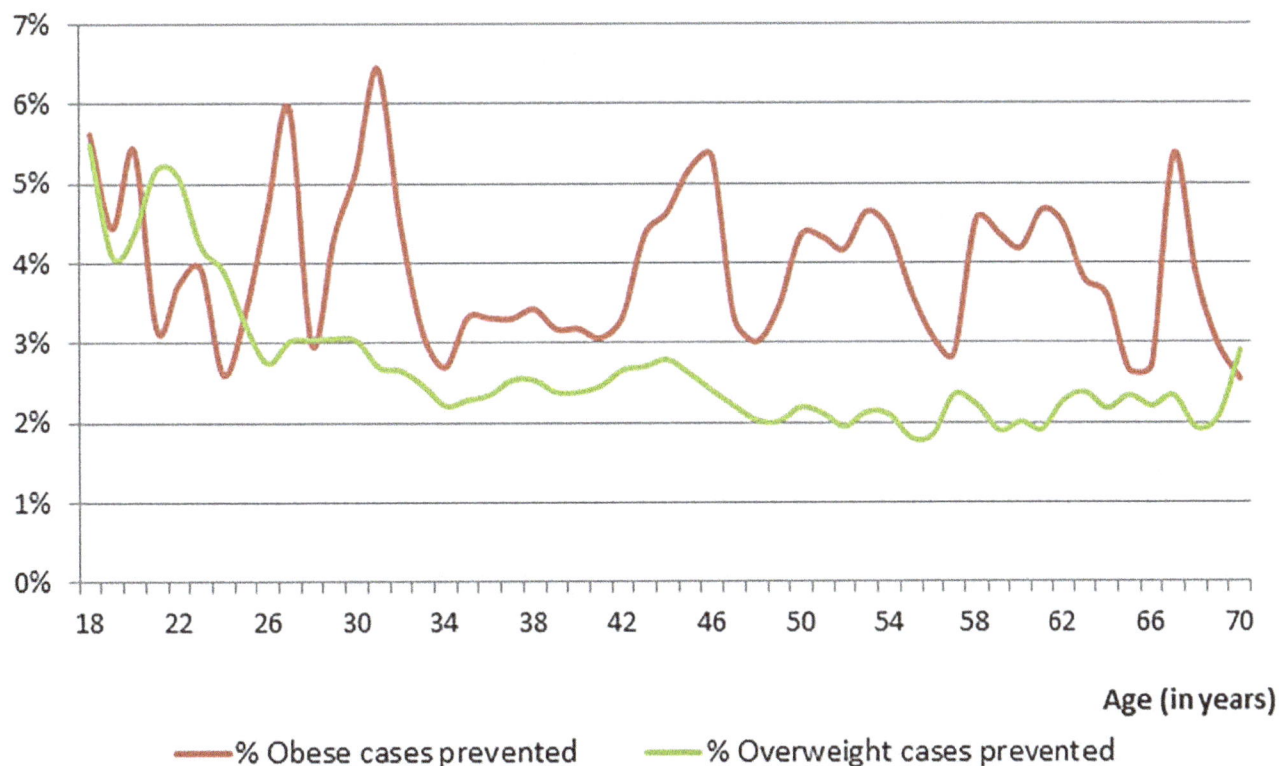

Figure 5. Life course projections of the percentage prevented overweight and obese cases.

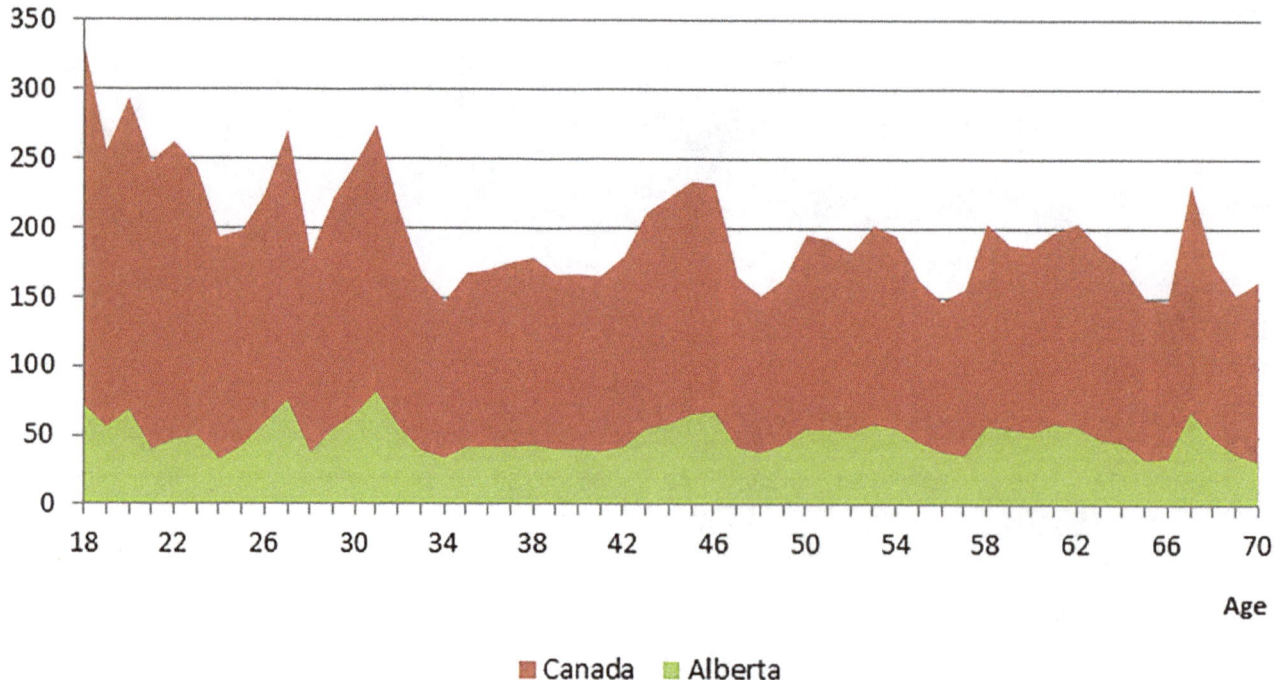

Figure 6. Life course projections of avoided health care costs for Canada and the province of Alberta (in million dollars).

projections assume that future developments follow patterns similar to the patterns in the observations on which the projection models are based. We acknowledge that future patterns may deviate from observed patterns which, in turn, may affect our estimates.

To conclude, preventing childhood obesity during their school years is forecasted to reduce obesity in adulthood which may lead to substantial savings in future health care costs at population level. Youth with healthy weights are less likely to develop overweight and obesity through their lives. Also, healthy habits and skills acquired in childhood may lend for life long healthy behaviors that further reduce the likelihood of weight gain [36]. Potential cost savings should encourage the allocation of resources towards school-based promotion of healthy eating and active living.

Acknowledgments

We thank all of the grade five students, parents and schools for their participation in the REAL Kids Alberta evaluation and APPLE Schools program, and the evaluation assistants, health promotion coordinators and school health facilitators for their contributions in data collection.

Author Contributions

Conceived and designed the experiments: PJV AO SK JAJ BXT. Performed the experiments: PJV AO BXT. Analyzed the data: BXT. Contributed reagents/materials/analysis tools: PJV AO SK JAJ BXT. Wrote the paper: PJV AO SK JAJ BXT.

References

1. Tran BX, Nair AV, Kuhle S, Ohinmaa A, Veugelers PJ (2013) Cost analyses of obesity in Canada: scope, quality, and implications. Cost Eff Resour Alloc 11: 3.
2. Trasande L (2011) Quantifying the economic consequences of childhood obesity and potential benefits of interventions. Expert Rev Pharmacoecon Outcomes Res 11: 47–50.
3. Saha AK, Sarkar N, Chatterjee T (2011) Health consequences of childhood obesity. Indian J Pediatr 78: 1349–1355.
4. Zenzen W, Kridli S (2009) Integrative review of school-based childhood obesity prevention programs. J Pediatr Health Care 23: 242–258.
5. Veugelers PJ, Fitzgerald AL (2005) Effectiveness of school programs in preventing childhood obesity: a multilevel comparison. Am J Public Health 95: 432–435.
6. Fung C, Kuhle S, Lu C, Purcell M, Schwartz M, et al. (2012) From "best practice" to "next practice": the effectiveness of school-based health promotion in improving healthy eating and physical activity and preventing childhood obesity. Int J Behav Nutr Phys Act 9: 27.
7. Greening L, Harrell KT, Low AK, Fielder CE (2011) Efficacy of a school-based childhood obesity intervention program in a rural southern community: TEAM Mississippi Project. Obesity (Silver Spring) 19: 1213–1219.
8. Verstraeten R, Roberfroid D, Lachat C, Leroy JL, Holdsworth M, et al. (2012) Effectiveness of preventive school-based obesity interventions in low- and middle-income countries: a systematic review. Am J Clin Nutr 96: 415–438.
9. Khambalia AZ, Dickinson S, Hardy LL, Gill T, Baur LA (2012) A synthesis of existing systematic reviews and meta-analyses of school-based behavioural interventions for controlling and preventing obesity. Obes Rev 13: 214–233.
10. Guyer B, Ma S, Grason H, Frick KD, Perry DF, et al. (2009) Early childhood health promotion and its life course health consequences. Acad Pediatr 9: 142–149 e141–171.
11. Asakawa K, Senthilselvan A, Feeny D, Johnson J, Rolfson D (2012) Trajectories of health-related quality of life differ by age among adults: results from an eight-year longitudinal study. J Health Econ 31: 207–218.
12. Orpana HM, Berthelot JM, Kaplan MS, Feeny DH, McFarland B, et al. (2010) BMI and mortality: results from a national longitudinal study of Canadian adults. Obesity (Silver Spring) 18: 214–218.
13. Katzmarzyk PT, Ardern CI (2004) Overweight and obesity mortality trends in Canada, 1985–2000. Can J Public Health 95: 16–20.
14. Ng C, Corey PN, Young TK (2012) Divergent body mass index trajectories between Aboriginal and non-Aboriginal Canadians 1994–2009–an exploration of age, period, and cohort effects. Am J Hum Biol 24: 170–176.
15. Pryor LE, Tremblay RE, Boivin M, Touchette E, Dubois L, et al. (2011) Developmental trajectories of body mass index in early childhood and their risk factors: an 8-year longitudinal study. Arch Pediatr Adolesc Med 165: 906–912.
16. Anis AH, Zhang W, Bansback N, Guh DP, Amarsi Z, et al. (2009) Obesity and overweight in Canada: an updated cost-of-illness study. Obes Rev 11: 31–40.
17. Kuhle S (2011) Forecasting the prevalence of overweight and obesity in Canada. Chapter 3 PhD thesis University of Alberta.

18. Wang YC, Colditz GA, Kuntz KM (2007) Forecasting the obesity epidemic in the aging U.S. population. Obesity (Silver Spring) 15: 2855–2865.

19. Finkelstein EA, Khavjou OA, Thompson H, Trogdon JG, Pan L, et al. (2012) Obesity and severe obesity forecasts through 2030. Am J Prev Med 42: 563–570.

20. Wu JF (2013) Childhood obesity: a growing global health hazard extending to adulthood. Pediatr Neonatol 54: 71–72.

21. Lehnert T, Sonntag D, Konnopka A, Riedel-Heller S, Konig HH (2012) The long-term cost-effectiveness of obesity prevention interventions: systematic literature review. Obes Rev 13: 537–553.

22. Moodie M, Haby MM, Swinburn B, Carter R (2011) Assessing cost-effectiveness in obesity: active transport program for primary school children–TravelSMART Schools Curriculum program. J Phys Act Health 8: 503–515.

23. McAuley KA, Taylor RW, Farmer VL, Hansen P, Williams SM, et al. (2010) Economic evaluation of a community-based obesity prevention program in children: the APPLE project. Obesity (Silver Spring) 18: 131–136.

24. Carter R, Moodie M, Markwick A, Magnus A, Vos T, et al. (2009) Assessing cost-effectiveness in obesity (ACE-obesity): an overview of the ACE approach, economic methods and cost results. BMC Public Health 9: 419.

25. Wang LY, Gutin B, Barbeau P, Moore JB, Hanes J, Jr., et al. (2008) Cost-effectiveness of a school-based obesity prevention program. J Sch Health 78: 619–624.

26. Brown HS, 3rd, Perez A, Li YP, Hoelscher DM, Kelder SH, et al. (2007) The cost-effectiveness of a school-based overweight program. Int J Behav Nutr Phys Act 4: 47.

27. Wang LY, Denniston M, Lee S, Galuska D, Lowry R (2010) Long-term health and economic impact of preventing and reducing overweight and obesity in adolescence. J Adolesc Health 46: 467–473.

28. Magarey AM, Daniels LA, Boulton TJ, Cockington RA (2003) Predicting obesity in early adulthood from childhood and parental obesity. Int J Obes Relat Metab Disord 27: 505–513.

29. Dietz WH, Robinson TN (2005) Clinical practice. Overweight children and adolescents. N Engl J Med 352: 2100–2109.

30. Park MH, Falconer C, Viner RM, Kinra S (2012) The impact of childhood obesity on morbidity and mortality in adulthood: a systematic review. Obes Rev 13: 985–1000.

31. Starc G, Strel J (2011) Tracking excess weight and obesity from childhood to young adulthood: a 12-year prospective cohort study in Slovenia. Public Health Nutr 14: 49–55.

32. Herman KM, Craig CL, Gauvin L, Katzmarzyk PT (2009) Tracking of obesity and physical activity from childhood to adulthood: the Physical Activity Longitudinal Study. Int J Pediatr Obes 4: 281–288.

33. Atkinson W (2008) Early intervention. Childhood obesity programs aim to put kids on a new, healthier path to adulthood. AHIP Cover 49: 26–28, 30, 32 passim.

34. Venn AJ, Thomson RJ, Schmidt MD, Cleland VJ, Curry BA, et al. (2007) Overweight and obesity from childhood to adulthood: a follow-up of participants in the 1985 Australian Schools Health and Fitness Survey. Med J Aust 186: 458–460.

35. Allman-Farinelli MA, King L, Bauman AE (2007) Overweight and obesity from childhood to adulthood: a follow-up of participants in the 1985 Australian Schools Health and Fitness Survey. Comment. Med J Aust 187: 314; author reply 314–315.

36. Lhachimi SK, Nusselder WJ, Lobstein TJ, Smit HA, Baili P, et al. (2013) Modelling obesity outcomes: reducing obesity risk in adulthood may have greater impact than reducing obesity prevalence in childhood. Obes Rev.

16

The "Sniffin' Kids" Test - A 14-Item Odor Identification Test for Children

Valentin A. Schriever[1]*, **Eri Mori**[3], **Wenke Petters**[1], **Carolin Boerner**[1], **Martin Smitka**[2], **Thomas Hummel**[1]

1 Smell & Taste Clinic, Department of Otorhinolaryngology, University Hospital Carl Gustav Carus, Technische Universität (TU) Dresden, Dresden, Germany, **2** Department of Neuropediatrics, University Hospital Carl Gustav Carus, Technische Universität (TU) Dresden, Dresden, Germany, **3** Department of Otorhinolaryngology, Jikei University, School of Medicine, Tokyo, Japan

Abstract

Tools for measuring olfactory function in adults have been well established. Although studies have shown that olfactory impairment in children may occur as a consequence of a number of diseases or head trauma, until today no consensus on how to evaluate the sense of smell in children exists in Europe. Aim of the study was to develop a modified "Sniffin' Sticks" odor identification test, the "Sniffin' Kids" test for the use in children. In this study 537 children between 6-17 years of age were included. Fourteen odors, which were identified at a high rate by children, were selected from the "Sniffin' Sticks" 16-item odor identification test. Normative date for the 14-item "Sniffin' Kids" odor identification test was obtained. The test was validated by including a group of congenital anosmic children. Results show that the "Sniffin' Kids" test is able to discriminate between normosmia and anosmia with a cutoff value of >7 points on the odor identification test. In addition the test-retest reliability was investigated in a group of 31 healthy children and shown to be $\rho = 0.44$. With the 14-item odor identification "Sniffin' Kids" test we present a valid and reliable test for measuring olfactory function in children between ages 6–17 years.

Editor: Matthieu Louis, Center for Genomic Regulation, Spain

Funding: This study received no external support. Internal funding was provided by the department of otolaryngology, TU Dresden. The funder had no role in study design, data collection and analysis, decision to publish, or preparation of the manuscript.

* Email: valentin.schriever@mac.com

Introduction

The evaluation of the chemical senses has gained more interest in recent years. The administration of smell tests is widely used in clinical routine, especially in ENT and neurological clinics [1]. Several tests have been established as instruments for measuring olfactory function. In Northern America the University of Pennsylvania Smell Identification Test (UPSIT) is broadly used [2], while in Europe the administration of the "Sniffin' Sticks" test battery is used more commonly [3,4]; in Japan the T&T olfactometer has been the standard for the last decades [5]. These tests were developed for distinguishing normosmia from hyposmia/anosmia in adults [2,3,6]. Despite the fact, that all tests have been used in children (e.g. [3,7]), they are not well suited for children, due to the lengths of the test and possible unfamiliarity of the odors to young children. Therefore many clinics and laboratories used self-made olfactory tests when evaluating and studying olfactory function of children [9–13]. Most of these tests were not well evaluated and therefore the study results were difficult to compare to each other. Only in recent years the development of olfactory tests, especially designed for the administration in children, has been undertaken [14–18]. The "smell wheel" and the olfactory test of the NIH Toolbox are based on the UPSIT and the scratch and sniff technique [14,16]. Both tests are for use in the USA or at least are aiming at English speaking children. Another odor identification test using squeeze bottles was developed in Australia [15]. None of these tests have

gained wide distribution in Europe. A few studies have been conducted in Europe addressing this issue. The short version of the "Sniffin' Sticks" odor identification test was evaluated in Dutch children between the age of 6 and 11 years [8]. To our knowledge this test was not evaluated in other countries for children. In a recent study conducted in Poland, a short 6-item odor identification test was developed. So far this test is only used in Poland due to its odor selection and self-development it is commercially unavailable [18]. Since the "Sniffin' Sticks" 16-item odor identification test is commonly used for assessing olfactory function of adults in Europe, the primary aim of the current study was the evaluation of this test in a population between age 6–17 years. Secondly a modification of the 16-item odor identification test was planned to make it more applicable to children, which we named "Sniffin' Kids" Test, establishing a feasible method for odor identification testing for children.

Material and Methods

Ethics statement

For all study protocols the approval of the local Ethics Board of the Faculty of Medicine of the TU of Dresden had been obtained and all aspects of the study were performed in accordance to the Declaration of Helsinki. The study was explained to the parents and children in great detail, including the study design, procedure, tasks and possible risks. In addition to the verbal information given to the children/parents, written study information was provided separately for children and parents. Children under 8 years of age received verbal information only. Written informed consent was obtained from the parents. All participants gave their assent to participate in this study.

This study consisted of two parts. In part one the original "Sniffin' Sticks" 16-item odor identification test was applied to children between age 6 and 17 years. In the second part the odor identification test was modified according to the results from part one. This modified version was named "Sniffin' Kids" test.

Part one

Participants. The data from 537 children, which underwent olfactory odor identification testing, was used for this study. The children were tested during the course of previously published [19,20] or still ongoing studies. Children were recruited for each study using advertising flyers at the University Campus in Dresden, therefore representing the local population. In addition data was collected at the University of Dresden science fairs. For all children normal sense of smell was self-reported or reported by their parents by questionnaire (Do you have any problems with your sense of smell? Did you notice any problems with your child's sense of smell? Did he/she did not perceive an odor others were able to perceive?). None of the children suffered from any disease linked to olfactory dysfunction (e.g. diabetes mellitus, epilepsy, renal failure etc.). All children included in the study grew up in Germany and were fluent in the German language.

The mean age of the children was 11.9 years (SD 3.1, range 6–17) with a gender distribution of 268 girls and 269 boys (Table 1).

Testing. Testing took place in a quiet environment in a well-ventilated room. Each child was tested alone. All children were tested using the original "Sniffin' Sticks" 16-item odor identification test [21]. The use of the "Sniffin' Sticks" for odor presentation has been well evaluated in several studies [3,4]. The "Sniffin' Sticks" are felt tip pens filled with odors. For odor presentation the cap is removed and each pen is presented approximately 2 cm under the nose for 3 seconds. The children were asked to identify the odors presented from four given descriptors, which were presented in writing and in pictures. In addition the descriptors were read to the children. The children were allowed to smell each odor as often as necessary but had to choose one of the four given descriptors (4 alternative forced choice). The sum of the correct answers was regarded as the odor identification score.

Part two

Two odors were excluded from the original odor identification test according to the results of part one. Thus resulting in the 14-item odor identification test ("Sniffin' Kids" test). Therefore the data analysis of the 537 children was repeated to obtain normative data for the 14-item odor identification test. The body mass index (BMI-Z-scores) was recorded to observe the influence of the BMI on the odor identification results in 81 children (45 girls, 36 boys).

Test validity. The validity of the test, to distinguish between normosmia and anosmia in children, was investigated by comparing

odor identification scores of children with isolated congenital anosmia (ICA) to the healthy control group (n = 537).

Anosmic children. Twenty-five children with ICA were included who were tested in our Smell & Taste Clinic between 2005 and 2010 with a mean age of 12 years (SD 2.7, range 8–17 years), (Table 1). All ICA subjects were referred to the Department of Otorhinolaryngology at the TU Dresden by other Departments of this University (e.g., Pediatrics and Neurology) or they presented themselves to the smell dysfunction clinic of the Department of Otorhinolaryngology. All subjects were in good health with no signs or symptoms except for anosmia. Upon careful questioning none of these patients could remember any odorous sensations apart from intranasal sensations likely to be mediated by the trigeminal nerves. All of the ICA subjects had MRI scans of the brain; none of them had any major cranial malformation as verified by T1- and T2-weighted MRI sequences. In addition to psychophysical testing most ICA subjects – whenever deemed necessary - also received electrophysiological testing using chemosensory event-related potentials; none of the tested ICA patients had electrophysiological responses to olfactory stimuli.

Test reliability. To test the reliability of the 14-item odor identification test, a subgroup of 31 children (19 girls, 12 boys; mean age 11.7 years, SD 1.33 years) was tested a second time 4-6 months after the first session.

Statistical analyses

Descriptive statistics were obtained for the odor identification scores. In addition the percentage of correct identification for each individual odor was calculated. The data was analyzed by means of SPSS 22.0 (SPSS Inc., Chicago, IL, USA). T-tests were used whenever appropriate. The data of the 16- as well as the 14-item odor identification test was not normally distributed as evaluated by the Kolmogorow-Smirnow-Test ($p < 0.0.001$ for both data sets). Therefore non-parametric tests (Cochran, Wilcoxon-Test, Mann-Whitney-U-Test and Kruskal-Walis-Test) were used whenever appropriate. In addition Spearman's correlations were used. The level of significance was set at 0.05. Degrees of freedom are written in subscript when indicated.

Results

Part one

In this study 537 children (268 girls, 269 boys) with an age range of 6-17 years (mean 11.9 years, SD 3.10 years) were included. The age distribution between girls and boys was not significantly different ($t_{535} = 0.19$, $p = 0.85$).

Children performed with a mean of 11.98 points (SD 2.07, range 2-16 points) on the 16-item odor identification test. The percentage of correct identification for each item was calculated to identify odors, which are not familiar to children. Listed from high to low mean percentage of correct identification: Peppermint: 97%, Banana: 93%, Fish: 92%, Orange: 86%, Cinnamon: 86%, Coffee: 83%, Cloves: 79%, Garlic: 78%, Pineapple: 76%, Rose 75%, Lemon: 75%, Liquorice: 70%, Aniseed: 69%, Shoe leather: 66%, Turpentine: 36%, Apple: 34% (Figure 1). A Cochran-test revealed significant differences between the identification of the 16 odors ($Q_{15} = 127.62$, $p < 0.001$). Multiple Bonferroni adjusted pairwise comparisons showed that the odors Apple and Turpentine were significantly less often correctly identified compared to all other odors (U between 8.56–17.77, all $ps < 0.001$). Because of that, the items Apple and Turpentine were excluded, forming a 14-item odor identification test, the "Sniffin' Kids" test (Figure 1).

Table 1. Descriptive statistics of participants.

Group	Participants	Girls/Boys	Age (mean, SD, range)
Control	537	268/268	11.9, 3.1, 6–17
Anosmic	25	18/7	12, 2.7, 8–17

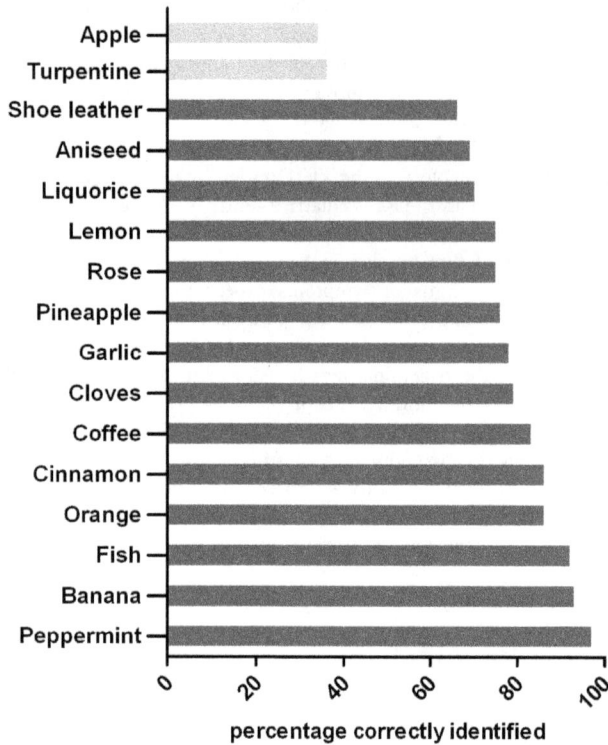

Figure 1. Percentage of correctly identified odors. Displayed are the percentages of correct identification of the 16-item odor identification test for all children (n=537). The odors, which were chosen for the 14-item "Sniffin' Kids" test are marked in dark grey. Odors, which were excluded were significantly less often correctly identified and are displayed in light grey.

Part two

The odors chosen for the "Sniffin' Kids" test are listed in Table 2. For all participants the mean odor identification score was 11.22 (SD 1.87, range 2–14). A detailed description of odor identification for each individual item can be found in Table 3. No sex difference ($U_{535} = 1.29$, p = 0.20) but a positive correlation between odor identification score and age was observed ($\rho_{537} = 0.29$, p<0.001). In addition to this correlation the age of children had a significant effect on odor identification performance ($X^2 = 59.26$, p<0.001) with older children reaching higher scores. Therefore we divided the sample into subgroups: group I (6–8 years), group II (9–14 years) and group III (15–17 years). A significant difference in odor identification performance was found between groups ($X^2 = 51.37$, p<0.001) (Figure 2), with mean sores increasing from group I to group III. Within each group the age did not affect the odor identification score (Group I: $X^2 = 0.59$, p = 0.74; II: $X^2 = 7.28$, p = 0.20; III: $X^2 = 0.23$, p = 0.89). In line with this, no correlation between age and odor identification score was found within the age groups (Group I: $\rho_{76} = 0.09$, p = 0.45; II: $\rho_{344} = 0.06$, p = 0.28; III: $\rho_{117} = 0.01$, p = 0.93).

The three groups scored on the 14-item odor identification test as followed: Group I (n = 76): mean odor identification score 10.09 points (SD 1.98, range 4–14 points). Group II (n = 344): mean odor identification score 11.19 points (SD 1.87, range 2–14 points). Group III (n = 117): mean odor identification score 12.05 points (SD 1.33, range 7–14 points). No sex differences were found in odor identification scores in all three groups (Table 4).

To separate normosmia from olfactory dysfunction with the "Sniffin' Sticks" test the 10th percentile was used [3]. We applied this cutoff to our data sample. According to the 10th percentile a score of >7 in age group I, a score of >8 in age group II and a score of > 10 in age group III is considered normosmic. Therefore scores below these values can be considered as hyposmic. According to this definition, 6 (7.9%) children in group I, 29 (8.4%) children in group II and 22 (11.1%) children in group III had olfactory dysfunction.

To evaluate the reliability of the olfactory test, a group of 31 children from age group II (mean age 11.7, SD 1.3 years, 12 girls, 19 boys) was tested again after a mean interval of 4–6 months. The mean odor identification score for the first testing was 11.58 points (SD 1.61) and for the second testing 12.23 points (SD 1.23). A test-retest reliability of $\rho = 0.44$ (p = 0.012) was observed.

Table 2. Items of the "Sniffin' Kids" test.

"Sniffin' Sticks" number	Odor	Descriptor 2	Descriptor 3	Descriptor 4
1	Orange	Blackberry	Strawberry	Pineapple
2	Leather	Smoke	Glue	Grass
3	Cinnamon	Honey	Vanilla	Chocolate
4	Peppermint	Chives	Wood	Onion
5	Banana	Coconut	Walnut	Cherry
6	Lemon	Peach	Apple	Grapefruit
7	Liquorice	Gummibears	Chewing gum	Cookies
9	Garlic	Onion	Sauerkraut	Carrot
10	Coffee	Cigarette	Wine	Candle smoke
12	Cloves	Pepper	Cinnamon	Mustard
13	Pineapple	Pear	Plum	Peach
14	Rose	Chamomile	Raspberry	Cherry
15	Aniseed	Rum	Honey	Wood
16	Fish	Bread	Cheese	Ham

The Table shows the 14 odors and their descriptors, which were selected for the "Sniffin' Kids" test from the "Sniffin' Sticks" 16-item odor identification test. The number is accordant to the 16-item odor identification test.

Table 3. Results of the odor identification test.

Odor		Control All ages	Group I (6–8)	Group II (9–14)	Group III (15–17)	Anosmic
Orange:	All	86 (83–89)	81 (73–91)	85 (81–88)	93 (89–98)	36 (16–56)
	Girls	88 (83–91)	89 (79–98)	85 (79–91)	94 (88–100)	39 (14–64)
	Boys	84 (80–88)	72 (55–88)	84 (79–90)	92 (85–100)	29 (0–74)
Leather	All	66 (62–70)	54 (43–65)	67 (62–72)	74 (65–82)	12 (0–26)
	Girls	67 (61–72)	48 (32–63)	67 (60–75)	77 (67–88)	17 (0–36)
	Boys	66 (60–72)	63 (45–80)	66 (59–73)	69 (55–82)	0 (0)
Cinnamon	All	86 (82–88)	91 (84–97)	86 (82–90)	81 (74–88)	28 (9–47)
	Girls	87 (82–90)	93 (85–100)	88 (83–93)	76 (69–89)	28 (5–51)
	Boys	85 (80–89)	88 (75–100)	84 (79–90)	84 (74–95)	27 (0–74)
Peppermint	All	97 (95–98)	91 (84–97)	97 (96–99)	99 (98–100)	48 (27–69)
	Girls	97 (94–99)	91 (82–100)	98 (96–100)	100 (100)	44 (19–70)
	Boys	96 (94–99)	91 (80–100)	97 (94–99)	98 (94–100)	57 (8–100)
Banana	All	93 (90–95)	84 (76–93)	93 (90–96)	97 (95–100)	20 (3–37)
	Girls	95 (90–96)	86 (76–97)	95 (92–98)	97 (93–100)	17 (0–36)
	Boys	91 (88–95)	81 (67–96)	91 (87–96)	98 (94–100)	29 (0–74)
Lemon	All	75 (70–78)	76 (67–86)	72 (67–77)	81 (74–88)	36 (16–56)
	Girls	71 (65–76)	77 (64–90)	65 (58–73)	80 (71–90)	28 (5–51)
	Boys	78 (74–83)	75 (60–91)	78 (72–84)	82 (72–93)	57 (8–100)
Liquorice	All	70 (66–74)	55 (44–67)	72 (67–77)	74 (65–82)	48 (27–69)
	Girls	70 (64–75)	54 (39–70)	74 (67–81)	71 (60–82)	44 (19–70)
	Boys	70 (64–75)	56 (38–74)	70 (64–77)	77 (64–89)	57 (8–100)
Garlic	All	78 (74–81)	55 (44–67)	80 (76–84)	86 (80–83)	44 (23–65)
	Girls	77 (71–82)	59 (44–74)	78 (71–84)	86 (78–95)	39 (14–64)
	Boys	78 (74–83)	50 (31–68)	81 (76–87)	86 (77–96)	57 (8–100)
Coffee	All	83 (79–85)	84 (76–93)	81 (77–85)	86 (80–93)	16 (0–31)
	Girls	81 (76–86)	80 (67–92)	79 (73–86)	88 (80–96)	6 (0–17)
	Boys	84 (79–88)	91 (80–100)	82 (77–88)	84 (74–95)	43 (0–92)
Cloves	All	79 (75–82)	65 (54–76)	81 (76–85)	82 (75–89)	16 (0–31)
	Girls	82 (76–86)	73 (59–86)	82 (76–88)	86 (78–95)	17 (0–36)
	Boys	76 (70–81)	53 (34–71)	79 (73–85)	77 (64–89)	14 (0–49)
Pineapple	All	76 (72–80)	68 (58–79)	74 (70–79)	87 (81–93)	28 (9–47)
	Girls	78 (72–82)	64 (48–78)	77 (70–83)	89 (82–97)	17 (0–36)
	Boys	75 (70–81)	75 (60–91)	72 (66–79)	84 (74–95)	57 (8–100)
Rose	All	75 (71–78)	63 (52–74)	74 (70–79)	84 (77–91)	32 (12–52)
	Girls	79 (74–84)	66 (51–81)	80 (73–86)	86 (78–95)	44 (19–70)
	Boys	71 (65–76)	60 41–77)	70 (63–77)	80 (69–92)	0 (0)
Aniseed	All	69 (64–72)	58 (47–69)	66 (61–71)	83 (76–90)	20 (3–37)
	Girls	69 (63–74)	61 (46–76)	66 (58–73)	82 (72–91)	28 (5–51)
	Boys	68 (62–74)	53 (35–71)	66 (59–73)	84 (74–95)	0 (0)
Fish	All	92 (89–94)	83 (74–92)	92 (89–95)	97 (95–100)	28 (9–47)
	Girls	91 (87–94)	86 (76–97)	91 (86–95)	97 (93–100)	33 (9–58)
	Boys	92 (89–95)	78 63–93)	93 (89–97)	98 (94–100)	14 (0–49)

Displayed are the mean percentage of correct identification for each odor for the control and anosmic children. The percentages are shown for all, girls, boys and each age group separately. In addition the 95% confidence interval is shown in brackets.

For validation of the 14-item odor identification test, results from a group of congenitally anosmic children (18 girls, 7 boys, no age difference to healthy group $(t_{560} = 0.49$, $p = 0.63)$) were compared to the above-mentioned results. Children in the anosmic group scored on average 4.12 points (SD 1.59; range 2–7 points) on the odor identification test. When compared to the group of healthy children (n = 537) a significant difference in olfactory performance was observed $(U_{560} = 8.46$; $p < 0.001)$

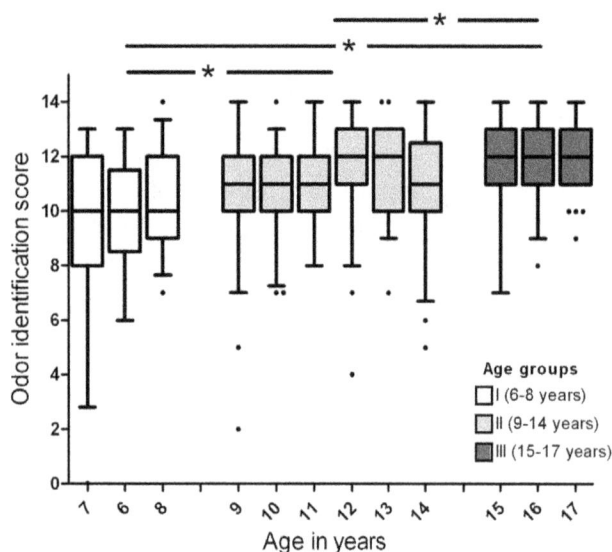

Figure 2. Odor identification score and age groups. The boxplot displays the mean odor identification score for all ages. The age groups I, II and III differ significantly by means of odor identification score, while no age difference was obtained within a group. (* = p<0.001).

(Figure 3). The group of anosmic children was too small to meaningfully divide it into the three age groups used above; only 2 children would be in group I, 16 in group II and 7 in group III. None the less all children in the anosmic group scored below 8 points, which is considered to indicate a reduced sense of smell in all three age groups.

Possible effects of BMI on the odor identification score were observed in a subgroup of healthy children (n = 81). For this the BMI-Z-scores were calculated. An average of 12.0 points (1.56, range 7–14 points) was achieved on the odor identification test. No correlation between BMI-Z-scores and odor identification was found (ρ = 0.06, p = 0.62).

Discussion

In the current study we evaluated the "Sniffin' Sticks" 16-item odor identification test in a large population of children. Results from part one shows that some odors of the test, especially Apple and Turpentine, are not familiar to children. Thus it was necessary to modify this test to be more suitable for children.

Although olfactory impairment is less common in children than in adults [22], recent studies have shown a reduced sense of smell in children due to several reasons like head trauma [11,23,24], adenoid hypertrophy [25], anorexia nervosa [26] or other psychiatric diseases [27]. Therefore there is need for a reliable, valid and

easy to use test for measuring olfactory function in children [28]. To date there are a few odor identification tests, which have been developed for children. The "Smell Wheel" and the odor identification test of the NIH Toolbox were developed for the USA. Children from Europe are not familiar with odors such as Play-Doh, which could lead to lower odor identification scores and/or increased variance when using these tests. Laing et al. developed an odor identification test in Australia for children aged 5-7 years using squeeze bottles for odor presentation [15]. In Europe a self-developed odor identification test was introduced to be used in a Polish population [18]. The first two tests are not commonly used in Europe and the later tests are not commercially available. The shorter 12-item "Sniffin' Sticks" odor identification test was evaluated in children in a Dutch population [8]. In our study we used the same odor presentation method – the "Sniffin' Sticks". The benefit of our current study is the odor selection and therefore choosing odors, which are well identified by children. The odors were selected from the original "Sniffin' Sticks" 16-item odor identification test resulting in a 14-item test. In addition two odors, Aniseed and Garlic, which are not included in the 12 odors tested in the Dutch population, have shown to be well known by children.

In the current study, a large group of 537 children between 6-17 years of age were included. We did not include children younger than six years, because previous studies have shown that odor identification is difficult and not reliable in children less than six years of age [20,29]. In contrast to that, children starting from age 3 years were included in one study [18]. Results from these children might be biased, because, if unknown, parents were allowed to explain the descriptors to the children. In our study all children understood the task and were able to perform the test. Due to unfamiliar items the odor identification test was modified excluding Apple and Turpentine. All other odors were identified at rates between 66-97%. Previous studies reported the validity of 12-item odor identification tests [30,31]. In an olfactory screening test a subset of odors were taken from the original "Sniffin' Sticks" test [31]. The 12-item cross-cultural smell identification test (CC-SIT) is a derivative of the UPSIT 40-item odor identification test [2,30]. Both tests have proven to be useful especially in a clinical setting. Thus, it is plausible that a 14-item odor identification test exhibits similar qualities. Whether women outperform men in odor identification tests has been controversially debated [3,8]. In line with previous studies no sex difference was found in the current study in odor identification scores [3,16,18,20]. It has been described that odor identification improves with age in children [14,16,20]. This was also the case in the current study. Therefore we created three age groups, which differed significantly in odor identification scores from one another. Within each group the odor identification score was not affected by age. For presenting normative values of an odor identification test it is necessary to obtain stable results within a population. This was achieved by

Table 4. Test results for different age groups.

Group	Participants	Girls/Boys	Age	Identification score	T-test, girls/boys	Kruskal-Wallis-Test effect of age
I (6–8)	76	44/32	7.3 (0.7)	10.09 (1.98)	t=0.93, p=0.36	X^2=0.56, p=0.74
II (9–14)	344	158/186	11.4 (1.8)	11.19 (1.87)	t=0.50, p=0.62	X^2=7.28, p=0.20
III (15–17)	117	66/51	16.3 (0.7)	12.05 (1.33)	t=0.79, p=0.43	X^2=0.23, p=0.89

Odor identification scores are shown for the three age groups in addition to descriptive data of the age groups. Displayed are mean (SD). No sex difference was found between girls and boys on the odor identification test for all three age groups. In addition no effect of age was observed within an age group.

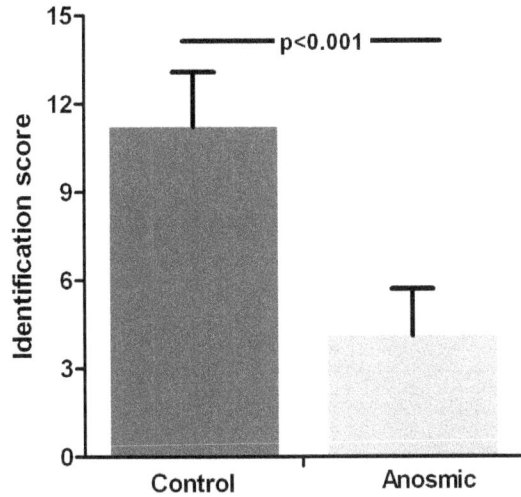

Figure 3. Comparing anosmic and healthy children. Odor identification scores of healthy children, dark grey, (n = 537) and congenital anosmic children, light grey, (n = 25) are shown (means, one standard deviation). Healthy children scored in average 11.22 (1.87) points on the "Sniffin' Kids" test, while congenital anosmic children scored 4.12 (1.59) points. This was significantly different with a p value <0.001.

forming the three age groups. This allowed us to establish normative data for each age group with a cut off value at the 10th percentile of odor identification scores, which separates normosmia from impaired olfactory function. The 10th percentile is an established value for separating normosmia from hyposmia in adults when using the "Sniffin' Sticks" test battery [3] or when using the UPSIT [2]. We were able to show that the "Sniffin' Kids" test is able to discriminate between normosmia and impaired olfactory function by including congenital anosmic children in the study. Interestingly, none of the above mentioned odor identification tests for children have been validated this way [8,14–18]. In our study all congenital anosmic children scored below the 10th percentile on the "Sniffin' Kids" test. In addition to this validation, the "Sniffin' Kids" test showed to be reliable for the tested age group with a reliability value of $\rho = 0.44$. This value is smaller when compared to the test-retest reliability of the "Sniffin' Sticks" 16-item odor identification test in adults [21]. It has to be considered that the population tested in this study was fairly small (n = 31) and that the number of items was reduced to 14. In addition, the small coefficient of correlation is also explained by the relative homogeneity of the group tested because no children with diminished or absent olfactory function had been

included here. Since the reliability was only tested in children from age group II (9-14 years) further studies are needed to evaluate the reliability especially in age group I (6–8 years). The interval between the first and second testing was between 4 to 6 months. The exact dates of testing were not available. Therefore it was not possible to study any effects of interval lengths on the outcome of the reliability. In line with previous findings the BMI (BMI-Z-score) of children had no effect on the odor identification performance [8]. It has to be considered that in our study only four children had a BMI-Z-score of ±2 from the mean. This is in contrast to a study reporting changed odor identification abilities in dependence of the BMI in children [9].

The "Sniffin' Kids" test is based on the original "Sniffin' Sticks" 16-item odor identification test, which is largely used in clinics and laboratories throughout Europe. We modified this test rather than creating a new test from scratch. Therefore it is possible to test children as well as adults with portions of the same test battery. This is considered an advantage compared to the "Smell Wheel" and the NIH Toolbox, which are not reusable and for the "Smell Wheel" not applicable in adults, making these tests much more costly than the "Sniffin' Kids" test.

The sample size of our study was fairly large to obtain normative data for the "Sniffin' Kids" test. Nonetheless further studies have to be conducted to strengthen these results, especially in the age group from 6-8 years of age. The original 16-item odor identification test was developed in Germany and evaluated in a number of other European countries. Children included in the study grew up in Germany. Both the NIH-toolbox and the "smell wheel" were administered to children, who grew up in the USA [14,16]. Additional studies are necessary to evaluate the "Sniffin' Kids" test in other countries especially countries outside of Europe.

Further studies are needed to evaluate possible influences of oral and nasal surgery on the outcome of odor identification score as has been shown previously [8]. A possible shortcoming of the study is that no cognitive test was conducted. Therefore the influence of cognition on odor identification ability could not been observed in the current study.

Conclusion

With the 14-item odor identification test, the "Sniffin' Kids" test, we propose a valid and reliable method for olfactory testing in children between 6–17 years of age. We provide normative data for three age groups from a large sample size.

Author Contributions

Conceived and designed the experiments: TH VAS. Performed the experiments: EM WP CB MS. Analyzed the data: VAS EM. Wrote the paper: VAS EM TH WP CB MS.

References

1. Gudziol V, Lotsch J, Hahner A, Zahnert T, Hummel T (2006) Clinical significance of results from olfactory testing. Laryngoscope 116: 1858–1863.
2. Doty RL, Shaman P, Dann M (1984) Development of the University of Pennsylvania Smell Identification Test: a standardized microencapsulated test of olfactory function. Physiol Behav 32: 489–502.
3. Hummel T, Kobal G, Gudziol H, Mackay-Sim A (2007) Normative data for the "Sniffin' Sticks" including tests of odor identification, odor discrimination, and olfactory thresholds: an upgrade based on a group of more than 3,000 subjects. Eur Arch Otorhinolaryngol 264: 237–243.
4. Kobal G, Hummel T, Sekinger B, Barz S, Roscher S, et al. (1996) "Sniffin' sticks": screening of olfactory performance. Rhinology 34: 222–226.
5. Kondo H, Matsuda T, Hashiba M, Baba S (1998) A study of the relationship between the T&T olfactometer and the University of Pennsylvania Smell Identification Test in a Japanese population. Am J Rhinol 12: 353–358.
6. Kobal G, Klimek L, Wolfensberger M, Gudziol H, Temmel A, et al. (2000) Multicenter investigation of 1,036 subjects using a standardized method for the

assessment of olfactory function combining tests of odor identification, odor discrimination, and olfactory thresholds. Eur Arch Otorhinolaryngol 257: 205–211.
7. Doty RL, Shaman P, Applebaum SL, Giberson R, Siksorski L, et al. (1984) Smell identification ability: changes with age. Science 226: 1441–1443.
8. van Spronsen E, Ebbens FA, Fokkens WJ (2013) Olfactory function in healthy children: normative data for odor identification. Am J Rhinol Allergy 27: 197–201.
9. Obrebowski A, Obrebowska-Karsznia Z, Gawlinski M (2000) Smell and taste in children with simple obesity. Int J Pediatr Otorhinolaryngol 55: 191–196.
10. Davidson TM, Freed C, Healy MP, Murphy C (1998) Rapid clinical evaluation of anosmia in children: the Alcohol Sniff Test. Ann N Y Acad Sci 855: 787–792.
11. Jacobi G, Ritz A, Emrich R (1986) Cranial nerve damage after paediatric head trauma: a long-term follow-up study of 741 cases. Acta Paediatr Hung 27: 173–187.
12. Roberts MA, Simcox AF (1996) Assessing olfaction following pediatric traumatic brain injury. Appl Neuropsychol 3: 86–88.

13. Monnery-Patris S, Rouby C, Nicklaus S, Issanchou S (2009) Development of olfactory ability in children: sensitivity and identification. Dev Psychobiol 51: 268–276.

14. Dalton P, Mennella JA, Maute C, Castor SM, Silva-Garcia A, et al. (2011) Development of a test to evaluate olfactory function in a pediatric population. Laryngoscope 121: 1843–1850.

15. Laing DG, Segovia C, Fark T, Laing ON, Jinks AL, et al. (2008) Tests for screening olfactory and gustatory function in school-age children. Otolaryngol Head Neck Surg 139: 74–82.

16. Cameron EL, Doty RL (2013) Odor identification testing in children and young adults using the smell wheel. Int J Pediatr Otorhinolaryngol 77: 346–350.

17. Murphy C, Anderson JA, Markison S (1994) Psychophysical assessment of chemosensory disorders in clinical populations. In: K. S. K Kunihara and H Ogawa, editors. Olfaction and Taste XI Tokyo: Springer-Verlag. pp. 609–613.

18. Dzaman K, Zielnik-Jurkiewicz B, Jurkiewicz D, Molinska-Glura M (2013) Test for screening olfactory function in children. Int J Pediatr Otorhinolaryngol 77: 418–423.

19. Chopra A, Bauer A, Hummel T (2008) Thresholds and chemosensory event-related potentials to malodors before, during and after puberty: differences related to sex and age. Neuroimage 40: 1257–1263.

20. Hummel T, Bensafi M, Nikolaus J, Knecht M, Laing DG, et al. (2007) Olfactory function in children assessed with psychophysical and electrophysiological techniques. Behav Brain Res 180: 133–138.

21. Hummel T, Sekinger B, Wolf SR, Pauli E, Kobal G (1997) 'Sniffin' sticks': olfactory performance assessed by the combined testing of odor identification, odor discrimination and olfactory threshold. Chem Senses 22: 39–52.

22. Oozeer NB, Forbes K, Clement AW, Kubba H (2011) Management of paediatric olfactory dysfunction: how we do it. Clin Otolaryngol 36: 494–499.

23. Bakker K, Catroppa C, Anderson V (2013) Olfactory dysfunction in pediatric traumatic brain injury: A systematic review. J Neurotrauma.

24. Schriever VA, Studt F, Smitka M, Grosser K, Hummel T (2014) Olfactory Function After Mild Head Injury in Children. Chem Senses.

25. Konstantinidis I, Triaridis S, Triaridis A, Petropoulos I, Karagiannidis K, et al. (2005) How do children with adenoid hypertrophy smell and taste? Clinical assessment of olfactory function pre- and post-adenoidectomy. Int J Pediatr Otorhinolaryngol 69: 1343–1349.

26. Roessner V, Bleich S, Banaschewski T, Rothenberger A (2005) Olfactory deficits in anorexia nervosa. Eur Arch Psychiatry Clin Neurosci 255: 6–9.

27. Schecklmann M, Schwenck C, Taurines R, Freitag C, Warnke A, et al. (2013) A systematic review on olfaction in child and adolescent psychiatric disorders. J Neural Transm 120: 121–130.

28. Moura RG, Cunha DA, Gomes AC, Silva HJ (2014) Quantitative instruments used to assess children's sense of smell: a review article. Codas 26: 96–101.

29. Hummel T, Smitka M, Puschmann S, Gerber JC, Schaal B, et al. (2011) Correlation between olfactory bulb volume and olfactory function in children and adolescents. Exp Brain Res 214: 285–291.

30. Doty RL, Marcus A, Lee WW (1996) Development of the 12-item Cross-Cultural Smell Identification Test (CC-SIT). Laryngoscope 106: 353–356.

31. Hummel T, Konnerth CG, Rosenheim K, Kobal G (2001) Screening of olfactory function with a four-minute odor identification test: reliability, normative data, and investigations in patients with olfactory loss. Ann Otol Rhinol Laryngol 110: 976–981.

17

Multi-Agent Chemotherapy Overcomes Glucocorticoid Resistance Conferred by a *BIM* Deletion Polymorphism in Pediatric Acute Lymphoblastic Leukemia

Sheila Xinxuan Soh[1]**, Joshua Yew Suang Lim**[2]**, John W. J. Huang**[1]**, Nan Jiang**[2]**, Allen Eng Juh Yeoh**[2,3,4,5]**, S. Tiong Ong**[1,6,7,8]*

1 Cancer and Stem Cell Biology Program, Duke-NUS Graduate Medical School, Singapore, Singapore, **2** Department of Paediatrics, Yong Loo Lin School of Medicine, National University of Singapore, Singapore, Singapore, **3** National University Cancer Institute, National University Health System, Singapore, Singapore, **4** Viva-University Children's Cancer Centre, University Children's Medical Institute, National University Health System, Singapore, Singapore, **5** Cancer Science Institute, National University of Singapore, Singapore, Singapore, **6** Department of Haematology, Singapore General Hospital, Singapore, Singapore, **7** Department of Medical Oncology, National Cancer Centre, Singapore, Singapore, **8** Division of Medical Oncology, Duke University Medical Center, Durham, North Carolina, United States of America

Abstract

A broad range of anti-cancer agents, including glucocorticoids (GCs) and tyrosine kinase inhibitors (TKIs), kill cells by upregulating the pro-apoptotic BCL2 family member, BIM. A common germline deletion in the *BIM* gene was recently shown to favor the production of non-apoptotic BIM isoforms, and to predict inferior responses in TKI-treated chronic myeloid leukemia (CML) and EGFR-driven lung cancer patients. Given that both *in vitro* and *in vivo* GC resistance are predictive of adverse outcomes in acute lymphoblastic leukemia (ALL), we hypothesized that this polymorphism would mediate GC resistance, and serve as a biomarker of poor response in ALL. Accordingly, we used zinc finger nucleases to generate ALL cell lines with the *BIM* deletion, and confirmed the ability of the deletion to mediate GC resistance *in vitro*. In contrast to CML and lung cancer, the *BIM* deletion did not predict for poorer clinical outcome in a retrospective analysis of 411 pediatric ALL patients who were uniformly treated with GCs and chemotherapy. Underlying the lack of prognostic significance, we found that the chemotherapy agents used in our cohort (vincristine, L-asparaginase, and methotrexate) were each able to induce ALL cell death in a BIM-independent fashion, and resensitize *BIM* deletion-containing cells to GCs. Together, our work demonstrates how effective therapy can overcome intrinsic resistance in ALL patients, and suggests the potential of using combinations of drugs that work via divergent mechanisms of cell killing to surmount *BIM* deletion-mediated drug resistance in other cancers.

Editor: Linda Bendall, University of Sydney, Australia

Funding: STO was supported by the Leukemia & Lymphoma Society Translational Research Program Grant (R913-302-026-597) www.lls.org. AEY was supported by the Singapore National Medical Research Council (NMRC/0582/2001, NMRC/CSA/003/2008). www.nmrc.gov.sg, and by A*STAR (SCS-POU98, NMRC/CSI/004/2005). www.a-star.edu.sg, and by Children's Cancer Foundation, Singapore. www.ccf.org.sg, and by VIVA Foundation for Children with Cancer, Singapore. www.viva.sg. The funders had no role in study design, data collection and analysis, decision to publish, or preparation of the manuscript.

Competing Interests: The authors have declared that no competing interests exist.

* Email: sintiong.ong@duke-nus.edu.sg

Introduction

Genome-wide profiling studies of acute lymphoblastic leukemia (ALL) have revealed it to be a highly heterogeneous disease [1]. In spite of this, the majority of ALL subtypes are treated with a remission-induction protocol that invariably consists of a glucocorticoid, vincristine and at least one other chemotherapy agent (L-asparaginase, an anthracycline, or both) [2]. Unfortunately, 15-20% of patients continue to relapse, and outcome remains poor for these individuals [3]. Consequently, there have been ongoing efforts to identify genetic factors that could account for this response heterogeneity and serve as prognostic markers for risk stratification or novel druggable targets in order to improve patient outcomes [4–6].

At the same time, recent reviews have underscored the notion that response heterogeneity can arise from not only somatic mutations but also germline polymorphisms [7,8]. A number of examples of the latter have been described, including genetic variants that influence the pharmacokinetic and pharmacodynamic phenotype of the host, as well as those affecting the underlying biology of the leukemic cell and thereby cell intrinsic drug resistance/sensitivity [9–15]. Notably, however, studies correlating genetic variants with clinical phenotypes have been largely based on genetic epidemiology data and lack experimental validation at a mechanistic level. Such mechanistic studies have been hampered in part by the difficulty and cost of generating isogenic cell lines that either possess or lack a mutation of interest. More recently, a variety of methods that enable genome engineering to faithfully recapitulate mutations of interest have been developed and these will aid the functional validation of these variants *in vitro* [16].

Using such an approach, we recently validated the functional consequences of a germline deletion in the *BIM* gene in chronic myeloid leukemia (CML) [17]. Unlike in ALL, a single causative lesion, the 9;22 translocation, is known to be present in >95% of chronic myeloid leukemia (CML) cases [18]. Despite the targeted nature of tyrosine kinase inhibitors (TKIs), response heterogeneity is also a significant challenge in CML [19]. From a group of TKI-resistant CML patients, we identified a 2.9 kb intronic deletion in the *BIM* gene, and later verified it to be a polymorphism found in 12.3% of East Asians [17]. *BIM* encodes a potent pro-apoptotic BH3-only protein that is required for specific anti-cancer therapies to induce apoptotic cell death [20–25]. When we introduced the deletion into a CML cell line using zinc finger nuclease-based technology, the polymorphism was sufficient to cause intrinsic resistance to tyrosine kinase inhibitors. Mechanistically, we showed that the *BIM* deletion biases splicing toward BIM isoforms that lack the BH3 domain encoded in exon 4, resulting in the expression of BIM isoforms incapable of inducing apoptosis. Consistent with the *in vitro* data, both CML and EGFR-driven lung cancer patients carrying the polymorphism experienced inferior responses to treatment with tyrosine kinase inhibitors.

Since BIM is required for GC-induced apoptosis in lymphoid lineage cells, including ALL cells [26–32], and both *in vitro* and *in vivo* GC response has been shown to predict favorable treatment outcome in ALL [33–37], we wondered if the polymorphism could contribute to response heterogeneity in ALL patients. If this were the case, we expect that pharmacological restoration of BIM function using drugs such as BH3 mimetics would enable us to improve response in patients with the polymorphism [17,25]. Furthermore, because multi-agent chemotherapy is essential to the long-term control of pediatric ALL, the clinical model of ALL could allow us to determine the interaction between a single germline variant and combination therapy.

Accordingly, we used zinc finger nucleases to generate *de novo* ALL cell lines with the *BIM* deletion polymorphism in both heterozygous and homozygous configurations. Using these lines, we found that the *BIM* deletion polymorphism was sufficient to confer GC resistance *in vitro*. However, analysis of a pediatric ALL cohort uniformly treated with GCs and chemotherapy [38] revealed that patients with the *BIM* deletion did not experience inferior response rates nor poorer clinical outcomes. Mechanistically, we determined that GC resistance conferred by the *BIM* polymorphism could be overcome with the addition of chemotherapeutic agents used in standard ALL protocols, and which likely act via a BIM-independent mechanism to cause cell death. Together, our data demonstrate that, whilst the *BIM* deletion is sufficient to confer resistance to GCs, the negative impact of polymorphic variants on single agent therapy can be overcome with multi-agent chemotherapy that kill cancer cells via divergent mechanisms. These results highlight the challenge of identifying genetic markers predictive of clinical outcome in populations treated with multi-agent therapy, the utility of genome editing technologies in the study of polymorphic variants, as well as the importance of using drug combinations that kill cancer cells via non-overlapping mechanisms.

Methods

Cell lines and culture conditions

CCRF-CEM was purchased from the American Type Culture Collection (Manassas, VA, USA). Cells were maintained in RPMI-1640 media (Nacalai Tesque, Japan) supplemented with 20% FBS, penicillin/streptomycin and L-glutamine (all from Thermo Scientific, Rockford, IL, USA). Dexamethasone (Rotexmedica, Ger-

many), methotrexate (ABIC Ltd, Israel), vincristine (Korea United Pharm Inc, Korea) and L-asparaginase (Kyowa Hakko Kirin, Japan) were used at the dosages and times indicated in the figure legends. All experiments using cell lines were performed at least 3 times.

Creation of genome-edited lines

The zinc finger nucleases (ZFNs) targeting the *BIM* gene were custom-made (Sigma-Aldrich, St Louis, MO, USA) and the repair template was generated as described in a previous paper [17]. Plasmids encoding the repair template and ZFNs were transfected into CCRF-CEM cells using the Neon system (Invitrogen, Carlsbad, CA, USA). Clones were isolated by dilution cloning and screened for presence of the deletion using the following primers: Forward (5'-GGCCTTCAACCACTATCTCAGTG-CAATGG-3') and Reverse (5'- GGTTTCAGAGACA-GAGCTGGGACTCC-3'). qPCR to determine exon 3 to exon 4 ratio was performed as previously described [17].

MTS assays

Cells were seeded at a density of 4×10^4 per well in a 96-well plate and incubated with the indicated drugs. In each experiment, every treatment condition was repeated in triplicate wells. After 48 h, CellTiter AQueous One Solution Cell Proliferation reagent (Promega, Fitchburg, WI, USA) was added to each well and incubated for 2 h before an absorbance reading at 490 nm was taken.

Immunoblotting

Cells were washed once in PBS and lysed in RIPA lysis buffer (Millipore, Billerica, MA, USA) containing proteinase inhibitor (Roche, Indianapolis, IN, USA). Protein concentrations were assayed using the Quick Start Bradford protein assay kit (Bio-Rad) and bovine serum albumin as a standard. The following antibodies were used at these concentrations: phospho-glucocorticoid receptor (S211) (Cell Signaling Technology, Danvers, MA, USA #4161, 1:1 000), glucocorticoid receptor (BD Transduction Laboratories, San Jose, CA, USA, 1:2 000), β-actin (Sigma-Aldrich, 1:10 000), PARP (Cell Signaling Technology #9542, 1:2 000), caspase 3 (Cell Signaling Technology #9663, 1:500) and BIM (Cell Signaling Technology #2819, 1:1 000). HRP-conjugated secondary antibodies against mouse or rabbit IgG (Santa Cruz Biotechnology, Santa Cruz, CA, USA) were used at 1:10 000. Western Lightning ECL reagent (PerkinElmer, Waltham, MA, USA) was used to visualize the protein bands. Any adjustments to contrast and intensity were applied uniformly to the images.

Patient recruitment

411 patients with newly-diagnosed ALL from the Malaysia-Singapore (Ma-Spore) acute lymphoblastic leukemia (ALL) 2003 study [38] were included on the basis of DNA availability. Written informed consent was obtained from the parents or the legal guardians of the patients. The study was approved by the National Healthcare Group Domain Specific Review Board (NHG DSRB). Since the *BIM* deletion is germline in nature, and will be present in both normal and leukemic samples, we were able to employ both remission (n = 362) and diagnostic (n = 49) samples for genotyping for this study. Patient risk stratification, details of the treatment protocol, minimal residual disease monitoring and molecular subgrouping were described previously [38].

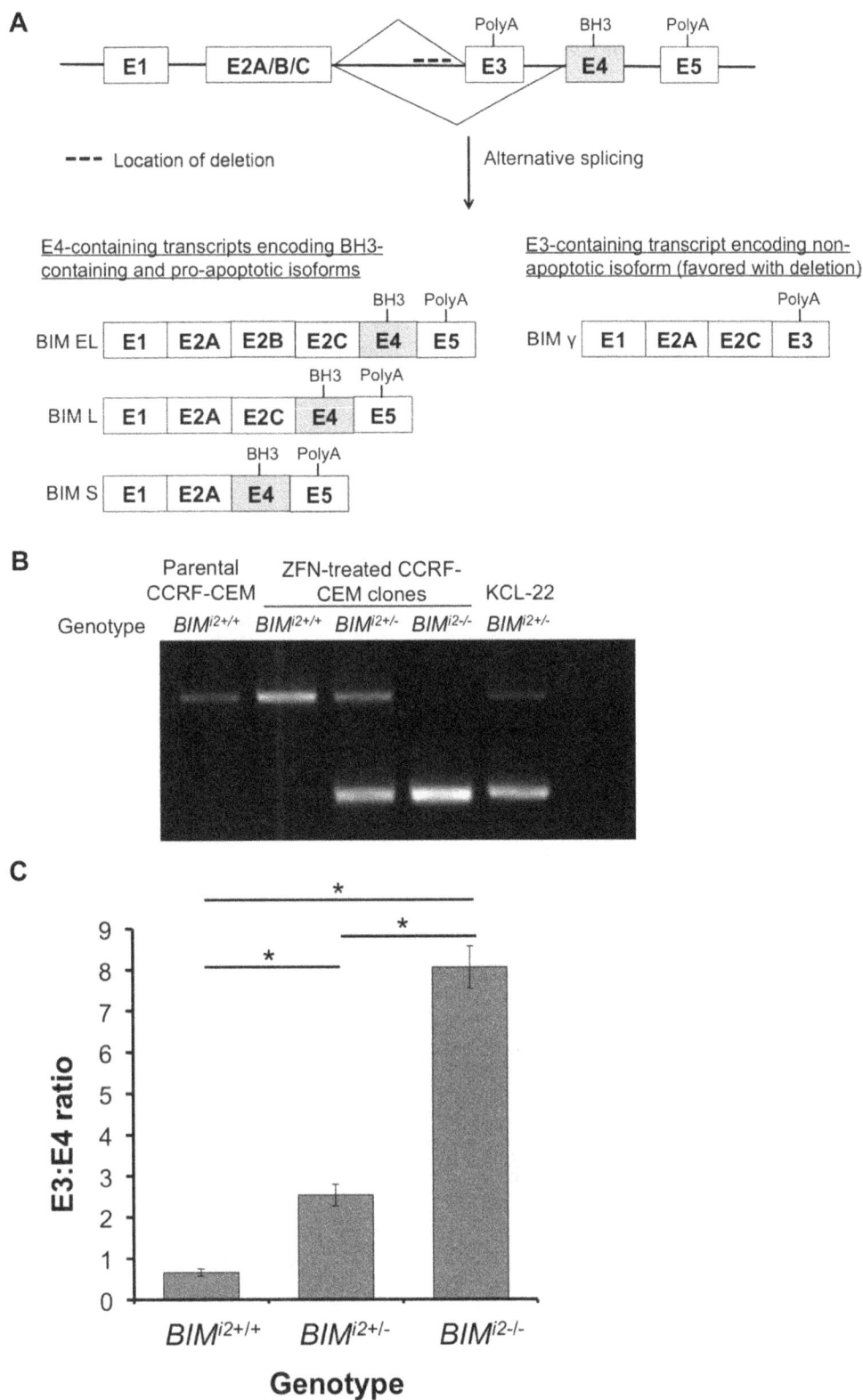

Figure 1. Generation of isogenic CCRF-CEM cell lines with the *BIM* deletion polymorphism. (A) Structure of the *BIM* gene and major splice isoforms. The *BIM* deletion polymorphism lies within intron 2 and upstream of exon 3, as indicated by the dashed line. Exon 4 contains the crucial BH3 domain required for apoptosis. Exon 3 (E3) and 4 (E4) are spliced in a mutually exclusive fashion, leading to the generation of either E4-containing isoforms with the BH3 domain (BIM EL, BIM L and BIM S) or E3-containing isoforms without the BH3 domain (BIM γ). When present, the deletion biases splicing towards E3-containing non-apoptotic isoforms. (B) Agarose gel of the products from a PCR reaction to detect the polymorphism in zinc finger nuclease (ZFN)-treated CCRF-CEM subclones, with the lower band indicating the presence of the deletion. Parental CCRF-CEM and KCL-22 cells (a CML cell line known to be heterozygous for the *BIM* deletion polymorphism) were included as controls. (C) The ratio of exon 3 to exon 4-

containing transcripts (E3:E4) in CCRF-CEM $BIM^{i2+/+}$, $BIM^{i2+/-}$ and $BIM^{i2-/-}$ clones as measured by qPCR. Error bars indicate mean $\pm$ SEM (n = 3). A student's t-test was performed for pairwise comparisons of E3:E4 ratio between genotypes. * indicates a significant difference with P<0.05.

Statistical analyses

Statistical analysis was performed using SPSS software (version 16.0 for Windows; IBM Corporation, Armonk, NY, USA). Comparisons between groups were examined by Fisher's exact test for categorical variables. A statistically significant difference was defined as a P value of <0.05. Survival curves were evaluated using Kaplan–Meier analysis. Event-free survival (EFS) was defined as the time from diagnosis to first recurrence of the disease, including induction failure, or death. Induction failure was defined as failure to achieve complete remission and considered as an event at one day after date of diagnosis. Overall survival (OS) was defined as the time from diagnosis to death. Patients who were alive and had no progression of disease or relapse were censored at the time of their last follow-up.

Results

De novo generation of ALL cell lines bearing the BIM deletion polymorphism

To determine if the *BIM* deletion polymorphism is sufficient to confer GC resistance to ALL cells, we used zinc finger nucleases to derive *de novo* ALL cell lines bearing the deletion. Because human cell lines vary in their amenability to transfection and genome editing by zinc fingers (personal communication, TK Ko and unpublished observations), we tested the ability of our approach to edit 3 different GC-sensitive ALL cell lines (CCRF-CEM, RS4;11, and PALL-2) [39–41] that did not have the polymorphism. Of these lines, we were only able to successfully generate clones containing the deletion in CCRF-CEM cells. The structure of the *BIM* gene and the location of the deletion in intron 2 are illustrated in Figure 1A. Using PCR primers that flank the deleted region, we identified subclones that either did not have the deletion (denoted $BIM^{i2+/+}$) or were heterozygous (denoted $BIM^{i2+/-}$) or homozygous (denoted $BIM^{i2-/-}$) for the deletion polymorphism (Figure 1B). The deleted region contains splicing elements that either promote the production of functional, exon 4-containing isoforms or suppress the production of non-apoptotic, exon 3-containing isoforms [42]. Consequently, when deleted, an increase in exon 3 to exon 4-containing transcripts is expected. To confirm that the deletion produced the expected changes in the splicing of *BIM*, we measured the ratio of exon 3- to exon 4-containing transcripts in clones of each genotype by exon-specific RT-PCR, and found that it was increased in a polymorphism-dosage-dependent manner (Figure 1C).

The BIM deletion polymorphism is sufficient to confer GC resistance in ALL cells

To determine if the deletion conferred resistance to GCs, we compared the effect of treating clones of each genotype with a range of dexamethasone concentrations. First, we quantified cell viability using the MTS assay and found that across the range tested, the deletion-containing clones exhibited increased cell viability in a polymorphism dosage-dependent manner (Figure 2A). Following this, we assessed the extent of apoptosis using the induction of cleaved poly ADP-ribose polymerase (PARP), as well as the level of cleaved caspase 3, using immunoblots performed on lysates of cells treated as in Figure 2A. We also probed for BIM using an antibody that only detects the pro-apoptotic E4-containing isoforms (BIM EL, L, and S). As a marker

of glucocorticoid receptor (GR) activation, we probed for phospho-GR (S211). As predicted, when compared to wildtype clones, upregulation of E4-containing BIM isoforms was impaired in a polymorphism dosage-dependent manner. Furthermore, apoptosis was attenuated in clones with the deletion, as evidenced by an increase in cleaved PARP, as well as cleaved caspase 3 (Figure 2B). Importantly, this occurred in spite of equivalent GR phosphorylation and auto-induction upon GC treatment across the genotypes (Figure 2C). These results indicate that GC resistance in the deletion-containing clones takes place downstream of the GR, and is consistent with our hypothesis that GC resistance results from impaired expression of BH3-containing BIM isoforms. Taken together, our data demonstrate that the presence of the *BIM* deletion polymorphism is sufficient to confer GC resistance in ALL cells.

Because prior work has shown that *in vitro* GC responses *per se* is an important prognostic factor in childhood ALL [33,34], we predicted that patients with the *BIM* deletion polymorphism would have inferior outcomes compared to those without.

The BIM deletion polymorphism does not predict inferior responses in pediatric ALL

To test our prediction that the *BIM* deletion polymorphism confers a poorer clinical outcome in pediatric ALL, we conducted a retrospective analysis correlating treatment outcome with the presence of the polymorphism in a group of uniformly-treated pediatric patients from the Malaysia-Singapore (Ma-Spore) ALL 2003 multicenter study. The Ma-Spore ALL 2003 protocol was based on a modified Berlin-Frankfurt-Münster regimen, where all patients received intrathecal methotrexate together with seven days of oral prednisolone at the point of diagnosis. Patients subsequently completed the rest of their induction regimen based on a common backbone of vincristine, L-asparaginase, and methotrexate, followed by risk-adapted consolidation and maintenance therapy as directed by their MRD status at day 33. Importantly, the design of this study allowed us to determine if the *BIM* deletion predicts for inferior clinical outcomes at three distinct assessment points: initial GC response (defined as absolute blast count $\geq 1000/\mu l$ at day 8), day 33 MRD following multi-agent induction chemotherapy, as well as overall survival (OS) and event-free survival (EFS) after consolidation and maintenance therapy.

Sufficient DNA from 411 individuals (out of a total of 556) from the Ma-Spore study was available for analysis for the *BIM* deletion polymorphism. Importantly, there was no difference in treatment outcome between this subgroup of 411 patients compared to the 556 patients in the full study (5-year EFS 82.0% vs 80.6%). Using this sample set, we determined the incidence of the *BIM* deletion to be 12.2%, which is consistent with the ethnic make up of the Ma-Spore cohort, as well as the incidence of the polymorphism in the normal population (Table 1, [17]). We also found that the *BIM* deletion polymorphism did not segregate according to any patient demographic except for Chinese ethnicity, which is as expected, or adverse prognostic indicators such as genetic subtype (Table 1).

We next determined if the *BIM* deletion predicted for inferior outcomes at each of the three response assessment points described above. Here, and to our surprise, we found that there was no significant difference between patients with or without the deletion for GC response at day 8 (P = 0.804), MRD response at day 33

A

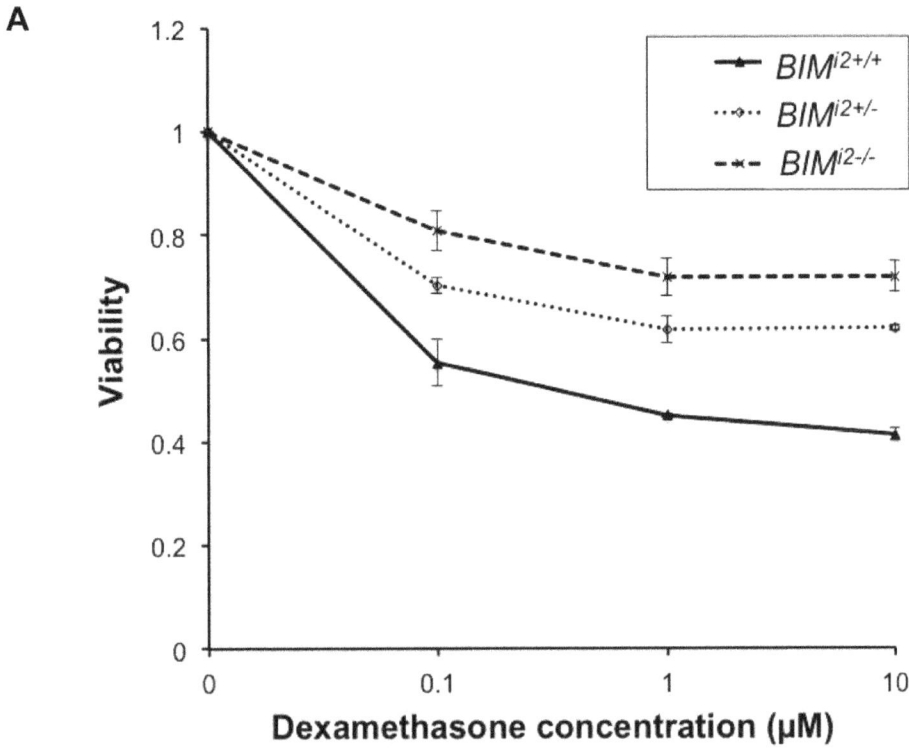

B

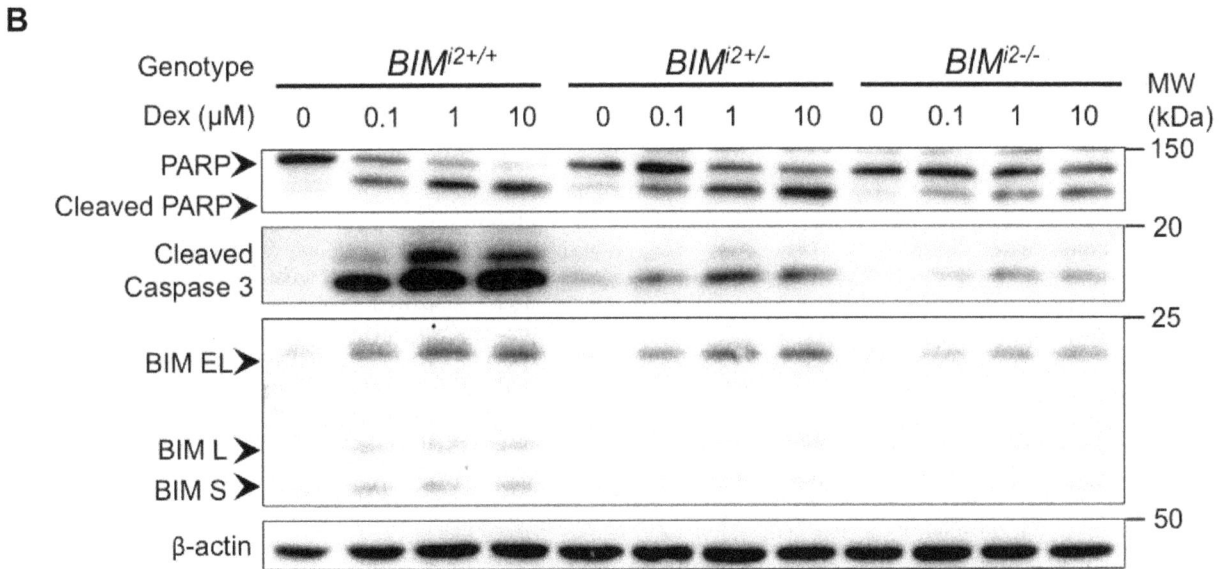

C

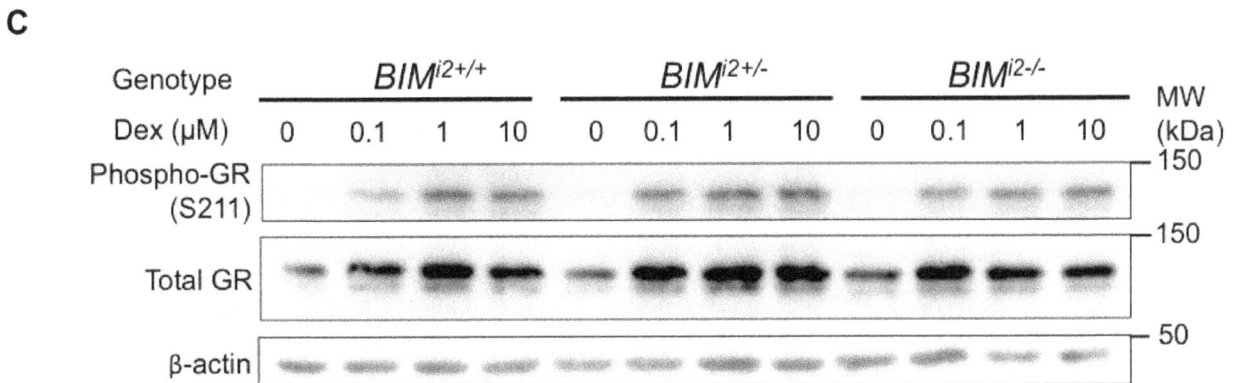

Figure 2. The *BIM* deletion confers dexamethasone resistance in CCRF-CEM cells. (A) Cell viability following exposure of CCRF-CEM subclones to increasing concentrations of dexamethasone. Viability was measured by MTS assay at 48 h. Error bars indicate mean $\pm$ SEM (n = 3) of 3 independent replicates. **(B)** Western blot of cell lysates from CCRF-CEM $BIM^{i2+/+}$, $BIM^{i2+/-}$ and $BIM^{i2-/-}$ clones following treatment with increasing doses of dexamethasone for 48 h. The induction of cleaved PARP and cleaved caspase 3 were used as readouts for apoptosis. An antibody that recognizes pro-apoptotic exon-4 containing BIM isoforms (BIM EL, L and S) was used to show the extent of BIM upregulation following GC exposure. β-actin was used as a loading control. **(C)** Western blot showing phosphorylation of the glucocorticoid receptor (Phospho-GR S211) in CCRF-CEM $BIM^{i2+/+}$, $BIM^{i2+/-}$ and $BIM^{i2-/-}$ clones upon treatment with dexamethasone.

($P = 0.970$), nor EFS ($P = 0.427$) or overall OS ($P = 0.646$) (Table 1, Figures 3A and 3B). Additionally, subgroup analysis by genetic subtype, race and risk category at diagnosis did not uncover any associations between the *BIM* deletion polymorphism and treatment outcome (data not shown). Together, these results demonstrate that the *BIM* deletion polymorphism does not predict for inferior outcomes following the administration of a modern GC-containing three-drug remission-induction regimen. Our clinical observations led us to propose that at least one or more of the chemotherapy agents employed during induction is able to overcome GC resistance conferred by the *BIM* deletion polymorphism.

Chemotherapy overcomes GC resistance conferred by the *BIM* deletion polymorphism

To determine if any of the chemotherapy agents used in the induction regimen was able to overcome *BIM* deletion-mediated GC resistance, we treated the *BIM* deletion-containing clones with methotrexate, vincristine, and L-asparaginase individually, and in combination with dexamethasone. Cells were then assessed for activation of apoptotic cell death, BIM protein induction, and cell viability.

First, using immunoblot, we found that each of the three chemotherapy agents was individually able to induce equivalent levels of apoptotic cell death (as measured by the production of cleaved PARP and caspase 3) in the absence and presence of the *BIM* deletion (Figures 4A–C, compare lanes 3, 7 and 11). Importantly, we also observed that chemotherapy-induced apoptosis occurred without significant induction of any of the three BIM isoforms (BIM EL, L, and S) reported to be important for GC-induced apoptosis [31]. These results demonstrate that methotrexate, vincristine, and L-asparaginase are each able to induce ALL cell death in a BIM-independent manner, and that this occurred regardless of the *BIM* deletion status of the cell line.

Next, we found that when dexamethasone was combined with methotrexate, vincristine or L-asparaginase, there was a consistent increase in the level of activated PARP and caspase 3 compared to GC alone (Figures 4A–C, lanes 4, 8 and 12). Similarly, when cell viability was assayed, the addition of methotrexate (Figure 5A), vincristine (Figure 5B), or L-asparaginase (Figure 5C) to dexamethasone augmented cell death in deletion-containing clones. Taken together, our *in vitro* data suggest that the ability of the *BIM* deletion polymorphism to confer GC resistance can be overcome by the co-administration of several of the cytotoxic components of the Ma-Spore regimen, including methotrexate, vincristine, and L-asparaginase.

Discussion

In the current work, we used a genome-editing approach to demonstrate that a common germline variant in the *BIM* gene is sufficient to confer GC resistance in ALL cell lines. Mechanistically, we confirm that cells harboring the deletion favor the splicing and expression of non-apoptotic isoforms of BIM, impairing the apoptotic response to GC exposure, and thereby promoting ALL cell survival. However, using a cohort of 411

uniformly-treated ALL patients, we also find that the deletion does not predict inferior responses to GC-containing multi-agent chemotherapy, and that this is associated with the ability of chemotherapy to induce BIM-independent cell death.

By generating CCRF-CEM subclones that were either wildtype, heterozygous or homozygous for the *BIM* polymorphism, we were able to demonstrate that the *BIM* deletion polymorphism is able to confer GC resistance in a T-ALL cell line. In these clones, the expected changes in splicing to favor the E3-containing, non-apoptotic splice variants were recapitulated in a polymorphism dose-dependent manner. We then showed that both upregulation of the E4-containing *BIM* isoforms and apoptosis upon GC treatment were impaired in the deletion-containing clones. Overall, our results are consistent with prior work demonstrating a critical role for BIM induction in GC-induced ALL cell death, particularly the EL, L, and S isoforms which harbor the E4- and BH3-containing isoforms capable of activating apoptosis [27,31]. One limitation of our *in vitro* studies is the use of a single cell line, CCRF-CEM, which is a T-ALL line. Although we were unable to generate deletion-containing lines of other lineages, we expect that introduction of the deletion, which phenocopies a BIM knock-down of BIM, will likely confer glucocorticoid resistance in other ALL cell lines [27,31,32].

The inability of the *BIM* deletion to segregate poor versus good risk patients was somewhat surprising given previous reports describing the ability of *in vitro* as well as clinical GC responses to predict long-term outcomes in pediatric ALL [33–37]. Importantly, because we were able to generate isogenic cell lines with and without the *BIM* deletion, we could explore the mechanisms underlying our clinical observations. Here, we found that three other agents employed in the Ma-Spore ALL 2003 regimen, methotrexate, vincristine, and L-asparaginase, are each individually able to overcome *BIM* deletion-associated GC resistance. Our *in vitro* results also indicate that each of these drugs activate apoptotic cell death in a largely BIM-independent manner, and that this is likely to underlie their clinical efficacy in overcoming *BIM* deletion-mediated GC resistance. While the precise mechanisms by which methotrexate and L-asparaginase induce apoptosis remain ill-defined [43], it is interesting to note that the mechanism of vincristine-induced apoptosis has recently been described [44]. Here [44], and consistent with our observations, vincristine-induced apoptosis was shown to occur via the depletion of the pro-survival protein MCL1, a factor that has itself been shown to mediate GC resistance in ALL [45].

It is also important to highlight that *in vitro* resistance to GC, which has been shown to correlate with clinical responses [33,34], may not necessarily readout for GC resistance *per se*. This is because such assays will also read out for more general mechanisms of resistance that would be expected to mediate cross-resistance among different drug classes, a conclusion that other studies have suggested [46,47]. More recent work has also implicated other germline *BIM* variants in mediating drug resistance [48,49]. Importantly, and reminiscent of our data, we note that it was the combination of a functional SNP in *BIM* with a SNP in the *MCL1* promoter (associated with increased *MCL1* expression) that best predicted OS in pediatric ALL [49,50].

Table 1. Biological and clinical features of patients from the Ma-Spore ALL 2003 trial genotyped for the *BIM* polymorphism.

Characteristics	Wildtype (n = 361)		*BIM* polymorphism present (n = 50)		P value
	No. %		No. %		
Age at diagnosis					1.000
<1 or >10	71	19.7	10	20	
1–10	290	80.3	40	80	
Sex					0.094
Male	213	59	23	46	
Female	148	41	27	54	
Molecular subtype^					0.127
ETV6-RUNX1	68	19	7	14.3	
TCF-PBX1	17	4.7	7	14.3	
BCR-ABL1	16	4.5	1	2	
MLL rearrangements	9	2.5	3	6.1	
Hyperdiploidy	65	18.2	12	24.5	
Hypodiploidy	4	1.1	0	0	
T-ALL	30	8.4	3	6.1	
Others	149	41.6	16	32.7	
NCI Risk					0.642
High	138	38.2	17	34	
Low	223	61.8	33	66	
Day 8 Prednisolone Response^					0.804
Good	320	88.9	44	91.7	
Poor	40	11.1	4	8.3	
Day 33 PCR MRD^					0.970
<0.01%	146	43.6	19	46.3	
0.01–1%	155	46.4	18	43.9	
≥1%	34	10	4	9.8	
PCR MRD Risk^					0.966
Standard	134	38.4	17	37	
Intermediate	194	55.6	27	58.7	
High	21	6	2	4.3	
Ma-Spore Risk^					0.463
Standard	109	30.2	14	28	
Intermediate	177	49	29	58	
High	75	20.8	7	14	
Ma-Spore Outcome					0.608
CCR	295	81.7	42	84	
Induction Failure	16	4.4	1	2	
Relapse	21	5.8	1	2	
Death	17	4.7	3	6	
Abandonment	12	3.3	3	6	
Race					<0.001
Chinese	156	43.2	35	70	
Malay	147	40.7	14	28	
Indian & Others	58	16.1	1	2	

Incidence of the *BIM* polymorphism is 50 out of 411 patients, or 12.2%. Abbreviations: Ma-Spore, Malaysia- Singapore; MRD, minimal residual disease; NCI, National Cancer Institute; PCR, polymerase chain reaction; CCR, continuous complete remission.
^indicates that data was unavailable for some patients.

A

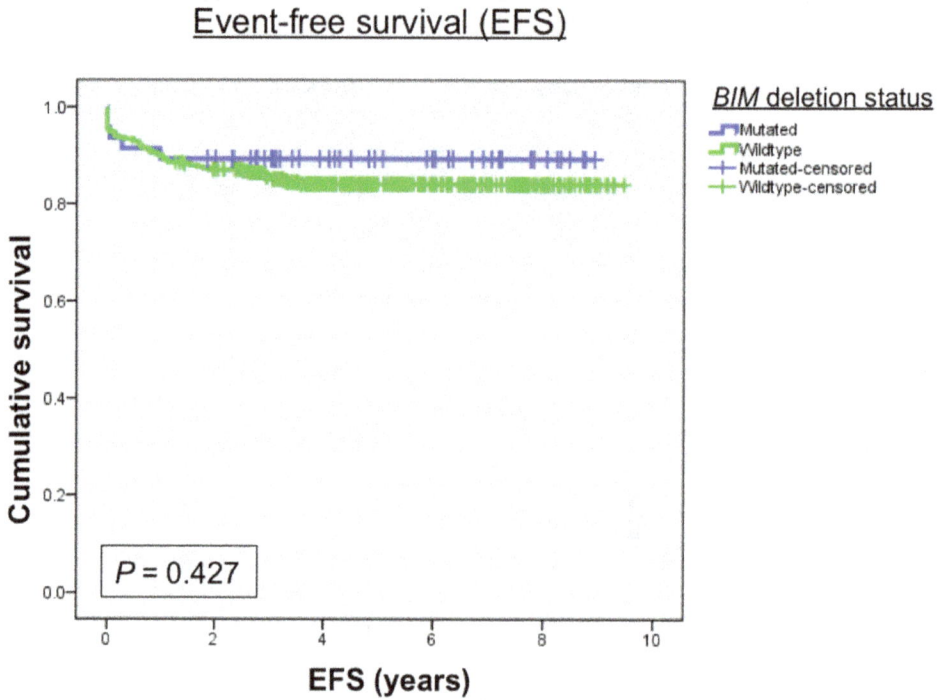

B

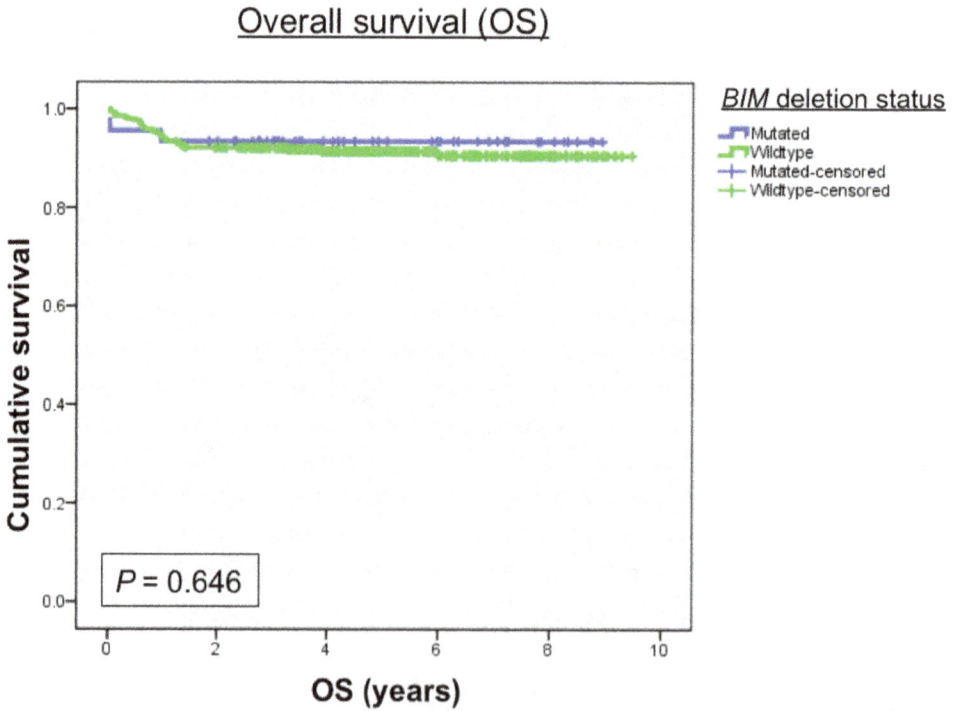

Figure 3. Retrospective analysis of the Ma-Spore ALL 2003 cohort according to the presence or absence of the *BIM* deletion polymorphism. Kaplan-Meier curves comparing event-free survival (**A**) or overall survival (**B**) in patients with or without the *BIM* deletion polymorphism are shown.

Together, our observations are consistent with a "BCL-2 rheostat" model where the cellular apoptotic threshold is set by the balance of pro-apoptotic BCL-2 family members such as BIM and anti-apoptotic members like MCL1 [27]. This model would predict

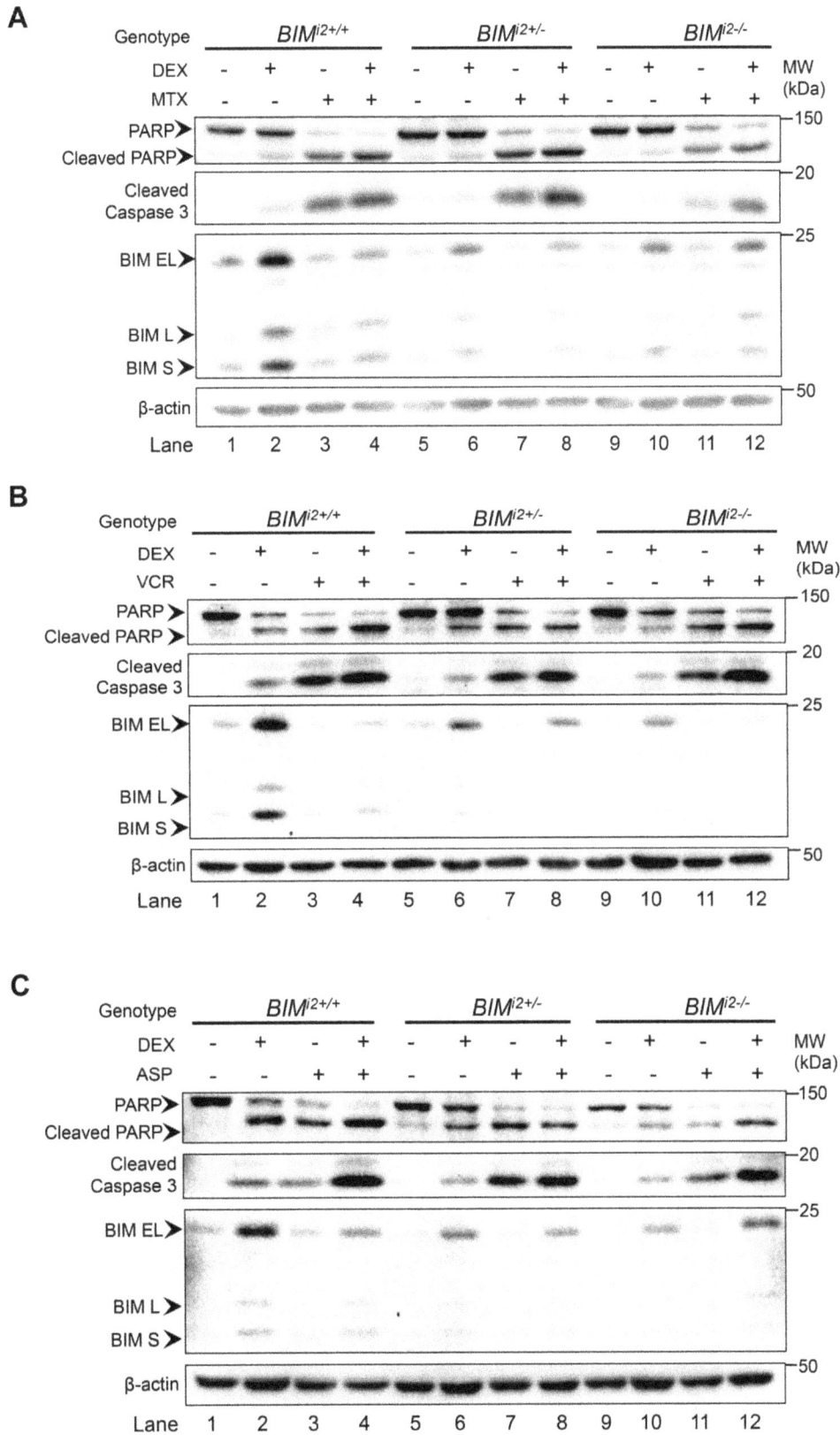

Figure 4. Methotrexate, vincristine, and L-asparaginase activate apoptosis in a BIM-independent manner, and overcome *BIM* deletion-mediated GC resistance. CCRF-CEM clones were treated with dexamethasone (DEX) (0.1 µM) with or without (**A**) methotrexate (MTX) (1 µM), (**B**) vincristine (VCR) (2 ng/ml), or (**C**) L-asparaginase (ASP) (0.5 IU/ml) for 48 h. Following incubation, cell lysates were obtained and analyzed for cleaved PARP and caspase 3, as well as BIM induction. β-actin was used as a loading control.

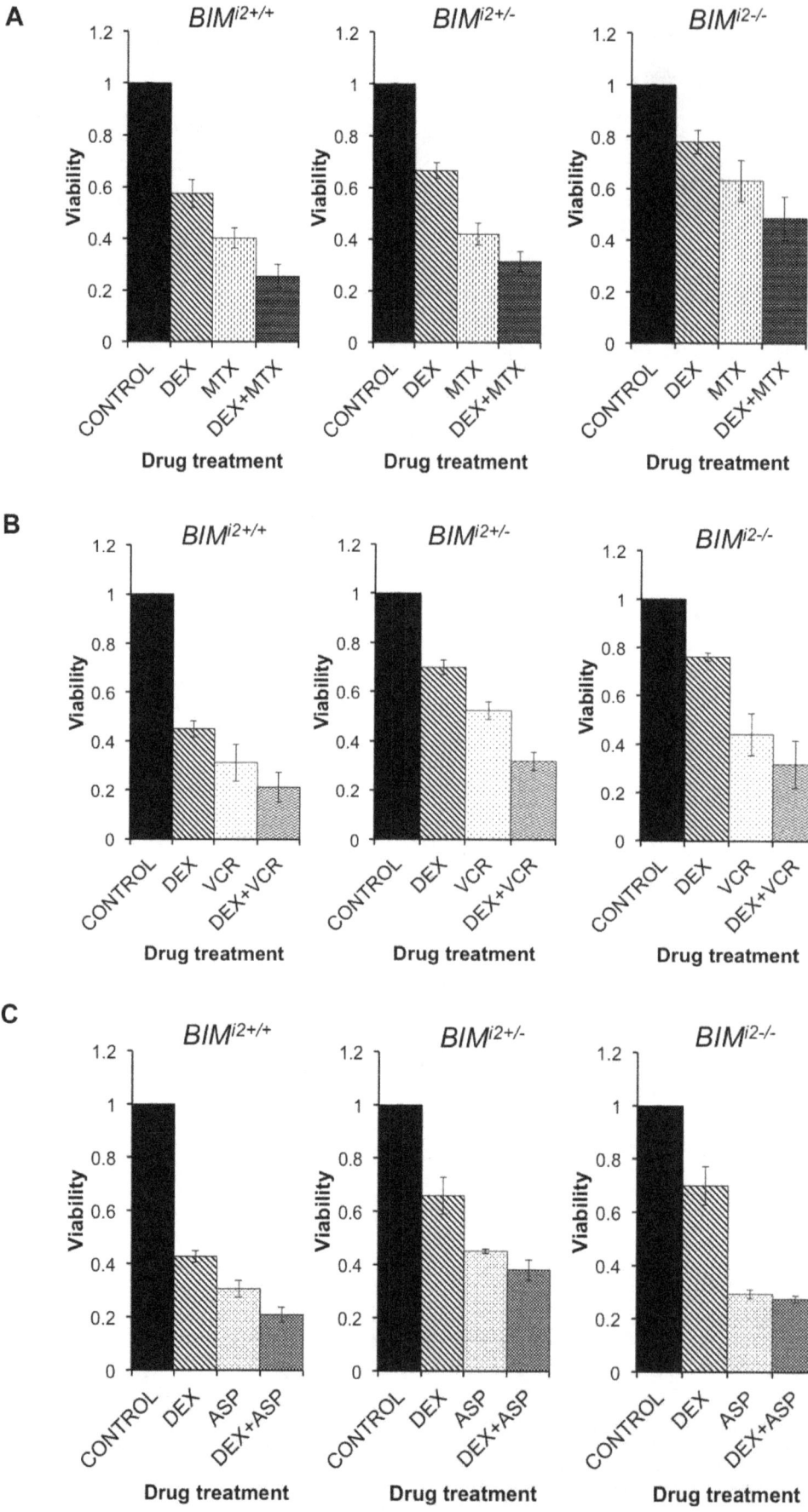

Figure 5. The addition of methotrexate, vincristine or L-asparaginase resensitizes *BIM* deletion-containing CCRF-CEM clones to dexamethasone. Cell viability was measured by MTS assay after (**A**) methotrexate (MTX) (1 μM), (**B**) vincristine (VCR) (2 ng/ml), or (**C**) L-asparaginase (ASP) (0.5 IU/ml) was used singly or in combination with dexamethasone (DEX) (0.1 μM) for 48 h. Values obtained for treated cells were normalized to the untreated control for the same genotype. Error bars indicate SEM (n =) of 3 independent replicates.

that genetic variants affecting BCL2 family members may only be clinically important when two or more act in concert to alter the apoptotic threshold.

While there is increasing evidence that germline polymorphisms contribute to clinical heterogeneity in ALL [13–15], it is likely that only those variants capable of conferring alterations in biological behavior and/or multi-drug resistance will be associated with clinically meaningful endpoints. Thus, as we have demonstrated with the *BIM* deletion, polymorphisms that confer single-drug resistance in the setting of modern multi-agent ALL therapy are less likely to be of clinical importance. Indeed, variants that have been shown to predict poor response are enriched for genes expected to confer a multi-drug resistance phenotype, and include those that influence systemic drug clearance and intracellular drug concentrations [9,12].

Finally, our observations also highlight the ability of at least three cytotoxic agents to induce apoptosis independently of BIM, and suggest that the success of modern day ALL regimens is due to the ability of individual agents to kill leukemia cells via targeting different components of the "BCL-2 rheostat". Indeed, this general lesson may be applied to cancers where we have found that the *BIM* deletion does play a part in clinical drug resistance [17], and supports the use of judiciously chosen combination therapies to overcome *BIM* deletion-mediated drug resistance in these patients.

Acknowledgments

The authors thank the collaborators and patients in the Ma-Spore ALL 2003 study, as well as TK Ko for advice on genome editing and SK Kham for technical assistance.

Author Contributions

Conceived and designed the experiments: STO AEJY. Performed the experiments: SXS JYL JWJH. Analyzed the data: SXS JYL NJ STO AEJY. Contributed to the writing of the manuscript: SXS STO.

References

1. Mullighan CG (2012) The molecular genetic makeup of acute lymphoblastic leukemia. Hematology Am Soc Hematol Educ Program 2012: 389–396.
2. Pui CH, Evans WE (2006) Treatment of acute lymphoblastic leukemia. N Engl J Med 354: 166–178.
3. Locatelli F, Schrappe M, Bernardo ME, Rutella S (2012) How I treat relapsed childhood acute lymphoblastic leukemia. Blood 120: 2807–2816.
4. Yeoh EJ, Ross ME, Shurtleff SA, Williams WK, Patel D, et al. (2002) Classification, subtype discovery, and prediction of outcome in pediatric acute lymphoblastic leukemia by gene expression profiling. Cancer Cell 1: 133–143.
5. Martinelli G, Iacobucci I, Storlazzi CT, Vignetti M, Paoloni F, et al. (2009) IKZF1 (Ikaros) deletions in BCR-ABL1-positive acute lymphoblastic leukemia are associated with short disease-free survival and high rate of cumulative incidence of relapse: a GIMEMA AL WP report. J Clin Oncol 27: 5202–5207.
6. Roberts KG, Morin RD, Zhang J, Hirst M, Zhao Y, et al. (2012) Genetic alterations activating kinase and cytokine receptor signaling in high-risk acute lymphoblastic leukemia. Cancer Cell 22: 153–166.
7. McLeod HL (2013) Cancer pharmacogenomics: early promise, but concerted effort needed. Science 339: 1563–1566.
8. Coate L, Cuffe S, Horgan A, Hung RJ, Christiani D, et al. (2010) Germline genetic variation, cancer outcome, and pharmacogenetics. J Clin Oncol 28: 4029–4037.
9. Radtke S, Zolk O, Renner B, Paulides M, Zimmermann M, et al. (2013) Germline genetic variations in methotrexate candidate genes are associated with pharmacokinetics, toxicity, and outcome in childhood acute lymphoblastic leukemia. Blood 121: 5145–5153.
10. Xu H, Cheng C, Devidas M, Pei D, Fan Y, et al. (2012) ARID5B genetic polymorphisms contribute to racial disparities in the incidence and treatment outcome of childhood acute lymphoblastic leukemia. J Clin Oncol 30: 751–757.
11. Trevino LR, Shimasaki N, Yang W, Panetta JC, Cheng C, et al. (2009) Germline genetic variation in an organic anion transporter polypeptide associated with methotrexate pharmacokinetics and clinical effects. J Clin Oncol 27: 5972–5978.
12. Rocha JC, Cheng C, Liu W, Kishi S, Das S, et al. (2005) Pharmacogenetics of outcome in children with acute lymphoblastic leukemia. Blood 105: 4752–4758.
13. Perez-Andreu V, Roberts KG, Harvey RC, Yang W, Cheng C, et al. (2013) Inherited GATA3 variants are associated with Ph-like childhood acute lymphoblastic leukemia and risk of relapse. Nat Genet 45: 1494–1498.
14. Yang JJ, Cheng C, Devidas M, Cao X, Campana D, et al. (2012) Genome-wide association study identifies germline polymorphisms associated with relapse of childhood acute lymphoblastic leukemia. Blood 120: 4197–4204.
15. Yang JJ, Cheng C, Yang W, Pei D, Cao X, et al. (2009) Genome-wide interrogation of germline genetic variation associated with treatment response in childhood acute lymphoblastic leukemia. JAMA 301: 393–403.
16. Gaj T, Gersbach CA, Barbas CF 3rd (2013) ZFN, TALEN, and CRISPR/Cas-based methods for genome engineering. Trends Biotechnol 31: 397–405.
17. Ng KP, Hillmer AM, Chuah CT, Juan WC, Ko TK, et al. (2012) A common BIM deletion polymorphism mediates intrinsic resistance and inferior responses to tyrosine kinase inhibitors in cancer. Nat Med 18: 521–528.
18. Morel F, Ka C, Le Bris MJ, Herry A, Morice P, et al. (2003) Deletion of the 5'ABL region in Philadelphia chromosome positive chronic myeloid leukemia: frequency, origin and prognosis. Leuk Lymphoma 44: 1333–1338.
19. Jabbour E, Cortes JE, Kantarjian HM (2009) Suboptimal response to or failure of imatinib treatment for chronic myeloid leukemia: what is the optimal strategy? Mayo Clin Proc 84: 161–169.
20. Aichberger KJ, Mayerhofer M, Krauth MT, Vales A, Kondo R, et al. (2005) Low-level expression of proapoptotic Bcl-2-interacting mediator in leukemic cells in patients with chronic myeloid leukemia: role of BCR/ABL, characterization of underlying signaling pathways, and reexpression by novel pharmacologic compounds. Cancer Res 65: 9436–9444.
21. Bouillet P, Metcalf D, Huang DC, Tarlinton DM, Kay TW, et al. (1999) Proapoptotic Bcl-2 relative Bim required for certain apoptotic responses, leukocyte homeostasis, and to preclude autoimmunity. Science 286: 1735–1738.
22. Cragg MS, Kuroda J, Puthalakath H, Huang DC, Strasser A (2007) Gefitinib-induced killing of NSCLC cell lines expressing mutant EGFR requires BIM and can be enhanced by BH3 mimetics. PLoS Med 4: 1681–1689; discussion 1690.
23. Gong Y, Somwar R, Politi K, Balak M, Chmielecki J, et al. (2007) Induction of BIM is essential for apoptosis triggered by EGFR kinase inhibitors in mutant EGFR-dependent lung adenocarcinomas. PLoS Med 4: e294.
24. Kuribara R, Honda H, Matsui H, Shinjyo T, Inukai T, et al. (2004) Roles of Bim in apoptosis of normal and Bcr-Abl-expressing hematopoietic progenitors. Mol Cell Biol 24: 6172–6183.
25. Kuroda J, Puthalakath H, Cragg MS, Kelly PN, Bouillet P, et al. (2006) Bim and Bad mediate imatinib-induced killing of Bcr/Abl+ leukemic cells, and resistance due to their loss is overcome by a BH3 mimetic. Proc Natl Acad Sci U S A 103: 14907–14912.
26. Erlacher M, Michalak EM, Kelly PN, Labi V, Niederegger H, et al. (2005) BH3-only proteins Puma and Bim are rate-limiting for gamma-radiation- and glucocorticoid-induced apoptosis of lymphoid cells in vivo. Blood 106: 4131–4138.
27. Ploner C, Rainer J, Niederegger H, Eduardoff M, Villunger A, et al. (2008) The BCL2 rheostat in glucocorticoid-induced apoptosis of acute lymphoblastic leukemia. Leukemia 22: 370–377.
28. Wang Z, Malone MH, He H, McColl KS, Distelhorst CW (2003) Microarray analysis uncovers the induction of the proapoptotic BH3-only protein Bim in multiple models of glucocorticoid-induced apoptosis. J Biol Chem 278: 23861–23867.
29. Schmidt S, Rainer J, Riml S, Ploner C, Jesacher S, et al. (2006) Identification of glucocorticoid-response genes in children with acute lymphoblastic leukemia. Blood 107: 2061–2069.
30. Bachmann PS, Piazza RG, Janes ME, Wong NC, Davies C, et al. (2010) Epigenetic silencing of BIM in glucocorticoid poor-responsive pediatric acute lymphoblastic leukemia, and its reversal by histone deacetylase inhibition. Blood 116: 3013–3022.
31. Abrams MT, Robertson NM, Yoon K, Wickstrom E (2004) Inhibition of glucocorticoid-induced apoptosis by targeting the major splice variants of BIM mRNA with small interfering RNA and short hairpin RNA. J Biol Chem 279: 55809–55817.

32. Jiang N, Koh GS, Lim JY, Kham SK, Ariffin H, et al. (2011) BIM is a prognostic biomarker for early prednisolone response in pediatric acute lymphoblastic leukemia. Exp Hematol 39: 321–329.

33. Kaspers GJ, Pieters R, Van Zantwijk CH, Van Wering ER, Van Der Does-Van Den Berg A, et al. (1998) Prednisolone resistance in childhood acute lymphoblastic leukemia: vitro-vivo correlations and cross-resistance to other drugs. Blood 92: 259–266.

34. Den Boer ML, Harms DO, Pieters R, Kazemier KM, Gobel U, et al. (2003) Patient stratification based on prednisolone-vincristine-asparaginase resistance profiles in children with acute lymphoblastic leukemia. J Clin Oncol 21: 3262–3268.

35. Lauten M, Moricke A, Beier R, Zimmermann M, Stanulla M, et al. (2012) Prediction of outcome by early bone marrow response in childhood acute lymphoblastic leukemia treated in the ALL-BFM 95 trial: differential effects in precursor B-cell and T-cell leukemia. Haematologica 97: 1048–1056.

36. Dordelmann M, Reiter A, Borkhardt A, Ludwig WD, Gotz N, et al. (1999) Prednisone response is the strongest predictor of treatment outcome in infant acute lymphoblastic leukemia. Blood 94: 1209–1217.

37. Schrappe M, Arico M, Harbott J, Biondi A, Zimmermann M, et al. (1998) Philadelphia chromosome-positive (Ph+) childhood acute lymphoblastic leukemia: good initial steroid response allows early prediction of a favorable treatment outcome. Blood 92: 2730–2741.

38. Yeoh AE, Ariffin H, Chai EL, Kwok CS, Chan YH, et al. (2012) Minimal residual disease-guided treatment deintensification for children with acute lymphoblastic leukemia: results from the Malaysia-Singapore acute lymphoblastic leukemia 2003 study. J Clin Oncol 30: 2384–2392.

39. Foley GE, Lazarus H, Farber S, Uzman BG, Boone BA, et al. (1965) Continuous Culture of Human Lymphoblasts from Peripheral Blood of a Child with Acute Leukemia. Cancer 18: 522–529.

40. Stong RC, Korsmeyer SJ, Parkin JL, Arthur DC, Kersey JH (1985) Human acute leukemia cell line with the t(4;11) chromosomal rearrangement exhibits B lineage and monocytic characteristics. Blood 65: 21–31.

41. Miyagi T, Ohyashiki J, Yamato K, Koeffler HP, Miyoshi I (1993) Phenotypic and molecular analysis of Ph1-chromosome-positive acute lymphoblastic leukemia cell lines. Int J Cancer 53: 457–462.

42. Juan WC, Roca X, Ong ST (2014) Identification of cis-Acting Elements and Splicing Factors Involved in the Regulation of BIM Pre-mRNA Splicing. PLoS One 9: e95210.

43. DeVita VT Jr, Lawrence TS, Rosenberg SA (2008) DeVita, Hellman, and Rosenberg's Cancer: Principles & Practice of Oncology. Philadelphia, PA, USA: Wolters Kluwer/Lippincott Williams & Wilkins. pp 427, 451, 490.

44. Wertz IE, Kusam S, Lam C, Okamoto T, Sandoval W, et al. (2011) Sensitivity to antitubulin chemotherapeutics is regulated by MCL1 and FBW7. Nature 471: 110–114.

45. Wei G, Twomey D, Lamb J, Schlis K, Agarwal J, et al. (2006) Gene expression-based chemical genomics identifies rapamycin as a modulator of MCL1 and glucocorticoid resistance. Cancer Cell 10: 331–342.

46. Pieters R, Kaspers GJ, van Wering ER, Huismans DR, Loonen AH, et al. (1993) Cellular drug resistance profiles that might explain the prognostic value of immunophenotype and age in childhood acute lymphoblastic leukemia. Leukemia 7: 392–397.

47. Kaspers GJ, Pieters R, Van Zantwijk CH, Van Wering ER, Veerman AJ (1995) Clinical and cell biological features related to cellular drug resistance of childhood acute lymphoblastic leukemia cells. Leuk Lymphoma 19: 407–416.

48. Augis V, Airiau K, Josselin M, Turcq B, Mahon FX, et al. (2013) A Single Nucleotide Polymorphism in cBIM Is Associated with a Slower Achievement of Major Molecular Response in Chronic Myeloid Leukaemia Treated with Imatinib. PLoS One 8: e78582.

49. Gagne V, Rousseau J, Labuda M, Sharif-Askari B, Brukner I, et al. (2013) Bim polymorphisms: influence on function and response to treatment in children with acute lymphoblastic leukemia. Clin Cancer Res 19(18): 5240–5249.

50. Sanchez R, St-Cyr J, Lalonde ME, Healy J, Richer C, et al. (2013) Impact of promoter polymorphisms in key regulators of the intrinsic apoptosis pathway in childhood acute lymphoblastic leukemia outcome. Haematologica. doi: 10.3324/haematol.2013.085340.

18

The Protective Effect of Adenoidectomy on Pediatric Tympanostomy Tube Re-Insertions: A Population-Based Birth Cohort Study

Mao-Che Wang[1,2], Ying-Piao Wang[2,3], Chia-Huei Chu[1], Tzong-Yang Tu[1], An-Suey Shiao[1], Pesus Chou[2]*

1 Department of Otolaryngology Head Neck Surgery, Taipei Veterans General Hospital, Taipei, Taiwan and School of Medicine, National Yang-Ming University, Taipei, Taiwan, 2 Institute of Public Health and Community Medicine Research Center, National Yang-Ming University, Taipei, Taiwan, 3 Department of Otolaryngology Head Neck Surgery, Mackay Memorial Hospital, Taipei, Taiwan and Department of Audiology and Speech Language Pathology and School of Medicine, Mackay Medical College, New Taipei City, Taiwan

Abstract

Objectives: Adenoidectomy in conjunction with tympanostomy tube insertion for treating pediatric otitis media with effusion and recurrent acute otitis media has been debated for decades. Practice differed surgeon from surgeon. This study used population-based data to determine the protective effect of adenoidectomy in preventing tympanostomy tube re-insertion and tried to provide more evidence based information for surgeons when they do decision making.

Study Design: Retrospective birth cohort study.

Methods: This study used the National Health Insurance Research Database for the period 2000–2009 in Taiwan. The tube reinsertion rate and time to tube re-insertion among children who received tympanostomy tubes with or without adenoidectomy were compared. Age stratification analysis was also done to explore the effects of age.

Results: Adenoidectomy showed protective effects on preventing tube re-insertion compared to tympanostomy tubes alone in children who needed tubes for the first time (tube re-insertion rate 9% versus 5.1%, $p = 0.002$ and longer time to re-insertions, $p = 0.01$), especially those aged over 4 years when they had their first tube surgery. After controlling the effect of age, adenoidectomy reduced the rate of re-insertion by 40% compared to tympanostomy tubes alone (aHR: 0.60; 95% CI: 0.41–0.89). However, the protective effect of conjunction adenoidectomy was not obvious among children with a second tympanostomy tube insertion. Children who needed their first tube surgery at the age 2–4 years were most prone to have tube re-insertions, followed by the age group of 4–6 years.

Conclusions: Adenoidectomy has protective effect in preventing tympanostomy tube re-insertions compared to tympanostomy tubes alone, especially for children older than 4 years old and who needed tubes for the first time. Nonetheless, clinicians should still weigh the pros and cons of the procedure for their pediatric patients.

Editor: Susanna Esposito, Fondazione IRCCS Ca' Granda Ospedale Maggiore Policlinico, Università degli Studi di Milano, Italy

Funding: This study was supported by the research grant of Taipei Veterans General Hospital (V102B-050). Website of Taipei Veterans General Hospital: www.vghtpe.gov.tw. The first author WANG MC received the funding. Taipei Veterans General hospital is a government owned hospital in Taiwan. WANG MC, CHU CH, TU TY, SHIAO AS are employees of Taipei Veterans General Hospital. The funder had no role in study design, data collection and analysis, decision to publish, or preparation of the manuscript.

Competing Interests: The authors have declared that no competing interests exist.

* Email: pschou@ym.edu.tw

Introduction

Acute otitis media (AOM) and otitis media with effusion (OME) are very common otologic problems in children. The middle ear cavity is filled with infected fluid and the mucosa is inflamed. Ninety percent of children experience AOM and OME before school age, most often between 6 months and 4 years of age [1,2]. Most OME resolve spontaneously within three months, but 30–40% may have recurrent OME and 5–10% of episodes may last for a year or longer [1,3,4]. Diagnosis of OME depends on history, including previous rhino-sinusitis or AOM, decreased hearing noted by the care giver, inattention at school, and aural fullness sensation as stated by the child. Physical examination is based mainly on pneumatic otoscopy, which is an inexpensive, accessible, and easily used diagnostic tool [3,5]. Diagnosis may be confirmed by telescopy, pure tone audiometry, and tympanometry [6]. Management includes conservative treatment and surgical intervention. The American Academy of Otolaryngology Head and Neck Surgery (AAO-HNS) set the clinical practice guidelines for OME in 2004. Based on the self-limiting nature of most OME,

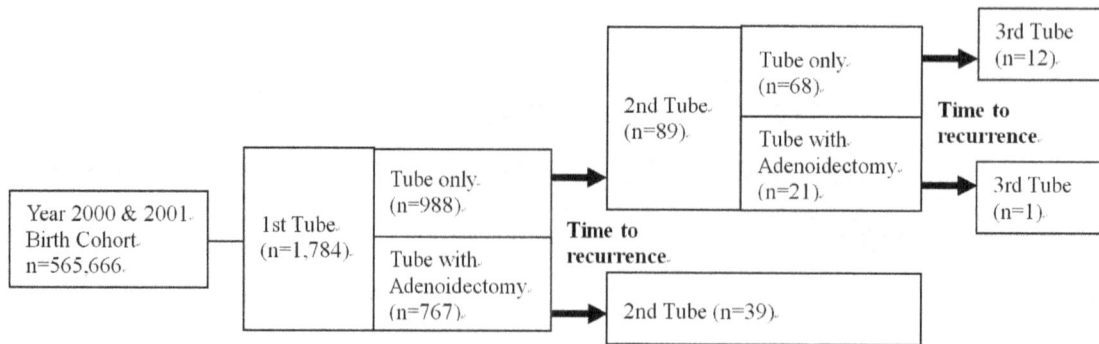

Figure 1. Study flow chart.

clinicians should manage children who are not at risk by watchful waiting for three months from the date of effusion onset (if known) or from the date of diagnosis (if onset is unknown). If a child becomes a surgical candidate, tympanostomy tube insertion is the preferred initial procedure. Adenoidectomy should only be performed when there is nasal obstruction or chronic adenoiditis, or in repeated tympanostomy tube insertions. Tonsillectomy or myringotomy alone should not be used [5]. The AAO-HNS also set clinical practice guidelines for tympanostomy tubes in children in 2013, recommending that clinicians offer bilateral tympanostomy tubes to children with bilateral chronic OME (OME last for 3 months or longer), and recurrent AOM with middle ear effusion. The guideline also recommended that clinicians should not offer tympanostomy tubes to children with single episode of OME lasting less than 3 months, and recurrent AOM without middle ear effusion [7].

For children with tympanostomy tubes, 20–50% may require repeated tympanostomy tubes after their initial tubes extruded [8–10]. Adenoidectomy has been proved to be effective in preventing recurrence of OME, recurrent AOM, or the need for repeated tympanostomy tubes in many studies in the past 30 years [11–20], and only a few demonstrated contrary data [21–24]. Adenoidectomy may reduce repeated tympanostomy tubes by 50% [15–19]. Why is adenoidectomy effective in preventing pediatric middle ear infection? The adenoids are considered an important factor in pediatric middle ear infection since it may be a reservoir of pathogens [25], while its size effect may block the Eustachian tube orifice [26,27]. Thus, it may play a role in middle ear inflammation or decreased ciliated mucosa [28–30]. However, it is not suggested as a regular procedure in treating chronic OME or recurrent AOM or in conjunction with primary tympanostomy tube insertions [5,31], for the possible complications of general anesthesia and the procedure itself like bleeding, nasopharyngeal stenosis, and injury to the orifice of Eustachian tubes [32–34]. Although the AAO-HNS practice guidelines for OME suggested adenoidectomy only for children requiring repeated tympanostomy tubes [5], many surgeons performed adenoidectomy in conjunction with tympanostomy tubes insertion as the initial treatment for chronic OME or recurrent AOM in recent years after the release of AAO-HNS practice guidelines [16,18,19]. When to perform adenoidectomy for children with chronic OME remains a major debatable issue. Another controversial issue is the age at which adenoidectomy will be beneficial to children with chronic OME. Many studies show that adenoidectomy is only beneficial to children of certain age groups. In three studies, Gates et al. and Maw showed that adenoidectomy was beneficial in children with OME older than 4 years [11,12,14], and one most

recent systemic review and metanalysis also concluded that adenoidectomy with primary tube insertion appears to provide a protective effect against repeated surgery in children older than 4 years [35], while Hammaren-Malmi et al. demonstrated that adenoidectomy did not reduce OME in children younger than 4 years old [21]. However, Coyte et al. found that adenoidectomy was beneficial to children older than 2 years old and that the benefits were more obvious among children older than 3 years old [15]. Thus, the results of these studies are not consistent. This population-based retrospective birth cohort study aimed to examine the protective effect of adenoidectomy for tube re-insertion using the National Health Insurance Research Database (NHIRD) in Taiwan. Specifically, this study examined the efficacy of adenoidectomy in conjunction with tympanostomy tube insertion for reducing the repeated tympanostomy tubes compared to tympanostomy tubes alone. We used Tympanostomy tube insertion as a surrogate for chronic OME and recurrent AOM because surgical procedures were usually for most serious and retractable cases. Besides, the reduction of tube insertion also means the reduction of the risk of general anesthesia and the procedure itself which were really burdens for both pediatric patients and their parents. The National Health Insurance (NHI) in Taiwan, established since 1995, has a nationwide coverage of more than 99% of legal residents. It is well known for its low fees and low reimbursement but high quality of service. All of the medical services and medication in Taiwan are paid for by NHI, which is also characterized by easy accessibility without a regulated referral system. Patients may go to any doctor or any hospital on their own will, with or without the referral of primary care physicians. All of the medical procedures and claims are recorded in the NHI database, which is the only buyer of medical service in Taiwan. The NHIRD is released for academic use yearly by the National Health Institute of Taiwan.

Materials and Methods

The study was reviewed and approved by the Institutional Review Board of Taipei Veterans General Hospital. (IRB number: 2013-02-019B) No inform consent was given because this study analyzed government released secondary data. The identification of every individual in the database was censored. This ten-year study (2000–2009) used the Taiwan NHIRD, a population-based data on approximately 23 million people covered by the NHI. Every admission and outpatient visit record was included in this database without sampling. All children born in the year 2000 and 2001 who had tympanostomy tube insertion before the end of the study period (end of the year 2009) were included. They were divided into two groups based on whether or not adenoidectomy

Table 1. Descriptions of 2000–2001 birth cohort who had undergone tympanostomy tubes before 9 years of age.

Characteristics	n	%
Total subjects	1755	100.0
Gender*		
Male	1065	60.7
Female	689	39.3
Age at 1st tube insertion*		
0–2 years	183	10.4
2–4 years	222	12.7
4–6 years	856	48.8
6–9 years	494	28.2
Number of chronic OME episodes		
1	1627	92.7
2	111	6.3
3	12	0.7
4+	5	0.3
Surgical operation		
Tube only	988	56.3
Tube + Adenoidectomy	767	43.7
Age at tube insertion†		
1st tube insertion	5.0	1.8
2nd tube insertion	5.9	1.5
3rd tube insertion	6.9	1.3
Age at adenoidectomy‡		
0–2 years	5	0.6
2–4 years	82	10.1
4–6 years	450	55.5
6–9 years	274	33.8

*One missing value.
†Shown by mean and standard deviation.
‡Only those who had undergone adenoidectomy were included (n = 767).

was done together with their first tympanostomy tube insertion. Data on these children was examined to determine if they received repeated tube insertions before the end of the study period.

Those with repeated tube insertions without adenoidectomy on their first tympanostomy tube insertion were further divided into two groups based on whether or not adenoidectomy was done together with their second tympanostomy tube insertion. Data on these children was further examined to determine if they received a third tube insertion before the end of the study period (Fig. 1). The repeat tube insertion rate and time to repeated tubes were compared between children who received adenoidectomy with tympanostomy tubes and those who received tube insertion alone.

The study population was obtained by retrieving all of the patients with the procedure code for myringotomy with ventilation tube insertion under a microscope from 2000 to 2009 from the claims data of the NHIRD, with a birthday between January 1, 2000 and December 31, 2001. That is a population-based data without any sampling. As such, a population based year 2000 and 2001 birth cohort for tympanostomy tube insertion was obtained and followed-up to 8 or 9 years old. Children with cleft palate with diagnosis codes in International Classification of Disease, 9th

Revision (ICD-9) 749.00~749.04 were excluded because they tended to have multiple tympanostomy tube insertions [36–38]. Adenoidectomy was also relatively contraindicated for children with cleft palate as it might lead to velo-pharyngeal incompetence [39]. Concurrent tympanostomy tube insertion and adenoidectomy was defined by identifying two procedure codes for myringotomy with ventilation tube insertion under a microscope, and for adenoidectomy on the same day in the claims data. Adenoidectomy done with tonsillectomy at the same time was also identified and was not included in this study.

The children were also stratified into four age groups in years in order to examine the effect of age ($0 \leq$ age < 2, $2 \leq$ age < 4, $4 \leq$ age < 6, and $6 \leq$ age < 9). The rate of repeated tympanostomy tube insertion and time to recurrence were examined in each age group to explore the protective effect of adenoidectomy on tube reinsertion. The age group with highest risk of tube re-insertion was further determined. The rate of post-adenoidectomy bleeding was also explored.

Statistical Analysis

The tube insertion rate between children with adenoidectomy and tympanostomy tubes and those with tympanostomy tubes alone in all age groups was compared using the Fisher's exact test. The time between the first tympanostomy tube insertion and repeated procedures in the study period was compared by log-rank test for failure time. The adjusted hazard ratio of recurrence between children with and those without adenoidectomy and among age groups was obtained by Cox proportional hazard model. The statistical results were obtained via the software SAS 9.1 (SAS Institute, Cary, NC, USA). Statistical significance was set at $p < 0.05$. All values were expressed as mean $\pm$ standard deviation (SD).

Results

According to the Taiwan National Statistics Report, there were 305,312 and 260,354 newborns in the year 2000 and 2001 respectively [40]. This study had a population-based birth cohort numbering 565,666 who were followed-up for 8 to 9 years. A total of 2221 children in the 2000 and 2001 birth cohorts had tympanostomy tube insertion before the age of 8 or 9 years. The cumulative incidence of tympanostomy tube insertion before 8 or 9 years of age was 0.393%. After excluding 437 children with cleft palate, and 29 children with adenotonsillectomy, 1755 were included in this study. Among them, 1627 cases had only one tube insertion before 8 or 9 years of age. There were 1065 males, or 60.7% of the total cases. Around 80% of children had their first tube surgery after 4 years of age. One hundred and eleven had two tubes insertions and 17 had more than two insertions. Additional adenoidectomy and age at tympanostomy tube insertions and adenoidectomy were shown in Table 1.

Of the 1755 cases included, 767 had adenoidectomy on their first tympanostomy tube insertion. The other 988 children had tube insertion alone, although 89 of them needed repeated tube insertions. There were 21 who had adenoidectomy on their second tubes insertion while 68 had tube insertion only. The age of children received adenoidectomy was 5.5 ± 1.3 (mean $\pm$ SD) years old. Children who received both adenoidectomy and tympanostomy tubes on their first tubes insertion had a lower recurrence rate than those who had tubes alone ($p = 0.002$). They also had a longer time to re-insertions ($p = 0.01$) (Fig. 2). However, the protective effect of adenoidectomy on the second tube insertion was not observed in terms of re-insertion rate and in time to re-insertions ($p = 0.29$ and $p = 0.22$, respectively) (Table 2).

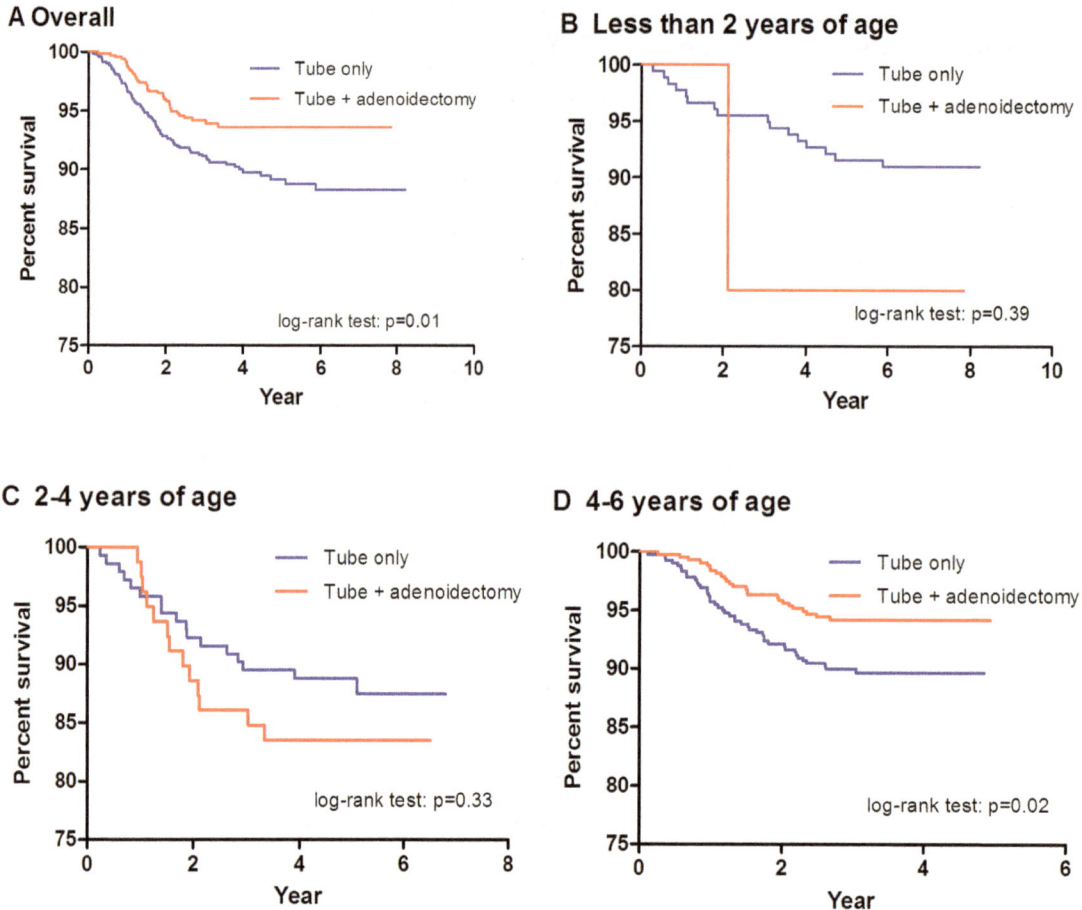

Figure 2. Survival curve of tube re-insertions. (A) Overall recurrence. (B) (C) and (D) Recurrence stratified by age.

Stratifying the children into four age groups (0–2 years, 2–4 years, 4–6 years, and 6–9 years), those older than 4 years old who received both adenoidectomy and tympanostomy tubes had statistically significant lower tube re-insertion rate and longer time to tube re-insertions than those who had tympanostomy tubes alone (Table 2 & Figure 2). ($p = 0.02$, $p<0.001$ for age group 4–6 and 6–9 respectively) There was no difference in tube re-insertions regardless of adenoidectomy in the age group 0–2 and 2–4 years (Table 2).

After controlling for age, adenoidectomy reduced the rate of tube re-insertion by 40% compared to tympanostomy tubes alone (aHR: 0.60; 95% CI: 0.41–0.89). After controlling for the effect of adenoidectomy, children who had their first tube surgery at the age of 2–4 years were most prone to tube re-insertions, followed by the 4–6 years age group (Table 3). Among 767 patients who received adenoidectomy, only two had severe post-operative bleeding that required intra-operative monitoring.

Discussion

The 2000 and 2001 birth cohort in Taiwan had 565,666 children. Among them, 2221 had tympanostomy tube insertion before the age of 8 or 9 years for a cumulative incidence of 0.393%. Compared to other reports, one study showed the tympanostomy tube insertion rate in United states was 6.8% before the age of 3 and another study revealed middle ear surgical procedure was 9% in Norway [41,42]. The rate of tube re-

insertion is about 20% to 50% [8–10,43]. The rate of tympanostomy tube insertion and tube re-sinsertion of children in Taiwan is low. This may be because Asian parents usually do not like their children to undergo surgery, leading to more conservative management or otolarygologists in Taiwan managed pediatric otitis media more conservatively under the suggestions of clinical practice guideline in comparison to surgeons in the United States [44–46].

This study demonstrates that adenoidectomy has a protective effect of preventing tube re-insertion in conjunction with the first tympanostomy tube insertion in children older than 4 years old compared to tube insertion alone. There were 849 cases in the 4–6 year old age group, which accounted for nearly half of the enrolled cases. Further stratifying this group into two groups of 4–5 years and 5–6 years for analysis, adenoidectomy had significant protective effects in the 4–5 year old age group but not in the 5–6 year old age group. The recurrence rate of children receiving adenoidectomy in the two age groups was 5.8% and 5.5%, respectively. The recurrence rates in tube only group was lower in the 5–6 year old age group (8.1%) than that in the 4–5 year old age group (12.1%). This may be due to the protective effect of age influencing the protective effect of adenoidectomy. We did not found the protective effect of adenoidectomy for children under 4 years old. Given small sample size for children under age of 4, post hoc power was calculated to examine whether the statistical power was large enough to detect differences in tube re-insertion rate between two surgical procedures. With an overall sample size of

Table 2. Tympanostomy tube re-insertions by previous surgical procedures and age groups.

Previous surgical procedures	Recurrence of chronic OME			Test for failure time
	n	%	P Value*	P Value[†]
All age groups				
First re-insertion				
Tube only (n = 988)	89	9.0	0.002	0.01
Tube+ adenoidectomy (n = 767)	39	5.1		
Second re-insertion				
Tube only (n = 68)	12	17.6	0.29	0.22
Tube+ adenoidectomy (n = 21)	1	4.8		
Age stratification at first tube insertion				
0–2 years				
Tube only (n = 178)	16	9.0	0.39	0.39
Tube+ adenoidectomy (n = 5)	1	20.0		
2–4 years				
Tube only (n = 143)	17	11.9	0.41	0.33
Tube+ adenoidectomy (n = 79)	13	16.5		
4–6 years				
Tube only (n = 422)	43	10.2	0.02	0.02
Tube+ adenoidectomy (n = 434)	25	5.8		
6–9 years				
Tube only (n = 245)	13	5.3	<0.001	<0.001
Tube+ adenoidectomy (n = 249)	0	0.0		

*Fisher's exact test was performed.
[†]Time to OME recurrence was tested by log-rank test.

183 0–2 years-old and 224 2–4 years-old children, the power achieves 37.1% and 33.6%, respectively, at a 0.05 significance level. This meant that there might be a protective effect which we could not detect due to small sample size for children under 4 years old.

After adjusting for the effect of age, adenoidectomy reduced the rate of tube re-insertion by 39%. These results are similar to those of most previous studies on this topic, most of them around 40% to 50% [10,15,17–19,35]. If a child requires tube insertion at the age of 2–4 years, he or she are more likely to have tube re-insertions. This may be due to children in this age group are more likely to have recurrent AOM episodes, attending day care services, or shorter tubes staying time. Clinicians should therefore pay more attention to this age group of patients with chronic OME because they are prone to have recurrence. On the other hand, adenoidectomy is not beneficial to patients in this age group. Education the parents to avoid exposure to risk factors [46], medical management of allergic rhinitis, and vaccination for

Table 3. Estimated hazard rations (HR) and 95% confidence intervals (95% CI) of tympanostomy tube re-insertions of 2000–2001 birth cohort of chronic OME who had undergone tympanostomy tubes before 9 years of age.

Variables	Recurrence of chronic OME			
	HR[†]	95% CI	aHR[†]	95% CI
Previous operation				
Tube only	1.00		1.00	
Tube+ adenoidectomy*	0.61	0.42–0.89*	0.60	0.41–0.89*
Age				
0–2 years	0.63	0.34–1.14	0.55	0.30–1.00*
2–4 years	1.00		1.00	
4–6 years	0.66	0.43–1.02	0.71	0.46–1.11
6–9 years	0.41	0.21–0.79*	0.44	0.23–0.86*

*p<0.05.
[†]HR = Hazard ratio; aHR = Adjusted hazard ratio; 95% CI = 95% confidence interval.

pneumococcal conjugate vaccine [47–49] are efforts that can be done in order to prevent the need for repeated tubes.

This study is the first to explore the problem using a population-based birth cohort. Every case born in the 2000 and 2001 were demonstrated and followed-up in this study without sampling to show what really happened to all these children in Taiwan who needed tympanostomy tube insertion before the age of 8 or 9 years. With the advantage of a population-based administrative database and the uniqueness a birth-cohort design, the numbers of tube insertions after birth of every case can be clearly defined and the concurrent surgical procedure (adenoidectomy or adeno-tonsillectomy) can be identified accurately without ambiguity in history.

To improve the internal validity of this study, tympanostomy tube insertion is used instead of diagnosis codes in ICD-9 as a surrogate of chronic OME and recurrent AOM for the accuracy of defining the study population. If there was a code for certain surgical procedures for a patient in the claims data, that patient definitely had the disease and underwent the surgical procedure for it on the date of the surgery. In contrast, if diagnosis codes in ICD-9 were used as a surrogate for the disease, the probability of miscoding by the physician might be much higher. Physicians might use a certain diagnosis code by misdiagnosis. They also might do this for prescribing antibiotics or laboratory test in order to pass the review of the insurance payer or to improve reimbursement.

The major limitation of this study is the limitation of the administrative claims data. Medical records and the operative notes of every patient could not be obtained. In the NHIRD, there was no clinical data like patient history, physical examination findings, laboratory data results, hearing level or surgical findings. Medical records could not be checked to identify if the patient had adenoid hypertrophy, adenitis, obstructive sleep apnea, or persistent purulent nasal discharge. The appearance of ear drum and culture results were also not known, which might lead to

selection bias because surgeons perform adenoidectomy for more severe cases. Disease severity in the adenoidectomy group might be higher than in the tube insertion alone group. In the real world, a population based randomized control trial for this problem is not feasible or ethical. This study does offer an alternative way to explore the protective effects of adenoidectomy on tympanostomy tube re-insertions without any ethical issue. Other unobserved confounders are very likely to be diluted in this population based birth cohort study design and may have little influence.

Although adenoidectomy has protective effects on preventing tube re-insertions for children who need tympanostomy tubes, especially those older than 4 years old, performing adenoidectomy for every kid who needs tubes is not being recommended. The complication rate may not be high but there are complications due to the general anesthesia or from the procedure itself, including post-operative bleeding and nasopharyngeal stenosis [32–34]. Surgeons should take consider both the benefits and harm for every individual patient and make the best decision accordingly.

Conclusions

Adenoidectomy has protective effect against the need for repeated tympanostomy tubes, especially for children older than 4 years. Children who need their first tube at the age of 2–4 years are most likely to have a tube re-insertion in the future. Surgeons should weigh the pros and cons for every individual patient before suggesting adenoidectomy to prevent recurrent chronic OME and AOM.

Author Contributions

Conceived and designed the experiments: MCW YPW CHC ASS PC. Performed the experiments: MCW YPW. Analyzed the data: MCW YPW. Contributed reagents/materials/analysis tools: MCW YPW TYT ASS. Contributed to the writing of the manuscript: MCW YPW CHC PC.

References

1. Tos M (1984) Epidemiology and natural history of secretory otitis. Am J Otol 5: 459–462.
2. Paradise JL, Rockette HE, Colborn DK, Bernard BS, Smith CG, et al (1997) Otitis media in 2253 Pittsburgh area infants: prevalence and risk factors during the first two years of life. Pediatrics 99: 318–333.
3. Stool SE, Berg AO, Berman S, Carney CJ, Cooley JR, et al. Otitis media with effusion in young children. Clinical Practice Guideline, Number 12. Rockville, MD: Agency for Health Care Policy and Research, Public Health Service, US Department of Health and Human Services; AHCPR Publication No. 94-0622, 1994.
4. Williamson IG, Dunleavy J, Baine J, Robinson D. (1994) The natural history of otitis media with effusion: a three-year study of the incidence and prevalence of abnormal tympanograms in four South West Hampshire infant and first schools. J Laryngol Otol 108: 930–934.
5. Rosenfeld RM, Culpepper L, Doyle KJ, Grundfast KM, Hoberman A, et al (2004) Clinical practice guideline: otitis media with effusion. Otolaryngol Head Neck Surg 130: S95–S118.
6. Shiao AS, Guo YC (2005) A comparison assessment of video-telescopy for diagnosis of pediatric otitis media with effusion. Int J Pediatr Otorhinolaryngol 69: 1497–1502.
7. Rosenfeld RM, Schwartz SR, Pynnonen MA, Tunkel DE, Hussey HM, et al (2013) Clinical practice guideline: tympanostomy tubes in children. Otolaryngol Head Neck Surg 149: S1–S35.
8. Mandel EM, Rockette HE, Bluestone CD, Paradise JL, Nozza RJ (1989) Myringotomy with or without tympanostomy tubes for chronic otitis media with effusion. Arch Otolaryngol Head Neck Surg 115: 1217–1224.
9. Mandel EM, Rockette HE, Bluestone CD, Paradise JL, Nozza RJ (1992) Efficiency of myringotomy with or without tympanostomy tubes for chronic otitis media with effusion. Pediat Infect Dis J 11: 270–277.
10. Boston M, McCook J, Burke B, Derkay C (2003) Incidence of and risk factors for additional tympanostomy tube insertion in children. Arch Otoloryngol Head Neck Surg 129: 293–296.
11. Gates GA, Avery CA, Prihoda TJ, Cooper JC Jr (1987) Effectiveness of adenoidectomy and tympanostomy tubes in the treatment of chronic otitis media with effusion. N Engl J Med 317: 1444–1451.
12. Maw AR (1983) Chronic otitis media with effusion (glue ear) and adenoid tonsillectomy: prospective randomized controlled study. Br Med J 287: 1586–1588.
13. Paradise JL, Bluestone CD, Rogers KD, Taylor FH, Colborn K, et al (1990) Efficacy of adenoidectomy for recurrent otitis media in children previously treated with tympanostomy-tube placement: Results of parallel randomized and non-randomized trials. J Am Med Assoc 263: 2066–2073.
14. Maw AR, Bawden R (1993) Spontaneous resolution of severe chronic glue ear in children and the effect of adenoidectomy, tonsillectomy and insertion of ventilation tube (grommets). Br Med J 306: 756–760.
15. Coyte PC, Croxford R, Mclsaac W, Feldman W, Friedberg J (2001) The role of adjuvant adenoidectomy and tonsillectomy in the outcome of insertion of tympanostomy tubes. N Engl J Med 344: 1188–1195.
16. MRC Multi-center Otitis Media Study Group (2012) Adjuvant adenoidectomy in persistent bilateral otitis media with effusion: hearing and revision surgery outcomes through 2 years in the TARGET randomized trial. Clin Otolaryngol 37: 107–116.
17. Black NA, Sanderson CFB, Freeland AP, Vessey MP (1990) A randomized controlled trial of surgery for glue ear. Br Med J 300: 1551–1556.
18. Kadhim AL, Spilsburry K, Semmens JB, Coates HL, Lannigan FJ (2007) Adenoidectomy for middle ear effusion: a study of 50,000 children over 24 years. Laryngoscope 117: 427–433.
19. Gleinser DM, Kriel HH, Mukerji S (2011) The relationship between repeat tympanostomy tube insertions and adenoidectomy. Int J Pediatr Otorhinolaryngol 75: 1247–1251.
20. Maw AR (1985) Factors affecting adenoidectomy for otitis media with effusion (glue ear). J R Soc Med 78: 1014–1018.
21. Hammaren-Malmi S, Saxen H, Tarkkanen J, Mattila PS (2005) Adenoidectomy does not significantly reduce the incidence of otitis media in conjunction with the insertion of tympanostomy tubes in children who are younger than 4 years: a randomized trial. Pediatrics 116: 185–189.
22. Kujala T, Alho OP, Luotonen J, Kristo A, Uhari M, et al (2012) Tympanostomy with and without adenoidectomy for the prevention of recurrence of acute otitis media: a randomized controlled trial. Pediatr Infect Dis J 31: 565–569.

23. Dempster JH, Browning GG, Gatehouse SG (1993) A randomized study of the surgical management of children with persistent otitis media with effusion associated with a hearing impairment. J Laryngol Otol 107: 284–289.

24. Casselbrant ML, Mandel EM, Rockette HE, Kurs-Lasky M, Fall PA, et al (2009) Adenoidectomy for otitis media with effusion in 2–3 year-old children. Int J Pediatr Otorhinolaryngol 73: 1717–1724.

25. Musher DM (2006) Pneumococcal vaccine-direct and indirect ("herd") effects. N Engl J Med 354: 1522–1524.

26. Wright ED, Alden JP, Manoukian JJ (1998) Laterally hypertrophic adenoids as a contributing factor in otitis media. Int J Pediatr Otorhinolaryngol 45: 207–214.

27. Nguyen LHP, Manoukian JJ, Yoskovitch A (2004) Adenoidectomy: selection criteria for surgical cases of otitis media. Larynogoscope 114: 863–866.

28. Yasan H, Dogru H, Tüz M, Candir O, Uygur K, et al (2003) Otitis media with effusion and histopathologic properties of adenoid tissue. Int J Pediatr Otorhinolaryngol 67: 1179–1183.

29. Cengel S, Akyol MU (2006) The role of topical nasal steroids in the treatment of children with otitis media with effusion and adenoid hypertrophy with otitis media with effusion and/or adenoid hypertrophy. Int J Pediatr Otorhinolaryngol 70: 639–645.

30. Abdullah B, Hassan S, Sidek D, Jaafar H (2006) Adenoid mast cell and their role in the pathogenesis of otitis media with effusion. J Laryngol Otol 120: 556–560.

31. Paradise JL, Bluestone CD, Colborn DK, Bernard BS, Smith CG, et al (1999) Adenoidectomy and adeno-tonsillectomy for recurrent acute otitis media: parallel randomized clinical trials in children not previously treated with tympanostomy tubes. J Am Med Assoc 282: 945–953.

32. van der Griend BF, Lister NA, McKenzie IM, Martin N, Ragg PG, et al (2011) Post-operative mortality in children after 101,885 anesthetics at a tertiary pediatric hospital. Anesth Anal 112: 1440–1447.

33. Randoll DA, Hoffer ME (1998) Complications of tonsillectomy and adenoidectomy. Otolaryngol Head Neck Surg 118: 61–68.

34. Thomas k, Boeger D, Buentzel J, Esser D, Hoffmann K, et al (2013) Pediatric adenoidectomy: A population-based regional study on epidemiology and outcome. Int J Pediatr Otorhinolaryngol 77: 1716–1720.

35. Mikals SJ, Brigger MT (2014) Adenoidectomy as an adjuvant to primary tympanostomy tube placement: a systematic review and meta-analysis. JAMA Otolaryngol Head Neck Surg 140: 95–101.

36. Sheahan P, Miller I, Sheahan JN, Earley MJ, Blayney AW (2003) Incidence and outcome of middle ear disease in cleft lip and/or cleft palate. Int J Pediatr Otorhinolaryngol 67: 785–793.

37. Kobayashi H, Sakuma T, Yamada N, Suzaki H (2012) Clinical outcomes of ventilation tube placement in children with cleft palate. Int J Pediatr Otorhinolaryngol 76: 718–721.

38. Marchica CL, Pitaro J, Daniel SJ (2013) Recurrent tube insertions for chronic otitis media with effusion in children over 6 years. Int J Pediatr Otorhinolaryngol 77: 252–255.

39. Kaufman FL (1991) Managing the cleft lip and palate patient. Pediatr Clin North Am 38: 1127–1147.

40. Taiwan National Statistics Report. Minister of the Interior. (Accessed December 31, 2013, at http://statis.moi.gov.tw/micst/stmain.jsp?sys = 100).

41. Kogan MD, Overpeck MD, Hoffman HJ, Casselbrant ML (2000) Factors associated with tympanostomy tube insertion among pre-school aged children in the United States. Am J Public Health 90: 245–250.

42. Kvaerner KJ, Nafstad P, Jaakkola JJK (2002) Otolaryngological surgery and upper respiratory tract infections in children: an epidemiological study. Ann Otol Rhinol Laryngol 111: 1034–39.

43. Spielmann PM, Adamson RM, Schenk D, Hussain SSM (2008) Follow up after middle ear ventilation tube insertion: what is needed and when. J Laryngol Otol 122: 580–583.

44. Wang MC, Huang CK, Wang YP, Chien CW (2012) Effects of increased payment for ventilation tube insertion on decision making for paediatric otitis media with effusion. J Eval Clin Pract 18: 919–922.

45. Keyhani S, Kleinman LC, Rothschild M, Bernstein JM, Anderson R, et al (2008) Clinical characteristics of New York City children who received tympanostomy tubes in 2002. Pediatrics 121: e24–33.

46. Keyhani S, Kleinman LC, Rothschild M, Bernestein JM, Anderson R, et al. (2008) Overuse of tympanostomy tubes in new York metropolitan area: evidence from five hospital cohort. Br Med J 337: a1067. doi:10.1136/bmj.a1607

47. Fireman B, Black SB, Shinefield HR, Lee J, Lewis E, et al (2003) Impact of the pneumococcal conjugate vaccine on otitis media. Pediatr Infect Dis J 22: 10–16.

48. Palmu AA, Verho J, Jokinen J, Karma P, Kilpi TM (2004) The seven-valent pneumococcal conjugate vaccine reduces tympanostomy tube placement in children. Pediatr Infect Dis J 23: 732–738.

49. Poehling KA, Szilagyi PG, Grijalva CG, Martin SW, LaFleur B, et al (2007) Reduction of frequent otitis media and pressure-equalizing tube insertions in children after introduction of pneumococcal conjugate vaccine. Pediatrics 19: 707–715.

19

The Immune System in Children with Malnutrition

Maren Johanne Heilskov Rytter[1]*, **Lilian Kolte**[2], **André Briend**[1,3], **Henrik Friis**[1], **Vibeke Brix Christensen**[4]

1 Department of Nutrition, Exercise and Sports, Faculty of Science, University of Copenhagen, Frederiksberg, Denmark, 2 Department of Infectious Diseases, Copenhagen University Hospital, Hvidovre, Denmark, 3 Department for International Health, University of Tampere, School of Medicine, Tampere, Finland, 4 Department of Paediatrics, Copenhagen University Hospital Rigshospitalet, Copenhagen, Denmark

Abstract

Background: Malnourished children have increased risk of dying, with most deaths caused by infectious diseases. One mechanism behind this may be impaired immune function. However, this immune deficiency of malnutrition has not previously been systematically reviewed.

Objectives: To review the scientific literature about immune function in children with malnutrition.

Methods: A systematic literature search was done in PubMed, and additional articles identified in reference lists and by correspondence with experts in the field. The inclusion criteria were studies investigating immune parameters in children aged 1–60 months, in relation to malnutrition, defined as wasting, underweight, stunting, or oedematous malnutrition.

Results: The literature search yielded 3402 articles, of which 245 met the inclusion criteria. Most were published between 1970 and 1990, and only 33 after 2003. Malnutrition is associated with impaired gut-barrier function, reduced exocrine secretion of protective substances, and low levels of plasma complement. Lymphatic tissue, particularly the thymus, undergoes atrophy, and delayed-type hypersensitivity responses are reduced. Levels of antibodies produced after vaccination are reduced in severely malnourished children, but intact in moderate malnutrition. Cytokine patterns are skewed towards a Th2-response. Other immune parameters seem intact or elevated: leukocyte and lymphocyte counts are unaffected, and levels of immunoglobulins, particularly immunoglobulin A, are high. The acute phase response appears intact, and sometimes present in the absence of clinical infection. Limitations to the studies include their observational and often cross-sectional design and frequent confounding by infections in the children studied.

Conclusion: The immunological alterations associated with malnutrition in children may contribute to increased mortality. However, the underlying mechanisms are still inadequately understood, as well as why different types of malnutrition are associated with different immunological alterations. Better designed prospective studies are needed, based on current understanding of immunology and with state-of-the-art methods.

Editor: Taishin Akiyama, University of Tokyo, Japan

Funding: The work was supported by a PhD grant from University of Copenhagen. The funders had no role in study design, data collection and analysis, decision to publish, or preparation of the manuscript.

Competing Interests: The authors have declared that no competing interests exist.

* Email: marenrytter@hotmail.com

Introduction

Malnutrition in children is a global public health problem with wide implications. Malnourished children have increased risk of dying from infectious diseases, and it is estimated that malnutrition is the underlying cause of 45% of global deaths in children below 5 years of age [1–2]. The association between malnutrition and infections may in part be due to confounding by poverty, a determinant of both, but also possibly due to a two-way causal relationship (**Figure 1**): malnutrition increases susceptibility to infections while infections aggravate malnutrition by decreasing appetite, inducing catabolism, and increasing demand for nutrients [3]. Although it has been debated whether malnutrition increases incidence of infections, or whether it only increases severity of disease [3], solid data indicates that malnourished children are at higher risk of dying once infected [2–4]. The increased susceptibility to infections may in part be caused by impairment of immune function by malnutrition [5]. The objective of this study was to investigate the associations of different types of malnutrition with immune parameters in children, through a systematic review of the literature.

Since most infections and deaths in malnourished children occur in low-income settings, the organisms causing disease are rarely identified. Therefore, little is known about whether these differ from pathogens infecting well-nourished children, and whether malnourished children are susceptible to opportunistic

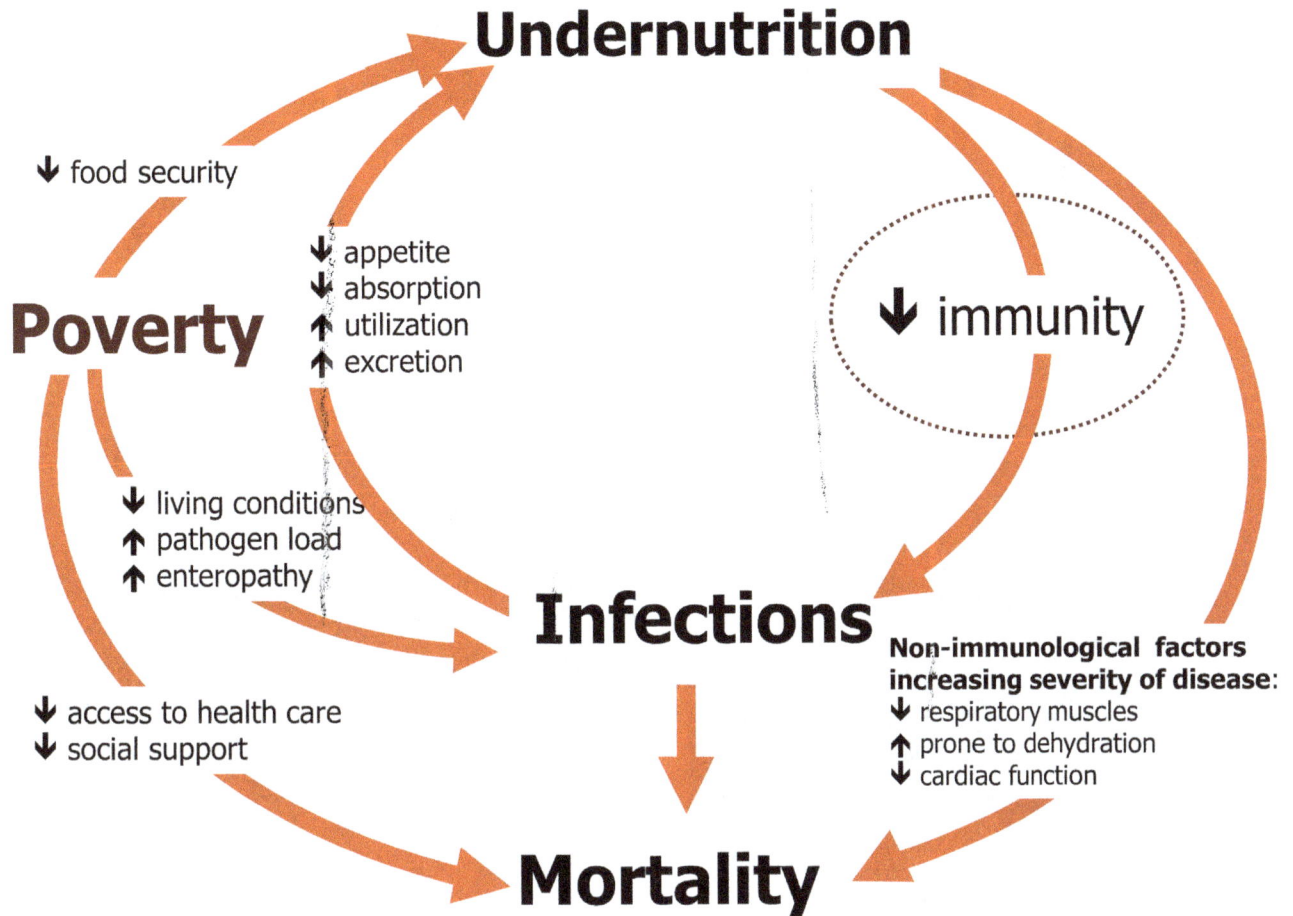

Figure 1. Conceptual framework on the relationship between malnutrition, infections and poverty.

infections. Although opportunistic infections like *Pneumocystis jirovecii* and severe varicella has been reported in malnourished children [6–7], these studies were carried out before the discovery of HIV, and may represent cases of un-diagnosed paediatric AIDS. More recent studies have found that *Pneumocystis jirovecii* pneumonia is not frequent in malnourished children not infected with HIV [8]. However, quasi-opportunistic pathogens like cryptosporidium and yeast are frequent causes of diarrhoea in malnourished children [9], and malnourished children have a higher risk of invasive bacterial infections, causing bacterial pneumonia [8], bacterial diarrhoea [10–11], and bacteraemia [12–14], with a predominance of gram negative bacteria. Due to the high prevalence of invasive bacterial infections, current guidelines recommend antibiotic treatment to all children with severe acute malnutrition, even though the evidence behind is not very strong [14].

Non-immunological factors may also contribute to increased mortality in malnourished children: reduced muscle mass may impair respiratory work with lung infections [15]; reduced electrolyte absorption from the gut [16] and impaired renal concentration capacity may increase susceptibility to dehydration from diarrhoea [5]; and diminished cardiac function may increase risk of cardiac failure [17]. Thus, immune function may only be one of several links between malnutrition, infections and increased mortality, but most likely an important one.

Definitions of malnutrition

This review considers childhood malnutrition in the sense of under-nutrition, causing growth failure or weight loss, or severe acute malnutrition, either oedematous, or non-oedematous.

Growth failure caused by malnutrition has commonly been defined by low weight-for-age (underweight), length-for-age (stunting), or weight-for-length (wasting) [5]. Generally, older studies diagnosed malnutrition using weight-for-age, while newer studies tend to use weight-for-length. Recently, mid-upper arm circumference (MUAC) has been promoted to diagnose severe acute malnutrition, because of its feasibility and because it predicts mortality risk better than other anthropometric indices [18]. Other definitions of malnutrition include specific micronutrient deficiencies, intra-uterine growth restriction, and obesity, but these conditions are outside the scope of this review.

Severe Acute Malnutrition

Two forms of severe acute malnutrition in children exist: non-oedematous malnutrition, also known as marasmus, characterized by severe wasting and currently defined by weight-for-length z-score <-3 of the WHO growth standard, or MUAC $<11,5$ cm; and oedematous malnutrition defined by bilateral pitting oedema (**Figure 2**) [19]. Kwashiorkor refers to a form of oedematous malnutrition, the fulminant syndrome including enlarged fatty liver, mental changes as well as skin and hair changes [20]. The term "marasmic kwashiorkor", has been used to describe children

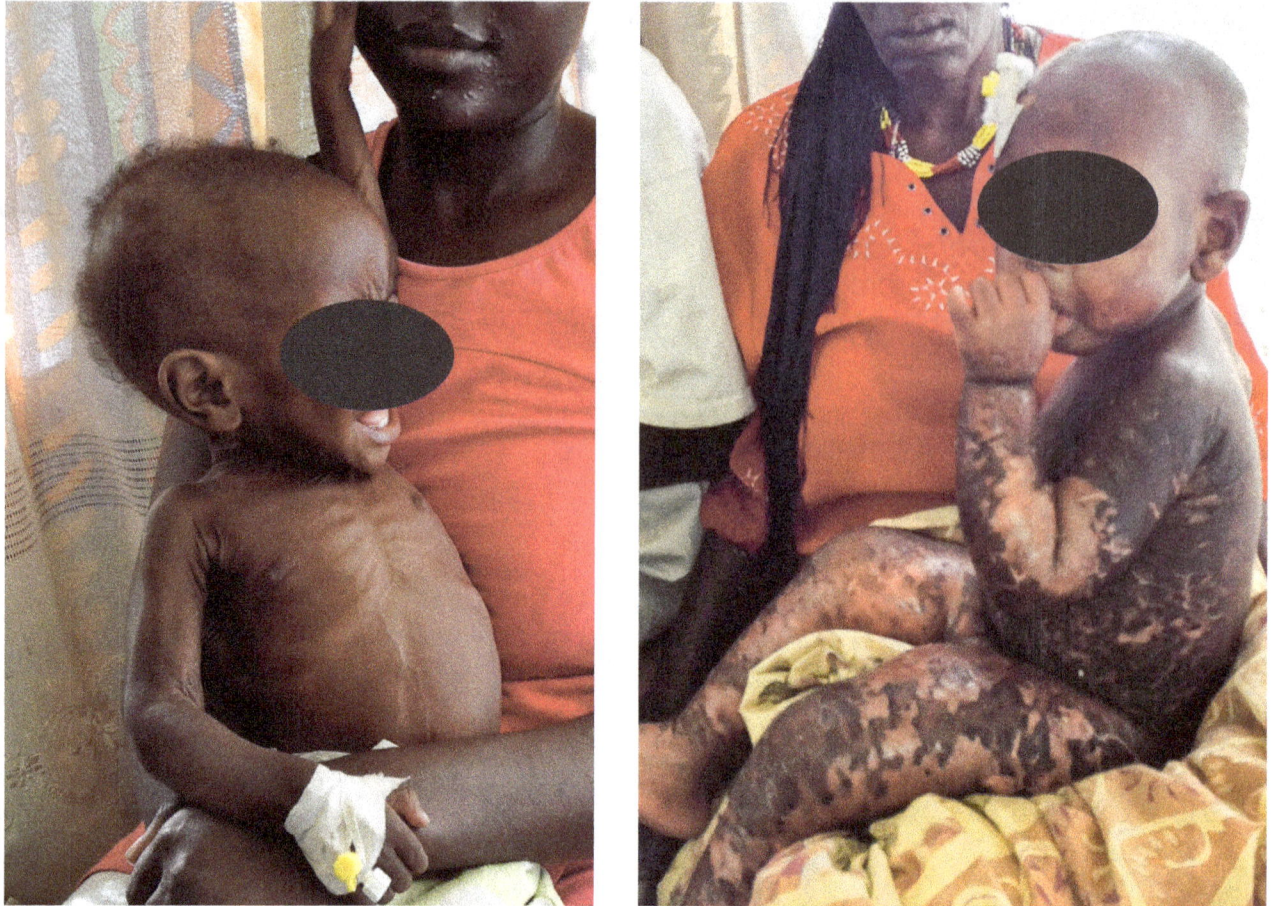

Figure 2. Clinical picture: two forms of severe acute malnutrition, oedematous and non-oedematous malnutrition.

with both wasting and oedema [21]. It is still unknown why some children develop oedematous malnutrition, and unclear whether this form of malnutrition is associated with a different degree of immune deficiency.

Materials and Methods

A systematic literature search was carried out in PubMed using combinations of the search terms related to malnutrition and immune parameters. The full search strategy and the search terms used are described in **Figure 3**.

Inclusion criteria were: studies presenting original clinical data regarding immune parameters in children, aged 1–60 months, where a comparison was made, either between malnourished and well-nourished children, or between malnourished children before and after nutritional rehabilitation. Exclusion criteria were studies of children with another primary diagnosis such as cancer, congenital heart disease or endocrine disease. Studies were accepted where children had co-morbid infections, since this is typically seen in malnourished children. Articles by RK Chandra were excluded, due to concerns about possible fraud [22]. Studies published in peer-reviewed scientific journals, as well as in books were included. Only articles in English were included.

The search was carried out in August 2013, and updated in December 2013. The search results were sorted by MJHR, based on titles, abstracts or full-text-articles. Additional literature was obtained from reference lists, text books and by personal communication with experts.

For data retrieval, studies were sorted according to whether they investigated barrier function (skin and gut), innate immunity or acquired immune system, and listed in tables based on the specific immune parameter studied. Some studies were included in more than one table. The following data was extracted from each article: year and country, number and age range of malnourished and well-nourished participants, type of malnutrition and whether included children fulfilled WHOs current diagnostic criteria for severe acute malnutrition, whether infections were present, immune parameter studied, methods used, how the parameter was associated with malnutrition, and whether children with oedematous and non-oedematous malnutrition were differentially affected.

The results of the included articles were summarized for each immune parameter. Due to the heterogeneous nature of study designs, participants and outcomes, it was not meaningful to synthesize the results in a meta-analysis. The main potential bias was presence of infection. For this reason, presence and effect of infection was considered for each study as well as for each outcome. The PRISMA (Preferred Reporting Items for Systematic Reviews and Meta-Analyses) guideline was followed, except for the items relating to meta-analysis (**Checklist S1**).

Search terms:

"malnutrition" OR "undernutrition" OR "marasmus" OR "kwashiorkor" OR "wasting" OR "stunting" OR "underweight"

AND

"immune" OR "antibodies" OR "thymus" OR "lymphatic" OR "delayed-type hypersensitivity" OR "leucocytes" OR "lymphocyte" OR "activation" OR "B-cell" OR "T-cell" OR "complement" OR "humoral" OR "cytokine" OR "chemotaxis"OR "acute phase response" OR "phagocytosis" OR "flow cytometry" OR "enteropathy" OR "barrier" OR "intestinal permeability" OR "microbiota" .

Filters: human studies, children from 0-18 years, and publications in English.

Figure 3. Full search strategy in PubMed, including search terms and filters.

Results

The search in PubMed yielded 3402 articles. By contacting experts in the field, an additional 631 papers were obtained. Reference list of all papers read were screened for relevant papers not included in the initial search. Of all the screened papers, 245 met the inclusion criteria (**Figure S1**). Another 49 articles were identified which, in addition to children 1–60 months old, also included older children. These studies were not included in the main analysis, but used in a sensitivity analysis in which all studies were included. The result of this additional analysis was essentially similar to the results obtained with studies only including children less than 60 month (results not shown). The studies were published between 1957–2014, mainly in the 1970s and 1980s. Only 33 studies were published after 2003 (**Figure 4**). The studies included 29 prospective studies that compared malnourished children to themselves after nutritional recovery, and 216 cross-sectional studies. Of the cross-sectional studies, 51 were community-based, comparing immune parameters in children according to nutritional status. The remaining 165 cross-sectional studies compared hospitalised malnourished children to well-nourished children, often recruited outside the hospital. In 53 studies, all children fulfilled WHOs diagnostic criteria for severe acute malnutrition [23]. The vast majority of these studies included children with oedematous malnutrition, while only two studies included children with non-oedematous malnutrition based on the new WHO growth standard.

The results of each immune parameter are summarized in **Table 1**, and the results of individual articles are summarized in **Tables S1–14**.

Epithelial barrier function

The barrier function of the skin and mucosal surfaces is considered the first-line defence of the immune system, upheld by the physical integrity of the epithelia, anti-microbial factors in secretions (e.g. lysozyme, secretory IgA and gastric acidity) and the commensal bacterial flora [24].

Of the articles describing barrier function in malnourished children, six described skin structure and function, 21 described structure and permeability of intestinal mucosa, 19 protective factors in secretions and 11 the microbial flora colonizing mucosal surfaces.

Skin. *Skin barrier* has mostly been studied in children with oedematous malnutrition, who may develop a characteristic dermatosis, characterized by hyper-pigmentation, cracking and scaling of the epidermis, resembling "peeling paint", providing a potential entry port for pathogens [25].

Six articles assessed barrier and immune function of the skin in malnourished children (**table S1**). Two articles describing histology reported atrophy of skin layers, but did not describe cutaneous immune cells [26–27]. Four articles described the "cutaneous inflammatory response": They made small abrasions in the skin, and placed microscopy slides over the sites. Similar or higher numbers of white blood cells migrated onto slides in malnourished children, predominantly granulocytes and a lower proportion of monocytes and macrophages [28–31]. This pattern was noted to resemble a neonatal immature immune response [30]. All four articles found this pattern in patients with oedematous malnutrition, while one study found that the response of non-oedematous children resembled that of well-nourished [30].

Structure and function of the intestinal mucosa. The intestinal mucosa of malnourished children was described in 21 articles (**table S2**). Autopsy-studies from as early as 1965 described a thin-walled intestine in malnourished children, and noted that "… the *tissue paper intestine* of kwashiorkor is well known to tropical pathologists." [32]. Small-intestinal biopsies showed thinning of the mucosa [33–36], decrease in villous height [37–43], altered villous morphology [32] [40] [44] and infiltration of lymphocytes [32] [34–38]. Electron-microscopy studies found sparse brush border with shortened microvilli and sparse endoplasmatic reticulum [42]. Others found increased intestinal permeability to lactulose [45–48]. Such an intestine may predispose to bacterial translocation, and likewise, one of the included articles described high levels of lipopolysaccharide in the blood of malnourished children, probably originating from gut bacteria translocating into the bloodstream [49]. However, the mucosal atrophy and functional changes did not only occur in malnourished children. Although sometimes found to be most severe in malnourished children [33] [35–36] [46–47], similar

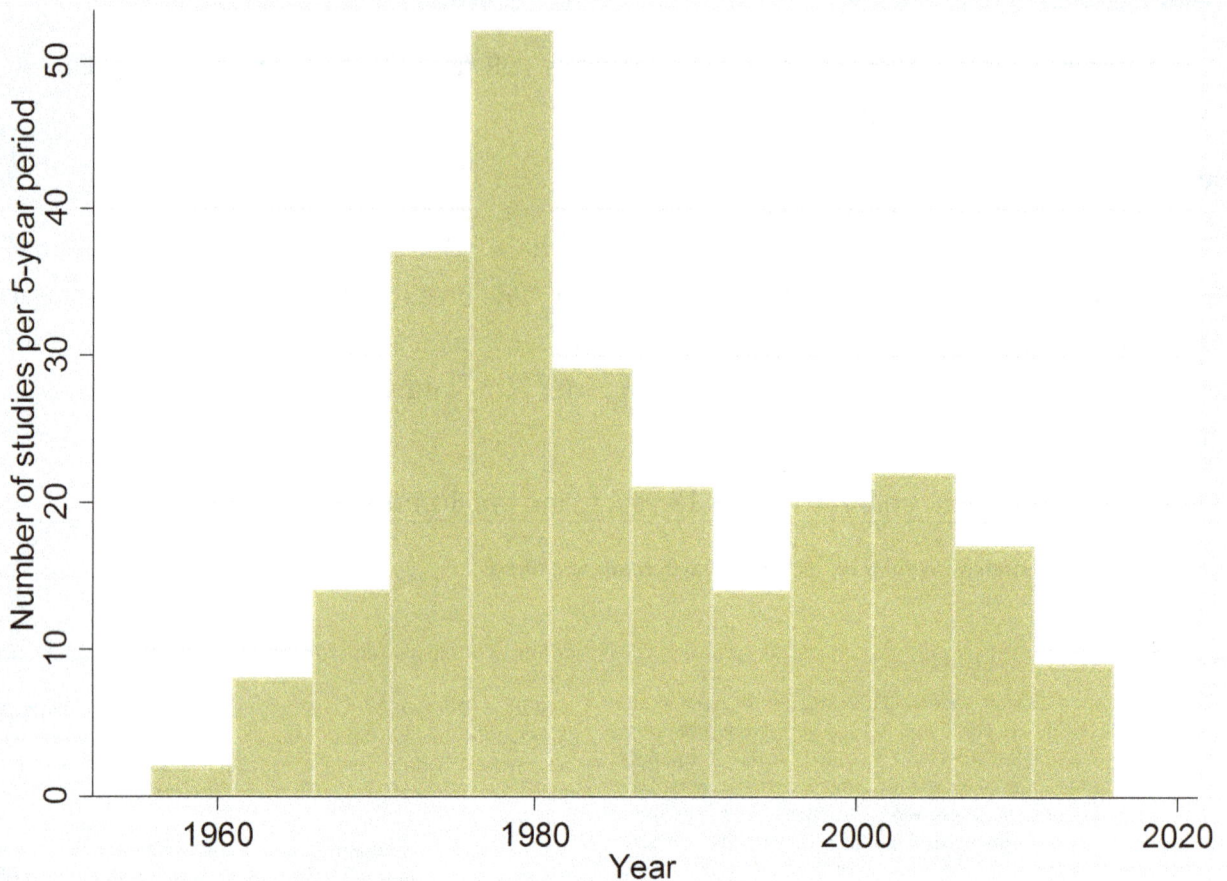

Figure 4. Number of studies published per 5-year period about immune function in malnourished children.

abnormalities were present in apparently well-nourished children from the same environment [38–40] [43] [50], and frequently persisted after nutritional recovery [34] [37] [51].

Two articles described immune cells in small intestinal biopsies from malnourished children in Gambia and Zambia: both reported increased lymphocyte infiltration, more T-cells, and cells expressing HLA-DR in malnourished children compared to English children [37–38]. However, it was similar to Gambian well-nourished children [38], and unaltered by nutritional recovery [37]. Both well-nourished and malnourished Gambian children had high levels of intestinal cytokine expression, but malnourished children had an increased ratio of cells expression pro-inflammatory to regulatory cytokines, compared to the well-nourished Gambian children [38].

The colon was only described in one article, reporting increased vascularity, atrophy of the mucosa and a tendency to rectal prolapse in children with oedematous malnutrition [52].

Four articles compared the intestine of children with oedematous and non-oedematous malnutrition: one study from South Africa found that the histological changes were most severe in those with oedema [40]. Two articles from Chile found that children with non-oedematous malnutrition had a thinner mucosa, whereas children with oedema had more villous atrophy and more cellular infiltration [35–36]. In contrast, a more recent study from Zambia found higher numbers of T-cells and cells expressing

HLA-DR in the intestines of children with non-oedematous than oedematous malnutrition, while the intestines of oedematous children were deficient in sulphated glycosaminoglycan [37].

Antimicrobial factors in mucosal secretions. Nineteen articles were published on anti-microbial factors in secretions from malnourished children (**table S3**). Secretory IgA (sIgA) was investigated in 15 studies, of which 11 investigated saliva, urine, tears, nasal washings and duodenal fluid [53–63] and three investigated small intestinal biopsies [39–40] [64].

SIgA in saliva, tears and nasal washings was frequently reduced in severely malnourished children [54–55] [57–58]. One article from Egypt reported increased levels in children with oedematous malnutrition [56], but may have overestimated sIgA, since saliva flow was reduced in malnourished children, and sIgA was expressed as g/l, whereas other articles expressed it as sIgA as % of protein content. Studies of sIgA in duodenal fluid showed conflicting results [57] [59], as did studies quantifying sIgA in small intestinal biopsies [39–40] [64]. The sIgA content of urine was increased or normal in severely malnourished children [60–61]. In mild to moderately underweight children, inconsistent results were found for sIgA in tears [63] and saliva [53–54] [62–63].

Tear lysozyme content was found to be reduced in malnourished children [54] [63], while saliva lysozyme was unaffected [53–54]. Gastric acid secretion was consistently reduced in severely

Table 1. Summary of results in studies of each immune parameter.

Immune parameter	Number of studies	Period	In children with severe malnutrition?	In children with moderate malnutrition?	Different in OM compared to NOM?	Comments	Listed in table
Skin	6	1968–1989	- Atrophy - Cells in skin abrasions: ↑ GRAN, ↓ monocytes	Not assessed	Cells in abrasions only affected in OM		S1
Gut function	21	1965–2013	Thin mucosa, shorter villi, infiltration of immune cells. Increased intestinal permeability.	No linear relationship	↑	Also in well-nourished children	S2
Factors in secretions	19	1968–2012	sIgA in saliva, tears, nasal washings: ↓ in duodenal fluids: ↕, in urine: 0 Lysozyme: ↕. Gastric juice and acidity: ↓	↕	Saliva flow ↓ in OM; sIgA ↑ in OM		S3
Microbial flora	11	1972–2014	Different pattern of stool micro-biota; bacterial growth in small intestine; ↑ yeast and g. neg. bact.	↑ yeast in mouth	Not assessed		S4
White blood cells	38	1964–2009	Leukocytes in blood: 0; Microbicidal activity ↓, Chemotaxis ↓; Phagocytosis: ↕	Leukocytes in blood: 0; NK cells: 0	Bactericidal activity ↓ in OM		S5
Acute phase	24	1970–2006	Positive APP ↑, negative APP ↓ with infection, sometimes also without clinical infection	Few studies	↑		S6
Complement	24	1973–2011	C3, C6, C1, C9, Factor B: ↓; C5, C activity: ↕; C4: 0	Not affected	All parameters ↓ in OM	Signs of in-vivo consumption in OM	S7
Lymphatic tissue	12	1956–2009	Thymic atrophy. Fewer lymphocytes in thymus cortex. Less atrophy of other lymphatic tissue.	Linear relationship of thymus size with nutritional status	↑	Also ↓ by infections and zinc deficiency	S8 and S9
DTHR	21	1965–2092	Mantoux after BCG vaccination: ↓; Reaction to other antigens: ↓	↓ ↕	↑	Also ↓ by infections and zinc deficiency	S10
Lymphocytes	58	1971–2009	Total lymphocytes 0; T-cells: 0/↑; CD4 count: 0/↑; B-cells: ↓; Response to PHA: ↓	Not affected	CD4 count ↑ in OM	Conflicting result by flow cytometry older methods	S11
Antibody levels	32	1962–2008	IgG: 0; IgM: 0; IgA ↑; IgE: ↕; IgD: ↑ in OM, ↓ in NOM	Not affected	IgA and IgD ↑ in OM		S12
Vaccination response	35	1957–2009	Antibody titre: ↓; Most acceptable sero-conversion; Possibly delay in antibody response	Antibody titre: 0; Sero-conversion: 0	Titres: ↓ in OM		S13
Cytokines	35	1975–2013	Th1-cytokines: IL1, IL2, IL12, IFN-γ: ↓; Th2 cytokines: IL10, IL14: ↑; Inflammatory cytokines (IL6, TNFα): ↕	Few studies: Same pattern as severe malnutrition	Th2-response ↑, IL6 ↑ in OM; Altered leukotrienes		S14

Legend: ↑ = higher in malnourished than well-nourished, ↓ = lower in malnourished than well-nourished, 0 = similar in malnourished and well-nourished; ↕ = inconsistent results; OM = Oedematous malnutrition, NOM = Non-oedematous malnutrition, GRAN = Granulocytes (Polymorph nuclear cells); slgA = secretory immunoglobulin A; NK = Natural killer; APP = Acute phase protein; C = Complement component, BCG = Bacille Calmette-Guérin, PHA: phyto-hemaglutinin; Ig = immunoglobulin; IL = Interleukin; IFNγ = Interferon-gamma; TNFα = Tumour-necrosis-factor-alpha.

malnourished children [65–68], and higher pH was associated with bacterial colonization of the stomach [65].

Microbial colonization. Microbes colonizing skin and mucosa may protect against infections by competing with pathogens, by producing specific antimicrobial substances, and by stimulating host immune function [69]. Despite much recent interest in the subject, of 11 articles describing the micro-flora in malnourished children, only four were published during the last ten years (**table S4**). All found malnourished children to host a different flora from well-nourished children. Their mouths and throats contained more yeast [70–72], and their stomach and duodenum, which in healthy children is considered to be almost sterile, contained a large number of microorganisms [72–75]. Although one study found similar degree of small intestinal bacterial overgrowth in diarrhoeal patients with and without malnutrition [75], another found more small intestinal bacteria in malnourished than in well-nourished children with diarrhoea [72]. While gram positive cocci predominated in the small intestine of well-nourished children, malnourished children hosted more gram negative bacteria [65] and yeast [74].

The colonic flora, containing the vast majority of commensal bacteria, was described by sequencing bacterial DNA from stool samples in four recent articles, which consistently found that the pattern of bacteria was different in malnourished and well-nourished children [76–79]. More bacteria with pathogenic potential were found in the malnourished children [77–78], and their flora was less mature [79] and less diverse [76] [78]. A twin study from Malawi suggested that micro-flora pattern could also play a role in developing malnutrition [76]. No articles have so far reported whether the intestinal flora is different in children with oedematous and non-oedematous malnutrition.

Innate immune system

The innate immune system delivers an unspecific response relying on leukocytes (like granulocytes, monocytes and macrophages), as well as soluble factors in blood (like acute phase proteins and the complement system) [24]. Of the articles describing innate immune response, 38 described number and function of leucocytes, 25 acute phase proteins and 24 complement components and activity.

White blood cells of the innate immune system. Thirty-eight articles described number and function of leukocytes of the innate immune system (**table S5**). Most reported similar or higher numbers of total leukocytes in blood of malnourished children [49] [80–92], and three found that granulocytes were higher in malnourished children [81] [86] [93].

Two studies from Nigeria and one from Ghana found no difference in the mean percentage of natural-killer-cells among malnourished or well-nourished children [94–96], although two reported that more malnourished children had abnormally low numbers of natural-killer cells. In Zambia, levels of dendritic cells were lower in blood from malnourished children before nutritional rehabilitation than after, and elevated inflammation markers were associated with a paradoxical lower level of dendritic cell activation. This was associated with endotoxin levels in the blood, and was interpreted as a type of immune-paralysis, related to inflammation and bacterial translocation [49]. Unfortunately, it was not assessed whether this was different from well-nourished children with severe infections.

Chemotaxis of granulocytes was reduced in malnourished children in three of five studies [80] [83] [97–99], and one study found a diminished ability to adhere to foreign material [100]. Results for phagocytosis were mixed: five of 12 studies found that leukocytes of malnourished children had reduced ability to ingest

particles or bacteria [81] [83] [88–89] [97–98] [101–106]. Microbicidal activity of granulocytes was reduced in malnourished children in five of seven studies [80] [83] [88] [97–98] [103] [107], while two of three studies found macrophages from malnourished children to have normal microbicidal activity [89] [108–109]. Neutrophils may kill microorganisms by producing reactive oxygen compounds; assessable by the Nitroblue Tetrazolenium (NBT) test, which, however, gave inconsistent results in malnourished children [83] [105] [110–114]. It has been hypothesized, that reactive oxygen production is involved in the pathogenesis of oedematous malnutrition [115]; however, the NBT test results did not show any clear pattern in children with oedematous compared to non-oedematous malnutrition.

One study found the levels of enzymes, like alkaline and acid phosphatase, to be increased in leukocytes from children with malnutrition [116]. More leukocytes of malnourished children were found to have markers of apoptosis (CD95) [92], and signs of DNA damage [117–118].

No articles have yet described the expression of pattern-recognition molecules, like Toll-like receptors in malnourished children, although these are fundamental to the function of the innate immune system.

Acute phase response. Acute phase responses is induced by infection or trauma, and mediated by cytokines like IL-6 and TNF-α. It involve temporal suppression of acquired, and amplification of innate immune responses, with secretion of positive acute phase proteins (APP) like C-reactive protein (CRP), serum-amyloid-A (SAA), complement factors, α-1-acid-glycoprotein or ferritin [119], while levels of other proteins are reduced, as albumin, pre-albumin, transferrin, α -2-HS-glycoprotein, and α -fetoprotein. These are sometimes called 'negative acute phase proteins', although it is not clear whether their reduced level are due to active down-regulation, or because of competition with production of positive acute phase proteins. Twenty-four articles described the levels of acute phase proteins in malnourished children with or without infection (**table S6**).

Acute phase response in children with infections. Most studies found elevated positive APP in malnourished children with infections. This included CRP [120–128], α-1 acid-glycoprotein [120–121] [129], haptoglobin [120–121] [125] [127] [129] while the results for ceruloplasmin [125] [130], and α-1-antitrysin were inconsistent [120–121] [125] [127–129]. Only one study found lower CRP levels in malnourished than well-nourished children with similar infections, despite higher levels of IL-6 [129]. So-called negative APP were uniformly low in children with malnutrition and infection, including transferrin [94] [127] [130–133], α-2-HS-glycoprotein [134–136], pre-albumin [122], fibronectin [132], and α-2-macroglobulin[127].

Acute phase response in children without infections. Three studies found elevated CRP in malnourished children without apparent infections [94] [124] [128], while two studies found similar CRP-levels in malnourished and well-nourished children [122] [137]. Results for α-1-antitrysin were inconsistent [128]. So-called negative acute phase proteins like transferrin [94] [130], α-2-HS-glycoprotein [135], fibronectin [133] [138] and pre-albumin [122] [138–139] were consistently reduced in malnourished children, even without infections.

Acute phase response to a controlled stressor. Four articles described the acute phase response induced by a vaccine. Two reported a normal [140] or increased [141] febrile response to measles vaccine in malnourished children. In another study, a similar rise in APP was seen in malnourished and well-nourished children [137], in response to a diphtheria-pertussis-tetanus-vaccination, but the increase in APP was greater when the vaccination was repeated after nutritional rehabilitation. The same was found for the febrile response to a repeated vaccine in malnourished children [142]. Since no repeated vaccine was given to well-nourished children, it is unknown whether they would also have had a stronger response to the second dose.

Complement. The complement system consists of plasma proteins secreted by the liver that, upon activation, react to recruit immune cells, opsonize and kill pathogens [24]. Three main pathways activate the complement system: the classical pathway, the alternative pathway and the lectin pathway [143], with the complement protein C3 playing a central role in all three pathways.

Twenty-four articles described levels or in-vitro activity of complement proteins (**table S7**). In 17 of 21 studies, levels of C3 were depressed in malnourished children [89] [94] [99] [106] [124–125] [127–130] [144–154]. Two studies found C3 to correlate with albumin [94] [148], and with one exception [94], C3 levels were lower in children with oedematous than non-oedematous malnutrition [89] [146] [149] [150–151] [153].

Few studies assessed C6, C9, and factor B, and most found reduced levels in malnourished children [145] [148–149] [151] [153], most so in oedematous malnutrition [148–149] [151] [153].

Levels of C1 and C4 were mostly normal in malnourished children [94] [99] [145] [148] [150–153], while two studies found reduced levels of C4 in patients with oedematous, but not non-oedematous malnutrition [89] [149]. Studies assessing C5 showed inconsistent results [145] [148–149] [151] [153].

Classical pathway activity was either unaffected [106] [145–146] [152], reduced [148] [155] [156], or reduced only in oedematous, but not in non-oedematous malnutrition [157]. Alternative pathway activity was reduced in two studies [145] [156] and unaffected in one [146]. General opsonic activity of serum was reduced in one study [156]. No articles reported the activity of the lectin pathway.

Both reduced production and increased consumption may explain the reduced levels of complement factors. Complement components are produced by the liver, and their levels correlated with albumin levels, the production of which is also impaired in malnutrition [158]. However, increased consumption is also supported by one study showing high levels of C3d, a by-product after activation of C3, in malnourished children, most pronounced in oedematous malnutrition [148].

Acquired immunity

Acquired immunity is characterized by specialized cellular and antibody-mediated immune responses, generated by T- and B-lymphocytes reacting with high specificity towards pathogens and creating long-lasting immunological memory. The acquired immune system also orchestrates tolerance to self and other non-pathogenic material like gut bacteria [24]. Of the articles describing acquired immunity, 12 described the thymo-lymphatic system, 21 delayed-type hypersensitivity responses (DTHR), 58 lymphocyte subsets in blood, 32 immunoglobulins in blood, 35 vaccination responses and 35 cytokines.

Thymus. The thymus gland is the central lymphatic organ in the acquired immune system, where maturation and proliferation of T-lymphocytes take place. The thymus is large at birth and undergoes gradual involution after childhood [159], with diminished output of T-lymphocytes [160].

Six articles reported autopsy studies of the thymo-lymphatic system in malnourished children, published between 1956 and 1988 [161–166] **table S8**). All reported thymus atrophy in malnourished children, to an extent termed "nutritional thymectomy" [164]. Histology revealed depleted thymocytes, replace-ment with connective tissue, and decreased cortico-medullar differentiation [163] [165–166].

Eight articles reported thymic size measured by ultrasound, in relation to nutritional status [91] [167–173] (**table S9**). Five of these studied children with severe malnutrition and found severe thymic atrophy [91] [167–170], reversible with nutritional rehabilitation, although thymic size did not reach normal levels as fast as anthropometric recovery [91] [170]. Thymic size was also measured by ultrasound in cohorts of children to determine patterns of thymic growth [159] [171], in a vaccination trial in Guinea Bissau [172] and in a pre-natal nutritional supplementation trial in Bangladesh [171]. These studies confirmed that thymus size was associated with nutritional status, even in mild malnutrition. Breastfed children often had a larger thymus than artificially fed children [174], possibly explained by IL-7 in breast milk [175], and children with a large thymus were found to have a higher chance of surviving than those with a small thymus [172] [176].

Other lymphatic tissue. Six articles reported investigations of other lymphatic tissue. Four autopsy studies found atrophy of lymph nodes, spleen, tonsils, appendix and Peyer's patches, although not as pronounced as in the thymus. Histology revealed a reduction in germinal centres and depletion of lymphocytes from para-cortical areas [161] [163–165]. Two studies in living children also found that the tonsils were smaller in malnourished than in well-nourished children [163] [177].

Delayed type hypersensitivity response (DTHR). Cellular immune function can be examined by dermal DTHR, the prototype of which is the Mantoux test. Intradermal application of substances like candida or phyto-hemaglutinin (PHA) are also used, as well as sensitizing skin with a local contact sensitizer such as 2-4-di-nitro-clorobenzene (DNCB). Twenty-one articles reported DTHR in relation to malnutrition (**table S10**).

The majority of studies found that malnourished children less frequently developed a positive Mantoux after BCG vaccination [154] [177–185]. Most also found diminished reactivity to *Candida*, PHA and other common antigens [29] [145] [179] [183] [186–190], and after sensitizing with DNCB [163] [177] [179] [183] [188] [191–192]. Conflicting results were found for DTHR in children with different types of severe malnutrition: Three studies found most impaired response in oedematous malnutrition [179] [181] [191], while one found that it was worst in non-oedematous malnutrition [184], and two studies found similar responses [186] [187].

The proportion of positive DTHR varied from study to study, both in well-nourished and malnourished children. Inconsistent results were found in moderately malnourished children [178] [180–181] [185–187] [193]. Other studies found that DTHR was improved with zinc supplementation [190] [194–195] diminished by infections [178] [181] [196], and in slightly older children, a strong interaction was seen between infections and nutritional status [197].

Lymphocytes in blood. Fifty-eight articles reported either total numbers of lymphocytes or lymphocyte subsets in blood (**table S11**). Of 16 articles, 13 reported similar or higher levels of lymphocytes in peripheral blood of malnourished children [80–83] [85–87] [90] [93] [101] [177] [179] [187] [191] [198] [199].

Three studies found that children with oedematous malnutrition had more atypical lymphocytes in blood, resembling plasma cells [81] [87] [93]. Other indicators of functional differences were higher density [200], different pattern of gene expression [201], and more markers of apoptosis in lymphocytes of malnourished children [92] [202].

T-lymphocytes in blood. Numbers of T-lymphocytes were described in 29 articles (**table S11**). Early studies identified T-lymphocytes as those forming rosettes with sheep red blood cells, while later studies used monoclonal antibodies to CD3. Using the rosette-method, 19 of 20 studies found lower levels of T-lymphocytes [28] [87] [93] [101] [128] [130] [144] [183] [186–187] [191] [199] [203–210]. Four studies using monoclonal CD3-antibodies and cell-counting by microscopy also found reduced levels of T-lymphocytes in malnourished children [144] [167–168] [207]. In contrast, only one flow cytometry study found lower levels of T-lymphocytes in malnourished children [211], while four did not [86] [94] [210] [212]. Accordingly, it seems like the rosette-based method identifies different T-lymphocytes than flow cytometry. Some studies found that the numbers of T-lymphocytes were reduced in acute infections [86] [90] [212].

Lymphocyte response to PHA stimulation. In healthy children, incubation of lymphocytes with PHA results in T-lymphocytes to proliferate. Seventeen out of 23 articles reported a reduced proliferative response to PHA in lymphocytes of malnourished children [93] [97–98] [101] [147] [154] [163] [177] [179] [186–187] [189–190] [192] [196] [203] [212–218]. Zinc supplementation improved the response in malnourished children [190].

CD4+ lymphocytes. With assessment of CD4 counts becoming widely available, it has been investigated whether the number of CD4+ lymphocytes was affected by malnutrition. In children without HIV, two of four studies using monoclonal antibodies and microscopy found reduced levels of CD4+ lymphocyte in malnourished children [144] [168] [219] [207], while all seven flow cytometry-studies except one [211] found similar or higher levels [86] [90] [91] [94] [198] [212]. Bacterial infections were noted to reduce the CD4-count [86]. For malnourished children infected with HIV, it was hoped that re-nutrition alone could increase their level of CD4+ lymphocytes. However, a study from Zambia found that CD4 counts declined during nutritional rehabilitation in HIV-infected malnourished children without anti-retroviral treatment [198]. Thus, a low level of CD4+ lymphocytes can probably not be attributed to malnutrition, regardless of whether the child has HIV or not.

Three studies noted that level of CD4+ lymphocytes were higher in children with oedematous than with non-oedematous malnutrition [91] [198] [220], and several studies have noted that children with HIV were less likely to develop oedematous malnutrition [198] [220] [221], suggesting that some level of CD4+ lymphocytes could be required to develop the syndrome.

Activation markers on T-lymphocytes. Most flow cytometry studies assessing surface markers on T-lymphocytes have been carried out in Mexico, all comparing malnourished infected children with similarly infected well-nourished children. Malnourished children were found to have fewer effector T-lymphocytes, identified as cells lacking the "naïve" markers CD62L and CD28 [90], fewer activated T-lymphocytes, with the markers CD69 and/or CD25 [212] [222] [223], and fewer memory T-lymphocytes identified by the marker CD45RO+ [86]. In contrast, a study from Ghana found similar numbers of activated T-lymphocytes, identified by HLA-DR, in malnourished and well-nourished children [94].

B-lymphocytes. Articles published before 1990 measured B-lymphocytes as those forming rosettes when incubated with sheep erythrocytes and C3, while more recent studies used monoclonal antibodies to CD20 and flow cytometry. All seven rosette-based studies found unaffected or higher B-lymphocyte counts in malnourished children [130] [186] [200] [204] [206] [213] [224], as did one study using anti-CD20 and microscopy [167].

In contrast, all four studies using flow cytometry found reduced numbers of B-lymphocytes in malnourished children [86] [94] [211] [212].

Antibody levels. Thirty-two articles described immunoglobulins in blood of malnourished children (**table S12**). Nineteen of 27 studies found no difference in IgG antibodies or total γ-globulin between malnourished and well-nourished children [94] [53] [63–64] [82] [130] [144] [147] [150] [154] [179] [186] [224–238]. Likewise, IgM levels were most frequently similar, or higher in malnourished than well-nourished children [94] [53] [63–64] [82] [130] [144] [147] [154] [179] [186] [224–225] [227–238].

IgA was elevated in malnourished children in 19 of 27 studies [94] [53] [55–56] [63–64] [82] [130] [144] [147] [150] [154] [179] [224–225] [227–238]. With a few exceptions [150] [232], all studies found elevated levels of IgA in oedematous malnutrition, while 11 of 19 studies found that IgA in non-oedematous or underweight children was normal [94] [53] [55–56] [63] [82] [130] [144] [150] [154] [179] [224] [227] [230] [233–238]. One study noted that levels of IgA correlated with the degree of dermatosis in children with Kwashiorkor [231].

IgE showed no clear pattern, but was elevated in malnourished children in three of six studies [82] [147] [211] [233] [238–239]. IgD, present in low amounts in healthy children, was elevated in children with malnutrition in two studies[130] [233], or elevated in oedematous but not non-oedematous malnutrition [179], while one study found that it was similar to well-nourished children [82].

Antibody vaccination responses. Thirty-five articles described vaccination responses to a specific antigen (**table S13**). The articles either reported *sero-conversion rates*, or *antibody titre* response. Studies assessing sero-conversion rates in children with severe malnutrition found mixed results: Six of 10 studies found reduced sero-conversion rates in children with severe malnutrition to typhoid [101] [240], diphtheria [101], tetanus[101] [206], tetanus-diphtheria-pertussis (DTP) [234], hepatitis B [241], measles [141] [149] [242] and yellow fever [243–244], and two studies found that sero-conversion was delayed in malnourished children [245] [238]. Ten of 11 studies found that severely malnourished children responded with reduced antibody titres [101] [141] [149] [206] [233–234] [238] [240–242] [246], despite some of the studies finding acceptable sero-conversion rates. No study found that children with oedematous malnutrition had a normal antibody response to vaccination. One study from 1964 found improved antibody response to DTP in children with oedematous malnutrition randomized to a high-protein diet [247]. There did not seem to be any specific vaccines whose antibody response was more affected than others by malnutrition, nor was there any pattern in terms of responses to live or dead vaccines.

In contrast, mild and moderately malnourished children were most often found to seroconvert normally when vaccinated against smallpox [248], diphtheria [101] [178] [249] [284] , DTP [178] [234], measles [139] [140] [178] [245] [250–255], polio [178] [256], meningococcus[178] [257], and hepatitis B [258], and 9 of 11 articles reported similar level of antibody titres response in moderately malnourished, as well-nourished children [101] [140] [154] [178] [234] [248–249] [252–253] [258–259].

Three of five articles reported similar adverse reactions to vaccination in malnourished as in well-nourished [140–141] [242] [245–255]. In contrast, one study found that malnourished children given measles vaccine frequently developed diarrhoea, pneumonia and fever, compared to well-nourished children, who, in turn, more often developed a rash [141].

Results were inconsistent for studies assessing levels of specific antibodies to non-vaccine antigens, like blood type antigens [260] malaria [261], H. *influenza*, E. *Coli* [235] [262], *Ascaris* [211],

Rotavirus and Lipopolysaccharide [262]. Most of these studies were done in children with moderate malnutrition.

Cytokines. Cytokines are signal molecules acting locally between immune cells, and sometimes with systemic effects. Thirty-five articles described cytokines in malnourished children (**table S14**).

Early works identified cytokines as factors in serum influencing various in-vitro functions of immune cells. Thus, three of five studies found that "Leucocyte Migration Inhibiting factor" was lower in malnourished children [84] [263–264], that serum from malnourished children contained an "E-rosette inhibiting substance" [128] [265], "lympho-cytotoxin" [266], and a substance inhibiting lymphocyte response to PHA [218] [147] [267–268], sometimes called IL-1 [269]. Similarly, Interferon (IFN) was quantified by the antiviral effect of plasma on a cell culture [95] [196]. In neither of these bioassays, the substance responsible for the effect was known. More recent studies assessed levels of cytokines by immunoassays, looking for structurally known cytokines in plasma [123] [270–272] or in cultured leucocytes [89], with flow cytometry staining for intracellular cytokines [222–223], or by identifying mRNA coding for the protein [273–274], with remarkably consistent results.

Cytokines commonly found to be low in malnourished children included IL- 1 and IL-2 [222–223] [269–270] [273–274], although one study found both cytokines to be normal in non-oedematous malnutrition and lower in oedematous malnutrition [89]. IFN-γ was low in malnourished children in six studies [49] [222–223] [273–275], unaltered in malnourished children in one [276], and elevated in one [272]. IL-12 [49] [274], IL-18 and IL-21 [274], and Granulocyte Macrophage Colony Stimulating Factor [270] were also found to be lower in malnourished children. Blunted cytokine response after in-vitro stimulation with LPS was found in malnourished children [276–278], while incubation with leptin normalized their pattern of intracellular cytokines [223].

Other cytokines were mostly found to be elevated in malnutrition: IL10 was elevated in four of five studies [49] [222–223] [272–273], so was IL-4 [211] [273] [276] and soluble receptors to Tumour Necrosis Factor-α [123]. IL-8 was elevated [277] or unaltered [272].

Tumour Necrosis Factor-α (TNFα) [49] [129] [271–273] [276] [279–280] and IL-6 [120] [122–123] [129] [271–273] [276–278] were mostly similar or higher compared to well-nourished, most often in studies of infected children.

Comparing cytokine pattern between children with oedematous and non-oedematous malnutrition, most found that the difference from well-nourished was greatest in children with oedematous malnutrition [84] [89] [123] [265] [269–270] [277], while two studies found no difference between oedematous and non-oedematous malnutrition [218] [271].

Leukotrienes (LT) are not strictly cytokines, but immune modulating molecules derived from long chain polyunsaturated fatty acids. Levels of LTC4 and LTE4 were higher, and LTB4 lower, in children with oedematous than with non-oedematous malnutrition, whose levels were similar to well-nourished [281], and prostaglandin E2 [282] was higher in children with oedematous malnutrition than in well-nourished.

Discussion

We identified and reviewed 245 articles about immune function in malnourished children. Some general problems apply to many of the studies, mostly related to their observational design. For this reason they can only describe associations, not causalities.

First, many studies were done in severely malnourished children from hospital settings, who were ill with infections, making it difficult to disentangle the immunological effect of malnutrition from the effect of infection. This problem has caused some to propose that there really is no immune impairment by malnutrition, and that all alterations seen are due to infections or underlying unknown immune deficiencies, which are also responsible for the poor growth [283]. Enteropathy could be an example of such an "invisible" condition, causing both immune deficiency and malnutrition. This hypothesis is difficult to test. However, some studies did try to account for this problem by selecting malnourished children without clinical infections, or by comparing them to well-nourished infected children. In studies from central Africa in the 1970s and 1980s, some malnourished children may have suffered from unrecognized paediatric HIV [284], giving obvious problems for interpretation.

Second, publication bias is a well-known problem, and may have occurred, particularly in older studies, where some small studies showed a dramatic effect.

Third, studies used different diagnostic criteria for malnutrition, making it difficult to determine the children's degree of malnutrition as defined by present-day criteria. While children in 52 of the studies fulfilled WHOs present criteria for severe acute malnutrition, only two diagnosed children based on the new WHO growth reference. Those defined as severely malnourished based on old growth references would most likely also be classified as severely malnourished today, since the new WHO standard tend to classify more children as severely malnourished, while some children then defined as moderately malnourished would be classified as severely malnourished today. The studies including children based on weight-for-age probably included children with stunting and wasting, without differentiating between the two.

Fourth, even using uniform criteria, malnourished children are a heterogeneous group. Anthropometric measurements are only crude markers of body composition, which - among other things - reflect nutrient deficiencies. It is unknown what specific nutrients were deficient, and to what extent infection contributed. Deficits in lean tissue and fat tissue are plausibly different physiologic conditions, and children appearing similarly malnourished may be so for entirely different reasons, with different immunological consequences. No articles have so far reported reliable measures of body composition, simultaneously with markers of immune function. Probably, the consequence of malnutrition on immune function may also depend on the pattern and load of infections. Although most studies were carried out in low-income settings with high infectious loads, a few were from middle- or high-income countries. This may also contribute to inconsistencies in the results.

In spite of these limitations, common patterns emerge from the studies, summarized below (**Figure 5**).

Immune parameters apparently not affected by malnutrition

Total white blood cell and lymphocyte counts in peripheral blood are not decreased in malnourished children, and granulocytes are frequently elevated. Likewise, T-lymphocytes and CD4 counts appear normal in malnourished children, when measured by flow cytometry, the gold standard for characterizing cell subsets. Their levels seem to be determined more by infections than by nutritional state, and do not reflect the degree of malnutrition-related immune deficiency, as high infectious mortality is seen in malnourished children, despite unaffected white blood cell counts [49].

Unaffected by malnutrition	Affected in severe malnutrition	Affected in moderate malnutrition

Total leukocytes in blood

Total lymphocytes in blood

T-cell count in blood

CD4 cell count in blood

Total immuloglobulins in blood

IgG and IgM in blood

Secretory IgA in urine and

duodenal fluid

CRP rise with infections

Inflammatory cytokines (IL6,

TNFα)

Gastric acid production↓
Flow of saliva ↓
Secretory IgA (saliva and tears)↓
Gut permeability ↑
Inflammatory cells in intestine ↑
Microbicidal activity of granulocytes ↓
Blood dendritic cells ↓
Blood complement factors ↓
Delayed type hypersensitivity ↓
Proliferative response to PHA ↓
Effector T-cells ↓
Apoptosis in lymphocytes ↑
B-cells in blood ↓
IgA in blood ↑
Vaccination titre response ↓

Thymus size ↓
Th2 cytokines (IL4, IL10) ↑
Th1 Cytokines (IL2, IL12, IFNγ)↓

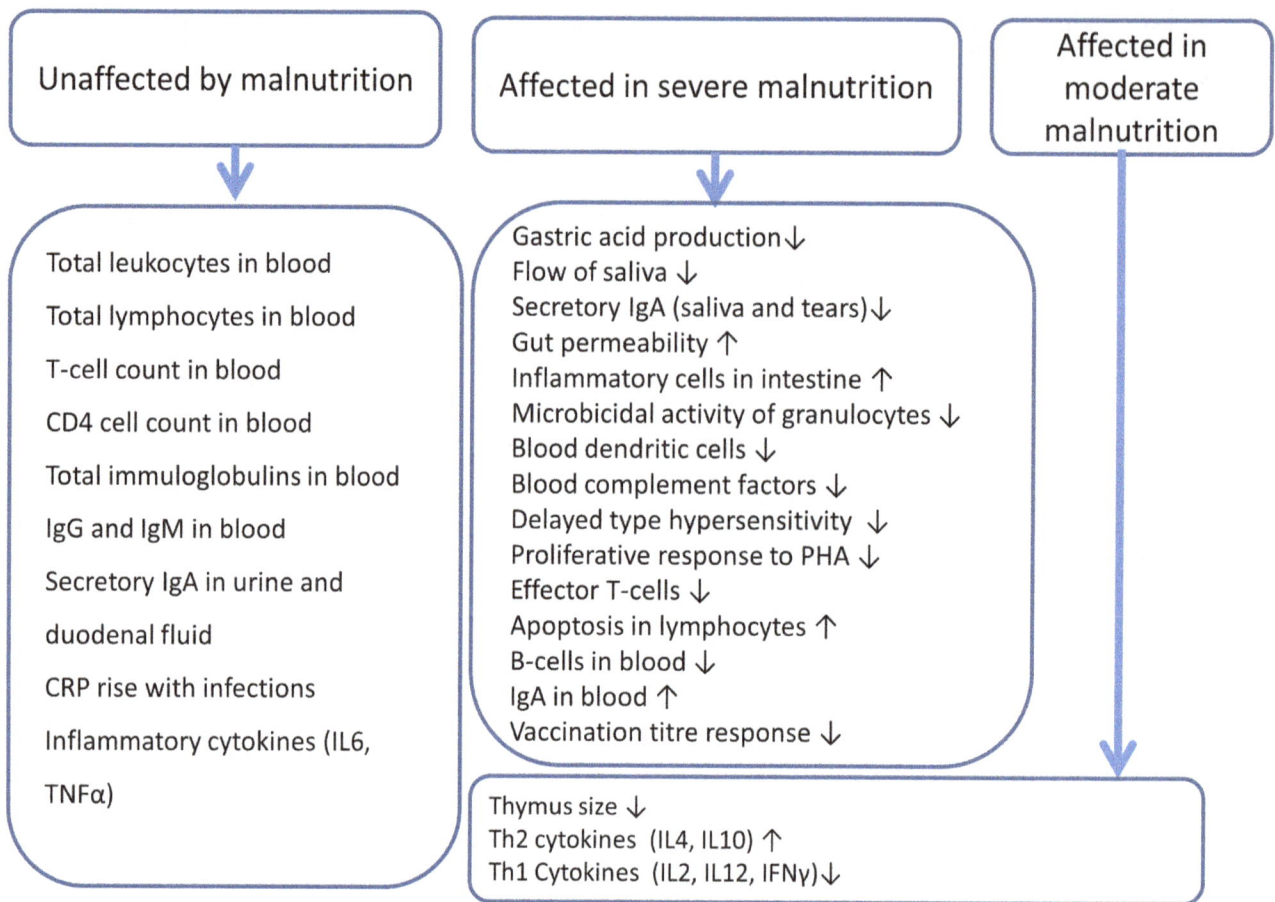

Figure 5. Summary of immune parameters affected and not affected by malnutrition.

Malnourished children can mount an acute phase response to infections, with elevated CRP and low negative acute phase reactants, and this can also be seen in absence of clinical infection. Thus, based on available evidence, the acute phase response, if anything, seems exaggerated rather than diminished. Levels of IgM and IgG are normal or elevated in malnourished children. Secretory IgA is not consistently lower in duodenal fluid, and frequently elevated in urine.

Immune parameters affected by malnutrition

The gut mucosa is atrophied and permeable in malnourished children. This enteropathy also affects well-nourished children in poor communities, but probably most severely in malnourished children. The condition appears similar to *tropical sprue* described in adults, and the term *enteropathy of malnutrition* has been replaced by the broader term *environmental enteropathy* [285]. At present, this condition is thought to result from high pathogen load rather than nutrient deficiencies, and thus primarily a cause of malnutrition, particularly stunting [286] [287].

Production of gastric acid and flow of saliva is reduced in malnourished children. Secretory IgA is also reduced in saliva, tears and nasal washings from children with severe, but not moderate malnutrition. The small bowel of malnourished children is often colonized with abundant bacteria, and their pattern of commensal flora is altered. Granulocytes kill ingested microorganisms less effectively. Levels of complement proteins are low in

blood from malnourished children, particularly in children with oedematous malnutrition, and less in children with moderate malnutrition.

Lymphatic tissue, particularly the thymus, undergoes atrophy in malnutrition in a dose-response fashion: thymic size depends on nutritional status even in milder degrees of malnutrition, and thymus size is a predictor of survival in children.

DTHR is diminished in malnourished children. Lymphocytes of malnourished children are less responsive to stimulation with PHA, fewer are activated and more cells have markers of apoptosis. Plasma IgA is mostly elevated in malnourished children, particular in those with oedema. Children with severe, but not moderate, malnutrition mount a lower specific antibody response to vaccination, although for most children sufficient to obtain protection. The lower titres seen in malnourished may be due to a delay in vaccination response.

Cytokines can be classified as those promoting a Th1 response of predominantly cellular immunity, and those promoting a Th2-response of humoral immunity [24]. Although this approach has somewhat been replaced by other classifications [288], it seems useful to describe the profile of malnourished children, whose immune system seems tuned towards a Th2 response, with high IL4 and IL10, and low levels of IL-2, IL-12 and IFN-γ. Elevated levels of IL-6 and TNFα may primarily be related to infections, and support the observation that induction of an acute phase response is intact in malnutrition. A more recent classification focuses on whether cytokines are predominantly inflammatory or anti-inflammatory [289]. Malnourished children appear to have high levels of anti-inflammatory cytokines and less clearly affected levels of pro-inflammatory cytokines in blood, in contrast to the predominantly pro-inflammatory cytokine expression in the gut of malnourished children.

Mechanisms

The mechanisms behind these immunological alterations are still not adequately understood. Some explain it by lack of energy and building blocks to synthesize the proteins required [290]. However, lack of building blocks does not explain why some immune parameters seem intact, or paradoxically elevated in malnutrition, such as plasma IgA, acute-phase proteins, leucocytes in blood, and production of Th2 cytokines. If it was simply a matter of lack of building blocks, all parameters of the immune system should be equally affected. The fact that the pattern of cytokines in malnourished children is tuned towards at Th2-response fits with their high levels of immunoglobulins, reduction in thymus size and diminished DTHR. Still, the pathophysiology behind this Th2 skewedness remains unexplained.

Infections could obviously contribute to the changes seen, and interactions have been noted between infection and malnutrition in their respective effects on immune parameters [197]. However, although many of the immunological changes appear to be synergistically affected by malnutrition and infections, malnutrition also seems to be independently associated with altered immune function.

Animal studies suggest hormonal factors to be involved in the immune profile of malnutrition. Leptin [291], prolactin [292] and growth hormone [293] all stimulate thymic growth and function, and their levels are low in malnourished children. In support of this, a recent study found that a low leptin level was associated with a higher risk of death in malnourished children [272]. Growth hormone therapy increased thymic size and output in adult HIV patients [294]. In contrast, cortisol and adrenalin induce thymic atrophy in mice [295–296], and cortisol is high in children with malnutrition and other forms of stress. It is plausible that this hormonal interplay is implicated in the immune deficiency in malnourished children.

This hormonal profile is similar to that of an acute phase response, where thymus atrophy also occurs, acquired immunity is temporarily suppressed and innate immunity takes over [296]. This could explain why some malnourished children have elevated positive APP and most have depressed negative APP in absence of clinical infections. Zinc deficiency causes thymic atrophy [297–298], and acute phase responses lower plasma zinc, so zinc status may contribute to the immune deficiency of both malnutrition and acute phase responses.

In HIV infection, persisting subclinical inflammation and immune activation is frequently present, and may be partly responsible for immune deficiency and disease manifestations [299]. Given the frequent finding of elevated acute phase proteins in malnourished children, it seems plausible that a similar state of subclinical inflammation could be involved in both the impairment of immune function, and in the vicious circle of catabolism and deterioration of the nutritional status. However, in spite of elevated acute phase proteins, most studies have reported unaffected or even paradoxically lowered levels of activated T-cell and dendritic cells in malnourished children.

The intracellular receptor, *mammalian target of Raptomycin* (mTOR), is present in most cells. It responds to concentrations of nutrients in the cell's surroundings, and to other signs of stress, such as hypoxia, enabling the cell to adapt its metabolism to locally available nutrients. Immune cells also use mTOR to regulate their state of activation. Nutrient availability may thereby determine whether an immune cell is activated [300], and whether T-cells differentiate towards a pro-inflammatory or a tolerance-inducing phenotype [301]. Some immune cells may even deplete the micro-environment of certain nutrients, to manipulate the activation of mTOR. Accordingly, the significance of nutrients in the micro-environment expands from simple building blocks to signal molecules. Obviously, this mechanism could be involved in the immunological profile in malnutrition. However, no articles have yet described the activity of mTOR in malnourished children.

A research group working with animal models of malnutrition has proposed a theory called the "tolerance hypothesis" [302]. This suggests that the depression of cellular immunity in malnutrition is an adaptive response to prevent autoimmune reactions, which would otherwise occur as a result of catabolism and release of self-antigens. Although adaptive in this sense, it happens at the price of increased susceptibility to infections [303]. However, if this tolerance hypothesis holds true, one would expect to see occasional break-through of auto-immune reactions in malnourished children. Such phenomena have apparently not been studied.

The pathogenesis of oedematous malnutrition is still unknown. Many immune parameters seem affected to a different degree in children with oedematous malnutrition, with higher levels of IgA, higher levels of abnormal antibodies like IgD, poorer vaccination responses and cytokines more skewed towards a Th2-response; their complement levels are lower, which may partly be caused by increased consumption of complement in-vivo. The pattern of leukotrienes is different in children with oedematous compared to non-oedematous malnutrition. This immunological profile resembles that seen in autoimmune diseases such as lupus erythematosus [304–305]. Moreover, elevated immunoglobulins in children with oedematous malnutrition seem to correlate with its unexplainable manifestations, like dermatosis and oedema [231] [233]. It could be speculated whether this syndrome could indeed represent some kind of autoimmune reaction to malnutrition, perhaps resulting from a failure to induce efficient tolerance.

Conclusion

In spite of the prevalence of malnutrition, and its fatal consequences, scientific interest in the immune deficiency of malnutrition seems dwindling, and little research has been carried out on the topic during the last ten years. For this reason, most evidence on the subject relies on immunological methods used 30 to 40 years ago, many of which are no longer in use, and little research has been done with modern methods, and with the present understanding of immunology. Moreover, most studies have looked at isolated aspects of immune function, despite the fact that the parameters are interdependent, and the division into innate and adaptive immune function seems to be a simplification. Thus, our understanding of immune function in malnutrition is still very limited.

This review illuminates the little that we know about the immunological alterations associated with malnutrition, and also points to significant gaps in our knowledge. Future well designed prospective cohort studies should examine how immune parameters are related to morbidity and mortality in malnourished children, with detailed characteristic of nutritional status, preferably body composition, of infections, enteropathy and of low-grade inflammation. When testing nutritional and medical interventions for malnutrition, immune parameters should be included as outcomes. Studies should investigate newer immunological parameters in malnutrition, like expression of innate pattern recognition receptors (as the Toll-like receptor), the lectin pathway of the complement system and mTOR expression and activity. It should be investigated whether a small thymus is associated with lower output of recent thymic-derived T-cells, and how it correlates with hormones like leptin, cortisol, insulin and Insulin Growth Factor-1. Innate and adaptive immune parameters should be assessed simultaneously, taking into account their dynamic interdependency. To understand whether malnutrition is indeed associated with active down-regulation of immune reactivity (as formulated in the "tolerance hypothesis"), the balance between regulatory T-lymphocytes and their counterparts, Th17 lymphocytes should be measured. Finally, prospective studies among children at risk should assess whether immune profiles differ in those who subsequently develop oedematous and non-oedematous malnutrition, and it should be investigated whether children with oedematous malnutrition have markers suggestive of auto-immune or inflammatory diseases. Such studies would reduce our current ignorance on the interplay between malnutrition and infectious diseases.

Supporting Information

Figure S1   PRISMA Flow diagram showing study retrieval and selection.

Table S1   Articles describing barrier and immune function of skin in malnourished children.

Table S2   Articles describing intestinal function and mucosal structure in children with malnutrition.

Table S3   Articles describing anti-microbial factors in mucosal secretions of malnourished children.

Table S4   Articles describing commensal flora in children with malnutrition.

Table S5   Articles describing function of innate immune cells: polymorph-nuclear cells and monocytes/macrophages in children with malnutrition.

Table S6   Articles describing acute phase response in malnourished children.

Table S7   Articles describing complement in malnourished children.

Table S8   Articles describing thymus and other lymphatic tissue in autopsies of malnourished children.

Table S9   Articles describing ultrasound scans of thymus in malnourished children.

Table S10   Articles describing delayed type hypersensitivity response in children with malnutrition.

Table S11   Articles describing lymphocyte subsets in children with malnutrition.

Table S12   Articles describing antibody levels in children with malnutrition.

Table S13   Articles describing humoral vaccination responses in children with malnutrition.

Table S14   Articles describing cytokines in malnourished children.

Checklist S1   PRISMA Checklist.

Acknowledgments

We are grateful to Dr Michael Golden for providing an extensive list of literature on the subject, and to Professor Kim Fleischer Michaelsen and Charlotte Gylling Mortensen for critically reviewing the manuscript.

Author Contributions

Conceived and designed the experiments: MJHR VBC. Performed the experiments: MJHR. Analyzed the data: MJHR. Contributed to the writing of the manuscript: MJHR LK AB HF VBC.

References

1. Black RE, Victora CG, Walker SP, Bhutta ZA, Christian P, et al. (2013) Maternal and child undernutrition and overweight in low-income and middle-income countries. Lancet 382: 427–451. doi:10.1016/S0140-6736(13)60937-X.
2. Pelletier DL, Frongillo EA Jr, Schroeder DG, Habicht JP (1995) The effects of malnutrition on child mortality in developing countries. Bull World Health Organ 73: 443–448.
3. Tomkins A, Watson F (1989) Malnutrition and Infection - A Review - Nutrition Policy Discussion Paper No. 5. United Nations - Administrative Commitee on Coordination - Subcommitee on Nutrition.
4. Chisti MJ, Tebruegge M, La Vincente S, Graham SM, Duke T (2009) Pneumonia in severely malnourished children in developing countries - mortality risk, aetiology and validity of WHO clinical signs: a systematic review. Trop Med Int Health TM IH 14: 1173–1189. doi:10.1111/j.1365-3156.2009.02364.x.
5. Waterlow JC (1992) Protein Energy malnutrition, 2nd ed. London: Hodder&Stouton.
6. Dutz W, Jennings-Khodadad E, Post C, Kohout E, Nazarian I, et al. (1974) Marasmus and Pneumocystis carinii pneumonia in institutionalised infants. Observations during an endemic. Z Für Kinderheilkd 117: 241–258.
7. Purtilo DT, Connor DH (1975) Fatal infections in protein-calorie malnourished children with thymolymphatic atrophy. Arch Dis Child 50: 149–152.
8. Ikeogu MO, Wolf B, Mathe S (1997) Pulmonary manifestations in HIV seropositivity and malnutrition in Zimbabwe. Arch Dis Child 76: 124–128.
9. Amadi B, Kelly P, Mwiya M, Mulwazi E, Sianongo S, et al. (2001) Intestinal and systemic infection, HIV, and mortality in Zambian children with persistent diarrhea and malnutrition. J Pediatr Gastroenterol Nutr 32: 550–554.
10. Mondal D, Haque R, Sack RB, Kirkpatrick BD, Petri WA Jr (2009) Attribution of malnutrition to cause-specific diarrheal illness: evidence from a prospective study of preschool children in Mirpur, Dhaka, Bangladesh. Am J Trop Med Hyg 80: 824–826.
11. Khatun F, Faruque ASG, Koeck JL, Olliaro P, Millet P, et al. (2011) Changing species distribution and antimicrobial susceptibility pattern of Shigella over a 29-year period (1980–2008). Epidemiol Infect 139: 446–452. doi:10.1017/S0950268810001093.
12. Berkley JA, Lowe BS, Mwangi I, Williams T, Bauni E, et al. (2005) Bacteremia among children admitted to a rural hospital in Kenya. N Engl J Med 352: 39–47. doi:10.1056/NEJMoa040275.
13. Aiken AM, Mturi N, Njuguna P, Mohammed S, Berkley JA, et al. (2011) Risk and causes of paediatric hospital-acquired bacteraemia in Kilifi District Hospital, Kenya: a prospective cohort study. Lancet 378: 2021–2027. doi:10.1016/S0140-6736(11)61622-X.
14. Alcoba G, Kerac M, Breysse S, Salpeteur C, Galetto-Lacour A, et al. (2013) Do children with uncomplicated severe acute malnutrition need antibiotics? A systematic review and meta-analysis. PloS One 8: e53184. doi:10.1371/journal.pone.0053184.

15. Soler-Cataluña JJ, Sánchez-Sánchez L, Martínez-García MA, Sánchez PR, Salcedo E, et al. (2005) Mid-arm muscle area is a better predictor of mortality than body mass index in COPD. Chest 128: 2108–2115. doi:10.1378/chest.128.4.2108.
16. Roediger WE (1990) The starved colon–diminished mucosal nutrition, diminished absorption, and colitis. Dis Colon Rectum 33: 858–862.
17. Faddan NHA, Sayh KIE, Shams H, Badrawy H (2010) Myocardial dysfunction in malnourished children. Ann Pediatr Cardiol 3: 113–118. doi:10.4103/0974-2069.74036.
18. Myatt M, Khara T, Collins S (2006) A review of methods to detect cases of severely malnourished children in the community for their admission into community-based therapeutic care programs. Food Nutr Bull 27: S7–23.
19. World Health Organization, United Nations Children's Fund (2009) WHO child growth standards and the identification of severe acute malnutrition in infants and children A Joint Statement. Available: http://www.who.int/maternal_child_adolescent/documents/9789241598163/en/. Accessed 2014 Aug 5.
20. Williams C (1935) Kwashiorkor - a nutritional disease in children associated with a maize diet. The Lancet nov 16, 1935: 1151–1152.
21. Wellcome Trust Working Party (1970) Classification of infantile malnutrition. The Lancet aug 8: 302–303.
22. Smith R (2005) Investigating the previous studies of a fraudulent author. BMJ 331: 288–291. doi:10.1136/bmj.331.7511.288.
23. WHO (2009) WHO child growth standards and the identification of severe acute malnutrition in infants and children. Geneva: WHO. Available: http://www.who.int/nutrition/publications/severemalnutrition/9789241598163_eng.pdf. Accessed 7 July 2013.
24. Murphy K (2012) Janeways's Immunobiology. 2012th ed. Garland Science, Taylor & Francis Group.
25. Heilskov S, Rytter MJH, Vestergaard C, Briend A, Babirekere E, et al. (2014) Dermatosis in children with oedematous malnutrition (Kwashiorkor): a review of the literature. J Eur Acad Dermatol Venereol JEADV. doi:10.1111/jdv.12452.
26. Sims RT (1968) The ultrastructure of depigmented skin in kwashiorkor. Br J Dermatol 80: 822–832.
27. Thavaraj V, Sesikeran B (1989) Histopathological changes in skin of children with clinical protein energy malnutrition before and after recovery. J Trop Pediatr 35: 105–108.
28. Kulapongs P, Edelman R, Suskind R, Olson RE (1977) Defective local leukocyte mobilization in children with kwashiorkor. Am J Clin Nutr 30: 367–370.
29. Bhaskaram P, Reddy V (1982) Cutaneous inflammatory response in kwashiorkor. Indian J Med Res 76: 849–853.
30. Freyre EA, Chabes A, Poémape O, Chabes A (1973) Abnormal Rebuck skin window response in kwashiorkor. J Pediatr 82: 523–526.
31. Edelman R, Suskind R, Olson RE, Sirisinha S (1973) Mechanisms of defective delayed cutaneous hypersensitivity in children with protein-calorie malnutrition. Lancet 1: 506–508.
32. Burman D (1965) The jejunal mucosa in kwashiorkor. Arch Dis Child 40: 526–531.
33. Brunser O, Castillo C, Araya M (1976) Fine structure of the small intestinal mucosa in infantile marasmic malnutrition. Gastroenterology 70: 495–507.
34. Schneider RE, Viteri FE (1972) Morphological aspects of the duodenojejunal mucosa in protein-calorie malnourished children and during recovery. Am J Clin Nutr 25: 1092–1102.
35. Brunser O, Reid A, Monckeberg F, Maccioni A, Contreras I (1968) Jejunal mucosa in infant malnutrition. Am J Clin Nutr 21: 976–983.
36. Brunser O, Reid A, Mönckeberg F, Maccioni A, Contreras I (1966) Jejunal biopsies in infant malnutrition: with special reference to mitotic index. Pediatrics 38: 605–612.
37. Amadi B, Fagbemi AO, Kelly P, Mwiya M, Torrente F, et al. (2009) Reduced production of sulfated glycosaminoglycans occurs in Zambian children with kwashiorkor but not marasmus. Am J Clin Nutr 89: 592–600. doi:10.3945/ajcn.2008.27092.
38. Campbell DI, Murch SH, Elia M, Sullivan PB, Sanyang MS, et al. (2003) Chronic T cell-mediated enteropathy in rural west African children: relationship between nutritional status and small bowel function. Pediatr Res 54: 306–311. doi:10.1203/01.PDR.0000076666.16021.5E.
39. Green F, Heyworth B (1980) Immunoglobulin-containing cells in jejunal mucosa of children with protein-energy malnutrition and gastroenteritis. Arch Dis Child 55: 380–383.
40. Kaschula RO, Gajjar PD, Mann M, Hill I, Purvis J, et al. (1979) Infantile jejunal mucosa in infection and malnutrition. Isr J Med Sci 15: 356–361.
41. Theron JJ, Wittmann W, Prinsloo JG (1971) The fine structure of the jejunum in kwashiorkor. Exp Mol Pathol 14: 184–199.
42. Shiner M, Redmond AO, Hansen JD (1973) The jejunal mucosa in protein-energy malnutrition. A clinical, histological, and ultrastructural study. Exp Mol Pathol 19: 61–78.
43. Römer H, Urbach R, Gomez MA, Lopez A, Perozo-Ruggeri G, et al. (1983) Moderate and severe protein energy malnutrition in childhood: effects on jejunal mucosal morphology and disaccharidase activities. J Pediatr Gastroenterol Nutr 2: 459–464.
44. Stanfield JP, Hutt MS, Tunnicliffe R (1965) Intestinal biopsy in kwashiorkor. Lancet 2: 519–523.
45. Behrens RH, Lunn PG, Northrop CA, Hanlon PW, Neale G (1987) Factors affecting the integrity of the intestinal mucosa of Gambian children. Am J Clin Nutr 45: 1433–1441.
46. Brewster DR, Manary MJ, Menzies IS, O'Loughlin EV, Henry RL (1997) Intestinal permeability in kwashiorkor. Arch Dis Child 76: 236–241.
47. Hossain MI, Nahar B, Hamadani JD, Ahmed T, Roy AK, et al. (2010) Intestinal mucosal permeability of severely underweight and nonmalnourished Bangladeshi children and effects of nutritional rehabilitation. J Pediatr Gastroenterol Nutr 51: 638–644. doi:10.1097/MPG.0b013e3181eb3128.
48. Boaz RT, Joseph AJ, Kang G, Bose A (2013) Intestinal permeability in normally nourished and malnourished children with and without diarrhea. Indian Pediatr 50: 152–153.
49. Hughes SM, Amadi B, Mwiya M, Nkamba H, Tomkins A, et al. (2009) Dendritic cell anergy results from endotoxemia in severe malnutrition. J Immunol Baltim Md 1950 183: 2818–2826. doi:10.4049/jimmunol.0803518.
50. Mishra OP, Dhawan T, Singla PN, Dixit VK, Arya NC, et al. (2001) Endoscopic and histopathological evaluation of preschool children with chronic diarrhoea. J Trop Pediatr 47: 77–80.
51. Sullivan PB, Lunn PG, Northrop-Clewes C, Crowe PT, Marsh MN, et al. (1992) Persistent diarrhea and malnutrition-the impact of treatment on small bowel structure and permeability. J Pediatr Gastroenterol Nutr 14: 208–215.
52. Redmond AO, Kaschula RO, Freeseman C, Hansen JD (1971) The colon in kwashiorkor. Arch Dis Child 46: 470–473.
53. McMurray DN, Rey H, Casazza LJ, Watson RR (1977) Effect of moderate malnutrition on concentrations of immunoglobulins and enzymes in tears and saliva of young Colombian children. Am J Clin Nutr 30: 1944–1948.
54. Watson RR, McMurray DN, Martin P, Reyes MA (1985) Effect of age, malnutrition and renutrition on free secretory component and IgA in secretions. Am J Clin Nutr 42: 281–288.
55. Sirisinha S, Suskind R, Edelman R, Asvapaka C, Olson RE (1975) Secretory and serum IgA in children with protein-calorie malnutrition. Pediatrics 55: 166–170.
56. Ibrahim AM, el-Hawary MF, Sakr R (1978) Protein-calorie malnutrition (PCM) in Egypt immunological changes of salivary protein in PCM. Z Für Ernährungswissenschaft 17: 145–152.
57. Reddy V, Raghuramulu N, Bhaskaram C (1976) Secretory IgA in protein-calorie malnutrition. Arch Dis Child 51: 871–874.
58. Yakubu AM (1982) Secretory IgA in nasal secretions of children with acute gastroenteritis and kwashiorkor. Ann Trop Paediatr 2: 139–142.
59. Bell RG, Turner KJ, Gracey M, Suharjono Sunoto (1976) Serum and small intestinal immunoglobulin levels in undernourished children. Am J Clin Nutr 29: 392–397.
60. Buchanan N, Fairburn JA, Schmaman A (1973) Urinary tract infection and secretory urinary IgA in malnutrition. South Afr Med J Suid-Afr Tydskr Vir Geneeskd 47: 1179–1181.
61. Marei MA, al-Hamshary AM, Abdalla KF, Abdel-Maaboud AI (1998) A study on secretory IgA in malnourished children with chronic diarrhoea associated with parasitic infections. J Egypt Soc Parasitol 28: 907–913.
62. Miller EM, McConnell DS (2012) Brief communication: chronic undernutrition is associated with higher mucosal antibody levels among Ariaal infants of northern Kenya. Am J Phys Anthropol 149: 136–141. doi:10.1002/ajpa.22108.
63. Watson RR, Reyes MA, McMurray DN (1978) Influence of malnutrition on the concentration of IgA, lysozyme, amylase and aminopeptidase in children's tears. Proc Soc Exp Biol Med Soc Exp Biol Med N Y N 157: 215–219.
64. Beatty DW, Napier B, Sinclair-Smith CC, McCabe K, Hughes EJ (1983) Secretory IgA synthesis in Kwashiorkor. J Clin Lab Immunol 12: 31–36.
65. Gilman RH, Partanen R, Brown KH, Spira WM, Khanam S, et al. (1988) Decreased gastric acid secretion and bacterial colonization of the stomach in severely malnourished Bangladeshi children. Gastroenterology 94: 1308–1314.
66. Shashidhar S, Shah SB, Acharya PT (1976) Gastric acid, pH and pepsin in healthy and protein calorie malnourished children. Indian J Pediatr 43: 145–151.
67. Gracey M, Cullity GJ, Suharjono S (1977) The stomach in malnutrition. Arch Dis Child 52: 325–327.
68. Adesola AO (1968) The influence of severe protein deficiency (kwashiorkor) on gastric acid secretion in Nigerian children. Br J Surg 55: 866.
69. Vael C, Desager K (2009) The importance of the development of the intestinal microbiota in infancy. Curr Opin Pediatr 21: 794–800. doi:10.1097/MOP.0b013e328332351b.
70. Scheutz F, Matee MI, Simon E, Mwinula JH, Lyamuya EF, et al. (1997) Association between carriage of oral yeasts, malnutrition and HIV-1 infection among Tanzanian children aged 18 months to 5 years. Community Dent Oral Epidemiol 25: 193–198.
71. Matee MI, Simon E, Christensen MF, Kirk K, Andersen L, et al. (1995) Association between carriage of oral yeasts and malnutrition among Tanzanian infants aged 6–24 months. Oral Dis 1: 37–42.
72. Omoike IU, Abiodun PO (1989) Upper small intestinal microflora in diarrhea and malnutrition in Nigerian children. J Pediatr Gastroenterol Nutr 9: 314–321.
73. Mata LJ, Jiménez F, Cordón M, Rosales R, Prera E, et al. (1972) Gastrointestinal flora of children with protein–calorie malnutrition. Am J Clin Nutr 25: 118–126.

74. Gracey M, Stone DE, Suharjono Sunoto (1974) Isolation of Candida species from the gastrointestinal tract in malnourished children. Am J Clin Nutr 27: 345–349.

75. Neto UF, Toccalino H, Dujovney F (1976) Stool bacterial aerobic overgrowth in the small intestine of children with acute diarrhoea. Acta Paediatr Scand 65: 609–615.

76. Smith MI, Yatsunenko T, Manary MJ, Trehan I, Mkakosya R, et al. (2013) Gut microbiomes of Malawian twin pairs discordant for kwashiorkor. Science 339: 548–554. doi:10.1126/science.1229000.

77. Monira S, Nakamura S, Gotoh K, Izutsu K, Watanabe H, et al. (2011) Gut microbiota of healthy and malnourished children in bangladesh. Front Microbiol 2: 228. doi:10.3389/fmicb.2011.00228.

78. Gupta SS, Mohammed MH, Ghosh TS, Kanungo S, Nair GB, et al. (2011) Metagenome of the gut of a malnourished child. Gut Pathog 3: 7. doi:10.1186/1757-4749-3-7.

79. Subramanian S, Huq S, Yatsunenko T, Haque R, Mahfuz M, et al. (2014) Persistent gut microbiota immaturity in malnourished Bangladeshi children. Nature. doi:10.1038/nature13421.

80. Rosen EU, Geefhuysen J, Anderson R, Joffe M, Rabson AR (1975) Leucocyte function in children with kwashiorkor. Arch Dis Child 50: 220–224.

81. Schopfer K, Douglas SD (1976) Fine structural studies of peripheral blood leucocytes from children with kwashiorkor: morphological and functional properties. Br J Haematol 32: 573–577.

82. Purtilo DT, Riggs RS, Evans R, Neafie RC (1976) Humoral immunity of parasitized, malnourished children. Am J Trop Med Hyg 25: 229–232.

83. Schopfer K, Douglas SD (1976) Neutrophil function in children with kwashiorkor. J Lab Clin Med 88: 450–461.

84. Fongwo NP, Arinola OG, Salimonu LS (1999) Leucocyte migration inhibition factor (L-MIF) in malnourished Nigerian children. Afr J Med Med Sci 28: 17–20.

85. Nájera O, González C, Toledo G, López L, Cortés E, et al. (2001) CD45RA and CD45RO isoforms in infected malnourished and infected well-nourished children. Clin Exp Immunol 126: 461–465.

86. Nájera O, González C, Toledo G, López L, Ortiz R (2004) Flow cytometry study of lymphocyte subsets in malnourished and well-nourished children with bacterial infections. Clin Diagn Lab Immunol 11: 577–580. doi:10.1128/CDLI.11.3.577-580.2004.

87. Keusch G, Urritia J, Guerrero O, Castenada G, Douglas S (1977) Rosette-Forming Lymphocytes in Guatemalan Children with Protein-Calorie Malnutrition. Malnutrition and the Immune Response, Edited by Robert M Suskind. New York: Raven Press, Vol. 1977.pp. 117–124.

88. Keusch G, Urrutia JJ, Fernandez R, Guerrero O, Casteneda G (1977) Humoral and Cellular Aspects of Intracellular Bactericidal killing in Guatemalan Children with Protein-Energy Malnutrition. Malnutrition and the Immune Response, Edited by Robert M Suskind. New York: Raven Press.pp. 245–251.

89. Lotfy OA, Saleh WA, el-Barbari M (1998) A study of some changes of cell-mediated immunity in protein energy malnutrition. J Egypt Soc Parasitol 28: 413–428.

90. Nájera O, González C, Cortés E, Toledo G, Ortiz R (2007) Effector T lymphocytes in well-nourished and malnourished infected children. Clin Exp Immunol 148: 501–506. doi:10.1111/j.1365-2249.2007.03369.x.

91. Nassar MF, Younis NT, Tohamy AG, Dalam DM, El Badawy MA (2007) T-lymphocyte subsets and thymic size in malnourished infants in Egypt: a hospital-based study. East Mediterr Health J Rev Santé Méditerranée Orient Al-Majallah Al-Ṣiḥḥīyah Li-Sharq Al-Mutawassiṭ 13: 1031–1042.

92. Nassar MF, El-Batrawy SR, Nagy NM (2009) CD95 expression in white blood cells of malnourished infants during hospitalization and catch-up growth. East Mediterr Health J Rev Santé Méditerranée Orient Al-Majallah Al-Ṣiḥḥīyah Li-Sharq Al-Mutawassiṭ 15: 574–583.

93. Schopfer K, Douglas SD (1976) In vitro studies of lymphocytes from children with kwashiorkor. Clin Immunol Immunopathol 5: 21–30.

94. Rikimaru T, Taniquchi K, Yartey J, Kennedy D, Nkrumah F (1998) Humoral and cell-mediated immunity in malnourished children in Ghana. Eur J Clin Nutr 1998 May; 52: 344–350.

95. Salimonu LS, Ojo-Amaize E, Williams AI, Johnson AO, Cooke AR, et al. (1982) Depressed natural killer cell activity in children with protein-calorie malnutrition. Clin Immunol Immunopathol 24: 1–7.

96. Salimonu LS, Ojo-Amaize E, Johnson AO, Laditan AA, Akinwolere OA, et al. (1983) Depressed natural killer cell activity in children with protein–calorie malnutrition. II. Correction of the impaired activity after nutritional recovery. Cell Immunol 82: 210–215.

97. Vásquez-Garibay E, Campollo-Rivas O, Romero-Velarde E, Méndez-Estrada C, García-Iglesias T, et al. (2002) Effect of renutrition on natural and cell-mediated immune response in infants with severe malnutrition. J Pediatr Gastroenterol Nutr 34: 296–301.

98. Vásquez-Garibay E, Méndez-Estrada C, Romero-Velarde E, García-Iglesias MT, Campollo-Rivas O (2004) Nutritional support with nucleotide addition favors immune response in severely malnourished infants. Arch Med Res 35: 284–288. doi:10.1016/j.arcmed.2004.03.002.

99. Rich K, Neumann C, Stiehm R (1977) Neutrophil Chemotaxis in Malnourished Ghanian Children. In: Suskind RM, editor.Malnutrition and the Immune Response.New York: Raven Press. pp. 271–275.

100. Goyal HK, Kaushik SK, Dhamieja JP, Suman RK, Kumar KK (1981) A study of granulocyte adherence in protein calorie malnutrition. Indian Pediatr 18: 287–292.

101. Reddy V, Jagadeesan V, Ragharamulu N, Bhaskaram C, Srikantia SG (1976) Functional significance of growth retardation in malnutrition. Am J Clin Nutr 29: 3–7.

102. Tejada C, Argueta V, Sanchez M, Albertazzi C (1964) Phagocytic and alkaline phosphatase activity of leucocytes in kwashiorkor. J Pediatr 64: 753–761.

103. Douglas SD, Schopfer K (1974) Phagocyte function in protein-calorie malnutrition. Clin Exp Immunol 17: 121–128.

104. Leitzmann C, Vithayasai V, Windecker P, Suskind R, Olson R (1977) Phagocytosis and Killing Function of Polymorphnuclear Leukocytes in Thai Children with Protein-Energy Malnutrition. In: Suskind RM, editor.Malnutrition and the Immune Response.New York: Raven Press. pp. 253–257.

105. Shousha S, Kamel K (1972) Nitro blue tetrazolium test in children with kwashiorkor with a comment on the use of latex particles in the test. J Clin Pathol 25: 494–497.

106. Forte WCN, Martins Campos JV, Leao RC (1984) Non specific immunological response in moderate malnutrition. Allergol Immunopathol (Madr) 12: 489–496.

107. Chhangani L, Sharma ML, Sharma UB, Joshi N (1985) In vitro study of phagocytic and bactericidal activity of neutrophils in cases of protein energy malnutrition. Indian J Pathol Microbiol 28: 199–203.

108. Bhaskaram P (1980) Macrophage function in severe protein energy malnutrition. Indian J Med Res 71: 247–250.

109. Bhaskaram P, Reddy V (1982) Macrophage function in kwashiorkor. Indian J Pediatr 49: 497–499.

110. Shilotri PG (1976) Hydrogen peroxide production by leukocytes in protein-calorie malnutrition. Clin Chim Acta Int J Clin Chem 71: 511–514.

111. Raman TS (1992) Nitroblue tetrazolium test in protein energy malnutrition. Indian Pediatr 29: 355–356.

112. Altay C, Dogramaci N, Bingol A, Say B (1972) Nitroblue tetrazolium test in children with malnutrition. J Pediatr 81: 392–393.

113. Machado RM, da Costa JC, de Lima Filho EC, Brasil MR, da Rocha GM (1985) Longitudinal study of the nitroblue tetrazolium test in children with protein-calorie malnutrition. J Trop Pediatr 31: 74–77.

114. Wolfsdorf J, Nolan R (1974) Leucocyte function in protein deficiency states. South Afr Med J Suid-Afr Tydskr Vir Geneeskd 48: 528–530.

115. Golden MH, Ramdath D (1987) Free radicals in the pathogenesis of kwashiorkor. Proc Nutr Soc 46: 53–68.

116. Shousha S, Kamel K, Ahmad KK (1974) Cytochemistry of polymorphonuclear neutrophil leukocytes in kwashiorkor. J Egypt Med Assoc 57: 298–308.

117. González C, Nájera O, Cortés E, Toledo G, López L, et al. (2002) Hydrogen peroxide-induced DNA damage and DNA repair in lymphocytes from malnourished children. Environ Mol Mutagen 39: 33–42.

118. González C, Nájera O, Cortés E, Toledo G, López L, et al. (2002) Susceptibility to DNA damage induced by antibiotics in lymphocytes from malnourished children. Teratog Carcinog Mutagen 22: 147–158.

119. Berczi I, Quintanar-Stephano A, Kovacs K (2009) Neuroimmune regulation in immunocompetence, acute illness, and healing. Ann N Y Acad Sci 1153: 220–239. doi:10.1111/j.1749-6632.2008.03975.x.

120. Reid M, Badaloo A, Forrester T, Morlese JF, Heird WC, et al. (2002) The acute-phase protein response to infection in edematous and nonedematous protein-energy malnutrition. Am J Clin Nutr 76: 1409–1415.

121. Morlese JF, Forrester T, Jahoor F (1998) Acute-phase protein response to infection in severe malnutrition. Am J Physiol 275: E112–117.

122. Malavé I, Vethencourt MA, Pirela M, Cordero R (1998) Serum levels of thyroxine-binding prealbumin, C-reactive protein and interleukin-6 in protein-energy undernourished children and normal controls without or with associated clinical infections. J Trop Pediatr 44: 256–262.

123. Sauerwein RW, Mulder JA, Mulder L, Lowe B, Peshu N, et al. (1997) Inflammatory mediators in children with protein-energy malnutrition. Am J Clin Nutr 65: 1534–1539.

124. Ekanem E, Umotong A, Raykundalia C, Catty D (1997) Serum C-reactive protein and C3 complement protein levels in severely malnourished Nigerian children with and without bacterial infections. Acta Pædiatrica 86: 1317–1320. doi:10.1111/j.1651-2227.1997.tb14905.x.

125. Razban SZ, Olusi SO, Ade-Serrano MA, Osunkoya BO, Adeshina HA, et al. (1975) Acute phase proteins in children with protein-calorie malnutrition. J Trop Med Hyg 78: 264–266.

126. El-Sayed HL, Nassar MF, Habib NM, Elmasry OA, Gomaa SM (2006) Structural and functional affection of the heart in protein energy malnutrition patients on admission and after nutritional recovery. Eur J Clin Nutr 60: 502–510. doi:10.1038/sj.ejcn.1602344.

127. McFarlane H (1977) Acute-Phase Proteins in Malnutrition. In: Suskind RM, editor.Malnutrition and the Immune Response.New York: Raven Press. pp. 403–405.

128. Salimonu LS (1985) Soluble immune complexes, acute phase proteins and E-rosette inhibitory substance in sera of malnourished children. Ann Trop Paediatr 5: 137–141.

129. Manary MJ, Yarasheski KE, Berger R, Abrams ET, Hart CA, et al. (2004) Whole-body leucine kinetics and the acute phase response during acute infection in marasmic Malawian children. Pediatr Res 55: 940–946. doi:10.1203/01.pdr.0000127017.44938.6d.

130. Nahani J, Nik-Aeen A, Rafii M, Mohagheghpour N (1976) Effect of malnutrition on several parameters of the immune system of children. Nutr Metab 20: 302–306.

131. Parent MA, Loening WE, Coovadia HM, Smythe PM (1974) Pattern of biochemical and immune recovery in protein calorie malnutrition. South Afr Med J Suid-Afr Tydskr Vir Geneeskd 48: 1375–1378.

132. Akenami FO, Koskiniemi M, Siimes MA, Ekanem EE, Bolarin DM, et al. (1997) Assessment of plasma fibronectin in malnourished Nigerian children. J Pediatr Gastroenterol Nutr 24: 183–188.

133. Hassanein el-S A, Assem HM, Rezk MM, el-Maghraby RM (1998) Study of plasma albumin, transferrin, and fibronectin in children with mild to moderate protein-energy malnutrition. J Trop Pediatr 44: 362–365.

134. Schelp FP, Thanangkul O, Supawan V, Pongpaew P (1980) α2HS-glycoprotein serum levels in protein–energy malnutrition. Br J Nutr 43: 381–383. doi:10.1079/BJN19800101.

135. Abiodun PO, Ihongbe JC, Dati F (1985) Decreased levels of alpha 2 HS-glycoprotein in children with protein-energy-malnutrition. Eur J Pediatr 144: 368–369.

136. Abiodun PO, Olomu IN (1987) Alpha 2 HS-glycoprotein levels in children with protein-energy malnutrition and infections. J Pediatr Gastroenterol Nutr 6: 271–275.

137. Doherty JF, Golden MH, Raynes JG, Griffin GE, McAdam KP (1993) Acute-phase protein response is impaired in severely malnourished children. Clin Sci Lond Engl 1979 84: 169–175.

138. Yoder MC, Anderson DC, Gopalakrishna GS, Douglas SD, Polin RA (1987) Comparison of serum fibronectin, prealbumin, and albumin concentrations during nutritional repletion in protein-calorie malnourished infants. J Pediatr Gastroenterol Nutr 6: 84–88.

139. Dao H, Delisle H, Fournier P (1992) Anthropometric status, serum prealbumin level and immune response to measles vaccination in Mali children. J Trop Pediatr 38: 179–184.

140. McMurray DN, Loomis SA, Casazza LJ, Rey H (1979) Influence of moderate malnutrition on morbidity and antibody response following vaccination with live, attenuated measles virus vaccine. Bull Pan Am Health Organ 13: 52–57.

141. Idris S, El Seed AM (1983) Measles vaccination in severely malnourished Sudanese children. Ann Trop Paediatr 3: 63–67.

142. Doherty JF, Golden MH, Griffin GE, McAdam KP (1989) Febrile response in malnutrition. West Indian Med J 38: 209–212.

143. Degn SE, Thiel S, Jensenius JC (2007) New perspectives on mannan-binding lectin-mediated complement activation. Immunobiology 212: 301–311. doi:10.1016/j.imbio.2006.12.004.

144. Ozkan H, Olgun N, Saşmaz E, Abacioğlu H, Okuyan M, et al. (1993) Nutrition, immunity and infections: T lymphocyte subpopulations in protein–energy malnutrition. J Trop Pediatr 39: 257–260.

145. Sakamoto M, Nishioka K (1992) Complement system in nutritional deficiency. World Rev Nutr Diet 67: 114–139.

146. Kumar R, Kumar A, Sethi RS, Gupta RK, Kaushik AK, et al. (1984) A study of complement activity in malnutrition. Indian Pediatr 21: 541–547.

147. Beatty DW, Dowdle EB (1978) The effects of kwashiorkor serum on lymphocyte transformation in vitro. Clin Exp Immunol 32: 134–143.

148. Haller L, Zubler RH, Lambert PH (1978) Plasma levels of complement components and complement haemolytic activity in protein-energy malnutrition. Clin Exp Immunol 34: 248–252.

149. Hafez M, Aref GH, Mehareb SW, Kassem AS, El-Tahhan H, et al. (1977) Antibody production and complement system in protein energy malnutrition. J Trop Med Hyg 80: 36–39.

150. Olusi SO, McFarlane H, Osunkoya BO, Adesina H (1975) Specific protein assays in protein-calorie malnutrition. Clin Chim Acta Int J Clin Chem 62: 107–116.

151. Olusi SO, McFarlane H, Ade-Serrano M, Osunkoya BO, Adesina H (1976) Complement components in children with protein-calorie malnutrition. Trop Geogr Med 28: 323–328.

152. Forte WC, Forte AC, Leão RC (1992) Complement system in malnutrition. Allergol Immunopathol (Madr) 20: 157–160.

153. Sirisinha S, Edelman R, Suskind R, Charupatana C, Olson RE (1973) Complement and C3-proactivator levels in children with protein-calorie malnutrition and effect of dietary treatment. Lancet 1: 1016–1020.

154. Kielman A (1977) Nutritional and Immune Responses of Subclinically Malnourished Indian Children. In: Suskind RM, editor. Malnutrition and the Immune Response. New York: Raven Press. pp. 429–440.

155. Abdulrhman MA, Nassar MF, Mostafa HW, El-Khayat ZA, Abu El Naga MW (2011) Effect of honey on 50% complement hemolytic activity in infants with protein energy malnutrition: a randomized controlled pilot study. J Med Food 14: 551–555. doi:10.1089/jmf.2010.0082.

156. Keusch GT, Torun B, Johnston RB Jr, Urrutia JJ (1984) Impairment of hemolytic complement activation by both classical and alternative pathways in serum from patients with kwashiorkor. J Pediatr 105: 434–436.

157. Suskind R, Edelman R, Kulapongs P, Pariyanonda A, Sirisinha S (1976) Complement activity in children with protein-calorie malnutrition. Am J Clin Nutr 29: 1089–1092.

158. Jahoor F, Badaloo A, Reid M, Forrester T (2008) Protein metabolism in severe childhood malnutrition. Ann Trop Paediatr 28: 87–101. doi:10.1179/146532808X302107.

159. Hasselbalch H, Ersbøll AK, Jeppesen DL, Nielsen MB (1999) Thymus size in infants from birth until 24 months of age evaluated by ultrasound. A longitudinal prediction model for the thymic index. Acta Radiol Stockh Swed 1987 40: 41–44.

160. Gui J, Mustachio LM, Su D-M, Craig RW (2012) Thymus Size and Age-related Thymic Involution: Early Programming, Sexual Dimorphism, Progenitors and Stroma. Aging Dis 3: 280–290.

161. Naeye RL (1965) Organ and cellular development in congenital heart disease and in alimentary malnutrition. J Pediatr 67: 447–458.

162. Watts T (1969) Thymus weights in malnourished children. J Trop Pediatr 15: 155–158.

163. Smythe PM, Brereton-Stiles GG, Grace HJ, Mafoyane A, Schonland M, et al. (1971) Thymolymphatic deficiency and depression of cell-mediated immunity in protein-calorie malnutrition. Lancet 2: 939–943.

164. Schonland M (1972) Depression of immunity in protein-calorie malnutrition: a post-mortem study. J Trop Pediatr Environ Child Health 18: 217–224.

165. Aref GH, Abdel-Aziz A, Elaraby II, Abdel-Moneim MA, Hebeishy NA, et al. (1982) A post-mortem study of the thymolymphatic system in protein energy malnutrition. J Trop Med Hyg 85: 109–114.

166. Jambon B, Ziegler O, Maire B, Hutin MF, Parent G, et al. (1988) Thymulin (facteur thymique serique) and zinc contents of the thymus glands of malnourished children. Am J Clin Nutr 48: 335–342.

167. Parent G, Chevalier P, Zalles L, Sevilla R, Bustos M, et al. (1994) In vitro lymphocyte-differentiating effects of thymulin (Zn-FTS) on lymphocyte subpopulations of severely malnourished children. Am J Clin Nutr 60: 274–278.

168. Chevalier P, Sevilla R, Zalles L, Sejas E, Belmonte G, et al. (1994) Study of thymus and thymocytes in Bolivian preschool children during recovery from severe acute malnutrition. J Nutr Immunol Vol 3, 1994: 27–39.

169. Chevalier P (1997) Thymic ultrasonography in children, a non-invasive assessment of nutritional immune deficiency. Nutr Res 17: 1271–1276. doi:10.1016/S0271-5317(97)00110-3.

170. Chevalier P, Sevilla R, Sejas E, Zalles L, Belmonte G, et al. (1998) Immune recovery of malnourished children takes longer than nutritional recovery: implications for treatment and discharge. J Trop Pediatr 44: 304–307.

171. Collinson AC, Moore SE, Cole TJ, Prentice AM (2003) Birth season and environmental influences on patterns of thymic growth in rural Gambian infants. Acta Paediatr Oslo Nor 1992 92: 1014–1020.

172. Garly M-L, Trautner SL, Marx C, Danebod K, Nielsen J, et al. (2008) Thymus size at 6 months of age and subsequent child mortality. J Pediatr 153: 683–688, 688.e1–3. doi:10.1016/j.jpeds.2008.04.069.

173. Moore SE, Prentice AM, Wagatsuma Y, Fulford AJC, Collinson AC, et al. (2009) Early-life nutritional and environmental determinants of thymic size in infants born in rural Bangladesh. Acta Paediatr Oslo Nor 1992 98: 1168–1175. doi:10.1111/j.1651-2227.2009.01292.x.

174. Hasselbalch H, Jeppesen DL, Engelmann MD, Michaelsen KF, Nielsen MB (1996) Decreased thymus size in formula-fed infants compared with breastfed infants. Acta Paediatr Oslo Nor 1992 85: 1029–1032.

175. Ngom PT, Collinson AC, Pido-Lopez J, Henson SM, Prentice AM, et al. (2004) Improved thymic function in exclusively breastfed infants is associated with higher interleukin 7 concentrations in their mothers' breast milk. Am J Clin Nutr 80: 722–728.

176. Moore SE, Fulford AJ, Wagatsuma Y, Persson LÅ, Arifeen SE, et al. (2013) Thymus development and infant and child mortality in rural Bangladesh. Int J Epidemiol. doi:10.1093/ije/dyt232.

177. McMurray DN, Loomis SA, Casazza LJ, Rey H, Miranda R (1981) Development of impaired cell-mediated immunity in mild and moderate malnutrition. Am J Clin Nutr 34: 68–77.

178. Greenwood BM, Bradley-Moore AM, Bradley AK, Kirkwood BR, Gilles HM (1986) The immune response to vaccination in undernourished and well-nourished Nigerian children. Ann Trop Med Parasitol 80: 537–544.

179. McMurray DN, Watson RR, Reyes MA (1981) Effect of renutrition on humoral and cell-mediated immunity in severely malnourished children. Am J Clin Nutr 34: 2117–2126.

180. Seth V, Kukreja N, Sundaram KR, Malaviya AN (1981) Delayed hypersensitivity after BCG in preschool children in relation to their nutritional status. Indian J Med Res 74: 392–398.

181. Satyanarayana K, Bhaskaram P, Seshu VC, Reddy V (1980) Influence of nutrition on postvaccinial tuberculin sensitivity. Am J Clin Nutr 33: 2334–2337.

182. Heyworth B (1977) Delayed hypersensitivity to PPD-S following BCG vaccination in African children–an 18-month field study. Trans R Soc Trop Med Hyg 71: 251–253.

183. Smith N, Khadroui S, Lopez V, Hamza B (1977) Cellular Immune Response in Tunisian Children with Severe Infantile Malnutrition. Malnutrition and the Immune Response, Edited by Robert Suskind. New York: Raven Press, Vol. 1977.

184. Abbassy AS, el-Din MK, Hassan AI, Aref GH, Hammad SA, et al. (1974) Studies of cell-mediated immunity and allergy in protein energy malnutrition. I. Cell-mediated delayed hypersensitivity. J Trop Med Hyg 77: 13–17.

185. Harland PS (1965) Tuberculin reactions in malnourished children. Lancet 2: 719–721.

186. Puri V, Misra PK, Saxena KC, Saxsena PN, Saxena RP, et al. (1980) Immune status in malnutrition. Indian Pediatr 17: 127–133.

187. Bhaskaram C, Reddy V (1974) Cell mediated immunity in protein-calorie malnutrition. J Trop Pediatr Environ Child Health 20: 284–286.

188. Edelman R (1973) Cutaneous hypersensitivity in protein-calorie malnutrition. Lancet 1: 1244–1245.

189. Geefhuysen J, Rosen EU, Katz J, Ipp T, Metz J (1971) Impaired cellular immunity in kwashiorkor with improvement after therapy. Br Med J 4: 527–529.

190. Castillo-Duran C, Heresi G, Fisberg M, Uauy R (1987) Controlled trial of zinc supplementation during recovery from malnutrition: effects on growth and immune function. Am J Clin Nutr 45: 602–608.

191. Fakhir S, Ahmad P, Faridi MA, Rattan A (1989) Cell-mediated immune responses in malnourished host. J Trop Pediatr 35: 175–178.

192. Schlesinger L, Stekel A (1974) Impaired cellular Immunity in marasmic infants. Am J Clin Nutr 27: 615–620.

193. Ziegler HD, Ziegler PB (1975) Depression of tuberculin reaction in mild and moderate protein-calorie malnourished children following BCG vaccination. Johns Hopkins Med J 137: 59–64.

194. Golden MH, Harland PS, Golden BE, Jackson AA (1978) Zinc and immunocompetence in protein-energy malnutrition. Lancet 1: 1226–1228.

195. Schlesinger L, Arevalo M, Arredondo S, Diaz M, Lönnerdal B, et al. (1992) Effect of a zinc-fortified formula on immunocompetence and growth of malnourished infants. Am J Clin Nutr 56: 491–498.

196. Schlesinger L, Ohlbaum A, Grez L, Stekel A (1977) Cell-mediated Immune studies in Marasmic Children from Chile: Delayed Hypersensitivity, Lymphocyte transformation, and Interferon Production. Suskind RM, editor. Malnutrition and the Immune Response. New York: Raven Press, Vol. 1977.

197. Wander K, Shell-Duncan B, Brindle E, O'Connor K (2013) Predictors of delayed-type hypersensitivity to Candida albicans and anti-Epstein-Barr virus antibody among children in Kilimanjaro, Tanzania. Am J Phys Anthropol 151: 183–190. doi:10.1002/ajpa.22250.

198. Hughes SM, Amadi B, Mwiya M, Nkamba H, Mulundu G, et al. (2009) CD4 counts decline despite nutritional recovery in HIV-infected Zambian children with severe malnutrition. Pediatrics 123: e347–351. doi:10.1542/peds.2008-1316.

199. Olusi SO, Thurman GB, Goldstein AL (1980) Effect of thymosin on T-lymphocyte rosette formation in children with kwashiorkor. Clin Immunol Immunopathol 15: 687–691.

200. Mahalanabis D, Jalan KN, Chatterjee A, Maitra TK, Agarwal SK, et al. (1979) Evidence for altered density characteristics of the peripheral blood lymphocytes in kwashiorkor. Am J Clin Nutr 32: 992–996.

201. González C, González H, Rodríguez L, Cortés L, Nájera O, et al. (2006) Differential gene expression in lymphocytes from malnourished children. Cell Biol Int 30: 610–614. doi:10.1016/j.cellbi.2006.02.011.

202. El-Hodhod MAA, Nassar MF, Zaki MM, Moustafa A (2005) Apoptotic changes in lymphocytes of protein energy malnutrition patients. Nutr Res 25: 21–29. doi:10.1016/j.nutres.2004.10.005.

203. Ferguson AC, Lawlor GJ Jr, Neumann CG, Oh W, Stiehm ER (1974) Decreased rosette-forming lymphocytes in malnutrition and intrauterine growth retardation. J Pediatr 85: 717–723.

204. Bang BG, Mahalanabis D, Mukherjee KL, Bang FB (1975) T and B lymphocyte rosetting in undernourished children. Proc Soc Exp Biol Med Soc Exp Biol Med N Y N 149: 199–202.

205. Rabson AR, Geefhuyzen J, Rosen EU, Joffe M (1975) Letter: Rosette-forming T-lymphocytes in malnutrition. Br Med J 1: 40.

206. Salimonu LS, Johnson AO, Williams AI, Adeleye GI, Osunkoya BO (1982) Lymphocyte subpopulations and antibody levels in immunized malnourished children. Br J Nutr 48: 7–14.

207. Joffe MI, Kew M, Rabson AR (1983) Lymphocyte subtypes in patients with atopic eczema, protein calorie malnutrition, SLE and liver disease. J Clin Lab Immunol 10: 97–101.

208. Cruz JR, Chew F, Fernandez RA, Torun B, Goldstein AL, et al. (1987) Effects of nutritional recuperation on E-rosetting lymphocytes and in vitro response to thymosin in malnourished children. J Pediatr Gastroenterol Nutr 6: 387–391.

209. Keusch GT, Cruz JR, Torun B, Urrutia JJ, Smith H Jr, et al. (1987) Immature circulating lymphocytes in severely malnourished Guatemalan children. J Pediatr Gastroenterol Nutr 6: 265–270.

210. Fakhir S, Ahmed P, Faridi MM, Rattan A (1988) Early rosette forming T cell–a marker of cellular immunodeficiency in PEM. Indian Pediatr 25: 1017–1018.

211. Hagel I, Lynch NR, Puccio F, Rodriguez O, Luzondo R, et al. (2003) Defective regulation of the protective IgE response against intestinal helminth Ascaris lumbricoides in malnourished children. J Trop Pediatr 49: 136–142.

212. Nájera O, González C, Cortés E, Betancourt M, Ortiz R, et al. (2002) Early Activation of T, B and NK Lymphocytes in Infected Malnourished and Infected Well-Nourished Children. J Nutr Immunol 5: 85–97. doi:10.1300/J053v05n03_07.

213. Kulapongs P, Suskind R, Vithayasai V, Olson R (1977) In Vitro Cell-Mediated Immune Response in Thai Children with Protein-Calorie Malnutrition. Malnutrition and the Immune Response, Edited by Robert M Suskind. New York: Raven Press, Vol. 1977.

214. Grace HJ, Armstrong D, Smythe PM (1972) Reduced lymphocyte transformation in protein calorie malnutrition. South Afr Med J Suid-Afr Tydskr Vir Geneeskd 46: 402–403.

215. Murthy PB, Rahiman MA, Tulpule PG (1982) Lymphocyte proliferation kinetics in malnourished children measured by differential chromatid staining. Br J Nutr 47: 445–450.

216. Ortiz R, Campos C, Gómez JL, Espinoza M, Ramos-Motilla M, et al. (1995) Effect of renutrition on the proliferation kinetics of PHA stimulated lymphocytes from malnourished children. Mutat Res 334: 235–241.

217. Moore DL, Heyworth B, Brown J (1974) PHA-induced lymphocyte transformations in leucocyte cultures from malarious, malnourished and control Gambian children. Clin Exp Immunol 17: 647–656.

218. Moore DL, Heyworth B, Brown J (1977) Effects of autologous plasma on lymphocyte transformation in malaria and in acute protein-energy malnutrition. Comparison of purified lymphocyte and whole blood cultures. Immunology 33: 777–785.

219. Noureldin MS, Shaltout AA, El Hamshary EM, Ali ME (1999) Opportunistic intestinal protozoal infections in immunocompromised children. J Egypt Soc Parasitol 29: 951–961.

220. Bachou H, Tylleskär T, Downing R, Tumwine JK (2006) Severe malnutrition with and without HIV-1 infection in hospitalised children in Kampala, Uganda: differences in clinical features, haematological findings and CD4+ cell counts. Nutr J 5: 27–27. doi:10.1186/1475-2891-5-27.

221. Ndagije F, Baribwira C, Coulter JBS (2007) Micronutrients and T-cell subsets: a comparison between HIV-infected and uninfected, severely malnourished Rwandan children. Ann Trop Paediatr 27: 269–275. doi:10.1179/146532807X245652.

222. Rodríguez L, González C, Flores L, Jiménez-Zamudio L, Graniel J, et al. (2005) Assessment by flow cytometry of cytokine production in malnourished children. Clin Diagn Lab Immunol 12: 502–507. doi:10.1128/CDLI.12.4.502-507.2005.

223. Rodríguez L, Graniel J, Ortiz R (2007) Effect of leptin on activation and cytokine synthesis in peripheral blood lymphocytes of malnourished infected children. Clin Exp Immunol 148: 478–485. doi:10.1111/j.1365-2249.2007.03361.x.

224. Fakhir S, Ahmad P, Faridi MM, Rattan A (1988) Serum immunoglobulins and B cell count in protein energy malnutrition. Indian Pediatr 25: 960–965.

225. Rosen EU, Geefhuysen J, Ipp T (1971) Immunoglobulin levels in protein calorie malnutrition. South Afr Med J Suid-Afr Tydskr Vir Geneeskd 45: 980–982.

226. Cohen S, Hansen JD (1962) Metabolism of albumin and gamma-globulin in kwashiorkor. Clin Sci 23: 351–359.

227. Najjar SS, Stephan M, Asfour RY (1969) Serum levels of immunoglobulins in marasmic infants. Arch Dis Child 44: 120–123.

228. Keet MP, Thom H (1969) Serum immunoglobulins in kwashiorkor. Arch Dis Child 44: 600–603.

229. Watson CE, Freesemann C (1970) Immunoglobulins in protein-calorie malnutrition. Arch Dis Child 45: 282–284.

230. el-Gholmy A, Helmy O, Hashish S, Ragan HA, el-Gamal Y (1970) Immunoglobulins in marasmus. J Trop Med Hyg 73: 196–199.

231. el-Gholmy A, Hashish S, Helmy O, Aly RH, el-Gamal Y (1970) A study of immunoglobulins in kwashiorkor. J Trop Med Hyg 73: 192–195.

232. Aref GH, el-Din MK, Hassan AI, Araby II (1970) Immunoglobulins in kwashiorkor. J Trop Med Hyg 73: 186–191.

233. Suskind R, Sirisinha S, Vithayasai V, Edelman R, Damrongsak D, et al. (1976) Immunoglobulins and antibody response in children with protein-calorie malnutrition. Am J Clin Nutr 29: 836–841.

234. Awdeh ZL, Kanawati AK, Alami SY (1977) Antibody response in marasmic children during recovery. Acta Paediatr Scand 66: 689–692.

235. Cripps AW, Otczyk DC, Barker J, Lehmann D, Alpers MP (2008) The relationship between undernutrition and humoral immune status in children with pneumonia in Papua New Guinea. P N G Med J 51: 120–130.

236. Casazza IJ, Sunoto S, Sugiono M (1972) Immunoglobulin levels in malnourished children. Paediatr Indones 12: 263–270.

237. Taddesse WW (1988) Immunoglobulins in kwashiorkor. East Afr Med J 65: 393–396.

238. Suskind R, Sirisinha S, Edelman R, Vithayasai V, Damrongsak D, et al. (1977) Immunoglobulins and Antibody Response in Thai Children with Protein-Calirie Malnutrition. Suskind RM, editor. Malnutrition and the Immune Response. New York: Raven Press, Vol. 1977.

239. Forte WCN, Santos de Menezes MC, Horta C, Carneiro Leão Bach R (2003) Serum IgE level in malnutrition. Allergol Immunopathol (Madr) 31: 83–86.

240. Pretorius PJ, De Villiers LS (1962) Antibody response in children with protein malnutrition. Am J Clin Nutr 10: 379–383.

241. el-Gamal Y, Aly RH, Hossny E, Afify E, el-Taliawy D (1996) Response of Egyptian infants with protein calorie malnutrition to hepatitis B vaccination. J Trop Pediatr 42: 144–145.

242. Powell GM (1982) Response to live attenuated measles vaccine in children with severe kwashiorkor. Ann Trop Paediatr 2: 143–145.

243. Brown RE, Katz M (1966) Failure of antibody production to yellow fever vaccine in children with kwashiorkor. Trop Geogr Med 18: 125–128.

244. Brown RE, Katz M (1965) Antigenic Stimulation in Undernourished Children. East Afr Med J 42: 221–232.

245. Wesley A, Coovadia HM, Watson AR (1979) Immunization against measles in children at risk for severe disease. Trans R Soc Trop Med Hyg 73: 710–715.

246. el-Molla A, el-Ghoroury A, Hussein M, Badr-el-Din MK, Hassen AH, et al. (1973) Antibody production in protein calorie malnutrition. J Trop Med Hyg 76: 248–250.

247. Reddy V, Srikantia SG (1964) Antibody Response in Kwashiorkor. Indian J Med Res 52: 1154–1158.

248. Brown RE, Katz M (1966) Smallpox vaccination in malnourished children. Trop Geogr Med 18: 129–132.

249. Paul S, Saini L, Grover S, Ray K, Ray SN, et al. (1979) Immune response in malnutrition–study following routine DPT immunization! Indian Pediatr 16: 3–10.

250. Ekunwe EO (1985) Malnutrition and seroconversion following measles immunization. J Trop Pediatr 31: 290–291.

251. Halsey NA, Boulos R, Mode F, Andre J, Bowman L, et al. (1985) Response to measles vaccine in Haitian infants 6 to 12 months old. Influence of maternal antibodies, malnutrition, and concurrent illnesses. N Engl J Med 313: 544–549. doi:10.1056/NEJM198508293130904.

252. Baer CL, Bratt DE, Edwards R, McFarlane H, Utermohlen V (1986) Response of mildly to moderately malnourished children to measles vaccination. West Indian Med J 35: 106–111.

253. Smedman L, Silva MC, Gunnlaugsson G, Norrby E, Zetterstrom R (1986) Augmented antibody response to live attenuated measles vaccine in children with Plasmodium falciparum parasitaemia. Ann Trop Paediatr 6: 149–153.

254. Smedman L, Gunnlaugsson G, Norrby E, Silva MC, Zetterström R (1988) Follow-up of the antibody response to measles vaccine in a rural area of Guinea-Bissau. Acta Paediatr Scand 77: 885–889.

255. Bhaskaram P, Madhusudan J, Radhrakrishna KV, Raj S (1986) Immunological response to measles vaccination in poor communities. Hum Nutr Clin Nutr 40: 295–299.

256. Chopra K, Kundu S, Chowdhury DS (1989) Antibody response of infants in tropics to five doses of oral polio vaccine. J Trop Pediatr 35: 19–23.

257. Greenwood BM, Bradley AK, Blakebrough IS, Whittle HC, Marshall TF, et al. (1980) The immune response to a meningococcal polysaccharide vaccine in an African village. Trans R Soc Trop Med Hyg 74: 340–346.

258. Asturias EJ, Mayorga C, Caffaro C, Ramirez P, Ram M, et al. (2009) Differences in the immune response to hepatitis B and Haemophilus influenzae type b vaccines in Guatemalan infants by ethnic group and nutritional status. Vaccine 27: 3650–3654. doi:10.1016/j.vaccine.2009.03.035.

259. Waibale P, Bowlin SJ, Mortimer EA Jr, Whalen C (1999) The effect of human immunodeficiency virus-1 infection and stunting on measles immunoglobulin-G levels in children vaccinated against measles in Uganda. Int J Epidemiol 28: 341–346.

260. Kahn E, Stein H, Zoutendyk A (1957) Isohemagglutinins and immunity in malnutrition. Am J Clin Nutr 5: 70–71.

261. Fillol F, Sarr JB, Boulanger D, Cisse B, Sokhna C, et al. (2009) Impact of child malnutrition on the specific anti-Plasmodium falciparum antibody response. Malar J 8: 116. doi:10.1186/1475-2875-8-116.

262. Brüssow H, Sidoti J, Dirren H, Freire WB (1995) Effect of malnutrition in Ecuadorian children on titers of serum antibodies to various microbial antigens. Clin Diagn Lab Immunol 2: 62–68.

263. Lomnitzer R, Rosen EU, Geefhuysen J, Rabson AR (1976) Defective leucocyte inhibitory factor (LIF) production by lymphocytes in children with kwashiorkor. South Afr Med J Suid-Afr Tydskr Vir Geneeskd 50: 1820–1822.

264. Heresi GP, Saitúa MT, Schlesinger L (1981) Leukocyte migration inhibition factor production in marasmic infants. Am J Clin Nutr 34: 909–913.

265. Salimonu LS, Johnson AO, Williams AI, Adeleye GI, Osunkoya BO (1982) The occurrence and properties of E rosette inhibitory substance in the sera of malnourished children. Clin Exp Immunol 47: 626–634.

266. Kobielowa Z, Turowski G, Szumera B, Lankosz-Lauterbach J (1979) Direct lymphocytotoxic test in protein-calorie malnutrition in infants. Acta Med Pol 20: 265–272.

267. Beatty DW, Dowdle EB (1979) Deficiency in kwashiorkor serum of factors required for optimal lymphocyte transformation in vitro. Clin Exp Immunol 35: 433–442.

268. Heyworth B, Moore DL, Brown J (1975) Depression of lymphocyte response to phytohaemagglutinin in the presence of plasma from children with acute protein energy malnutrition. Clin Exp Immunol 22: 72–77.

269. Bhaskaram P, Sivakumar B (1986) Interleukin-1 in malnutrition. Arch Dis Child 61: 182–185.

270. Aslan Y, Erduran E, Gedik Y, Mocan H, Okten A, et al. (1996) Serum interleukin-1 and granulocyte-macrophage colony-stimulating factor levels in protein malnourished patients during acute infection. Cent Afr J Med 42: 179–184.

271. Dülger H, Arik M, Sekeroğlu MR, Tarakçioğlu M, Noyan T, et al. (2002) Pro-inflammatory cytokines in Turkish children with protein-energy malnutrition. Mediators Inflamm 11: 363–365. doi:10.1080/0962935021000051566.

272. Bartz S, Mody A, Hornik C, Bain J, Muehlbauer M, et al. (2014) Severe acute malnutrition in childhood: hormonal and metabolic status at presentation, response to treatment, and predictors of mortality. J Clin Endocrinol Metab 99: 2128–2137. doi:10.1210/jc.2013-4018.

273. González-Martínez H, Rodríguez L, Nájera O, Cruz D, Miliar A, et al. (2008) Expression of cytokine mRNA in lymphocytes of malnourished children. J Clin Immunol 28: 593–599. doi:10.1007/s10875-008-9204-5.

274. González-Torres C, González-Martínez H, Miliar A, Nájera O, Graniel J, et al. (2013) Effect of malnutrition on the expression of cytokines involved in Th1 cell differentiation. Nutrients 5: 579–593. doi:10.3390/nu5020579.

275. Solis B, Samartín S, Gómez S, Nova E, de la Rosa B, et al. (2002) Probiotics as a help in children suffering from malnutrition and diarrhoea. Eur J Clin Nutr 56 Suppl 3: S57–59. doi:10.1038/sj.ejcn.1601488.

276. Palacio A, Lopez M, Perez-Bravo F, Monkeberg F, Schlesinger L (2002) Leptin levels are associated with immune response in malnourished infants. J Clin Endocrinol Metab 87: 3040–3046.

277. Abo-Shousha SA, Hussein MZ, Rashwan IA, Salama M (2005) Production of proinflammatory cytokines: granulocyte-macrophage colony stimulating factor, interleukin-8 and interleukin-6 by peripheral blood mononuclear cells of protein energy malnourished children. Egypt J Immunol Egypt Assoc Immunol 12: 125–131.

278. Doherty JF, Golden MH, Remick DG, Griffin GE (1994) Production of interleukin-6 and tumour necrosis factor-alpha in vitro is reduced in whole blood of severely malnourished children. Clin Sci Lond Engl 1979 86: 347–351.

279. Giovambattista A, Spinedi E, Sanjurjo A, Chisari A, Rodrigo M, et al. (2000) Circulating and mitogen-induced tumor necrosis factor (TNF) in malnourished children. Medicina (Mex) 60: 339–342.

280. Hemalatha R, Bhaskaram P, Balakrishna N, Saraswathi I (2002) Association of tumour necrosis factor alpha & malnutrition with outcome in children with acute bacterial meningitis. Indian J Med Res 115: 55–58.

281. Mayatepek E, Becker K, Hoffmann G, Leichsenring M, Gana L (1993) Leukotrienes in the pathophysiology of kwashiorkor. The Lancet 342: 958–960. doi:10.1016/0140-6736(93)92003-C.

282. Iputo JE, Sammon AM, Tindimwebwa G (2002) Prostaglandin E2 is raised in kwashiorkor. South Afr Med J Suid-Afr Tydskr Vir Geneeskd 92: 310–312.

283. Morgan G (1997) What, if any, is the effect of malnutrition on immunological competence? Lancet 349: 1693–1695. doi:10.1016/S0140-6736(96)12038-9.

284. Saxinger WC, Levine PH, Dean AG, de Thé G, Lange-Wantzin G, et al. (1985) Evidence for exposure to HTLV-III in Uganda before 1973. Science 227: 1036–1038.

285. Prendergast A, Kelly P (2012) Enteropathies in the developing world: neglected effects on global health. Am J Trop Med Hyg 86: 756–763. doi:10.4269/ajtmh.2012.11-0743.

286. Keusch GT, Rosenberg IH, Denno DM, Duggan C, Guerrant RL, et al. (2013) Implications of acquired environmental enteric dysfunction for growth and stunting in infants and children living in low- and middle-income countries. Food Nutr Bull 34: 357–364.

287. Campbell DI, Elia M, Lunn PG (2003) Growth faltering in rural Gambian infants is associated with impaired small intestinal barrier function, leading to endotoxemia and systemic inflammation. J Nutr 133: 1332–1338.

288. Basso AS, Cheroutre H, Mucida D (2009) More stories on Th17 cells. Cell Res 19: 399–411. doi:10.1038/cr.2009.26.

289. Opal SM, DePalo VA (2000) Anti-inflammatory cytokines. Chest 117: 1162–1172.

290. Manary MJ, Yarasheski KE, Smith S, Abrams ET, Hart CA (2004) Protein quantity, not protein quality, accelerates whole-body leucine kinetics and the acute-phase response during acute infection in marasmic Malawian children. Br J Nutr 92: 589–595.

291. Howard JK, Lord GM, Matarese G, Vendetti S, Ghatei MA, et al. (1999) Leptin protects mice from starvation-induced lymphoid atrophy and increases thymic cellularity in ob/ob mice. J Clin Invest 104: 1051–1059. doi:10.1172/JCI6762.

292. De Mello-Coelho V, Savino W, Postel-Vinay MC, Dardenne M (1998) Role of prolactin and growth hormone on thymus physiology. Dev Immunol 6: 317–323.

293. Savino W, Postel-Vinay MC, Smaniotto S, Dardenne M (2002) The thymus gland: a target organ for growth hormone. Scand J Immunol 55: 442–452.

294. Hansen BR, Kolte L, Haugaard SB, Dirksen C, Jensen FK, et al. (2009) Improved thymic index, density and output in HIV-infected patients following low-dose growth hormone therapy: a placebo controlled study. AIDS Lond Engl 23: 2123–2131. doi:10.1097/QAD.0b013e3283303307.

295. Barone KS, O'Brien PC, Stevenson JR (1993) Characterization and mechanisms of thymic atrophy in protein-malnourished mice: role of corticosterone. Cell Immunol 148: 226–233. doi:10.1006/cimm.1993.1105.

296. Haeryfar SM, Berczi I (2001) The thymus and the acute phase response. Cell Mol Biol Noisy-Gd Fr 47: 145–156.

297. Golden MH, Jackson AA, Golden BE (1977) Effect of zinc on thymus of recently malnourished children. Lancet 2: 1057–1059.

298. Chevalier P (1995) Zinc and duration of treatment of severe malnutrition. Lancet 345: 1046–1047.

299. Miedema F, Hazenberg MD, Tesselaar K, van Baarle D, de Boer RJ, et al. (2013) Immune Activation and Collateral Damage in AIDS Pathogenesis. Front Immunol 4: 298. doi:10.3389/fimmu.2013.00298.

300. Cobbold SP (2013) The mTOR pathway and integrating immune regulation. Immunology. doi:10.1111/imm.12162.

301. Peter C, Waldmann H, Cobbold SP (2010) mTOR signalling and metabolic regulation of T cell differentiation. Curr Opin Immunol 22: 655–661. doi:10.1016/j.coi.2010.08.010.

302. Monk JM, Steevels TAM, Hillyer LM, Woodward B (2011) Constitutive, but not challenge-induced, interleukin-10 production is robust in acute pre-

pubescent protein and energy deficits: new support for the tolerance hypothesis of malnutrition-associated immune depression based on cytokine production in vivo. Int J Environ Res Public Health 8: 117–135. doi:10.3390/ijerph8010117.

303. Monk JM, Richard CL, Woodward B (2011) A non-inflammatory form of immune competence prevails in acute pre-pubescent malnutrition: new evidence based on critical mRNA transcripts in the mouse. Br J Nutr: 1–5. doi:10.1017/S0007114511004399.

304. Lo MS, Zurakowski D, Son MB, Sundel RP (2013) Hypergammaglobulinemia in the pediatric population as a marker for underlying autoimmune disease: a retrospective cohort study. Pediatr Rheumatol Online J 11: 42. doi:10.1186/1546-0096-11-42.

305. Chen M, Daha MR, Kallenberg CGM (2010) The complement system in systemic autoimmune disease. J Autoimmun 34: J276–J286. doi:10.1016/j.jaut.2009.11.014.

20

Understanding Inequalities in Child Health in Ethiopia: Health Achievements Are Improving in the Period 2000–2011

Eirin Krüger Skaftun[1]*, Merima Ali[2], Ole Frithjof Norheim[1]

1 Department of Global Public Health and Primary Care, University of Bergen, Bergen, Norway, **2** Chr. Michelsen Institute, Bergen, Norway

Abstract

Objective: In Ethiopia, coverage of key health services is low, and community based services have been implemented to improve access to key services. This study aims to describe and assess the level and the distribution of health outcomes and coverage for key services in Ethiopia, and their association with socioeconomic and geographic determinants.

Methods: Data were obtained from the 2000, 2005 and 2011 Ethiopian Demographic and Health Surveys. As indicators of access to health care, the following variables were included: Under-five and neonatal deaths, skilled birth attendance, coverage of vaccinations, oral rehydration therapy for diarrhoea, and antibiotics for suspected pneumonia. For each of the indicators in 2011, inequality was described by estimating their concentration index and a geographic Gini index. For further assessment of the inequalities, the concentration indices were decomposed. An index of health achievement, integrating mean coverage and the distribution of coverage, was estimated. Changes from 2000 to 2011 in coverage, inequality and health achievement were assessed.

Results: Significant pro-rich inequalities were found for all indicators except treatment for suspected pneumonia in 2011. The geographic Gini index showed significant regional inequality for most indicators. The decomposition of the 2011 concentration indices revealed that the factor contributing the most to the observed inequalities was different levels of wealth. The mean of all indicators improved from 2000 to 2011, and the health achievement index improved for most indicators. The socioeconomic inequalities seem to increase from 2000 to 2011 for under-five and neonatal deaths, whereas they are stable or decreasing for the other indicators.

Conclusion: There is an unequal socioeconomic and geographic distribution of health and access to key services in Ethiopia. Although the health achievement indices improved for most indicators from 2000 to 2011, socioeconomic determinants need to be addressed in order to achieve better and more fairly distributed health.

Editor: Claire Thorne, UCL Institute of Child Health, University College London, United Kingdom

Funding: This study was funded through the Medical Students Research Program/the Norwegian Research Council, a NORAD/Norwegian Research Council grant (#218694) and the University of Bergen. The funders had no role in study design, data collection and analysis, decision to publish, or preparation of the manuscript.

Competing Interests: The authors have declared that no competing interests exist.

* Email: eirin.skaftun@igs.uib.no

Introduction

Evidence from low and middle income countries worldwide shows that health outcomes and access to key services are unevenly distributed across different subgroups of the population. Children from socioeconomically disadvantaged households have higher mortality rates and lower coverage of key services than children from more affluent households [1–4]. Geographic factors such as region of residence and distance to health facilities also influence mortality rates and coverage of health services [5–8]. The majority of child deaths occur from causes that are easily prevented or treated; they are therefore unnecessary and may be considered unfair [9].

Inequalities across socioeconomic groups are generally considered to be unfair, but the standardly reported measures of mean levels of health and health service coverage in the population do not tell us enough to assess the overall distribution. There is therefore a need to go beyond averages measures [10,11].

An increase of the mean level of health and coverage may be accompanied by decreasing inequalities across the population [12], but an improvement of the mean level may also be associated with increasing inequalities [13,14]. Policy makers may be willing to trade off equality against improvements of the mean level; a small increase of inequality may be acceptable if the mean increases, while a small increase of the mean and a large increase in inequality is not acceptable. It is therefore important to monitor health and access to key services, as well as the distribution of these in the population in order to develop and evaluate policies aimed at health and reducing inequities in health.

The per capita health expenditure in Ethiopia has increased substantially since 2000. The World Health Statistics published by the World Health Organization (WHO) estimates that the total per capita health expenditure in 2000 was 20 $ int. PPP, of which 11 were government expenditures [15]. In 2010 the total health expenditure per capita has increased to50 $ int. PPP, of which 26 were paid by the government.

In 2003 the Ethiopian government started the implementation of the Health Extension Programme to increase primary health care coverage on the community level. This is the basic level of health care in Ethiopia, consisting of one health post and two associated health extension workers. On average, one health post serves a *Kebele* (county) of 5000 inhabitants. The goals of this programme include improving access to key preventive and curative health services for everyone, with a special focus on maternal and child health [16].

According to the WHO's African Health Observatory, the under-five mortality rate in Ethiopia decreased from 198 to 77 deaths per 1000 live births from 1990 to 2011, corresponding to an annual rate of reduction of 4.5 per cent [17]. Over the same period improvements are also seen for key services such as coverage of measles vaccinations for one-year-olds, increasing from 38 per cent to 57 per cent. However, coverage of key services in Ethiopia remains among the lowest in Africa, as seen in skilled birth attendance, where Ethiopia has the lowest coverage of all the countries included in the African Health Observatory.

Child health outcomes and access to essential maternal and child health services are not equally distributed across all parts of the Ethiopian population. Studies have shown regional differences in coverage for maternal and child health services, and the services are more likely to be used by mothers with formal education, those living in urban areas and the richer parts of the population [18–21]. Hosseinpoor et al. found substantial wealth-related inequalities in coverage for several maternal and child health services in Ethiopia [22], and a study on the trends and determinants of neonatal mortality in Ethiopia finds, among other factors, the mother's level of education and region of residence to be associated with the probability of survival [23].

To develop policies aiming at reducing inequality in health outcomes and access to key services, it is important for policy makers to better understand the existing inequalities. There is limited evidence on the combined trends in level and distribution of child health and the underlying factors, that is, information that is necessary to address these challenges in a national context. The objective of this study is to describe the combined level and distribution of coverage for key child health services and outcomes in Ethiopia, and to analyse their association with socioeconomic and geographic determinants.

Methods

Data and variables

Data were obtained from the Ethiopian Demographic and Health Surveys (DHS) conducted in 2000, 2005 and 2011 [24–26]. These surveys are nationally representative, with sample sizes of 14072, 13721 and 16702 households respectively. For the respective surveys, information was collected on 10873, 9861 and 11654 children. Six different indicators capturing health outcomes and preventive and curative key services were selected for the analysis: Under-five deaths, neonatal deaths, coverage of skilled birth attendance, coverage of basic vaccinations, coverage of oral rehydration therapy for diarrhoea and coverage of antibiotics for suspected pneumonia. Under-five and neonatal deaths are defined as the proportion of live born children who die before the age of five years and four weeks respectively. Skilled birth attendance is defined as the proportion of women reporting that they were assisted by a doctor or a nurse during delivery. Vaccination

coverage is defined as the proportion of children aged 12 to 23 months who, at the time of the survey, had received the following vaccines: three doses of DPT, three doses of polio, BCG and measles. Treatment for diarrhoea and suspected pneumonia is defined as the proportion of those reporting symptoms in the past two weeks who have been given oral rehydration therapy (oral rehydration solution or recommended home solution) and antibiotics respectively. The data from the DHS are complimented by the 2007 Population and Housing Census of Ethiopia to obtain population data [27].

Geographic inequality

The degree of geographic inequality was measured for each of the health indicators in 2011 by what we call the geographic Gini index. The Gini index is closely related to the Lorenz curve, which plots the cumulative proportion of the outcome variable against the cumulative proportion of people ranked by the outcome. The Gini index is defined as twice the area between the Lorenz curve and the diagonal line, called the "line of equality". The geographic Gini index was calculated for each of the indicators in 2011 based on each region ranked from worst to best achievement of the indicator, and weighed by population size, using the following formula [28]:

$$G = \frac{2}{\mu} \sum_{t=1}^{T} \mu_t \times f_t \times R_t - 1 \qquad (1)$$

Where μ is the mean of the health variable in the entire population, T the number of groups, μ_t the mean of the health variable in the tth region ant f_t its population share. R_t is the relative rank of the tth region ranked by the health variable.

Socioeconomic inequality

The degree of socioeconomic inequality for each of the indicators in 2011 was quantified by the concentration index. The concentration index is analogous to the Gini index, but uses a measure of socioeconomic status for ranking the observations. The concentration index is related to the concentration curve, which plots the cumulative proportion of the outcome variable against the cumulative proportion of the population ranked by a measure of socioeconomic status [28,29]. The DHS does not contain data on household income or consumption, but the dataset contains a wealth index which was used as a measure of socioeconomic position. This index is calculated by principal component analysis, based on information on household assets (table, radio, refrigerator etc.) and household characteristics (building material, source of drinking water, toilet facilities etc.) [30].

The concentration index equals twice the area between the concentration curve and the line of equality, and for a health variable y it can be expressed as follows [28]:

$$C = \frac{2}{n \times \mu} \sum_{i=1}^{n} y_i \times R_i - 1 \qquad (2)$$

Where C denotes the concentration index, n is the number of observations, μ is the mean of the health variable y, and R is the fractional rank of the individuals by the household's socioeconomic status. The concentration index takes a value between -1 and 1. By convention, the concentration index will take a positive value if the variable in question is more prevalent among the rich, and conversely, a negative value if the variable is more prevalent among the poor. If there is no socioeconomic inequality, the concentration index will take the value 0.

Decomposition of the concentration index

The concentration indices of the health indicators in 2011 were decomposed in order to determine the contribution of different factors to the overall socioeconomic inequality. The factors included in the decomposition analysis were: mother's education, region of residence, and household's wealth. The factors were chosen on the basis of the conceptual framework used by the WHO and the Commission on Social Determinants of Health [31]. Education was included as a continuous variable, corresponding to the numbers of years of schooling the respondent reported having completed, ranging from zero to eight years. The household's wealth was included as a continuous variable, using the wealth index estimated by the DHS. The 11 regions were included as binary variables in the analysis, with one region chosen as reference on the basis of progress towards the United Nations fourth Millennium Development Goal. The United Nation's fourth Millennium Development Goal calls for a reduction of the under-five mortality by two thirds from 1990 to 2015, which for Ethiopia signifies a reduction from 204 to 68 deaths per 1000 live births over this period. The capital region, Addis Ababa, had already reached this goal in 2011 with 53 deaths per 1000 live births according to the estimates done by the DHS [26], but as this region is not representative for the country, it was not chosen as reference region. The region, apart from Addis Ababa, that is closest to achieving the Millennium Goal is Tigray, with an under-five mortality rate of 85 per 1000 live births. The Tigray region was therefore selected as a reference region for the analysis.

The decomposition of the concentration index has been explained in detail elsewhere [29,32]. In summary, a decomposition of the concentration index links the different indicators of child health to a set of K determinants, $x_1, ..., x_k$, by linear regression:

$$y = \alpha + \sum_{k=1}^{K} \beta_k x_k + \varepsilon \tag{3}$$

Where y is the indicator in question and ε is an error term. Given the relationship between y_i and x_{ki} in equation (3), we get:

$$C = \sum_{k=1}^{K} \frac{\beta_k \overline{x}_k}{\mu} C_k + \frac{GC_\varepsilon}{\mu} \tag{4}$$

Where C is the concentration index, β_k is the regression coefficient in equation (3), is the mean of the determinant k, μ is the mean of the outcome variable y and C_k is the concentration index of the determinant k. The last term is the unexplained part calculated as a residual, where GC_ε is the cumulative concentration index of the error term. Equation (4) is basically made up of two components, the explained component giving the contribution of each determinant, and an unexplained component or residual.

However, this method is developed for continuous outcomes where linear regression is appropriate, and does not allow for binary outcome variables that require non-linear regression models. Van Doorslaer et al. proposed a modification of the standard decomposition method for use in non-linear situations [33]. They propose a probit regression followed by estimation of

the marginal effects for each of the explanatory variables evaluated at the sample's mean. The marginal effects go into equation (4) instead of the regression coefficients β_k and the linearity required for the decomposition is re-established. The modification proposed by Van Doorslaer et al. was used for the decomposition analysis of all the indicators in this study.

The health achievement index

The mean level of the indicator and the distributional pattern of the indicator, as estimated by either the concentration index or the geographic Gini index, can be combined into an index of health achievement. The health achievement index was calculated for the socioeconomic distribution of all indicators in 2000, 2005 and 2011, using the following formula [34]:

$$I = \mu(1 - C) \tag{5}$$

Where I is the health achievement, μ is the mean of the health variable and C it's concentration index.

Time trends

The mean level, concentration index and health achievement index were estimated for all indicators in 2000, 2005 and 2011. The change in the mean level was assessed by logistic regression, with the indicator in question as dependent variable and the time of the surveys as independent variable.

All statistical analysis was performed using STATA IC version 12.0, taking the sample design into account.

Results

Descriptive statistics

Summary statistics of the 2011 indicators as well as a breakdown by maternal and household characteristics is provided in **Table 1**. The neonatal and under-five mortality, as reported by the DHS, was 37 and 88 per 1000 live born children respectively [26]. The proportion of women giving birth assisted by a skilled birth attendant was 10 per cent. 24 per cent of the children aged 12–23 months at the time of the survey had received all basic vaccinations. 30 per cent of the children who reported cases of diarrhoea in the two weeks preceding the survey had been given oral rehydration therapy, and 11 per cent of the children with suspected pneumonia in the two weeks preceding the survey had received antibiotics. The level of coverage and mortality differed according to wealth quintile, level of mother's education and region of residence.

Geographic inequality

The geographic Gini indices estimating the inequality between the regions can be found in **Table 1**. The geographic Gini indices ranged from 0.047 (95 per cent confidence interval $((-0.0068) - 0.10)$ for under-five deaths to 0.33 $((-0.043) -0.70)$ for skilled birth attendance. **Figure 1** displays the geographic Lorenz curve for under-five deaths and skilled birth attendance.

Socioeconomic inequality

The concentration indices for each of the indicators in 2011 can be found in **Table 1**. For all indicators except treatment for suspected pneumonia, the concentration indices were significantly different from zero at a 95 per cent significance level. The absolute values of the concentration indices were above or equal to 0.10 for all indicators. The lowest degree of socioeconomic inequality was

Table 1. Summary statistics of the indicators (2011).

	Under-five mortality*	Neonatal mortality*	Skilled birth attendance	Vaccination	Treatment for diarrhoea	Treatment for pneumonia	Number of children
Wealth quintile							
Poorest	137	50	1.7%	16.8%	21.7%	7.1%	3625
Poorer	121	48	2.9%	18.2%	24.5%	14.7%	2114
Middle	96	35	3.2%	18.2%	31.7%	7.6%	1872
Richer	100	39	7.4%	24.9%	31.2%	14.2%	1870
Richest	86	37	45.6%	50.5%	50.9%	15.8%	2173
Mother's education							
No education	121	46	4.6%	20.1%	25.9%	10.7%	8142
Primary	88	35	15.3%	28.3%	36.1%	11.2%	2930
Secondary	46	31	72.0%	57.0%	57.5%	**	386
Higher	24	8	74.0%	57.7%	**	**	196
Region							
Tigray	85	44	11.6%	58.9%	37.1%	7.8%	1202
Affar	127	33	7.1%	8.6%	40.0%	5.8%	1130
Amhara	108	54	10.1%	26.3%	30.4%	9.8%	1294
Oromiya	112	40	8.1%	15.6%	26.1%	11.4%	1761
Somali	122	34	8.2%	16.6%	35.1%	4.8%	1027
Benishangul-Gumuz	169	62	8.9%	23.6%	38.5%	12.7%	1020
SNNP	116	38	6.1%	24.1%	29.0%	14.3%	1614
Gambela	123	39	27.0%	15.5%	48.7%	16.1%	851
Harari	94	35	32.5%	34.1%	44.9%	**	659
Addis Ababa	53	21	83.9%	78.7%	54.4%	**	400
Dire Dawa	97	30	40.3%	58.6%	47.8%	5.1%	696
National average	**88**	**37**	**10.0%**	**24.3%**	**29.9%**	**11.0%**	**11654**
Concentration index	**−0.12**	**−0.10**	**0.65**	**0.23**	**0.14**	**0.10**	
95% CI	(−0.17)−(−0.064)	(−0.18)−(−0.022)	0.60−0.70	0.15−0.30	0.081−0.20	(−0.065)−0.27	
Geographic Gini index	**0.047**	**0.092**	**0.33**	**0.29**	**0.091**	**0.14**	
95% CI	(−0.0068)−0.10	0.029−0.16	(−0.043)−0.70	0.11−0.47	0.026−0.16	0.030−0.25	

*Estimates from the Ethiopia DHS 2011 Final Report [26]. The mortality rates are reported as number of deaths per thousand live births.

**The figure is based on fewer than 25 cases and has been supressed.

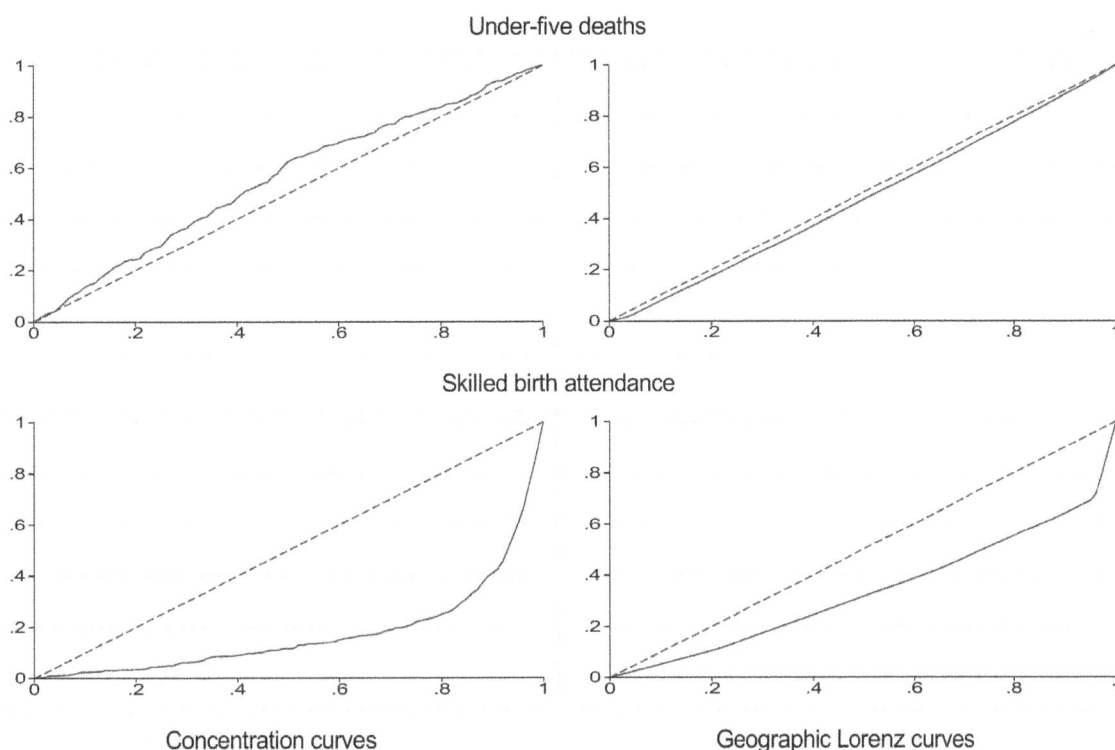

Figure 1. Concentration curves and geographic Lorenz curves for under-five deaths and skilled birth attendance in 2011. The two figures to the left are concentration curves, with the cumulative proportion of the individuals ranked by wealth on the x-axis and the cumulative proportion of the outcome variable on the y-axis. The two figures to the right are geographic Lorenz curves, with the cumulative proportion of the regions ranked from worst to best achievement of the indicator, and weighed by population size on the x-axis. The cumulative proportion of the outcome variable is on the y-axis. The solid red lines represent the concentration and Lorenz curves, and the dashed blue lines represent the "line of equality".

found for neonatal deaths and antibiotics, with concentration indices of -0.10 $((-0.18)-(-0.022))$ and 0.10 $((-0.065) -0.27)$ respectively. The indicator revealing the largest degree of socioeconomic inequality was skilled birth attendance, with a concentration index of 0.65 $(0.60-0.70)$. For under-five and neonatal deaths, the concentration indices were negative, indicating that a disproportionate fraction of these deaths occurs in children of poor families. The concentration indices for coverage of skilled birth attendance, vaccinations, oral rehydration therapy for diarrhoea and antibiotics for suspected pneumonia were positive; these services were therefore more prevalent among the wealthier part of the population. **Figure 1** displays the concentration curve for under-five deaths and skilled birth attendance.

Decomposition analysis

The results of the decomposition of the indicators' concentration indices in 2011 are presented in **Table 2** and graphically in **Figure 2**. The wealth factor alone accounts for the majority of the explained inequalities for all indicators, with a contribution ranging from 13.6 per cent of the total inequality in neonatal deaths to 84.8 per cent for coverage of basic vaccinations. The percentage contribution of wealth in the decomposition analysis is an estimate of the pure effect of wealth on the total inequality, adjusting for other relevant factors. Education accounts for a smaller proportion of the inequalities, with a contribution ranging from 5.1 per cent of the total inequality in skilled birth attendance to 24.6 per cent in treatment of suspected pneumonia. The proportion of the inequalities not explained by systematic

variations in the explanatory variables is captured by the residual, the lowest is found for coverage of vaccinations where 6.4 per cent of the inequality is not explained by the model, and the highest is found for neonatal deaths with a residual of 73.8 per cent.

Time trends

The mean level, concentration indices and health achievement index for all variables in 2000, 2005 and 2011 can be found in **Table 3**. Since geographic inequality as measured here accounts for very little of the explained inequalities, we did not include a geographic achievement index. The mean of all indicators improved from 2000 to 2011. The concentration indices revealed increasing socioeconomic inequalities for under-five and neonatal deaths, and somewhat decreasing or unchanged inequalities for the remaining indicators. The health achievement index shows an improvement for all indicators except neonatal deaths. The change over time in mean level and health achievement is shown graphically in **Figure 3**.

Discussion

This study demonstrates the presence of geographic inequalities and pro-rich inequalities for all indicators in 2011. The major contributor to the observed socioeconomic inequality in access to key services and health outcomes is wealth. The mean level of all indicators improved from 2000 to 2011. Socioeconomic inequalities seem to decrease for most but not all indicators from 2000 to 2011, while the health achievement index shows improvement for all the indicators except neonatal deaths.

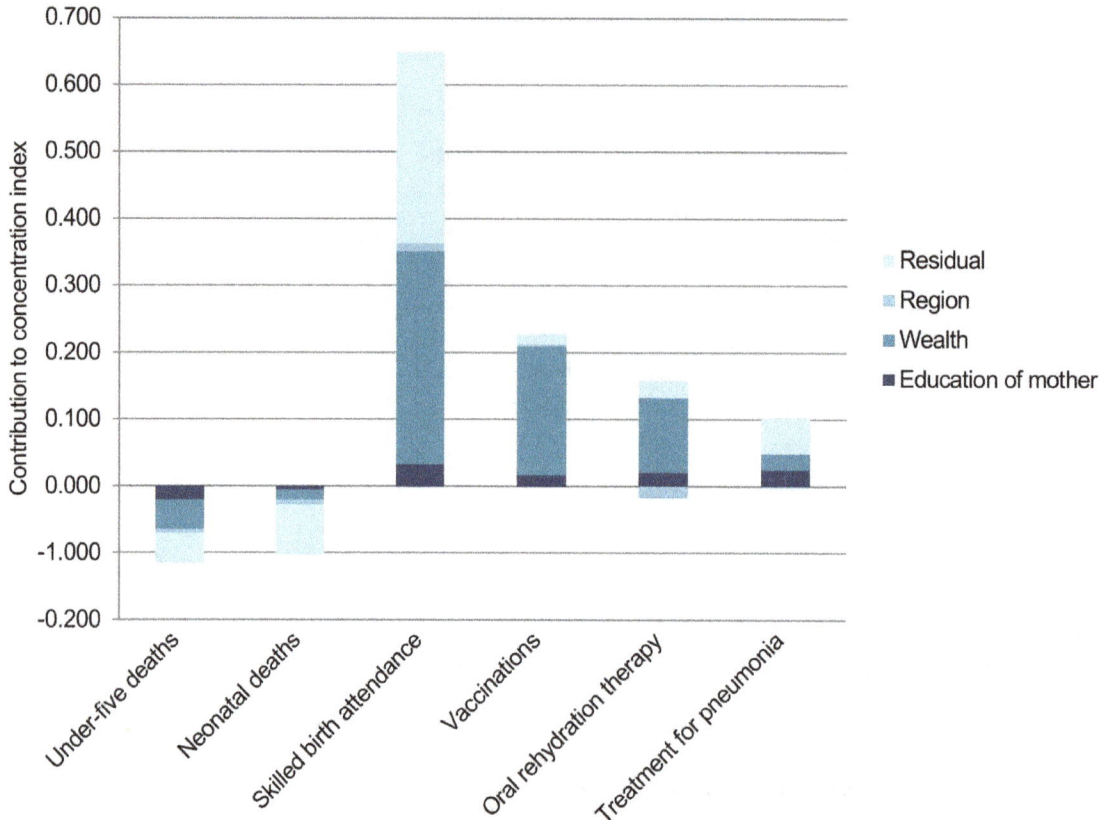

Figure 2. Factors contributing to socioeconomic inequality. Contribution of wealth, the mother's education and region of residence to the total socioeconomic inequality, as measured by the concentration index, for each of the indicators in 2011.

Other studies have found mother's educational level, wealth and region of residence to be important determinants for child health and access to health services in Ethiopia [21–23], which is in line with this study. However, in this study a combination of different methods for assessing inequalities is used, which leads to a better and more nuanced understanding of the current situation and changes over time. Quantifying inequalities using the concentration index provides a useful tool for comparing the magnitude of the inequalities for different services, and for assessing the changes in inequality over time. The health achievement index, that incorporates socioeconomic inequality and the average level in the population into one metric, gives useful additional evidence to policymakers concerned with both of these aspects.

Previous studies decomposing socioeconomic inequalities in child mortality and skilled birth attendance in low and middle income countries have found that the mother's education and wealth are the main contributors to overall socioeconomic inequalities [1,3,35]. The proportion of total inequality that is attributable to education is higher in these studies than the results of our study indicate. This may be explained by the low coverage of key services in Ethiopia. Few people have access to the services; it is therefore not unexpected that there are large disparities in access across the population and that wealth is the most important determinant for accessing key services. A review comparing inequalities in several low and middle income countries finds that the coverage in the lower wealth quintiles are subject to more variability than coverage in the richest quintile [4], suggesting that the richest part of the population have the means to receive

needed services irrespective of how the country's health system is functioning.

The lowest degree of socioeconomic inequality is found for neonatal deaths and treatment for suspected pneumonia. Wealth contributes to a comparatively smaller degree of the socioeconomic inequality for neonatal deaths than for the other indicator, and a large proportion of the inequalities is not explained by the decomposition. This might be due to the large impact of biological factors, health system factors and other factors that are not included in our model.

Access to antibiotics for pneumonia was included as a binary variable indicating whether children presenting symptoms in the two weeks preceding the survey had received antibiotics. The weakness of this classification is that those who seek medical care, but for whom antibiotics are not needed, are classified as not having access to treatment. However, the alternative indicator measuring access to treatment of pneumonia by whether medical advice was sought, will not take account of the quality of the consultation or the availability of drugs.

When decomposing inequalities in health outcomes and access to key services, the geographic determinants account for a relatively small proportion of the inequalities. The geographic determinants are included as regions, and one possible explanation of the relatively small contribution of the regions may be that the major part of the geographic inequality is due to factors on a more detailed level than the regional level that we measure, for example, walking distance to the closest health facility. A study from a rural area in north-western Ethiopia found that children who had more than one and a half hour travel time to the nearest health centre

Table 2. Absolute and percentage contribution of mother's education. wealth and region of residence to the concentration indices (C): results of the decomposition analysis.

	Under-five deaths		Neonatal deaths		Skilled birth attendance		Vaccination		ORS		Antibiotics	
	Absolute	%	Absolute	%	Absolute	%	Absolute	%	Absolute	%	Absolute	%
Education of mother	-0.020	17.5	-0.006	5.7	0.033	5.1	0.017	7.4	0.022	15.3	0.025	24.6
Wealth	-0.045	39.0	-0.014	13.6	0.318	48.9	0.193	84.8	0.111	77.6	0.024	23.5
Region												
Tigray	Ref.	Ref.	Ref.	Ref.	Ref.	Ref.	Ref.	Ref.	Ref.	Ref.	Ref.	Ref.
Affar	0.000	0.4	0.003	-2.6	0.001	0.1	0.006	2.6	0.000	-0.2	0.001	0.6
Amhara	0.001	-0.5	-0.001	0.8	-0.004	-0.6	0.017	7.6	0.002	1.3	-0.001	-1.2
Oromiya	0.000	0.0	-0.003	2.7	0.002	0.3	-0.027	-12.0	-0.013	-9.3	0.006	5.8
Somali	0.000	0.0	0.002	-1.6	0.001	0.1	0.004	1.5	0.000	-0.3	0.003	3.3
Benishangul-Gumuz	0.000	0.3	0.000	0.2	-0.001	-0.1	0.001	0.4	0.000	-0.2	0.001	0.5
SNNP	-0.001	0.8	0.002	-1.5	0.001	0.2	0.015	6.7	0.002	1.5	-0.002	-1.7
Gambela	0.000	0.1	0.000	0.0	0.000	-0.1	0.001	0.4	0.000	-0.2	-0.001	-0.9
Harari	0.000	-0.1	0.000	0.0	0.001	0.1	-0.001	-0.7	0.000	0.0	*	*
Addis Ababa	-0.004	3.6	-0.008	8.2	0.011	1.6	-0.012	-5.3	-0.006	-4.5	-0.007	-7.1
Dire Dawa	0.000	0.2	-0.001	0.9	0.001	0.1	0.000	-0.01	0.000	-0.002	0.000	-0.1
Residual	-0.045	38.8	-0.076	73.8	0.287	44.1	0.015	6.4	0.027	18.9	0.054	52.6
Total	**-0.116**	**100.0**	**-0.103**	**100.0**	**0.650**	**100.0**	**0.228**	**100.0**	**0.142**	**100.0**	**0.102**	**100.0**

*The contribution of the region Harari to the inequality in use of antibiotics was omitted in the regression analysis because ALL = 0.

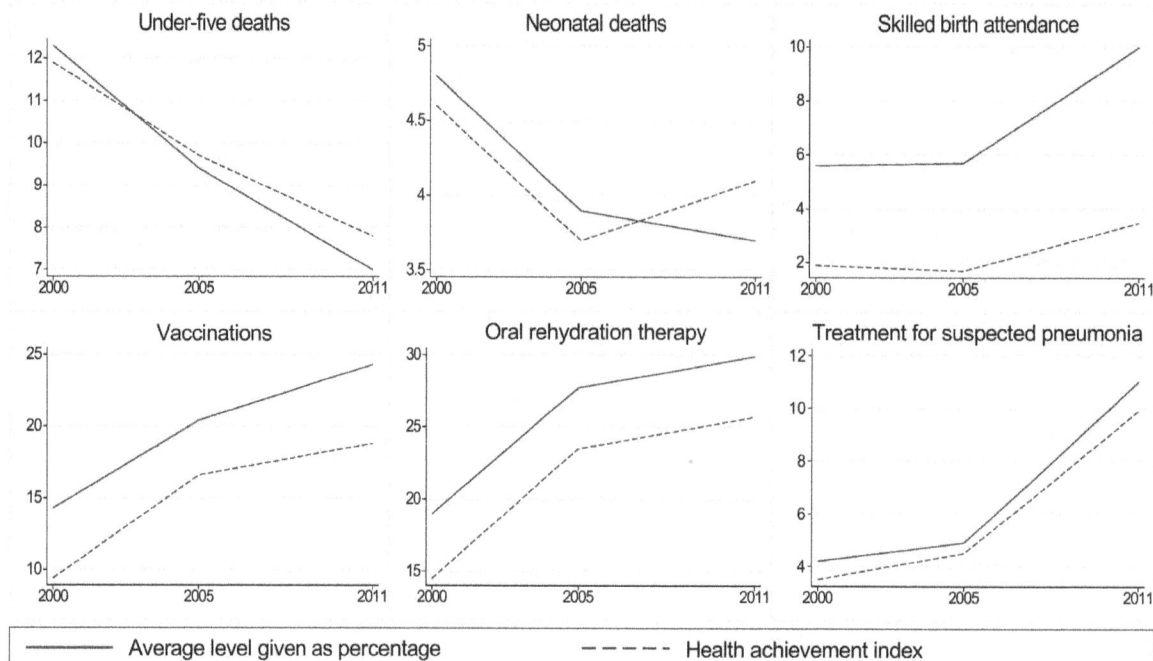

Figure 3. Changes in average level (given as percentage) and health achievement index from 2000 to 2011. Change from 2000 to 2011 in average level and health achievement index for each of the indicators. The time is on the x-axis, and the health achievement index and average level or coverage are on the y-axis.

had a two- to threefold greater risk of dying before the age of five than children living within one and a half hour from the health centre [7]. A study from Burkina Faso reports similar findings [8].

Assessing whether the situation is improving for each of the indicators depends on the measure used. If one is only concerned with the mean level in the population, there has been a positive evolution for all indicators from 2000 to 2011. If

Table 3. Change in average level and health achievement index from 2000 to 2011.

	Average/ coverage	Concentration index (95% CI)	Health achievement index	Average/ coverage	Concentration index (95% CI)	Health achievement index
	Under-five deaths			**Neonatal deaths**		
2000	12.3%	0.029 ((−0.010) −0.067)	11.9%	4.8%	0.037 ((−0.028) −0.10)	4.6%
2005	9.4%	−0.030 ((−0.071) −0.012)	9.7%	3.9%	0.052 ((−0.016) −0.13)	3.7%
2011	7.0%	−0.12 ((−0.17)–(−0.064))	7.8%	3.7%	−0.10 ((−0.18)–(−0.022))	4.1%
p for trend	<0.001			0.008		
	Skilled birth attendance			**Oral rehydration therapy**		
2000	5.6%	0.66 (0.61–0.72)	1.9%	19.0%	0.24 (0.16–0.31)	14.5%
2005	5.7%	0.70 (0.65–0.75)	1.7%	27.7%	0.15 (0.082–0.22)	23.5%
2011	10.0%	0.65 (0.60–0.70)	3.5%	29.9%	0.14 (0.081–0.20)	25.7%
p for trend	<0.001			<0.001		
	Vaccination			**Treatment for suspected pneumonia**		
2000	14.3%	0.34 (0.26–0.43)	9.4%	4.2%	0.17 (0.037–0.30)	3.5%
2005	20.4%	0.18 (0.10–0.27)	16.6%	4.9%	0.088 (0.088–0.088)	4.5%
2011	24.3%	0.23 (0.15–0.30)	18.8%	11.0%	0.10 ((−0.065) −0.27)	9.9%
p for trend	<0.001			<0.001		

one is only concerned with the distribution across socioeconomic groups, the results are more diverse, indicating increased inequality for some indicators and reduced inequality for others. This has been shown for several other countries as well [12,14]. However, we argue that it is crucial to achieve both a higher mean level and more fairly distributed health and coverage of key services. The health achievement index is a way of incorporating both of these concerns into one metric. The health achievement index improved for all indicators from 2000 to 2011, except neonatal deaths. This means that even where the concentration index is worsening, the increase in inequality is outweighed by improvement of the mean level. To date, few studies have combined the information available on coverage and on distribution into a single metric such as the health achievement index. A study from Nigeria uses the health achievement index to assess malnutrition, and emphasises the importance of including both inequality and the mean level, because subgroups of the population that do well in one dimension often do less well in the other dimension [36]. A study that uses the health achievement index to assess time trends in measles vaccination in 21 low and middle income countries finds both increasing and decreasing health achievement indices [13].

The changes in mean level, inequality and health achievement are assessed from 2000 to 2011 in our study. This corresponds to the time period when the Health Extension Programme was implemented [16]. The Health Extension Programme focuses on community based services, with the aim of improving health outcomes and coverage of key services and making key services universally accessible. Studies evaluating the impact of the Health Extension Programme in Ethiopia find that the programme has contributed to increased coverage of vaccinations, improved maternal and neonatal health care practices and improvement of health-promoting and care-seeking behaviour, but the programme does not seem to have impacted coverage of skilled birth attendance and postnatal care [37–40]. Our study has not assessed the effects of the Health Extension Programme, but the results of our study should be seen in relation to the implementation of the Health Extension Programme.

This study is based on data from the Demographic and Health Surveys. These surveys are conducted in many low and middle income countries with standardised questionnaires. The surveys are nationally representative with a relatively large sample size. However, the estimates done by the Ethiopian Ministry of Health differ somewhat from the DHS' estimates for some indicators. For example, the 2011 report on health and health related indicators published by the Ethiopian Ministry of Health estimates measles coverage to be 82 per cent [41], whereas it is estimated at 56 per cent by the 2011 Ethiopian DHS [26].

There are several limitations to this study. First, the decomposition analysis is based on regression analysis with varying degree of statistical significance. The results of the decomposition analysis should therefore be interpreted with caution. Second, factors other than those incorporated into the models may exclude people from receiving health care. Supply side factors, such as the presence of health facilities, quality of care and the availability of drugs may be important reasons why people are not receiving needed health care. This is not fully accounted for in the model, although it is partly explained through the geographic inequalities. Demand side factors, such as cultural barriers, costs of receiving health care and time available to seek medical care, are not explicitly incorporated into the model due to data limitations.

Conclusion

Socioeconomic and geographic inequalities exist in the distribution of access to key services and health outcomes in Ethiopia. Wealth is the major determinant of socioeconomic inequality in child health, and there are widening inequalities for some of the indicators included in this study. However, the mean level of health outcomes and coverage of key services is improving, and the health achievement indices show improvements for all indicators with the exception of neonatal deaths.

Acknowledgments

We thank the Global Health Priorities research group at the University of Bergen for valuable feedback and support.

Author Contributions

Conceived and designed the experiments: EKS OFN. Analyzed the data: EKS MA OFN. Wrote the paper: EKS MA OFN.

References

1. Zere E, Oluwole D, Kirigia JM, Mwikisa CN, Mbeeli T (2011) Inequities in skilled attendance at birth in Namibia: a decomposition analysis. BMC Pregnancy Childbirth 11: 34.

2. Houweling TAJ, Kunst AE (2010) Socio-economic inequalities in childhood mortality in low- and middle-income countries: a review of the international evidence. British Medical Bulletin 93: 7–26.

3. Pradhan J, Arokiasamy P (2010) Socio-economic inequalities in child survival in India: A decomposition analysis. Health Policy 98: 114–120.

4. Barros AJD, Ronsmans C, Axelson H, Loaiza E, Bertoldi AD, et al. (2012) Equity in maternal, newborn, and child health interventions in Countdown to 2015: a retrospective review of survey data from 54 countries. The Lancet 379: 1225–1233.

5. Hertel-Fernandez AW, Giusti AE, Sotelo JM (2007) The Chilean infant mortality decline: improvement for whom? Socioeconomic and geographic inequalities in infant mortality, 1990–2005. Bulletin of the World Health Organization 85: 798–804.

6. Fang P, Dong S, Xiao J, Liu C, Feng X, et al. (2010) Regional inequality in health and its determinants: Evidence from China. Health Policy 94: 14–25.

7. Okwaraji YB, Cousens S, Berhane Y, Mulholland K, Edmond K (2012) Effect of Geographical Access to Health Facilities on Child Mortality in Rural Ethiopia: A Community Based Cross Sectional Study. PLoS ONE 7: e33564.

8. Schoeps A, Gabrysch S, Niamba L, Sié A, Becker H (2011) The Effect of Distance to Health-Care Facilities on Childhood Mortality in Rural Burkina Faso. American Journal of Epidemiology 173: 492–498.

9. Kinney MV, Kerber KJ, Black RE, Cohen B, Nkrumah F, et al. (2010) Sub-Saharan Africa's Mothers, Newborns, and Children: Where and Why Do They Die? PLoS Med 7: e1000294.

10. Ruhago G, Ngalesoni F, Norheim O (2012) Addressing inequity to achieve the maternal and child health millennium development goals: looking beyond averages. BMC Public Health 12: 1119.

11. Tranvag E, Ali M, Norheim O (2013) Health inequalities in Ethiopia: modeling inequalities in length of life within and between population groups. International Journal for Equity in Health 12: 52.

12. Victora CG, Barros AJD, Axelson H, Bhutta ZA, Chopra M, et al. (2012) How changes in coverage affect equity in maternal and child health interventions in 35 Countdown to 2015 countries: an analysis of national surveys. The Lancet 380: 1149–1156.

13. Meheus F, Van Doorslaer E (2008) Achieving better measles immunization in developing countries: does higher coverage imply lower inequality? Social Science & Medicine 66: 1709–1718.

14. Moser KA, Leon DA, Gwatkin DR (2005) How does progress towards the child mortality millennium development goal affect inequalities between the poorest and least poor? Analysis of Demographic and Health Survey data. BMJ 331: 1180–1182.

15. World Health Organization (2013) World Health Statistics 2013.

16. Federal Ministry of Health of Ethiopia (2007) Health Extension Program in Ethiopia Profile. Addis Ababa, Ethiopia: Health Extension and Education Center, Federal Ministry of Health.

17. World Health Organization Regional Office for Africa (2012) Atlas of African Health Statistics 2012– Health situation analysis of the African Region.

18. Wilunda C, Putoto G, Manenti F, Castiglioni M, Azzimonti G, et al. (2013) Measuring equity in utilization of emergency obstetric care at Wolisso Hospital in Oromiya, Ethiopia: a cross sectional study. International Journal for Equity in Health 12: 27.

19. Wirth M, Sacks E, Delamonica E, Storeygard A, Minujin A, et al. (2008) "Delivering" on the MDGs?: equity and maternal health in Ghana, Ethiopia and Kenya. East Afr J Public Health 5: 133–141.

20. Bayou NB, Gacho YH (2013) Utilization of clean and safe delivery service package of health services extension program and associated factors in rural kebeles of Kafa Zone, Southwest Ethiopia. Ethiop J Health Sci 23: 79–89.

21. Sullivan M-C, Tegegn A, Tessema F, Galea S, Hadley C (2010) Minding the Immunization Gap: Family Characteristics Associated with Completion Rates in Rural Ethiopia. Journal of Community Health 35: 53–59.

22. Hosseinpoor AR, Victora CG, Bergen N, Barros AJ, Boerma T (2011) Towards universal health coverage: the role of within-country wealth-related inequality in 28 countries in sub-Saharan Africa. Bulletin of the World Health Organization 89: 881–889.

23. Mekonnen Y, Tensou B, Telake D, Degefie T, Bekele A (2013) Neonatal mortality in Ethiopia: trends and determinants. BMC Public Health 13: 483.

24. Central Statistical Authority [Ethiopia] and ORC Macro (2001) Ethiopia Demographic and Health Survey 2000 [Dataset]. Addis Ababa, Ethiopia and Claverton, Maryland, USA: Central Statistical Authority and ORC Macro.

25. Central Statistical Agency [Ethiopia] and ORC Macro (2006) Ethiopia Demographic and Health Survey 2005 [Dataset]. Addis Ababa, Ethiopia and Claverton, Maryland, USA: Central Statistical Agency and ORC Macro.

26. Central Statistical Agency of Ethiopia and ICF International (2012) Ethiopia Demographic and Health Survey 2011. Addis Ababa, Ethiopia and Calverton, Maryland, USA: Central Statistical Agency and ICF International.

27. Central Statistical Agency of Ethiopia (2007) Population and Housing Census Report 2007.

28. Kakwani N, Wagstaff A, van Doorslaer E (1997) Socioeconomic inequalities in health: Measurement, computation, and statistical inference. Journal of Econometrics 77: 87–103.

29. O'Donnell O, van Doorslaer E, Wagstaff A, Lindelow M (2008) Analyzing Health Equity Using Household Survey Data: A Guide to Techniques and Their Implementation: The World Bank, Washington D.C.

30. Shea Oscar Rutstein and Kiersten Johnson MD, ORC Macro, Calverton Maryland, USA (2004) The DHS Wealth index.

31. Commission on Social Determinants of Health (2008) Closing the gap in a generation: Health equity through action on the social determinants of health. Final Report of the Commission on Social Determinants of Health. Geneva, World Health Organization.

32. Wagstaff A, van Doorslaer E, Watanabe N (2003) On decomposing the causes of health sector inequalities with an application to malnutrition inequalities in Vietnam. Journal of Econometrics 112: 207–223.

33. Doorslaer Ev, Koolman X, Jones AM (2004) Explaining income-related inequalities in doctor utilisation in Europe. Health Economics 13: 629–647.

34. Wagstaff A (2002) Inequality aversion, health inequalities and health achievement. Journal of Health Economics 21: 627–641.

35. Hosseinpoor AR, Van Doorslaer E, Speybroeck N, Naghavi M, Mohammad K, et al. (2006) Decomposing socioeconomic inequality in infant mortality in Iran. Int J Epidemiol 35: 1211–1219.

36. Uthman OA (2009) Using extended concentration and achievement indices to study socioeconomic inequality in chronic childhood malnutrition: the case of Nigeria. International Journal for Equity in Health 8: 22–22.

37. Admassie A, Abebaw D, Woldemichael AD (2009) Impact evaluation of the Ethiopian Health Services Extension Programme. Journal of Development Effectiveness 1: 430–449.

38. Karim AM, Admassu K, Schellenberg J, Alemu H, Getachew N, et al. (2013) Effect of Ethiopia's Health Extension Program on Maternal and Newborn Health Care Practices in 101 Rural Districts: A Dose-Response Study. PLoS ONE 8: e65160.

39. Medhanyie A, Spigt M, Kifle Y, Schaay N, Sanders D, et al. (2012) The role of health extension workers in improving utilization of maternal health services in rural areas in Ethiopia: a cross sectional study. BMC Health Services Research 12: 352.

40. Bilal NK, Herbst CH, Zhao F, Soucat A, Lemiere C (2011) Health Extension Workers in Ethiopia: Improved Access and Coverage for the Rural Poor. In: Chuhan-Pole P, Angwafo M, editors. Yes Africa Can: Success Stories from a Dynamic Continent. The World Bank, Washington D.C., USA. pp. 433–443.

41. Federal Ministry of Health of Ethiopia (2011) Health and Health Related Indicators 2003 E.C. (2010/11 G.C.). In: Directorate PP, editor.

21

Isolated Assessment of Translation or Rotation Severely Underestimates the Effects of Subject Motion in fMRI Data

Marko Wilke[1,2]*

1 Department of Pediatric Neurology and Developmental Medicine, Children's Hospital, University of Tübingen, Tübingen, Germany, **2** Experimental Pediatric Neuroimaging group, Pediatric Neurology & Department of Neuroradiology, University Hospital, Tübingen, Germany

Abstract

Subject motion has long since been known to be a major confound in functional MRI studies of the human brain. For resting-state functional MRI in particular, data corruption due to motion artefacts has been shown to be most relevant. However, despite 6 parameters (3 for translations and 3 for rotations) being required to fully describe the head's motion trajectory between timepoints, not all are routinely used to assess subject motion. Using structural (n = 964) as well as functional MRI (n = 200) data from public repositories, a series of experiments was performed to assess the impact of using a reduced parameter set (translation$_{only}$ and rotation$_{only}$) versus using the complete parameter set. It could be shown that the usage of 65 mm as an indicator of the average cortical distance is a valid approximation in adults, although care must be taken when comparing children and adults using the same measure. The effect of using slightly smaller or larger values is minimal. Further, both translation$_{only}$ and rotation$_{only}$ severely underestimate the full extent of subject motion; consequently, both translation$_{only}$ and rotation$_{only}$ discard substantially fewer datapoints when used for quality control purposes ("motion scrubbing"). Finally, both translation$_{only}$ and rotation$_{only}$ severely underperform in predicting the full extent of the signal changes and the overall variance explained by motion in functional MRI data. These results suggest that a comprehensive measure, taking into account all available parameters, should be used to characterize subject motion in fMRI.

Editor: Qiyong Gong, West China Hospital of Sichuan University, China

Funding: This study was funded in part by the German Research Council (DFG, WI3630/1-2) as well as the H.W. & J. Hector Foundation, Mannheim (M66). Neither sponsor had any role in study design, in the collection, analysis and interpretation of data, in the writing of the report, or in the decision to submit the article for publication.

* Email: marko.wilke@med.uni-tuebingen.de

Introduction

Subject motion has long since been known to be a major confound in functional MRI studies of the human brain [1]. For resting-state functional MRI (rsfMRI) and functional connectivity analyses in particular, even minimal motion was recently found to be highly problematic [2–5]. Both prospective [6–8] and retrospective approaches [9,10] to motion correction have been suggested, but the most commonly-used approach still is retrospective "motion correction" by using a rigid-body translation [11,12]. However, even after such a procedure, motion still explains substantial variance in the data [1,14,15]. Motion correction (a.k.a. realignment) is usually performed using the first (or mean) image of a dataset as the reference, providing a measure of absolute motion over a functional run [16]. However, it was suggested that the scan-to-scan (relative) motion may be more relevant, as slow motion may be both easier to correct and less detrimental to data quality [17]. As the thus-detected extent of subject motion is commonly used to identify and remove bad datasets ("motion scrubbing" [4,18,19]), accurately describing motion is most important.

During realignment, the aim is to find the combination of parameters that minimizes the difference between consecutive images, which may be defined using different cost functions [20]. The result of this rigid-body approach to motion correction is a set of 6 parameters. It is important to notice that these parameters are jointly optimized to achieve a final result; hence, only in their combination do they fully describe the motion trajectory detected by the realignment algorithm. However, assessing subject motion is only straightforward in the case of translations, which is described by 3 parameters (one for each dimension in space) and is provided in millimeters [mm]. In contrast to this, the assessment of subject rotation, (again described by 3 parameters but provided in degrees or radians), requires knowledge about the distance from the origin around which rotation was performed; only then are degrees/radians convertible to an absolute distance. It was suggested previously that the length of the vector resulting from these 6 transformations in space is an appropriate representation of subject motion ([15,21,22]; see Figure 1 for an illustration). This requires a definition of "at what distance" this motion is assessed, which may be the corner of the volume [22], set empirically (to 50 [4] or 65 mm [21]) or calculated individually [15]. This obstacle likely is responsible for many researchers qualifying "subject motion" by only inspecting absolute/relative translation, often applying a rule-of-thumb of "motion exceeding one voxel size" [12,13,23,24]. As using only a subset of the complete realignment parameter set may systematically under- or overestimate motion and its effects, this study was aimed at addressing the following questions: I) what is a representative measure of cortical distance, and what is the effect of modifying it; II) to what extent does the isolated assessment of translation$_{only}$ or rotation$_{only}$ reflect true subject motion, as defined by total displacement; III) to what extent does the isolated assessment of translation$_{only}$ or rotation$_{only}$ affect data scrubbing procedures, i.e., when setting thresholds of acceptable subject motion; IV) to what extent does the isolated assessment of translation$_{only}$ or rotation$_{only}$ predict signal changes in the data; and V) to what extent does the isolated assessment of translation$_{only}$ or rotation$_{only}$ explain variance in the data, when compared with the complete assessment. This manuscript was not aimed to address these issues in such a way that solutions are presented, but rather to explore the presence, and potentially the magnitude, of the problem.

Methods

To address the research questions posited above, both structural and functional MRI data was obtained from public data repositories. Structural MRI data was obtained from children (MRI dataset 1; The NIH study on normal brain development; n = 401 [25]) and adults (MRI dataset 2; IXI Study; n = 563 [26]); details of both datasets are described in Table 1 and are given in the Supplements S1 and S2. Functional MRI data (resting-state fMRI series) from adults was obtained by randomly picking 20 subjects each from 10 randomly selected participating sites' datasets from the fcon_1000 project (MRI dataset 3; n = 200 [27,28]); details of this dataset are described in Table 2 and are given in the Supplement S3. All data processing steps and analyses were carried out in Matlab (version 8.2, The Mathworks, Natick, MA, USA), using custom scripts and functions as well as functionality provided within the SPM8 software package (Wellcome Trust Centre for Neuroimaging, University College London, UK). For all calculations, a 7th order B-spline interpolation was used whenever possible [29] in order to avoid interpolation artefacts [30].

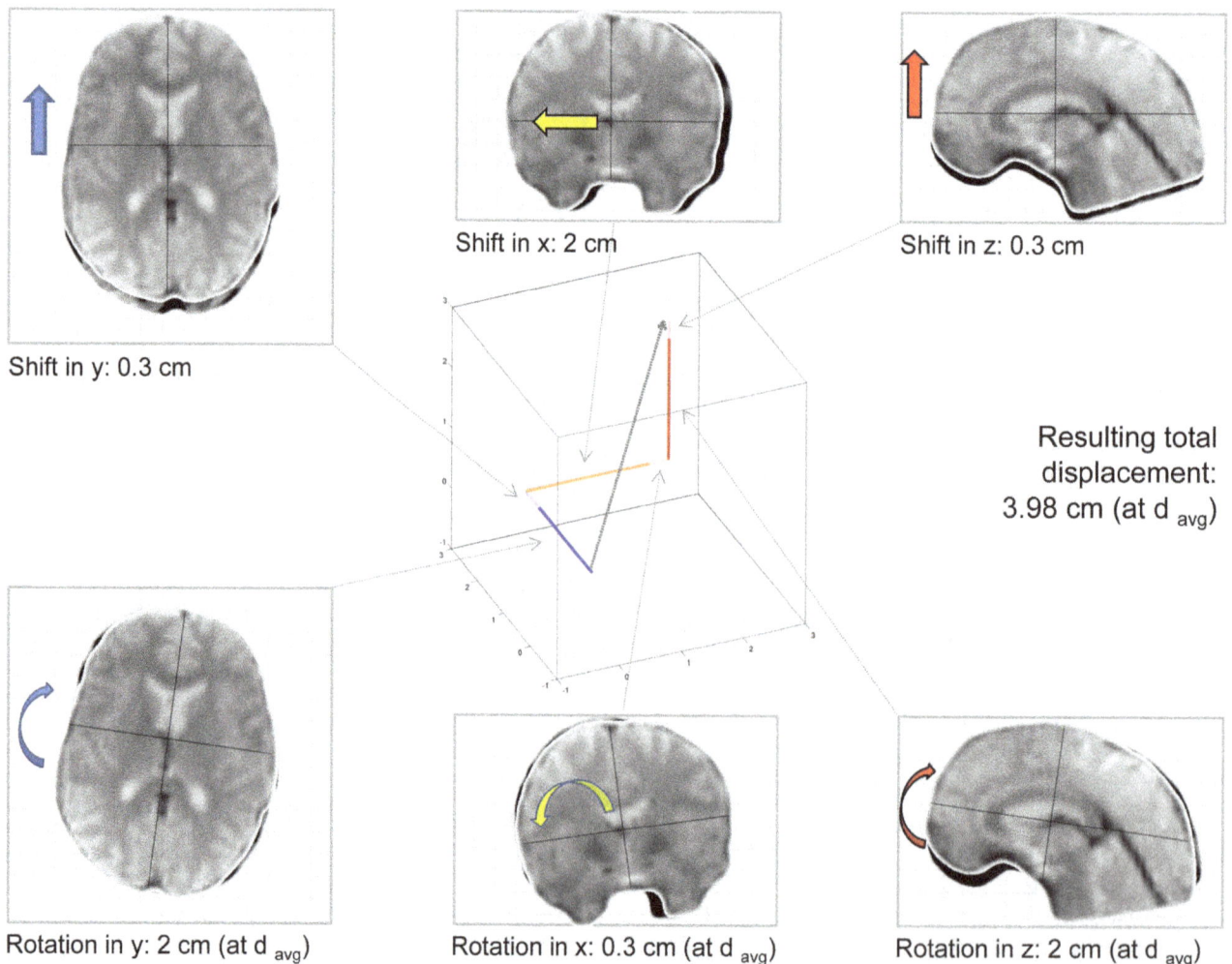

Figure 1. Illustration of the non-linear effects of combining translations (top row) and rotations (bottom row) into a single measure of total displacement (resulting gray arrow in the Cartesian coordinate system, middle). The values provided are only examples. Note that in this example, all displacements are additive, which is not always the case (see manuscript for more details). Note: d$_{avg}$ is a measure of the average cortical distance, required to transform rotations to absolute distances.

Table 1. Core characteristics of dataset 1 and 2 (structural MRI).

Dataset	Center	Subjects [n]	Voxel size [mm³]	Sex [M/F]	Ages [min-max]
Dataset 1 (NIH)	East	126	1.32±.61	61/65	4–17
	West	126	1.60±.48	62/64	4–18
	Midwest	149	1.43±.62	69/80	4–18
	Total Sample:	401	1.45±.59	192/209	10.6±3.48
Dataset 2 (IXI)	Guy's	313	1.025±.002	137/176	20–88
	IOP	70	1.025±0	24/46	20–81
	Hammersmith	180	1.025±0	87/93	20–86
	Total Sample:	563	1.025±.002	248/315	48.6±16.46

All data was acquired on scanners with a field strength of 1.5 Tesla, except for the Hammersmith Hospital data. Note that age is provided in years here, but was converted to "months at date of scan" for all calculations. Guy's, Guy's Hospital, London; IOP, Institute of Psychiatry, London; Hammersmith, Hammersmith Hospital, London. For more information on these datasets, see also Supplements S1 and S2.

Experiment 1

The first experiment was aimed to address question I, what is a representative measure of cortical distance, and what is the effect of modifying it. For this experiment, MRI datasets 1 & 2 were used. The starting point here was the previously-suggested measure of average cortical distance [15,21]. This indicator aims to provide a single number (distance from rotation origin) for which rotation can be converted to an absolute distance ([15,21]; cf. Figure 1). In the motion fingerprint algorithm, it is calculated from each dataset individually [15], whereas in a commonly-used toolbox to assess motion effects in fMRI timeseries [31], this value is set empirically to 65 mm. While it is unclear as to whether this value is representative for a normal adult population, the situation is even less clear in the setting of developing brains, where substantial changes occur [25,32–34]. To this effect, the combined structural MRI dataset of children and adults (total n = 964) was segmented into tissue classes using the unified segmentation approach implemented in SPM8 [35]. To rule out partial volume effects of different voxel sizes, the resulting native space gray matter tissue partitions were resliced to 1×1×1 mm isotropic resolution. Thereafter, all voxels on the outer cortical surface were identified and their absolute distance (in mm) to the image

volume's point of origin was determined using a 3D extension of Pythagoras's theorem, as done before [15], yielding the Euclidian norm. These values were averaged, resulting in one value (average cortical distance, d_{avg}) for each subject. These were then plotted according to age (in month at the time of data acquisition), and correlations with age were assessed as described below. Further, the effect of a difference in d_{avg} was investigated by modifying it in steps of .5 mm within a range of 50–80 mm as different values are used in the literature [4,15,31]. These values were then used to recalculate total displacement as well as scan-to-scan displacement (absolute and relative motion, respectively; see also below), for all subjects, using the results from d_{avg} = 65 mm as a reference.

Experiment 2

The second experiment was aimed to address question II, to what extent does the isolated assessment of translation$_{only}$ or rotation$_{only}$ reflect true subject motion, as defined by total displacement. To this effect, MRI dataset 3 was used (resting state fMRI series, n = 200). Initially, a rigid-body realignment procedure was performed [11] as implemented in SPM8. Total displacement was calculated from the realignment parameters, as described above. Here, the spatial trajectory that minimizes the

Table 2. Core characteristics of dataset 3 (resting state functional MRI).

Dataset	Center	TR [msec]	Slices [n]	Volumes [n]	Sex [M/F/U]	Ages [min-max]
Dataset 3 (fcon_1000)	Atlanta, GA, USA	2000	20	205	6/14/1	22–54
	Baltimore, MD, USA	2500	47	123	7/13/0	20–40
	Bangor, UK	2000	34	265	20/0/0	19–38
	Beijing, China	2000	33	225	11/9/0	18–25
	Berlin, Germany	2300	34	195	12/8/0	23–44
	Cambridge, MA, USA	3000	47	119	3/17/0	18–24
	Cleveland, OH, USA	2800	31	127	8/12/0	24–57
	Dallas, TX, USA	2000	36	115	11/9/0	20–71
	ICBM, Montreal, Canada	2000	23	128	10/10/0	19–85
	Leiden, Netherlands	2180	38	215	16/4/0	20–27
					104/95/1	30.67±13.43

From each center, 20 subjects were selected at random (total n = 200); all data was acquired on scanners with a field strength of 3 Tesla. Note that age is provided in years here, but was converted to months at date of scan for all calculations. M, male; F, female; U, unknown. For more information on this dataset, see also Supplement S3.

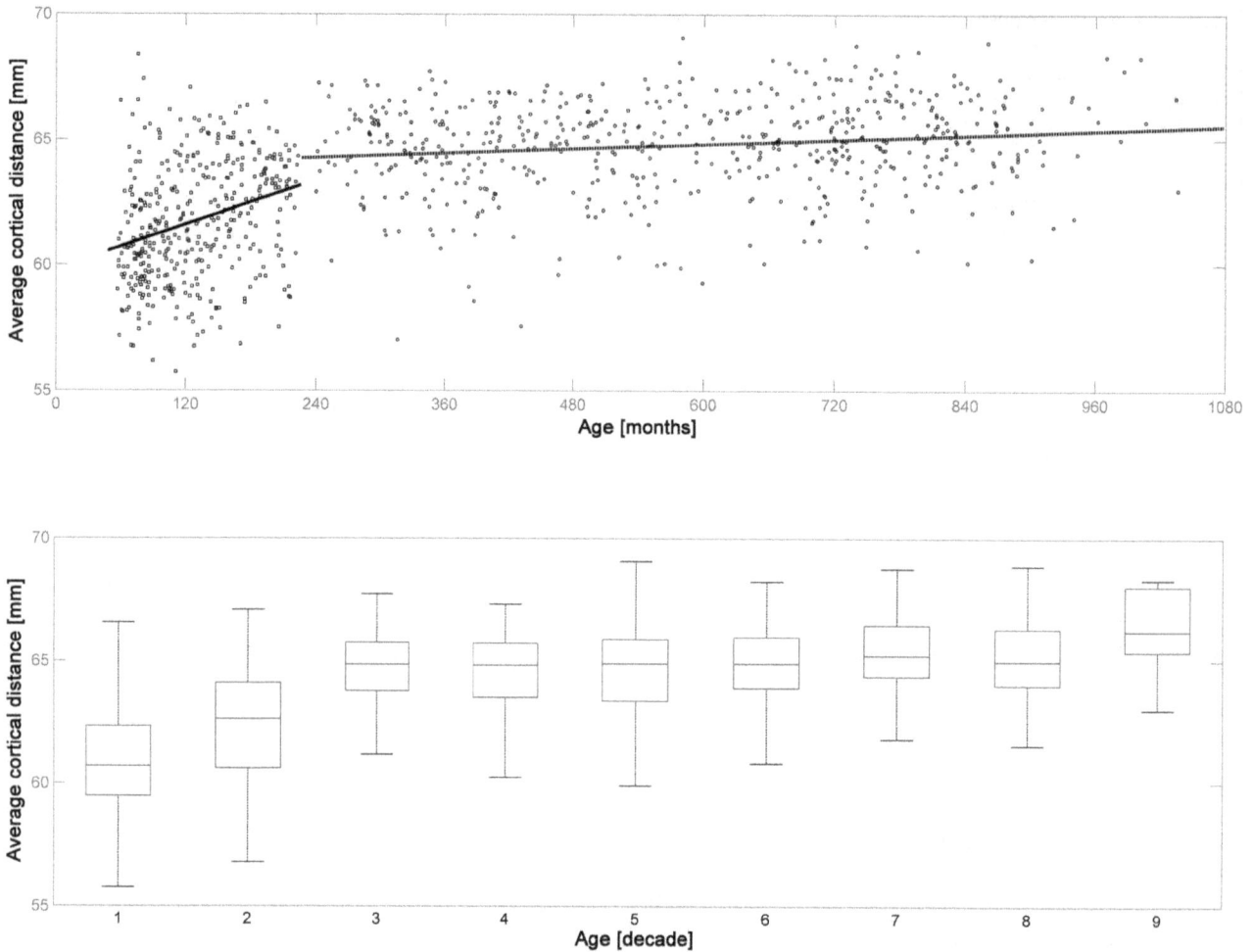

Figure 2. Illustration of the average cortical distance of all subjects in datasets 1 & 2 (structural MRI, n = 964). Note steep increase in childhood and adolescence (dataset 1, solid trendline in upper panel) and much more shallow increase in adulthood (dataset 2, dashed trendline in upper panel). Lower panel: illustration of the same results per decade of life. The difference between datasets 1 & 2 and of the first two decades with all other decades is significant (see manuscript for more details).

difference between the images and thus "corrects for" the individual subject's head motion is effectively recreated from the parameter set. From these 6 values, a vector in space is determined, the length of which (a.k.a. the Euclidian norm of the resulting 3-dimensional vector [22]) describes total displacement ([15,21]; cf. Figure 1). The motion fingerprint algorithm [15] was used to assess absolute motion (total displacement, relative to the first volume) as well as relative motion (scan-to-scan displacement, relative to the previous volume) at the average cortical distance (d_{avg}), here derived from the functional images. First, the original realignment parameters (6 parameters) were used; thereafter, values for either translation or rotation were set to 0, and calculations were repeated. This results in three displacement datasets (complete assessment [used as reference], translation$_{only}$, and rotation$_{only}$) and two resulting indicators (absolute and relative motion).

Experiment 3

The third experiment was aimed to address question III, to what extent does the isolated assessment of translation$_{only}$ or rotation$_{only}$ affect data scrubbing procedures, when compared with the complete assessment dataset. This was explored by setting

thresholds of acceptable subject motion, as done routinely in fMRI studies [4,12,13,19,24]. To this effect, cutoff values of.5/1/1.5/2/ 2.5/3 mm admissible motion were applied, again for both absolute and relative motion. Absolute and relative total displacement was calculated from the complete (used as reference) as well as the reduced (translation$_{only}$, and rotation$_{only}$) parameter sets. The number of datapoints exceeding these cutoff values was recorded and, for the reduced assessments, was related to the results from the complete assessment.

Experiment 4

The fourth experiment was aimed to address question IV, to what extent does the isolated assessment of translation$_{only}$ or rotation$_{only}$ induce signal changes in the data. This was explored by again using the complete set of realignment parameters as well as the two reduced parameter sets (translation$_{only}$ or rotation$_{only}$) to recreate the subject's motion in a phantom timeseries. This timeseries is created by copying the first image in the timeseries n times and by then applying the inverted motion parameters from the n images to them (while simultaneously accounting for motion * B0 effects; [36]); this allows to assess the signal changes occurring as a function of motion. These signal changes are derived from 9

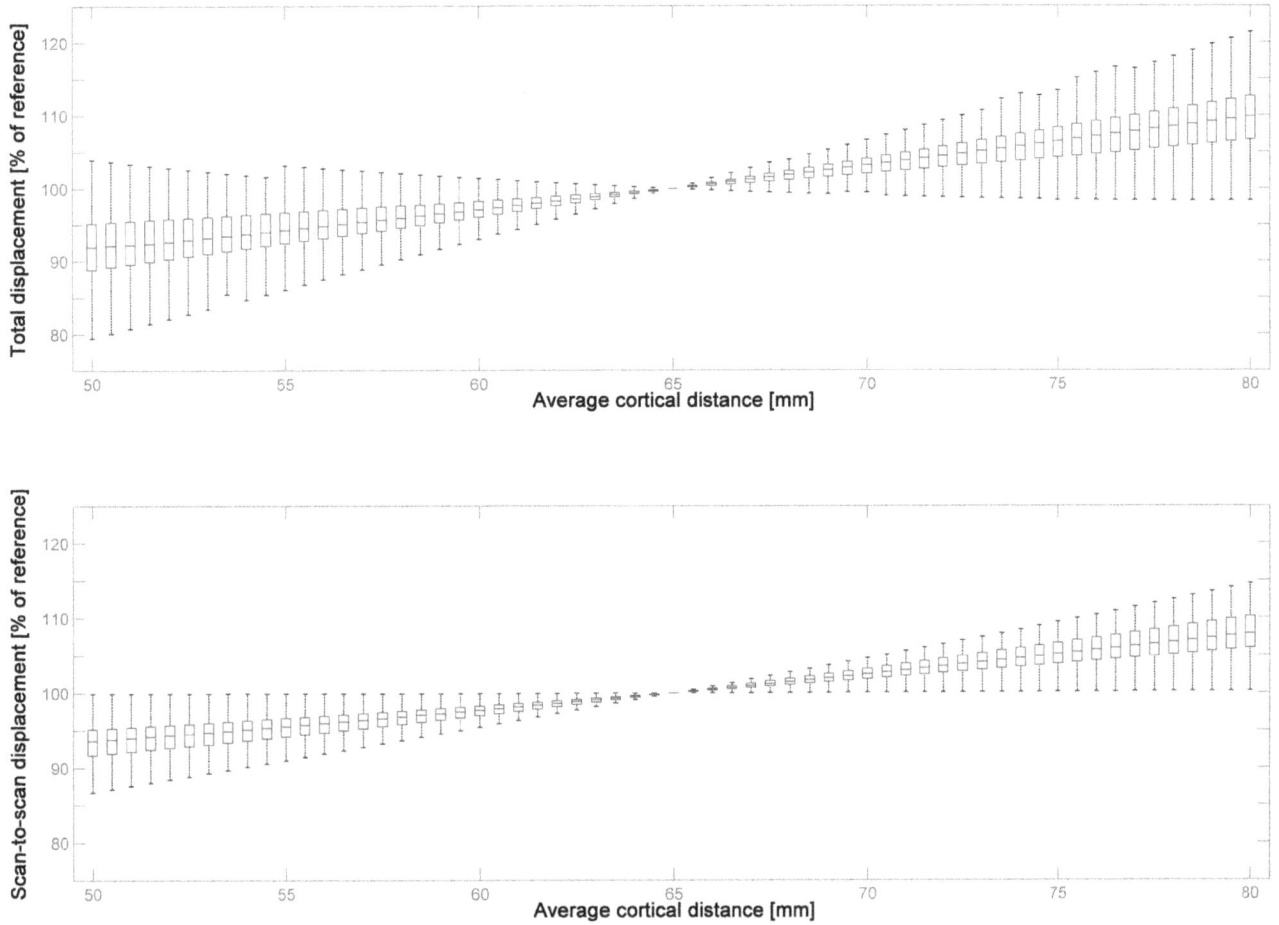

Figure 3. Illustration of the effect of varying average cortical distance on the resulting measure of absolute (total displacement, upper panel) and relative motion (scan-to-scan displacement, lower panel) in dataset 3 (n = 200), using 65 mm as a reference. Note systematic, but overall small effect, and substantial variability between subjects, underlining the inter-individual variation in ultimate motion trajectory composition.

automatically-derived regions of interest in the brain [15,37]; briefly, these are individually determined to be at the interface of brain and non-brain near the 8 corners of the image volume, as well as in the center of the brain. For this analysis, an average of the (absolute) timecourses from all 9 regions was used. The signal changes observable as a result of applying the reduced parameter sets were then again related to the changes resulting from applying the complete parameter set.

Experiment 5

The fifth experiment was aimed to address question V, to what extent does the isolated assessment of translation$_{only}$ or rotation$_{only}$ explain variance in the data, when compared with the complete assessment parameter set. To this effect, different combinations of the reduced and complete assessment parameter sets were used as explanatory variables in a series of general linear model analyses (GLM [38]). The following parameter combinations were assessed: all realignment parameters from the complete assessment (rps$_{complete}$), all realignment parameters from the translation$_{only}$ assessment (rps$_{to}$), and all realignment parameters from the rotation$_{only}$ assessment (rps$_{ro}$). For comparison purposes and following up on the results from experiment 4 (see below), the motion fingerprint (3 original and 3 traces, shifted back in time by one timepoint) from the complete assessment (mfp$_{complete}$) as well

as from both reduced assessments (mfp$_{to}$ and mfp$_{ro}$) was also included. These GLM-analyses were performed for every functional series in dataset 3. Thereafter, an omnibus F-test was used to assess the amount of variance explained by a given set of parameters [1,15,34]. It should be noted that this experiment is aimed to explore the relation of the variance explained by the complete and the reduced parameter sets; it is not aimed to exhaustively of formally compare the explanatory power of either approach. As a reference, the complete assessment set including two modifications (known as "Volterra expansions") was used; to this effect, the original 6 realignment parameters were shifted back in time, and squared versions of each parameter were included, resulting in 24 parameters [1,17]. This modified set was recently shown to explain the largest amount of variance in the data [15] and is therefore used as a reference (i.e., is set to 100%). Possible effects of loss of detection power [39,40] and the fact that more parameters will by default explain more variance were not considered here.

Statistics

Owing to considerations regarding non-linear interactions between parameters and non-normally distributed data, statistical comparisons were done using the non-parametrical Mann-Whitney-U-Test. Correlations were likewise assessed using Spear-

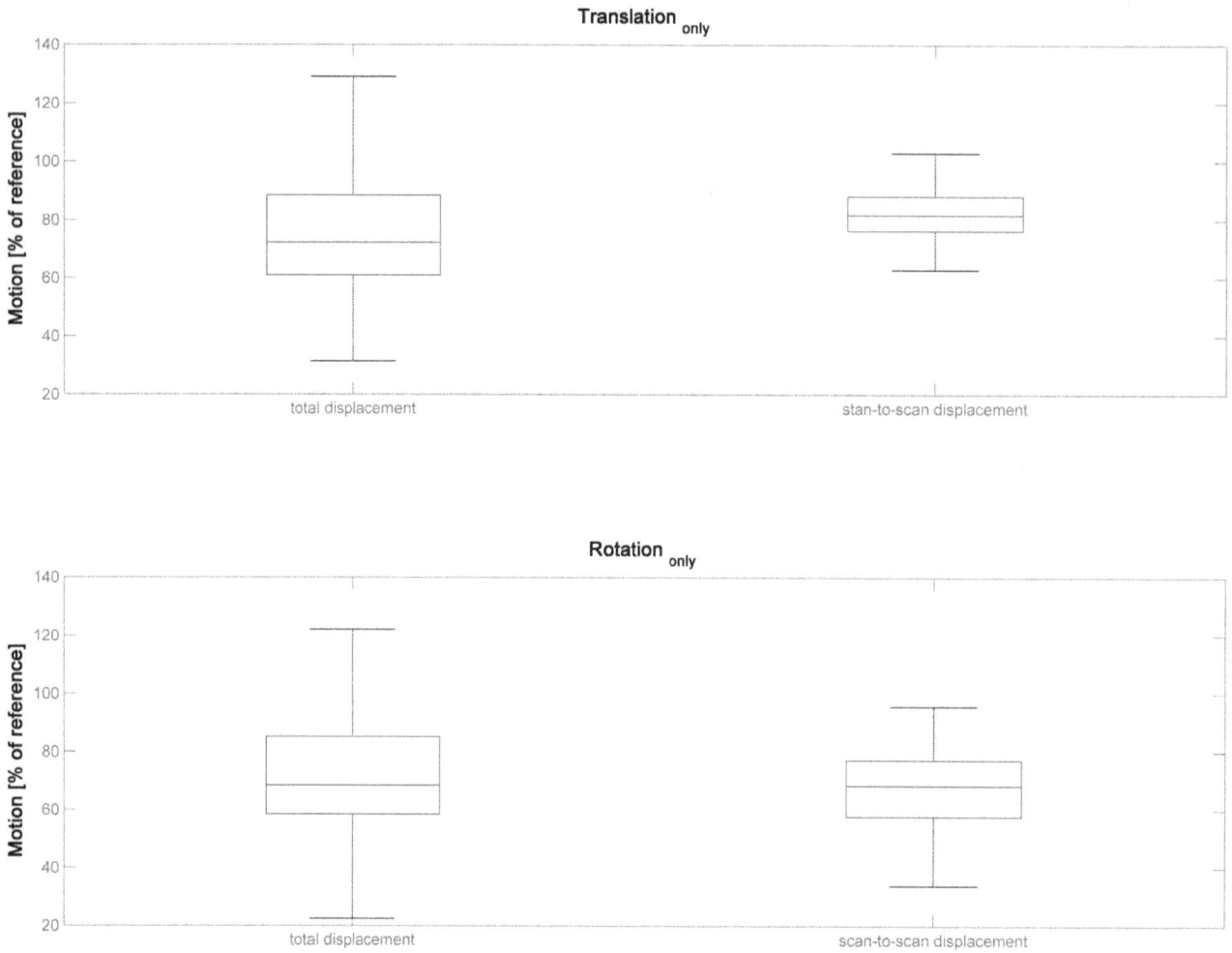

Figure 4. Illustration of estimated subject motion in dataset 3 (n = 200) for the two reduced parameter sets (translation$_{only}$, top panels, and rotation$_{only}$, bottom panels), for both indicators (total displacement, left panels, and scan-to-scan displacement, right panels). Note severe underestimation of total subject motion when compared with the full parameter set (= 100%).

man's rank correlation. In order to avoid being vulnerable to the impact of unequal variances, heteroscedasticity was assessed using Henze-Zirkler's multivariate normality test, as implemented in the robust correlation toolbox [41]. In the presence of inhomogeneous variances, a skipped Spearman's correlation was calculated instead. Bootstrapped confidence intervals (CI) are given, providing further evidence that the correlation is not due to outliers alone. Significance was assumed at $p \leq .05$, Bonferroni-corrected for multiple comparisons where appropriate.

Results

Experiment 1

When assessing the average cortical distance d_{avg} in the structural MR images in dataset 1 and 2, it is apparent that there is a clear developmental trend in childhood & adolescence (Figure 2), with d_{avg} increasing significantly with age (increase of .18 mm/year of age; skipped Spearman's r = .367 with CI = [.285–.452], $p \leq .001$). Interestingly, there is a further increase in adulthood across the age range studied, but the slope is much less steep (increase of .015 mm/year of age; skipped Spearman's r = .1508 with CI = [.075–.232], $p \leq .001$; Figure 2). When comparing the two datasets, there is a significant difference in d_{avg} in

dataset 1 (children & adolescents, median = 61.58 mm) vs. dataset 2 (adults; median 64.95 mm; corrected $p \leq .001$, Mann-Whitney-U-Test), as well as between the datasets from the first and second vs. all other decades (corrected $p \leq .05$, Mann-Whitney-U-Test). The impact of systematically varying d_{avg} on both absolute and relative motion is illustrated in Figure 3.

Experiment 2

When comparing total displacement resulting from the complete assessment parameter set with the isolated assessment of translation$_{only}$, it is apparent that the whole extent of subject motion is severely underestimated, for absolute (median = 72.3%, range 31.5–275.9) as well as for relative motion (median = 81.9%, range, 54.1–102.9; Figure 4). For both cases, this is significantly different from the complete parameter set (set to 100%; corrected $p \leq .001$, Mann-Whitney-U-Test). A similar picture emerges when assessing total displacement resulting from rotation$_{only}$ (absolute motion, median = 68.5%, range, 13.8–279.4; relative motion, median = 68.4%, range, 20.2–108.4). Again and for both cases, this is significantly different from the complete parameter set (set to 100%; corrected $p \leq .001$, Mann-Whitney-U-Test).

Table 3. Summary of discarded datapoints per approach (from dataset 3, with total n = 34.340) and threshold, providing the relation to the assessment using the complete parameter set (= 100%) as well as the corresponding absolute number of datapoints exceeding the threshold (n, values in parentheses).

		0.5 mm	1 mm	1.5 mm	2 mm	2.5 mm	3 mm
Complete assessment	absolute	100% (16.921)	100% (6.989)	100% (3.122)	100% (1.602)	100% (798)	100% (17)
	relative	100% (757)	100% (184)	100% (90)	100% (53)	100% (36)	100% (30)
Translation only	absolute	69.4% (11.749)	41.2% (2.881)	27.8% (870)	26.5% (425)	27.6% (221)	576.5% (98)
	relative	65.6% (497)	66.8% (123)	50% (45)	45.3% (24)	30.6% (11)	20% (6)
Rotation only	absolute	69.1% (11.693)	53.7% (3.760)	39.1% (1.221)	28.9% (463)	12.3% (98)	317.6% (54)
	relative	31.1% (236)	42.3% (78)	53.3% (48)	0% (0)	0% (0)	0% (0)

Experiment 3

When introducing a cutoff value to remove datapoints with unacceptable motion, both isolated assessments discard substantially less datapoints when compared with the results using the complete parameter set (Table 3). The effect initially becomes more pronounced at higher thresholds such that, on average, $\sim$31% (absolute motion) and $\sim$52% (relative motion) less voxels are discarded at a lower threshold (.5 mm), but $\sim$72% (absolute motion) and $\sim$77% (relative motion) less at a higher threshold (2 mm). Interestingly, the pattern reverses at the highest threshold (absolute motion, cutoff of 3 mm), such that the isolated assessment of both translation$_{only}$ and rotation$_{only}$ discard more datapoints then when using the complete parameter set.

Experiment 4

When assessing the signal changes induced in the functional series in dataset 3 by re-applying the complete as well as the reduced parameter sets to a phantom timeseries, it is again apparent that there is no linear cause-effect relation (Figure 5). When assessing the signal changes induced by translation$_{only}$, there is a notable increase in the observable signal changes over all subjects (median = 124.17%, range, 49.18–664.92). In contrast to this, the single changes induced by the rotation$_{only}$ approach are substantially lower, albeit again with a wide spread (median = 71.98%, range, 4.68–627.86). For both cases, the difference is significant, as is the difference between the results from the two reduced parameter sets (all corrected $p \leq .001$, Mann-Whitney-U-Test).

Experiment 5

When assessing the variance explained in the functional series by the complete as well as the reduced parameter sets, it is apparent that all complete and reduced parameter sets explain substantially and significantly less variance than the reference, Volterra-expanded complete parameter set (set to 100%; all corrected $p \leq .001$, Mann-Whitney-U-Test; Figure 6). Further, the differences between the complete and the reduced realignment parameters sets also reach significance (corrected $p \leq .001$, Mann-Whitney-U-Test). Interestingly, the difference between the complete and the reduced motion fingerprint parameter sets is much lower and does not reach significance.

Discussion

This technical note was aimed at addressing the question of how well the effects of subject motion can be predicted when using a reduced parameter set (such as translation$_{only}$).

The first experiment was aimed at assessing whether a representative value of the average cortical distance (d_{avg}) could be derived from MRI data of both children and adults, to allow for the conversion of rotations into an absolute distance. As could be expected [25,33], there is a clear developmental trend in children and adolescents, with a significant increase in d_{avg} (Figure 2). However, this finding is not as trivial as it may sound as brain size does not change substantially anymore [42] and linear scaling during spatial normalization does not correlate with age, in the age range studied [43]. Hence, global and local changes in tissue volume and shape as well as in gyrification could be to blame, with evidence for simultaneous progressive and regressive trends in either [32,33,44,45]. The correlation of this distance parameter with age is actually also significant over the whole cohort in adults, but with a rather shallow slope and a low amount of explained variance. However, it is interesting to note that this correlation is likely brought about by an increase at the older end of the age

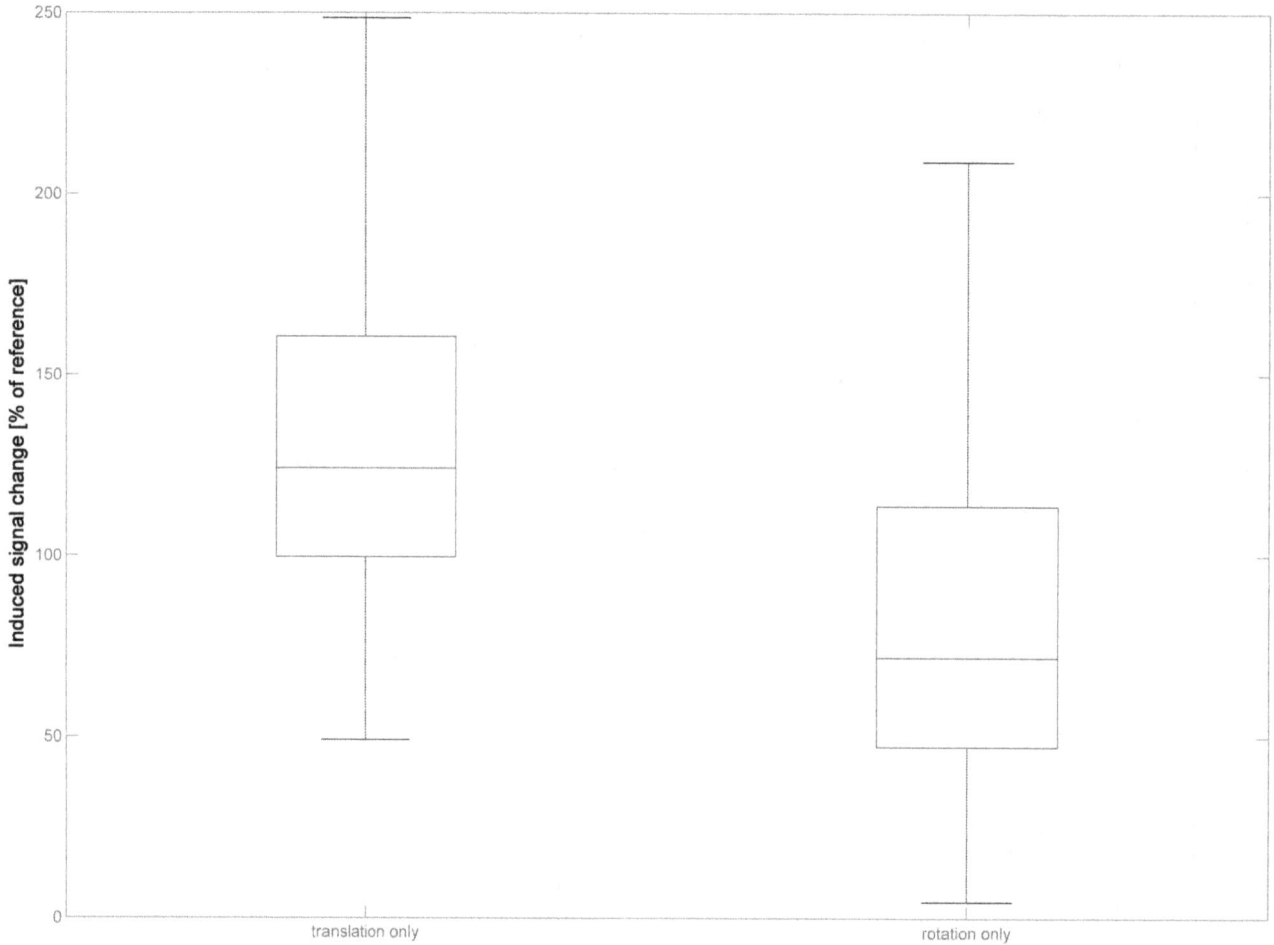

Figure 5. Illustration of the induced signal changes in dataset 3 (n = 200) for the two reduced parameter sets (translation$_{only}$, left panel, and rotation$_{only}$, right panel). Note severe deviation from expected observable signal changes when compared with the signal changes induced by the full parameter set (= 100%).

spectrum, most prominently when comparing the 8th and the 9th decade (Figure 2), although it must be admitted that the individual numbers are small here. It is well known that local and global atrophy as well as changes in gyrification are also hallmarks or normal ageing [46–48]. One explanation for these two, seemingly contradictory observations could be that the predominating, opposing processes (increases in complexity in youth and cortical atrophy in ageing) lead to the same observable phenomena due to their impact on cortical morphology. However, it was felt that a further exploration of the underlying mechanisms was beyond the scope of this manuscript; hence, no further analyses were carried out.

When assessing the influence of modifying d_{avg}, Figure 3 illustrates that the effect is, as expected, systematic, but surprisingly small. For example, when using $d_{avg} = 60$ mm instead of 65 mm, median absolute motion is 97.07% of the original, over all subjects; similarly, when using $d_{avg} = 70$ mm, it is 103.15%. These differences are slightly lower (97.69% and 102.50%, respectively), and less variable, for relative motion. Among the adults included here, 98.8% were within the range of 60–70 mm, and still 73% of the children and adolescents. While these median differences are small, there is a certain variability, which becomes wider when moving further away from the suggested value of 65 mm. This increase in variability can only be due to rotations and underlines

that the relation between translations and rotations is highly individual to each subject, as seen before [23]. Hence, a systematic bias may indeed result when comparing subjects with a systematically differing d_{avg}, such as children vs. adults, as motion will either be slightly underestimated in children or slightly overestimated in adults. On the other hand, these results also suggest that the magnitude of the imprecision induced by using a single, empirically derived value of 65 mm [21] will be rather small, even when assessing a wide range of normal (adult or pediatric) subjects (cf. Figure 2). Using a single indicator has the advantage of making results more comparable between subjects and populations, and it precludes being vulnerable to miscalculations from the actual data [15], for example when the available fMRI data only covers part of the brain, as in high-resolution studies [49,50]. Consequently, this value can be considered to be both useful and representative.

The second experiment was aimed to address the relation of subject motion when using the complete parameter set versus when assessing translation or rotation in isolation. The results demonstrate that the true extent of subject motion is underestimated by a median of ~20–30% when looking at translation$_{only}$ or rotation$_{only}$ (Figure 4). This effect can be observed for both absolute and relative motion. Interestingly, motion is not exclusively underestimated in both reduced parameter sets: while

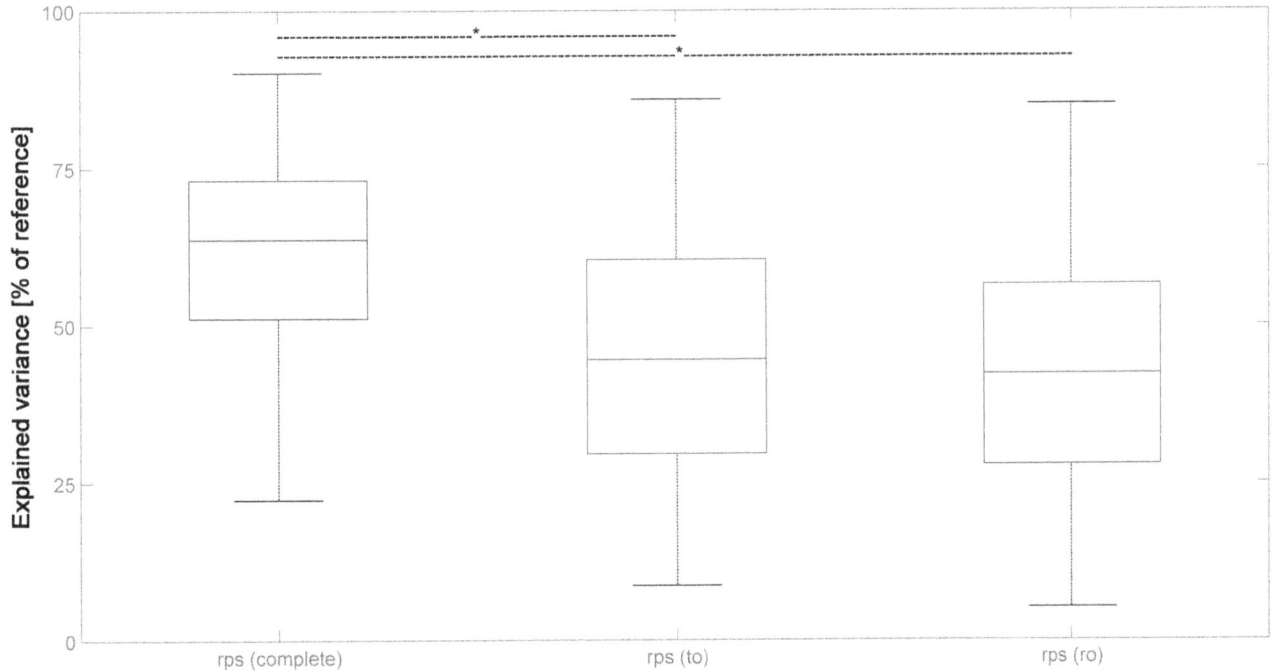

Figure 6. Illustration of the variance explained in dataset 3 (n = 200) by different parameter combinations: complete set of realignment parameters [rps (complete)], realignment parameters from translation$_{only}$ [rps (to)] and rotation$_{only}$ [rps (ro)]. Note increasingly severe underestimation of total motion-induced variance when compared with the full parameter set including Volterra expansion (= 100%); see text for details.

the median is substantially lower, there are also several datapoints exceeding 100% in both analyses. This underlines that the relation of both sets of parameters is not simply additive: accounting for rotation may mean that the motion estimated from translation$_{only}$ is actually reduced, and vice versa. In fact, when assessing the corresponding dimensions (shifts & rotations in x, y, and z) in the whole functional MRI dataset, every single subject shows a substantial number of datapoints with opposite signs between these two parameters. Specifically, in 16.044 [x], 15.641 [y], and 15.385 [z], respectively, of the 34.340 datapoints [per dimension], a shift with a positive sign was accompanied by a rotation with a negative sign, or vice versa. It is therefore important to notice that this complex interrelation precludes an extrapolation of total motion from either factor (as in "total motion≈translation * x", with x representing a fixed factor). This further argues for a combined assessment.

The effect of using a reduced parameter set for quality control purposes was addressed in experiment 3. As can be seen from Table 3, substantially fewer datapoints are discarded when applying a cutoff value in the isolated analyses of translation$_{only}$ or rotation$_{only}$ in almost all scenarios, when compared with using the full parameter set. However, the effect may actually reverse, as can be seen at higher thresholds (Table 3, right-most column). This further underlines the non-linear nature of the interaction of the two reduced parameter sets and again suggests that using translation$_{only}$ or rotation$_{only}$ to assess data quality in functional MRI studies is of only limited applicability, and may be misleading.

In order to assess the effects of motion on the actual fMRI data, the signal change induced by motion can be estimated by reproducing motion in phantom timeseries [15]. This was investigated here in experiment 4, again using the complete parameter set as the reference for the two reduced sets. It is

interesting to notice that translation$_{only}$ actually leads to stronger signal changes in the data, while rotation$_{only}$ induces significantly weaker signal changes, when compared with signal changes induced by the complete parameter set (Figure 5). This again points toward the non-linear interrelation of both reduced parameter sets: while they may in some cases be additive, they may also be subtractive (which, as laid out above, is the case in ~45% of datapoints). It should be noted that the signal changes resulting from the interaction of the head with the static magnetic field (motion * B0 interaction [36,51]) are automatically computed in our motion fingerprint approach. The impact of using a reduced parameter set on this procedure has not been evaluated here. Irrespective of the exact contribution of the different sources, though, these results suggest that the extent of either parameter in isolation is not reliably predictive of the to-be-expected signal change in functional MRI data.

When assessing the amount of variance explained by the different parameter sets in experiment 5, the lower variance explained by the 6 realignment parameters when compared with the Volterra-expanded version confirms previous results [1,15,17]. However, the reduced parameter sets (translation$_{only}$ and rotation$_{only}$) explain significantly less variance again (Figure 6). The difference between the original motion fingerprint approach and the complete realignment parameter set is not significant, again in line with previous results [15]. It is interesting to note, though, that the variance explained by the motion fingerprint does not change as much when using the reduced parameter sets. This is likely due to the fact that, although the reduced parameter sets underestimate subject motion per se (cf. Figure 4), they may both over- and underestimate the resulting signal changes (cf. Figure 5). These discrepancies seem to cancel out to the effect that, overall, the variance explained in the reduced analyses does not differ significantly from the original analysis. On a side note and again confirming previous results [15], the variance explained by a complete motion fingerprint (9 traces) including shifted versions was not significantly lower (median = 93.93%, data not shown) than the variance explained by the reference dataset (Volterra-expanded motion parameters; [1,17]). Taken together, these results suggest that either reduced parameter set in isolation does not reliably predict the variance explained by subject motion in functional MRI data.

Limitations

For this study, several large datasets were used, providing a robust assessment of the resulting metrics, but as always, there are limitations. For one, segmentation of pediatric imaging data should ideally not be performed using adult reference data [34,52]; in order to allow comparability of results over both (adult & pediatric) datasets in experiment 1, the potentially resulting inaccuracies were considered to be secondary. Further, the isolation of the realignment parameters for translation$_{only}$ and rotation$_{only}$ was done post-hoc, and it could be argued that the realignment algorithm should be constrained *a priori* to only perform motion correction using either in isolation. Alternatively, a completely synthetic motion effects simulator approach could be used [51]. On the other hand, the current manuscript investigates a realistic scenario, and being closer to a real-life setting was ultimately judged to be more important. It should also be noted that only one approach to motion correction (the one implemented in SPM8) was used here, while several other implementations are available, e.g. [20,53–55]; however, this manuscript was aimed at highlighting the different shortcomings of using a reduced parameter set to assess subject motion, and the main results are likely independent of the technical implementation of the algorithm, and thus generalizable. Also, no fMRI data acquired in special settings (such as high-motion datasets from patients [17], tasks involving overt speech [56], or data from children [15]) was investigated here. In fact, no dataset using task-based functional MRI was investigated here, which disallows assessing the impact of using different strategies on the resulting statistical maps; however, this was done before [1,15,17,19,54]; besides, using resting-state fMRI data has the added benefit of avoiding the potential interaction of task-induced activation with motion correction [23].

Conclusions

Subject motion is "corrected for" by using a rigid body procedure, which is described in full only by all 6 translation *and* rotation parameters. The results presented here suggest that these two reduced parameter sets (translation$_{only}$ and rotation$_{only}$) can be combined in a meaningful way, using 65 mm as a representative and useful approximation of the average cortical distance. The thus-resulting total displacement cannot be reliably approximated using either reduced parameter set. Therefore, motion censoring procedures relying on a reduced parameter set do not seem appropriate, and both signal changes induced and variance explained by subject motion are severely underestimated. Consequently, a comprehensive measure, taking into account all parameters, should be used to characterize subject motion in fMRI.

Supporting Information

Supplement S1 Includes the detailed listing of all subject IDs from dataset 1 that were used in this study.

Supplement S2 Includes the detailed listing of all subject IDs from dataset 2 that were used in this study.

Supplement S3 Includes the detailed listing of all subject IDs from dataset 3 that were used in this study.

Acknowledgments

I am grateful to those organizations and individuals advancing the field of imaging neuroscience by making their collective datasets publicly available. To this effect, I want to thank all contributors to dataset 1 (the *NIH Study of normal brain development* (NIH, Bethesda, MD, USA), to dataset 2 (the *Biomedical Image Analysis Group* (Imperial College, London, UK), and to dataset 3 (*The 1000 Functional Connectomes Project*), particularly those from Atlanta, Baltimore, Bangor, Beijing, Berlin, Cambridge, Cleveland, Dallas, Montreal, and Leiden. Further details on the exact study participants can be found in the accompanying Supplements S1, S2, and S3.

Disclaimer: The following official disclaimer applies for dataset 1: This manuscript reflects the views of the author and may not reflect the opinions or views of the Brain Development Cooperative Group Investigators or the NIH. The contract numbers for the NIH MRI study of normal brain development were N01-HD02-3343, N01-MH9-0002, and N01-NS-9-2314, 2315, 2316, 2317, 2319 and 2320. A listing of the participating sites and a complete listing of the study investigators can be found at the website of the data coordinating center at www.bic.mni.mcgill.ca/nihpd/info/participating_centers.html.

Author Contributions

Conceived and designed the experiments: MW. Performed the experiments: MW. Analyzed the data: MW. Contributed reagents/materials/analysis tools: MW. Wrote the paper: MW.

References

1. Friston KJ, Williams SR, Howard R, Frackowiak RSJ, Turner R (1996) Movement-related effects in fMRI time-series. Magn Reson Med 35: 346–355.
2. Fair DA, Nigg JT, Iyer S, Bathula D, Mills KL, et al. (2013) Distinct neural signatures detected for ADHD subtypes after controlling for micro-movements in resting state functional connectivity MRI data. Front Syst Neurosci 6: 80.
3. Hallquist MN, Hwang K, Luna B (2013) The nuisance of nuisance regression: spectral misspecification in a common approach to resting-state fMRI preprocessing reintroduces noise and obscures functional connectivity. NeuroImage 82: 208–225.
4. Power JD, Barnes KA, Snyder AZ, Schlaggar BL, Petersen SE (2012) Spurious but systematic correlations in functional connectivity MRI networks arise from subject motion. NeuroImage 59: 2142–2154.
5. Van Dijk KR, Sabuncu MR, Buckner RL (2012) The influence of head motion on intrinsic functional connectivity MRI. NeuroImage 59: 431–438.
6. Brown TT, Kuperman JM, Erhart M, White NS, Roddey JC, et al. (2010) Prospective motion correction of high-resolution magnetic resonance imaging data in children. NeuroImage 53: 139–145.

7. Lee CC, Grimm RC, Manduca A, Felmlee JP, Ehman RL, et al. (1998) A prospective approach to correct for inter-image head rotation in fMRI. Magn Reson Med 39: 234–243.
8. Schulz J, Siegert T, Bazin PL, Maclaren J, Herbst M, et al. (2014) Prospective slice-by-slice motion correction reduces false positive activations in fMRI with task-correlated motion. NeuroImage 84: 124–132.
9. Glover GH, Li TQ, Ress D (2000) Image-based method for retrospective correction of physiological motion effects in fMRI: RETROICOR. Magn Reson Med 44: 162–167.
10. Loktyushin A, Nickisch H, Pohmann R, Schölkopf B (2013) Blind retrospective motion correction of MR images. Magn Reson Med 70: 1608–18.
11. Ashburner J, Friston KJ (2003) Rigid body registration. In Frackowiak RSJ, Friston KJ, Frith C, Dolan R, Price CJ, Zeki S, Ashburner J, Penny WD, editors: Human Brain Function. Academic Press, 2nd edition.
12. Johnstone T, Ores Walsh KS, Greischar LL, Alexander AL, Fox AS, et al. (2006) Motion correction and the use of motion covariates in multiple-subject fMRI analysis. Hum Brain Mapp 27: 779–788.

13. Nemani AK, Atkinson IC, Thulborn KR (2009) Investigating the consistency of brain activation using individual trial analysis of high-resolution fMRI in the human primary visual cortex. NeuroImage 47: 1417–1424.

14. Lund TE, Nørgaard MD, Rostrup E, Rowe JB, Paulson OB (2005) Motion or activity: their role in intra- and inter-subject variation in fMRI. NeuroImage 26: 960–964.

15. Wilke M (2012) An alternative approach towards assessing and accounting for individual motion in fMRI timeseries. NeuroImage 59: 2062–2072.

16. Friston KJ, Ashburner J, Frith CD, Poline JB, Heather JD, et al. (1995) Spatial registration and normalization of images. Hum Brain Mapp 2: 165–189.

17. Lemieux L, Salek-Haddadi A, Lund TE, Laufs H, Carmichael D (2007) Modelling large motion events in fMRI studies of patients with epilepsy. Magn Reson Imaging 25: 894–901.

18. Murphy K, Birn RM, Bandettini PA (2013) Resting-state fMRI confounds and cleanup. NeuroImage 80: 349–359.

19. Siegel JS, Power JD, Dubis JW, Vogel AC, Church JA, et al. (2014) Statistical improvements in functional magnetic resonance imaging analyses produced by censoring high-motion data points. Hum Brain Mapp 35: 1981–1996.

20. Jenkinson M, Bannister P, Brady M, Smith S (2002) Improved optimization for the robust and accurate linear registration and motion correction of brain images NeuroImage 17: 825–841.

21. Mazaika PK, Glover GH, Reiss AL (2011) Rapid Motions in Pediatric and Clinical Populations. Abstract #4535, presented at HBM-conference, Quebec City.

22. Yuan W, Altaye M, Ret J, Schmithorst V, Byars AW, et al. (2009) Quantification of head motion in children during various fMRI language tasks. Hum Brain Mapp 30: 1481–1489.

23. Churchill NW, Oder A, Abdi H, Tam F, Lee W, et al. (2012) Optimizing preprocessing and analysis pipelines for single-subject fMRI. I. Standard temporal motion and physiological noise correction methods. Hum Brain Mapp 33: 609–627.

24. Wilke M, Lidzba K, Staudt M, Buchenau K, Grodd W, et al. (2005) Comprehensive language mapping in children, using functional magnetic resonance imaging: what's missing counts. Neuroreport 16: 915–919.

25. Evans AC, Brain Development Cooperative Group (2006) The NIH MRI study of normal brain development. NeuroImage 30: 184–202.

26. Biomedical Image Analysis Group (2014); IXI - Information eXtraction from Images (EPSRC GR/S21533/02), available at http://biomedic.doc.ic.ac.uk/brain-development/index.php?n=Main.Datasets; last accessed February 4th, 2014.

27. fcon_1000 (2014) The 1000 Functional Connectomes Project resting-state fMRI repository, available at http://fcon_1000.projects.nitrc.org/index.html, last accessed February 4th, 2014.

28. Biswal BB, Mennes M, Zuo XN, Gohel S, Kelly C, et al. (2010) Toward discovery science of human brain function. Proc Natl Acad Sci USA 107: 4734–4739.

29. Unser M (1999) Splines: A Perfect Fit for Signal and Image Processing. IEEE Sign Proc Mag 16: 22–38.

30. Grootoonk S, Hutton C, Ashburner J, Howseman AM, Josephs O, et al. (2000) Characterization and correction of interpolation effects in the realignment of fMRI time series. NeuroImage 11: 49–57.

31. ArtRepair (2014) ArtRepair Software, available at http://cibsr.stanford.edu/tools/human-brain-project/artrepair-software.html, last accessed February 6th, 2014.

32. Brain Development Cooperative Group (2012) Total and regional brain volumes in a population-based normative sample from 4 to 18 years: the NIH MRI Study of Normal Brain Development. Cereb Cortex 22: 1–12.

33. Wilke M, Krägeloh-Mann I, Holland SK (2007) Global and local development of gray and white matter volume in normal children and adolescents. Exp Brain Res 178: 296–307.

34. Wilke M, Holland SK, Altaye M, Gaser C (2008) Template-O-Matic: a toolbox for creating customized pediatric templates. NeuroImage 41: 903–913.

35. Ashburner J, Friston KJ (2005) Unified segmentation. NeuroImage 26: 839–851.

36. Andersson JL, Hutton C, Ashburner J, Turner R, Friston K (2001) Modeling geometric deformations in EPI time series. NeuroImage 13: 903–919.

37. Wilke M, Rose DF, Holland SK, Leach JL (2014) Multidimensional Morphometric 3D MRI Analyses for Detecting Brain Abnormalities in Children: Impact of Control Population. Hum Brain Mapp 35: 3199–3215.

38. Friston KJ, Holmes AP, Worsley KJ, Poline JB, Frith C, et al. (1995) Statistical Parametric Maps in Functional Imaging: A General Linear Approach. Hum Brain Mapp 2: 189–210.

39. Josephs O, Turner R, Friston KJ (1997) Event-related fMRI. Hum. Brain Mapp 5: 243–248.

40. Liu TT, Frank LR, Wong EC, Buxton RB (2001) Detection power, estimation efficiency, and predictability in event-related fMRI. NeuroImage 13: 759–773.

41. Pernet CR, Wilcox R, Rousselet GA (2913) Robust correlation analyses: false positive and power validation using a new open source matlab toolbox. Front Psychol 3: 606.

42. Huttenlocher PR (1979) Synaptic density in human frontal cortex - developmental changes and effects of aging. Brain Res 163: 195–205.

43. Wilke M, Schmithorst VJ, Holland SK (2002) Assessment of spatial normalization of whole-brain magnetic resonance images in children. Hum Brain Mapp 17: 48–60.

44. Vannucci RC, Barron TF, Lerro D, Antón SC, Vannucci SJ (2011) Craniometric measures during development using MRI. NeuroImage 56: 1855–1864.

45. White T, Su S, Schmidt M, Kao CY, Sapiro G (2010) The development of gyrification in childhood and adolescence. Brain Cogn 72: 36–45.

46. Magnotta VA, Andreasen NC, Schultz SK, Harris G, Cizadlo T, et al. (1999) Quantitative in vivo measurement of gyrification in the human brain: changes associated with aging. Cereb Cortex 9: 151–160.

47. Rettmann ME, Kraut MA, Prince JL, Resnick SM (2006) Cross-sectional and longitudinal analyses of anatomical sulcal changes associated with aging. Cereb Cortex 16: 1584–1594.

48. Ziegler G, Dahnke R, Jäncke L, Yotter RA, May A, et al. (2012) Brain structural trajectories over the adult lifespan. Hum Brain Mapp 33: 2377–2389.

49. Besle J, Sánchez-Panchuelo RM, Bowtell R, Francis S, Schluppeck D (2013) Single-subject fMRI mapping at 7 T of the representation of fingertips in S1: a comparison of event-related and phase-encoding designs. J Neurophysiol 109: 2293–2305.

50. Carr VA, Engel SA, Knowlton BJ (2013) Top-down modulation of hippocampal encoding activity as measured by high-resolution functional MRI. Neuropsychologia 51: 1829–1837.

51. Drobnjak I, Gavaghan D, Süli E, Pitt-Francis J, Jenkinson M (2006) Development of a functional magnetic resonance imaging simulator for modeling realistic rigid-body motion artifacts. Magn Reson Med 56: 364–380.

52. Wilke M, Schmithorst VJ, Holland SK (2003) Normative pediatric brain data for spatial normalization and segmentation differs from standard adult data. Magn Reson Med 50: 749–757.

53. Cox RW, Hyde JS (1997) Review Software tools for analysis and visualization of fMRI data. NMR Biomed 10: 171–178.

54. Morgan VL, Dawant BM, Li Y, Pickens DR (2007) Comparison of fMRI statistical software packages and strategies for analysis of images containing random and stimulus-correlated motion. Comput Med Imaging Graph 31: 436–446.

55. Oakes TR, Johnstone T, Ores Walsh KS, Greischar LL, Alexander AL, et al. (2005) Comparison of fMRI motion correction software tools. NeuroImage 28: 529–543.

56. Vannest J, Rasmussen J, Eaton KP, Patel K, Schmithorst V, et al. (2010) FMRI activation in language areas correlates with verb generation performance in children. Neuropediatrics 41: 235–239.

22

Lactate and Choline Metabolites Detected *In Vitro* by Nuclear Magnetic Resonance Spectroscopy Are Potential Metabolic Biomarkers for PI3K Inhibition in Pediatric Glioblastoma

**Nada M. S. Al-Saffar[1]*, Lynley V. Marshall[2,3,4], L. Elizabeth Jackson[1], Geetha Balarajah[1¤],
Thomas R. Eykyn[1,5], Alice Agliano[1], Paul A. Clarke[3,6], Chris Jones[2,3], Paul Workman[3,6],
Andrew D. J. Pearson[3,4], Martin O. Leach[1]**

1 Cancer Research UK and EPSRC Cancer Imaging Centre, Division of Radiotherapy and Imaging, The Institute of Cancer Research and The Royal Marsden NHS Foundation Trust, London, United Kingdom, 2 Division of Molecular Pathology, The Institute of Cancer Research and The Royal Marsden NHS Foundation Trust, London, United Kingdom, 3 Division of Cancer Therapeutics, The Institute of Cancer Research and The Royal Marsden NHS Foundation Trust, London, United Kingdom, 4 Division of Clinical Studies. The Institute of Cancer Research and The Royal Marsden NHS Foundation Trust, London, United Kingdom, 5 Division of Imaging Sciences and Biomedical Engineering, King's College London, St Thomas' Hospital, London, United Kingdom, 6 Cancer Research UK Cancer Therapeutics Unit, The Institute of Cancer Research, London, United Kingdom

Abstract

The phosphoinositide 3-kinase (PI3K) pathway is believed to be of key importance in pediatric glioblastoma. Novel inhibitors of the PI3K pathway are being developed and are entering clinical trials. Our aim is to identify potential non-invasive biomarkers of PI3K signaling pathway inhibition in pediatric glioblastoma using *in vitro* nuclear magnetic resonance (NMR) spectroscopy, to aid identification of target inhibition and therapeutic response in early phase clinical trials of PI3K inhibitors in childhood cancer. Treatment of SF188 and KNS42 human pediatric glioblastoma cell lines with the dual pan-Class I PI3K/mTOR inhibitor PI-103, inhibited the PI3K signaling pathway and resulted in a decrease in phosphocholine (PC), total choline (tCho) and lactate levels ($p<0.02$) as detected by phosphorus (^{31}P)- and proton (^{1}H)-NMR. Similar changes were also detected using the pan–Class I PI3K inhibitor GDC-0941 which lacks significant mTOR activity and is entering Phase II clinical trials. In contrast, the DNA damaging agent temozolomide (TMZ), which is used as current frontline therapy in the treatment of glioblastoma postoperatively (in combination with radiotherapy), increased PC, glycerophosphocholine (GPC) and tCho levels ($p<0.04$). PI-103-induced NMR changes were associated with alterations in protein expression levels of regulatory enzymes involved in glucose and choline metabolism including GLUT1, HK2, LDHA and CHKA. Our results show that by using NMR we can detect distinct biomarkers following PI3K pathway inhibition compared to treatment with the DNA-damaging anti-cancer agent TMZ. This is the first study reporting that lactate and choline metabolites are potential non-invasive biomarkers for monitoring response to PI3K pathway inhibitors in pediatric glioblastoma.

Editor: Ramón Campos-Olivas, Spanish National Cancer Center, Spain

Funding: This work was supported by The Brain Tumour Charity [www.thebraintumourcharity.org] (6/54) to NMSA, GB and AA; The Oak Foundation [www.oakfnd.org] (OCay-04-169) to LVM; Cancer Research UK and EPSRC Cancer Imaging Centre in association with the MRC and Department of Health (England) (C1060/A10334, C1060/6916) to MOL, NMSA, LEJ and TE; Cancer Research UK Life Chair and Programme Grant included within a Cancer Research UK ICR Core Award (C347/A15403) to AP; Cancer Research UK (C309/A2187, C309/A8274) to PW and PAC. PW is a Cancer Research UK Life Fellow; MOL is an NIHR senior investigator. The Institute of Cancer Research co-authors acknowledge National Health Service funding to the Biomedical Research Centre. The funders had no role in study design, data collection or analysis, decision to publish, or preparation of the manuscript.

Competing Interests: The authors of this manuscript have the following competing interests: NMSA, LEJ, GB, TRE, AA, PAC, CJ, ADJP, PW and MOL are employees of the Institute of Cancer Research, which has a commercial interest in the development of PI3K inhibitors, and operates a Rewards to Inventors scheme. PW and PAC have been involved in a commercial collaboration with Yamanouchi (now Astellas Pharma) and with Piramed Pharma and intellectual property arising from the program has been licensed to Genentech. Genentech and Piramed Pharma were acquired by Roche. PW was a founder of, consultant to, and Scientific Advisory Board member of Piramed Pharma (acquired by Roche); was a founder of, consultant to and Scientific Advisory Board and Main Board member of Chroma Therapeutics; is a Consultant/Scientific Advisory Board member to Nextech Ventures, Astex Pharmaceuticals and Wilex Oncology; and w a s formerly an employee of AstraZeneca.

* Email: Nada.Al-Saffar@icr.ac.uk

¤ Current address: Cancer Research UK Cancer Therapeutics Unit, The Institute of Cancer Research, London, United Kingdom

Introduction

Approximately 40% of all pediatric brain tumors are astrocytomas (gliomas), and of these some 15–20% are malignant gliomas, i.e. high-grade (WHO grade III and IV) tumors [1,2]. High-grade gliomas (HGGs) are very aggressive tumors and are one of the leading causes of cancer-related deaths in children with a median survival of just 12–15 months for children with glioblastoma [1,3]. Although these tumors are morphologically similar to malignant gliomas that arise in adults, the molecular pathways of gliomagenesis in children differ substantially from those in adults, resulting in tumors that may arise at differing incidences in different anatomical sites compared to adults and which have a distinct underlying biology [3–8].

As well as numerous qualitative and quantitative differences in DNA copy number abnormalities between pediatric and adult HGG [3], childhood tumors are defined in part by the presence of specific somatic mutations in the gene encoding the histone H3.3 variant, *H3F3A* [7]. These mutations result in amino acid substitutions at two critical positions within the histone tail: the K27M mutation results in a lysine to methionine substitution and the G34R or G34V mutations result in glycine to arginine or valine substitutions. The K27 mutations are typically seen in younger pediatric patients with tumors arising in central locations e.g. brainstem or thalamus, whereas the G34 mutations arise in older pediatric/adolescent patients with tumors arising in the supratentorial (typically cerebral hemispheric) locations [3,7,8]. These histone H3 mutations are not seen in adult HGG beyond approximately 30 years of age and are mutually exclusive with the high frequency of *IDH1* mutations seen in adult populations between 35–45 years of age.

Despite these substantial molecular differences, both adult and childhood malignant gliomas are generally treated similarly with a combination of surgery, irradiation and alkylator-based chemotherapy, using agents such as temozolomide (TMZ), with the classic drug treatment being the Stupp regimen of postoperative radiotherapy with concomitant and adjuvant TMZ [9]. Even with the best protocols, these current treatment strategies provide dismal cure rates for pediatric glioblastoma patients, with TMZ adding only modest survival benefit at best [10,11]. Therefore, research is continuing to unravel the key molecules and signaling pathways responsible for the oncogenesis of different childhood brain tumors with the aim that a new era of molecular based therapies will deliver major benefits for pediatric gliomas [1].

There is mounting evidence that the PI3K/AKT/mTOR signaling pathway is activated in pediatric glioblastoma and contributes to resistance to TMZ [12,13], thus providing key targets for the treatment of pediatric glioblastoma. Numerous small-molecule inhibitors of the PI3K signaling pathway are being developed [14–16] and are progressing through Phase I/II clinical trials in adults with solid tumors, including glioma, and we are currently planning a first-in-child pediatric Phase I trial with an expansion cohort in pediatric glioblastoma.

For the clinical development and evaluation of new molecularly targeted therapies that inhibit signaling pathways, new methods for the assessment of changes in biological properties are required [17]. Non-invasive methods are of particular clinical importance in the study of childhood brain tumors, as they may avoid the need for (repeated) biopsy whilst still providing pharmacodynamic evidence of target or pathway inhibition. A recent study demonstrated the feasibility of [^{18}F]FDG PET to monitor response to PI3K inhibition in adult patients with advanced solid tumors [18]. However, radiation exposure is a potential limitation of PET radioisotopes, particularly in children [19].

Magnetic resonance spectroscopy (MRS) offers the opportunity to investigate metabolic components of cells and tissues in physiological environments, non-invasively and without the use of radioactive reagents. The data are represented by a spectrum, in which the peaks correspond to different metabolites wherein peak areas can be measured and metabolite concentrations quantified [20]. MRS is a powerful tool for the assessment of brain tumors including pre-surgical diagnosis of tumor type and grade, monitoring of treatment response, and evaluation of tumor recurrence [21–23]. There are a number of metabolites that can be identified by standard brain proton (^{1}H)-MRS, but only a few of them have a clinical significance in gliomas including N-acetylaspartate, choline-containing metabolites, creatine, myo-inositol, lactate, and lipids [21]. Our goal is to define the utility of *in vitro* nuclear magnetic resonance (NMR) and subsequently *in vivo* MRS in providing non-invasive pharmacodynamic biomarkers for the inhibition of the PI3K signaling pathway and to aid identification of target inhibition and therapeutic response in early phase clinical trials of PI3K pathway inhibitors in children with glioblastoma.

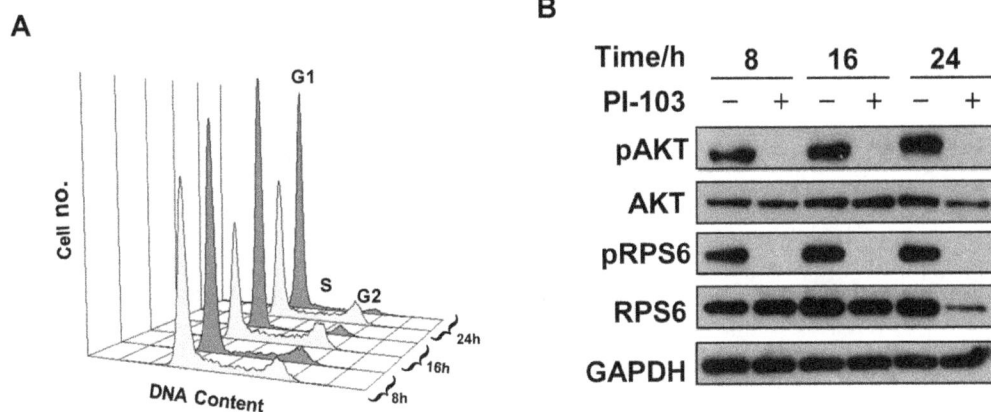

Figure 1. Molecular changes following treatment of SF188 pediatric glioblastoma cells with PI-103. (A) Representative flow cytometry analysis histograms showing cell cycle distribution of cells following vehicle treatment (DMSO, control, light grey), or treatment with PI-103 (5×GI$_{50}$, dark grey) at 8, 16 or 24 hours post treatment. (B) Representative Western blots showing inhibition the PI3K signaling pathway as indicated by decreased phosphorylation of AKT (Ser473) and RPS6 (Ser240/244) at selected time points post treatment with PI-103 (5×GI$_{50}$).

Table 1. Time-response analysis of cell cycle effects following treatment of SF188 pediatric glioblastoma cells with PI-103 ($5 \times GI_{50}$).

Time/hour	8		16		24	
	C	T	C	T	C	T
G1	61±2	75±3*	51±4	85±3**	55±3	86±3***
S	29±3	17±3*	37±5	9±1**	32±1	11±4**
G2	10±1	8±1	12±2	6±2*	13±3	3±2*

Data are expressed as % total cell count and presented as the mean ± SD, n≥3.
Two-tailed unpaired *t* test was used to compare results in treated cells to controls.
*P<0.05,
**P<0.005,
***P<0.0005.

Using NMR, we have previously reported altered choline metabolism in response to inhibition of the PI3K signaling pathway with LY294002, wortmannin and the selective dual pan-Class I PI3K/mTOR inhibitor PI-103 in adult human cancer cell models [24,25]. In this work, we have utilized *in vitro* ^{1}H- and phosphorus (^{31}P)-NMR to monitor metabolic changes following PI3K pathway inhibition by PI-103 and pan–Class I PI3K inhibitor GDC-0941 which lacks significant mTOR activity and is entering Phase II clinical trials, using the pediatric glioblastoma cell lines SF188 and KNS42. Metabolic changes were compared to biomarkers of treatment with the standard of care cytotoxic drug TMZ. We have also investigated potential mechanisms underlying the observed metabolic changes. We report distinct metabolic changes including a decrease in the levels of lactate, phosphocholine (PC) and total choline (tCho) following PI3K pathway inhibition with PI-103 or GDC-0941, whereas there was an increase in PC, glycerophosphocholine (GPC) and tCho following treatment with TMZ. Furthermore, the decrease in PC levels was associated with a decrease in the protein levels of choline kinase alpha (CHKA), the enzyme responsible for choline phosphorylation to form PC. A decrease in the protein expression levels of the facilitative glucose transporter (GLUT1) and the glycolytic enzymes hexokinase II (HK2) and lactate dehydrogenase alpha (LDHA) as well as a decrease in glucose uptake were also observed following PI3K pathway inhibition, suggesting reduced glycolytic flux as a mechanism for depletion of lactate.

Materials and Methods

Cell culture and treatment

The human pediatric glioblastoma (WHO grade IV) cell lines SF188 (a kind gift from Dr. Daphne Haas-Kogan, University of California San Francisco, San Francisco, CA, USA [26]) and KNS42 (obtained from Japan Cancer Research Resources cell bank [27]), have been extensively characterized previously [28]. Both cell lines are wildtype for *PTEN* and *PIK3CA* [13,28] (data not shown). KNS42 is histone H3.3 (H3F3A) G34V mutant and SF188 is wildtype [4]. Cells were grown as monolayers in DMEM/F12 Ham's medium+10% FCS in 5% CO2. Cell viability was routinely >90%, as judged by trypan blue exclusion. Both cell lines routinely tested negative for mycoplasma by PCR.

The two cell lines were treated with the dual pan-Class I PI3K/mTOR inhibitor PI-103 [14–16] (Sigma) and the pan–Class I PI3K inhibitor GDC-0941 [14–16] (Genentech) which lacks significant mTOR activity. SF188 cells were also treated with the cytotoxic drug TMZ (Sigma). GI_{50} values (concentrations causing 50% inhibition of proliferation of tumor cells) were determined using the MTS assay [29] following continuous

exposure to compounds for 3 doubling times. Preliminary experiments were performed on both pediatric cell lines to measure levels of PC per cell at different cell number. This was to establish the cell number to be used for setting up the experiments such that the availability of PC per cell is similar in control and treated cells over the time course of treatment. The final time point was based on the length of the doubling time for the cell lines used (SF188 doubling time 26 hours and KNS42 doubling time 48 hours) and intermediate time points were selected to assess early detection of biomarkers. At the required time points, cells underwent trypsinization and trypan blue exclusion assay [30]. The effect of treatment on cell number was monitored by counting the number of viable attached cells in a treated flask and comparing that number with the number of attached cells in a control flask.

Flow cytometry

Cell cycle analysis was performed as previously described [30]. Control and treated cells were harvested by trypsinization, washed in PBS and fixed in 70% ethanol. Fixed cells were washed and resuspended in PBS supplemented with 10 mg/ml RNase A (Sigma) and 40 mg/mL propidium iodide (Sigma). After 30 minutes of incubation at 37°C, cells were analyzed using BD LSRII flow cytometer (BD, San Jose, CA, USA). The cytometry data were analyzed using the WinMdi and Cylchred software (University of Wales College of Medicine, Cardiff, UK).

Immunoblotting

Western blotting was performed as previously described [25]. Cells were lysed in lysis buffer (Cell Signaling) supplemented with a complete mini protease inhibitor cocktail (Roche Diagnostics). Protein concentration was determined using a BIO-RAD assay. Total protein extracts (30 µg/lane) were separated electrophoretically in 10% SDS-polyacrylamide gel and transferred onto immobilon-P membranes (Millipore). Immunodetection was performed using antibodies against pAKT (Ser473), total AKT, pRPS6 (Ser240/244), total RPS6, HK2 (Cell Signaling), CHKA (Sigma), GLUT1, LDHA (Santa Cruz Biotechnology) and GAPDH (Chemicon). Blots were revealed with peroxidase-conjugated secondary anti-rabbit or anti-mouse antibodies (Cell Signaling) followed by ECL chemiluminescence solution (Amersham Biosciences).

In vitro ^{1}H- and ^{31}P-NMR of cell extracts

To obtain an NMR spectrum, an average of 3×10^7 cells in logarithmic phase were extracted from cell culture using the dual phase extraction method, as previously described [30,31]. Briefly,

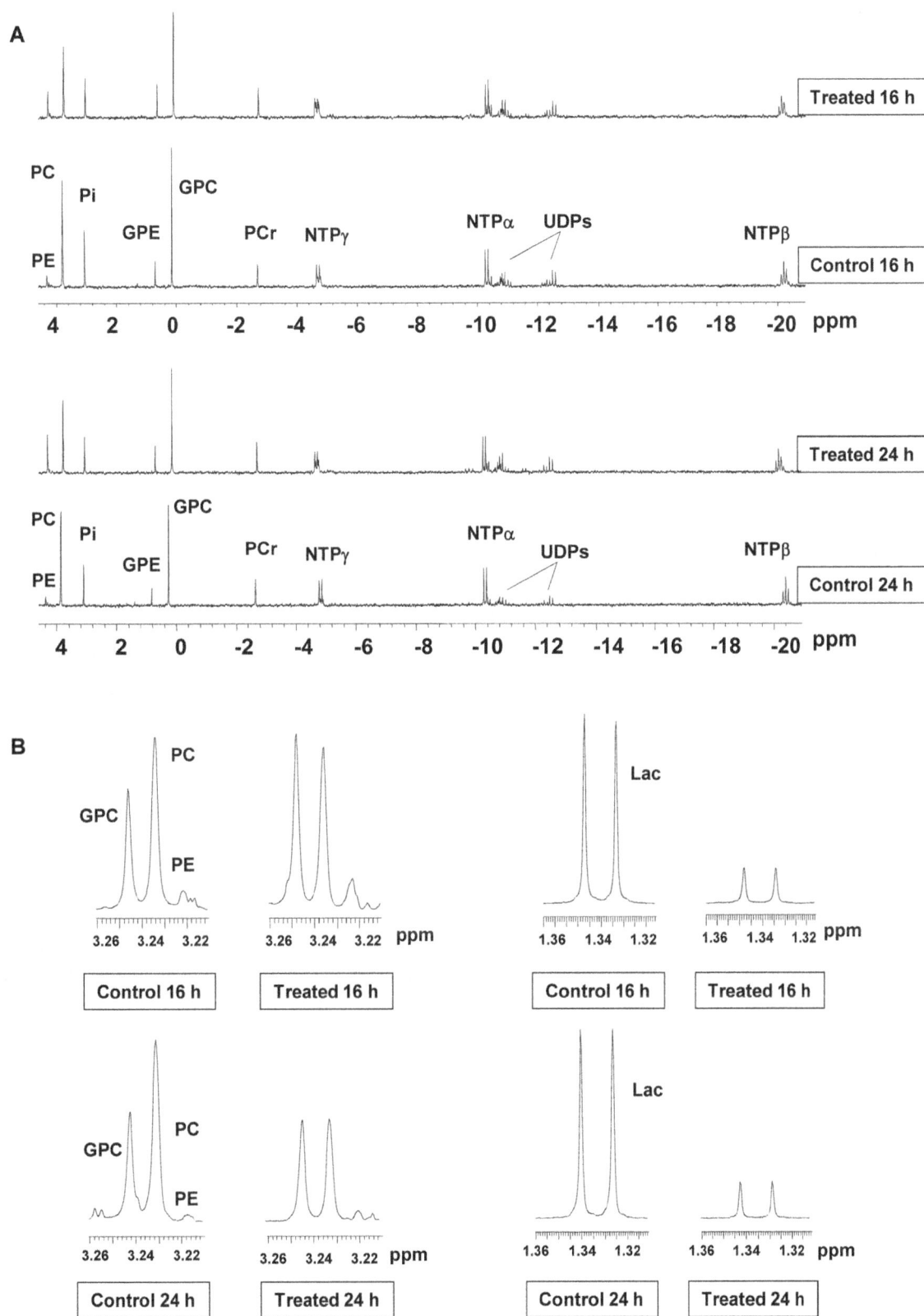

Figure 2. Metabolic changes following treatment of SF188 pediatric glioblastoma cells with PI-103. Representative *in vitro* (A) ^{31}P-NMR spectra and (B) expansion of ^{1}H-NMR spectra regions representing choline–containing metabolites (left) or lactate (Lac; right) of SF188 aqueous cell extracts following 16 or 24 hours treatment with PI-103 ($5 \times GI_{50}$) compared to vehicle (DMSO) treated control. UDPs = UDP sugars.

Table 2. Time-response analysis showing percentage changes in ^{31}P-NMR-detected metabolite levels following treatment of SF188 pediatric glioblastoma cells with PI-103 ($5 \times GI_{50}$).

Time/hour	8	16	24
PE	90±21	183±53*	306±82*
PC	56±6**	70±17*	60±10*
GPC	74±11*	138±58	110±53
NTP	75±9*	106±31	94±15

Data are expressed as percentage of treated to control (% T/C) and presented as the mean ± SD, n≥3.
Glycerophosphoethanolamine (GPE) level was not affected by treatment with PI-103.
Two-tailed unpaired t test was used to compare results in treated cells to controls.
*P<0.05,
**P<0.005.

cells were rinsed with ice-cold saline and fixed with 10 ml of ice-cold methanol. Cells were then scraped off the surface of the culture flask and collected into tubes. Ice-cold chloroform (10 ml) was then added to each tube followed by an equal volume of ice-cold deionized water. Following phase separation, the solvent in the upper methanol/water phase was removed by lyophilization. Prior to acquisition of the NMR spectra, the water-soluble metabolites were resuspended in deuterium oxide (D_2O) for ^{1}H-NMR or D_2O with 10 mM EDTA (pH 8.2) for ^{31}P-NMR. ^{1}H-NMR and ^{1}H-decoupled ^{31}P-NMR spectra were acquired at 25°C on a 500 MHz Bruker spectrometer (Bruker Biospin, Coventry, UK) using a 90-degree flip angle, a 1-second relaxation delay, spectral width of 12 ppm, 64 K data points, and HDO resonance suppression by presaturation for ^{1}H-NMR and a 30-degree flip angle, a 1-second relaxation delay, spectral width of 100 ppm, and 32 K data points for ^{31}P. Metabolite contents were determined by integration and normalized relative to the peak integral of an internal reference [TSP (0.15%) for ^{1}H-NMR, and MDPA (2 mmol/L) for ^{31}P-NMR] and corrected for signal intensity saturation and the number of cells extracted per sample.

In vitro Dynamic Nuclear Polarization (DNP) and Carbon (^{13}C)-NMR

Real-time pyruvate-lactate exchange was measured in live cells at 37°C with a DNP-based assay as previously described [32,33]. Live SF188 cells were studied in control or post treatment with PI-103. Cells ($3.4 \pm 1 \times 10^7$) were suspended in 500 µl of FCS free media containing DMSO (control) or PI-103 (treated) within 10 minutes of cell harvesting. [1-^{13}C]pyruvic acid (99% isotopically enriched (Sigma) containing 15 mM trityl free radical OX63 (Oxford Instruments, UK) was polarized in a HyperSense® DNP polarizer (Oxford Instruments Molecular Biotools Ltd, UK) for 1 hour. The polarized sample was dissolved in 4 ml aqueous buffer (50 mM sodium lactate, 50 mM NaOH, 1 mM EDTA) resulting in a 50 mM pyruvate solution at pH 7, 37°C. A solution of 100 µl, 50 mM hyperpolarized [1-^{13}C]pyruvate was mixed with 500 µl cell suspension to yield a final concentration 8 mM hyperpolarized pyruvate, 8 mM unpolarized lactate. ^{13}C spectra were acquired every 2 seconds using a single scan and a 10° flip angle. Spectra were phase and baseline corrected, and peak areas integrated over the time-course of the experiment. Kinetic modeling was carried out in Matlab (Mathworks®, UK) by fitting the time-series of peak areas with the modified Bloch equations using maximum likelihood estimation. The time-courses of integrals from hyperpolarized lactate and pyruvate signals were summed and the ratios of the total lactate/total pyruvate curves were calculated to give the area under the curve metric (AUC).

Statistical analysis

Data are presented as the mean ± SD and n ≥ 3. Statistical significance of differences was determined by unpaired two-tailed Student's standard t-tests with a p-value of ≤0.05 considered to be statistically significant.

Table 3. Time-response analysis showing percentage changes in ^{1}H-NMR-detected metabolite levels following treatment of SF188 pediatric glioblastoma cells with PI-103 ($5 \times GI_{50}$).

Time/hour	8	16	24
Lac	35±5***	39±11**	27±6**
PC	63±4***	69±13*	71±9*
GPC	88±8	125±43	105±12
tCho	65±18*	89±17	85±9

Data are expressed as percentage of treated to control (% T/C) and presented as the mean ± SD, n≥3.
Two-tailed unpaired t test was used to compare results in treated cells to controls.
*P<0.05,
**P<0.005,
***P<0.0005.

A

B

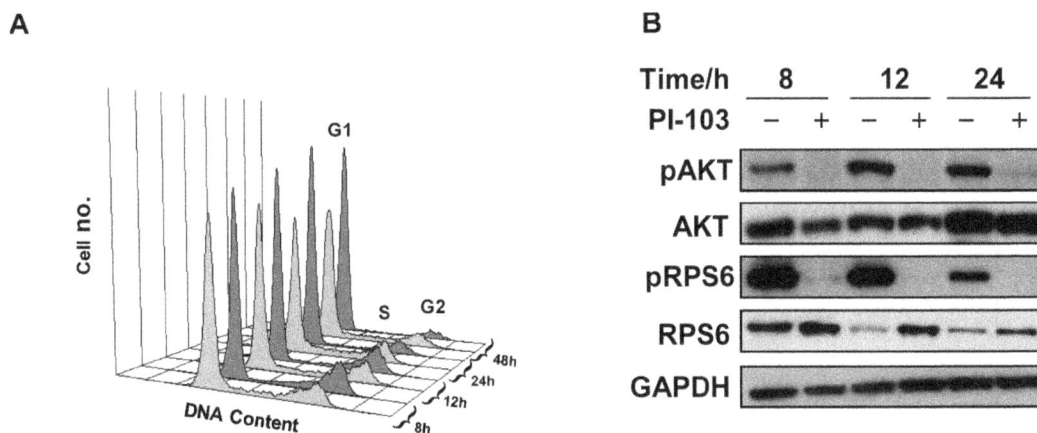

Figure 3. Molecular changes following treatment of KNS42 pediatric glioblastoma cells with PI-103. (A) Representative flow cytometry analysis histograms showing cell cycle distribution of cells with vehicle treatment (DMSO, control, light grey), or following treatment with PI-103 ($5 \times GI_{50}$, dark grey) at 8, 12, 24 or 48 hours post treatment. (B) Representative Western blots showing inhibition of the PI3K signaling pathway as indicated by decreased phosphorylation of AKT (Ser473) and RPS6 (Ser240/244) at selected time points post treatment with PI-103 ($5 \times GI_{50}$).

Results

^{1}H- and ^{31}P-NMR detect metabolic changes following inhibition of the PI3K signaling pathway in pediatric glioblastoma cell lines

Treatment of the pediatric glioblastoma cell line SF188 with the dual pan-Class I PI3K/mTOR inhibitor PI-103 [14–16] for 8, 16 and 24 hours at pharmacologically active concentrations corresponding to $5 \times GI_{50}$ ($GI_{50} = 0.2$ μM) resulted in an increase in G1 cell population and a decrease in S phase relative to control cells (Figure 1A, Table 1). This led to a decrease in the number of treated cells per flask compared to controls (down to $82 \pm 2\%$, $p = 0.001$ and $63 \pm 4\%$, $p = 0.0004$ at 16 hours and 24 hours post treatment, respectively). Inhibition of signaling downstream of PI3K was confirmed by immunoblotting as indicated by decreased phosphorylation of AKT (Ser473) and RPS6 (Ser240/244) in treated cells compared to their controls (Figure 1B).

NMR spectroscopy of aqueous extracts from cells treated *in vitro* with PI-103 was used to identify potential biomarkers of PI3K pathway inhibition. Examples of the ^{31}P-NMR spectra of control and PI-103 treated SF188 cells are illustrated in Figure 2A (16 and 24 hour time points). ^{31}P-NMR spectra showed that PI-103 treatment caused a decrease in PC levels compared to controls starting from 8 hours following treatment (from 24.4 ± 5.1 fmol/cell to 13.4 ± 2.3 fmol/cell, $p = 0.03$) and these were further reduced from 17.5 ± 1.3 fmol/cell to 9.8 ± 1.8 fmol/cell ($p = 0.01$) at 24 hours post treatment. A decrease in GPC was also observed (from 18.3 ± 1.4 fmol/cell to 13.4 ± 1.7 fmol/cell, $p = 0.009$) at 8 hours post PI-103 treatment while an increase in phosphoethanolamine (PE) levels was detected at 16 hours and further increased at 24 hours from 1.6 ± 0.3 fmol/cell to 5.4 ± 0.8 fmol/cell ($p = 0.01$). Time-course changes in the levels of PC and other ^{31}P-NMR detected metabolites relative to their controls are summarized in Table 2.

^{1}H-NMR spectra of extracts from control and PI-103 treated SF188 cells were also investigated at several time points (Figure 2B shows the 16 & 24 hour time points). As had been seen with ^{31}P-NMR, a decrease in PC levels was observed by ^{1}H-NMR starting from 8 hours following treatment with PI-103 (Table 3). Furthermore, levels of tCho (PC+GPC+choline+ethanolamine metabolites) decreased at 8 hours but recovered to control levels from 16 hours post treatment (Table 3). The apparent recovery at 16 hours

and later is due to the increase in PE peaks (NCH_2, 3.22 ppm) that reside close to the tCho peaks area ($N^+(CH_3)_3$, 3.21–3.24 ppm) within the ^{1}H-NMR spectrum and is included in the summed tCho peak [20] (Figure 2B). Moreover, treatment with PI-103 caused a highly significant ($p < 0.004$) reduction in lactate levels over the time course of treatment (Figure 2B, Table 3). No significant changes were observed in other ^{1}H-NMR-detected metabolites.

To test for the consistency of the NMR detected data, we also treated the pediatric glioblastoma cell line KNS42 with PI-103 for 8, 12, 24 and 48 hours at a pharmacologically active concentration corresponding to $5 \times GI_{50}$ ($GI_{50} = 1.4$ μM). As for SF188, PI-103 caused a G1 arrest in KNS42 cells (Figure 3A, Table 4), resulting in a decrease in the proliferation of treated cells compared to controls (down to $49 \pm 8\%$, $p = 0.002$, 48 hours). Inhibition of PI3K signaling was confirmed by decreased phosphorylation of AKT (Ser473) and RPS6 (Ser240/244) in treated cells compared to their controls (Figure 3B).

Analysis of ^{31}P-NMR spectra of control and PI-103 treated KNS42 cells showed a decrease in PC levels relative to controls that was similar to that observed with SF188, starting from 8 hours but in this case reaching significance at 12 hours following treatment from 40.2 ± 2.0 fmol/cell to 26.3 ± 7.9 fmol/cell ($p = 0.02$) and was down from 37.8 ± 5.9 fmol/cell to 20.5 ± 6.1 fmol/cell ($p = 0.02$) following 48 hours of incubation with PI-103 (Figure 4A shows the 12 & 24 hour time points). Time-course changes in the levels of PC and other ^{31}P-NMR detected metabolites relative to their controls are summarized in Table 5. ^{1}H-NMR confirmed changes detected by ^{31}P-NMR and further showed a significant ($p < 0.01$) decrease in levels of tCho and lactate (Figure 4B, Table 6).

Treatment of the pediatric glioblastoma cell lines with the pan-Class I PI3K inhibitor GDC-0941 results in similar metabolic changes compared to the dual pan-Class I PI3K/mTOR inhibitor PI-103

We see consistent and significant changes in PC, tCho and lactate in two different pediatric cell lines. Hence we tried a different PI3K inhibitor to assess the potential relevance of the NMR-detectable metabolic changes to inhibition of the PI3K signaling pathway. Both pediatric glioblastoma cell lines were

Table 4. Time-response analysis of cell cycle effects following treatment of KNS42 pediatric glioblastoma cells with PI-103 (5×GI$_{50}$).

Time/hour	8		12		24		48	
	C	T	C	T	C	T	C	T
G1	60±5	63±4	62±2	70±4*	60±4	84±1*	69±3	89±2***
S	30±4	26±4	26±2	18±3**	27±8	10±3	22±1	5±2***
G2	10±3	11±1	12±3	12±2	13±4	6±2	9±3	6±2

Data are expressed as % total cell count and presented as the mean ± SD, n≥3.
Two-tailed unpaired t test was used to compare results in treated cells to controls.
*P<0.05,
**P<0.005,
***P<0.0005.

treated with the selective pan-Class I PI3K inhibitor GDC-0941 [14–16] which does not significantly inhibit mTOR and is entering Phase II clinical trials. Treatment with GDC-0941 at 5×GI$_{50}$ for 24 hours (SF188 GI$_{50}$ = 1.2 μM, KNS42 GI$_{50}$ = 1.8 μM), decreased cell number to 60±10% (p = 0.00003) and 81±11% (p = 0.03) in SF188 and KNS42, respectively. Inhibition of PI3K signaling was confirmed by decreased phosphorylation of AKT (Ser473) and RPS6 (Ser240/244) in treated cells compared to their controls (Figure 5A & B).

NMR analysis showed decreases in PC, tCho and lactate levels in both cell lines, similar to that observed following PI-103 treatment (Figure 5C & D). Again like PI-103, treatment with GDC-0941 caused a significant increase in PE levels in SF188 cells (up to 145±27%, p = 0.03) but not with KNS42 cells (124±48%, p = 0.4). However, the effects of GDC-0941 on GPC levels were different to that of PI-103, with an increase (up to 133±23%, p = 0.05) in SF188 cells and no change (119±37%, p = 0.4) in KNS42 cells.

Treatment of SF188 pediatric glioblastoma cells with the cytotoxic drug TMZ results in metabolic changes distinct from those seen with the PI3K pathway inhibitors PI-103 and GDC-0941

To further assess specificity of our NMR-detected metabolic changes to PI3K inhibition rather than anti-proliferative effects, the SF188 pediatric glioblastoma cell line was treated with PI-103 or the cytotoxic drug TMZ. TMZ was selected as this is the standard frontline treatment for patients with glioblastoma [10,11]. Concentrations equivalent to 2×GI$_{50}$ were selected for this comparison in order to be more representative of clinical conditions and to assess whether the metabolic changes could be detected even at lower drug concentrations than previously tested. Treatment of SF188 cells with PI-103 at 2×GI$_{50}$ for 24 hours decreased cell number to 58±8%, p = 0.00007 relative to controls and inhibited PI3K signaling (Figure 6A). Our NMR-detected changes were still observed when PI-103 concentration was reduced to 2×GI$_{50}$ (Figure 6B) compared to 5×GI$_{50}$ (Figure 5C). Treatment of SF188 cells with TMZ at 2×GI$_{50}$ for 24 hours (GI$_{50}$ = 0.46 mM) decreased cell number to 66±17%, p = 0.008 and as expected, TMZ did not affect PI3K signaling (Figure 6A). In direct contrast to the decrease in PC and tCho consistently observed with PI-103 and GDC-0941, ^{1}H-NMR spectra showed that TMZ significantly (p≤0.04) increased levels of PC, GPC and tCho. TMZ had no effect on lactate levels (Figure 6B).

Inhibition of the PI3K signaling pathway in SF188 pediatric glioblastoma cells results in altered expression of enzymes involved in choline and glucose metabolism

We used different techniques to explore the mechanisms underlying the metabolic changes observed with NMR. The SF188 cell line treated with PI-103 (5×GI$_{50}$) was selected as a model. Previously [24], we have shown a direct correlation between changes in PC levels detected with NMR and changes in protein expression levels of CHKA, the enzyme responsible for phosphorylating choline and generating PC. To find out whether this applies to the pediatric cell line SF188, CHKA protein levels were analyzed by immunoblotting. A decrease in CHKA protein expression was detectable from 8 hours following treatment of SF188 cells with PI-103, and was maintained over the time course of treatment (Figure 7A).

Immunoblotting was also used to assess mechanisms underlying the decrease in lactate following PI3K pathway inhibition; protein expression levels of the facilitative glucose transporter GLUT1 and

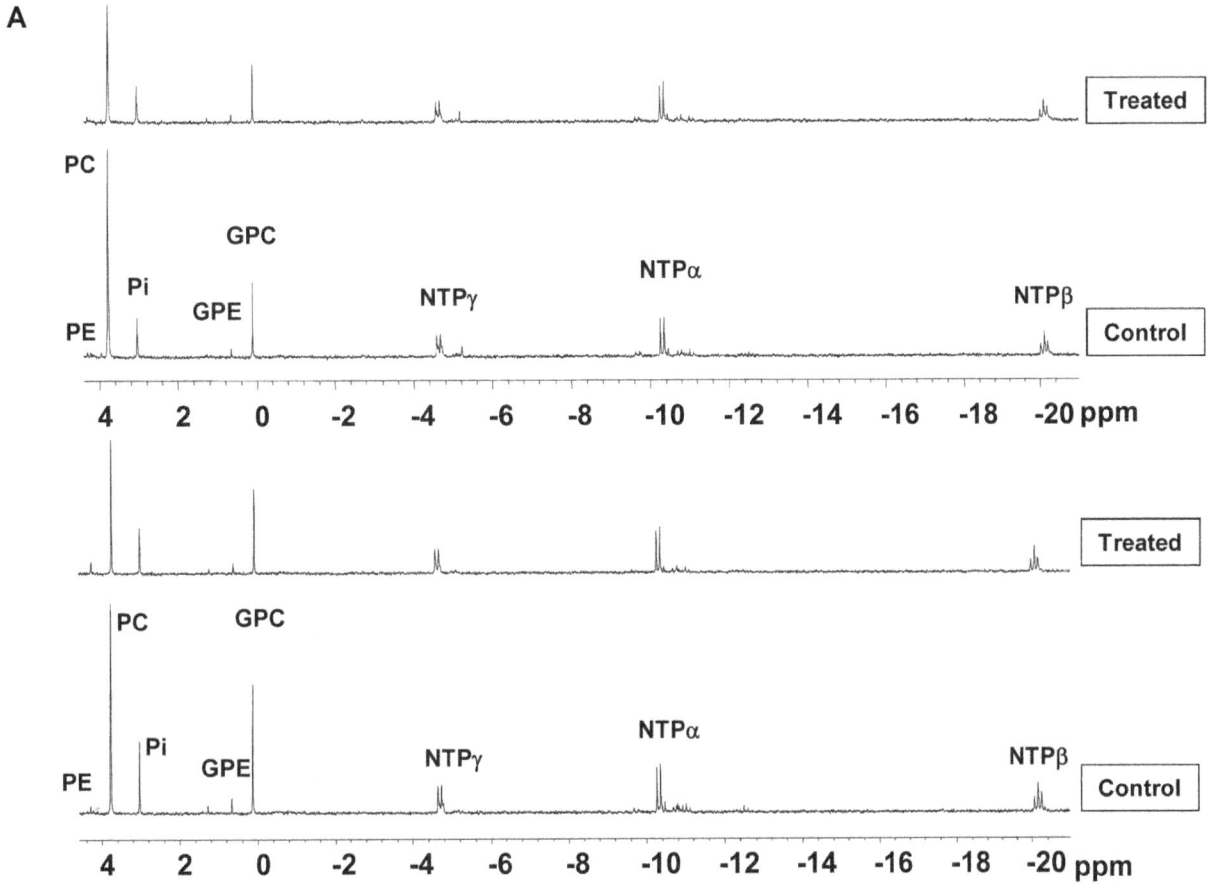

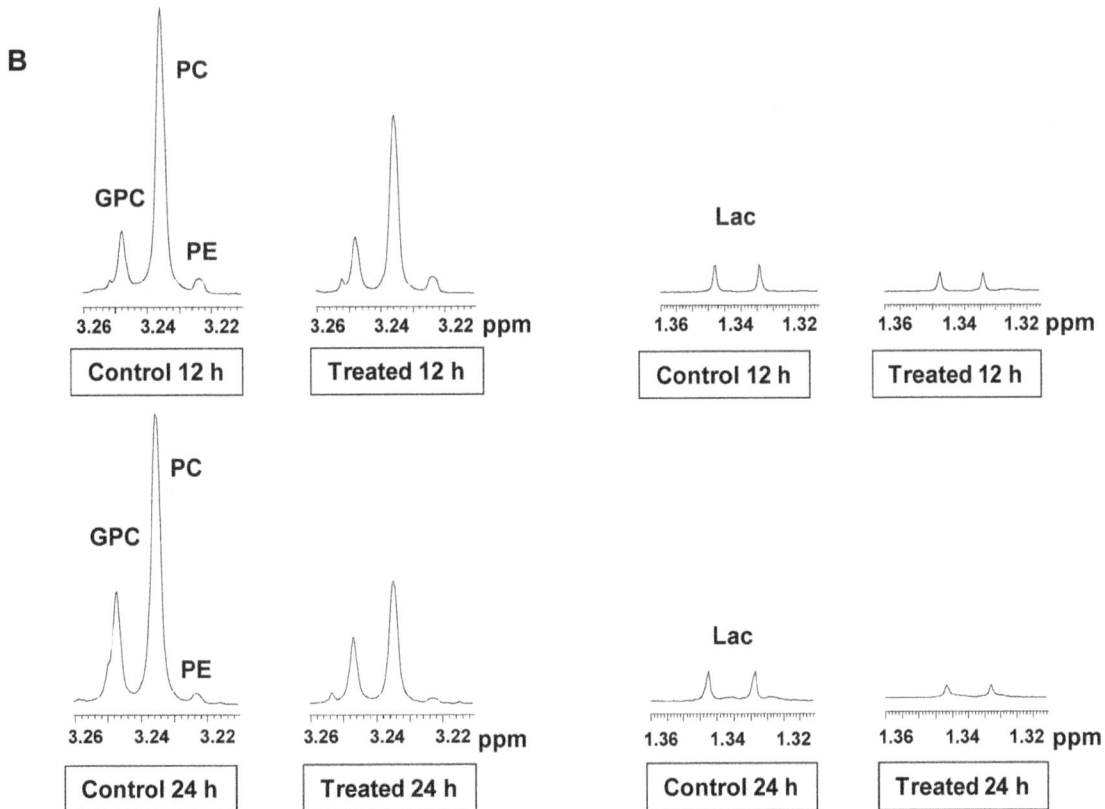

Figure 4. Metabolic changes following treatment of KNS42 pediatric glioblastoma cells with PI-103. Representative *in vitro* (A) ^{31}P-NMR spectra and (B) expansion of ^{1}H-NMR spectra regions representing choline–containing metabolites (left) or lactate (Lac; right) of KNS42 aqueous cell extracts following 12 or 24 hours treatment with PI-103 ($5 \times GI_{50}$) compared to vehicle (DMSO) treated control.

the glycolytic enzymes HK2 and LDHA were reduced over the time course of treatment with PI-103 (Figure 7A). Interestingly, protein expression levels of the glycolytic enzyme GAPDH was not affected by PI-103 treatment allowing its use as a loading control.

To determine whether the decrease in intracellular lactate could be due to the efflux of lactate into the tissue culture medium, we used ^{1}H-NMR to measure levels of lactate in the growth media of control and PI-103 treated SF188 cells. Similar amounts of lactate were detected in the medium of treated compared to control cells. However, analysis of glucose showed higher glucose levels in media from the 16 and 24 hours PI-103 treated cells relative to controls (Figure 7B), indicating a decrease in glucose uptake by the PI-103 treated cells.

Hyperpolarized pyruvate-lactate ^{13}C exchange assay

Finally, we used the DNP technique to measure the exchange kinetics of hyperpolarized lactate from hyperpolarized pyruvate in PI-103 treated compared to control live SF188 cells. Sum ^{13}C-NMR spectra over the entire time-series are displayed in Figure 7C with peaks corresponding to lactate, pyruvate and pyruvate hydrate for the SF188 cell line in either control (top) or PI-103 treated groups (bottom), from which a decrease in the lactate peak intensity can be appreciated. The time-series of the lactate peak integral normalized to cell number is shown pre and post treatment in Figure 7D with inset showing the pyruvate time dependence. Rate constants for the forwards exchange reaction from pyruvate to lactate were derived from non-linear least squares fitting of the bi-exponential time dependence of the hyperpolarized lactate and pyruvate curves and normalized to cell number in both control and treated cells [32,33].

A decrease in the rate of pyruvate-lactate exchange rate constants (Figure 7E) was detected in PI-103 treated cells (0.285 ± 0.018 nmol s^{-1} 10^{-6} cells) compared to controls (0.400 ± 0.039 nmol s^{-1} 10^{-6} cells), p = 0.02. A decrease in the area under the curve was also observed (Figure 7F) in PI-103 treated cells ($3.84 \pm 0.44 \times 10^{-9}$ cells) compared to controls ($5.83 \pm 0.25 \times 10^{-9}$ cells), p = 0.005.

Discussion

There is substantial evidence to suggest that activation of the PI3K signaling pathway is of major importance in pediatric

glioblastoma [12,13]. Numerous small-molecule inhibitors of the PI3K signaling pathway have been developed [14–16], and early phase clinical studies of these inhibitors are planned for children with glioblastoma. Identification of non-invasive biomarkers of target and pathway inhibition and potentially of tumor response to this novel treatment would be of great value in the clinical development of PI3K inhibitors. The challenges of obtaining pharmacodynamic biomarker information is especially challenging in childhood brain tumors, where repeated biopsy is typically too invasive and therefore not routinely carried out. Other potential functional imaging techniques such as [18] FDG-PET have the disadvantage of requiring exposure to ionizing radiation, preferably avoided in pediatric patients where possible. In this study, we used NMR spectroscopy to search for potential non-invasive biomarkers for the effects of the dual pan-Class I PI3K/mTOR inhibitor PI-103 [14–16] and the pan–Class I PI3K inhibitor GDC-0941 lacking significant mTOR activity [14–16] in two pediatric glioblastoma cell lines, SF188 and KNS42, *in vitro*. This was with a view to informing future *in vivo* validation of such biomarkers.

Using ^{1}H- and ^{31}P-NMR, a significant decrease in PC concentrations was detected in both cell lines following treatment with either PI-103 or GDC-0941. Furthermore, both treatments resulted in a significant increase in PE levels in SF188 cells but not in KNS42 cells. Treatment with GDC-0941 also caused an increase in GPC in SF188 but not in KNS42 cells. This and our previously published results, using different adult cancer models [24,25], indicate that the decrease in PC levels is likely to be related to the action of LY294002, wortmannin, PI-103 and GDC-0941 on their common target PI3K. In contrast, the increase in PE or GPC was less consistent over a range of PI3K pathway inhibitors and was cell line dependent and, moreover, was seen only after longer inhibition periods (≥ 16 hours) and when higher concentrations of PI3K pathway inhibitors were used ($5 \times GI_{50}$). This may be related to specific functions of these metabolites in those particular cell lines or to non-specific effects triggered by prolonged PI3K pathway inhibition. Interestingly, despite the difference in response of some choline- and ethanol-containing metabolites, the sum of these metabolites represented by the tCho peak in the ^{1}H-NMR spectra generally decreased following treatment with both PI-103 and GDC-0941 in both pediatric glioblastoma cell lines. This indicates that the effect of

Table 5. Time-response analysis showing percentage changes in ^{31}P-NMR-detected metabolite levels following treatment of KNS42 pediatric glioblastoma cells with PI-103 ($5 \times GI_{50}$).

Time/hour	8	12	24	48
PC	76±32	65±10*	50±11*	56±5*
GPC	84±32	78±22	69±12	168±70
NTP	86±28	87±35	81±9	111±31

Data are expressed as percentage of treated to control (% T/C) and presented as the mean ± SD, n≥3.
PE in KNS42 cells was not consistently detectable due to the low levels of this metabolite and was not affected by treatment with PI-103.
Glycerophosphoethanolamine (GPE) level was not affected by treatment with PI-103.
Two-tailed unpaired *t* test was used to compare results in treated cells to controls.
*P<0.05.

Table 6. Time-response analysis showing percentage changes in ^{1}H-NMR-detected metabolite levels following treatment of KNS42 pediatric glioblastoma cells with PI-103 ($5 \times GI_{50}$).

Time/hour	8	12	24	48
Lac	73±32	70±10*	42±11*	36±5***
PC	77±20	62±10**	49±6*	50±8**
GPC	84±22	75±9*	62±6*	133±25
tCho	81±21	65±10**	54±9*	64±10*

Data are expressed as percentage of treated to control (% T/C) and presented as the mean ± SD, n≥3.
Two-tailed unpaired t test was used to compare results in treated cells to controls.
*P<0.05,
**P<0.005,
***P<0.0005.

both PI3K pathway inhibitors may be monitored *in vivo* or clinically in future, using either ^{31}P-MRS by following changes in PC levels or the composite tCho peak with ^{1}H-MRS. Clinically, we and others have shown that these metabolites can be measured non-invasively in spectra from a range of tumors in adult and pediatric subjects [22,34–36].

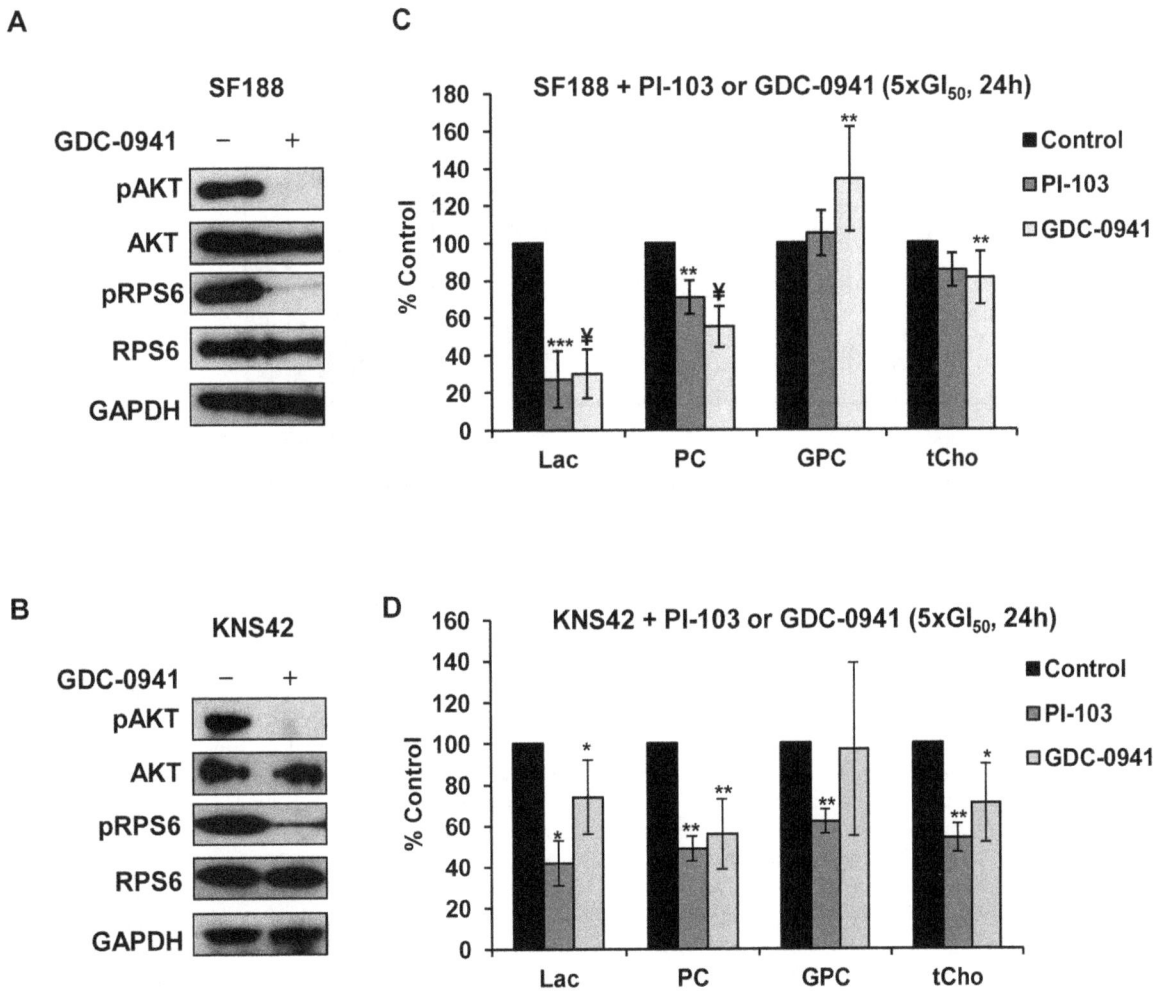

Figure 5. Molecular and metabolic percentage changes caused by treatment of pediatric glioblastoma cells with GDC-0941 or PI-103 ($5 \times GI_{50}$, 24 hours). Representative Western blots showing inhibition of the PI3K signaling pathway as indicated by decreased phosphorylation of AKT (Ser473) and RPS6 (Ser240/244) post-treatment with GDC-0941 in: (A) SF188 or (B) KNS42 cells. Comparison of ^{1}H-NMR detected metabolite percentage changes caused by treatment with PI-103 or GDC-0941 in: (C) SF188 or (D) KNS42 cells. Results are expressed as percentage of treated to control and presented as the mean ± SD (error bars) of at least three separate experiments. Statistically significantly different from the control *p≤ 0.05, **p≤0.01, ***p<0.005, ¥p<0.0005; two-tailed unpaired t test was used for all comparisons.

A

B

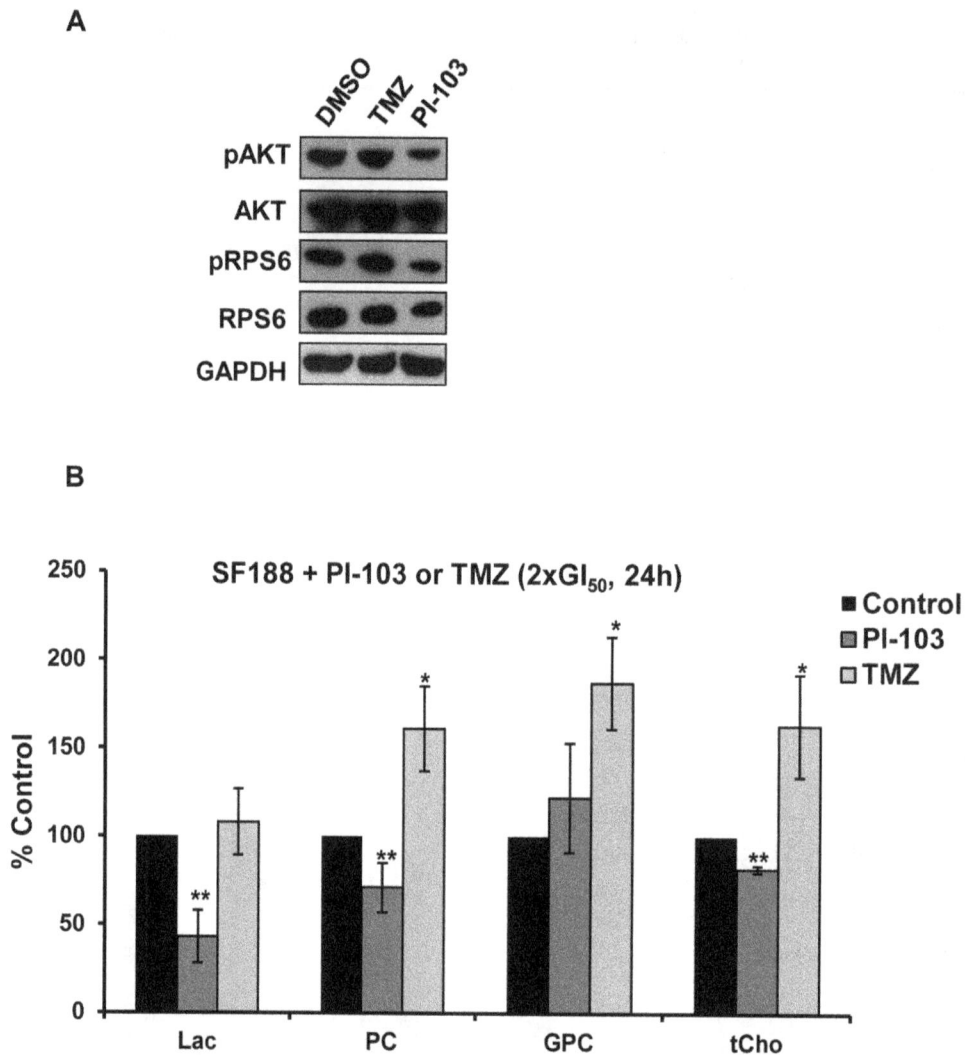

Figure 6. Comparison of molecular and metabolic changes caused by 24 hours treatment of SF188 pediatric glioblastoma cells with PI-103 or TMZ at $2\times GI_{50}$. (A) Representative Western blots showing inhibition of the PI3K signaling pathway as indicated by decreased phosphorylation of AKT (Ser473) and RPS6 (Ser240/244) following treatment with PI-103 but not with TMZ. (B) Quantification of ^{1}H-NMR detected metabolite changes. Results are expressed as percentage of treated to control and presented as the mean $\pm$ SD (error bars) of at least three separate experiments. Statistically significantly different from the control *$p \leq 0.05$, **$p \leq 0.01$, ***$p < 0.005$, $^{\yen}p < 0.0005$; two-tailed unpaired t test was used for all comparisons.

In direct contrast to the decrease in PC and tCho levels observed with PI3K pathway inhibitors, treatment of the pediatric glioblastoma cell line SF188 with the standard-of-care DNA damaging agent TMZ resulted in an increase in PC, GPC and tCho levels. This is in line with the increase in GPC levels we previously reported following treatment with various cytotoxic anti-cancer drugs [30,37]. Together, these results are consistent with the NMR-detected decreases in PC and tCho being a consequence of the inhibition of PI3K pathway signaling and not due to anti-proliferative effects associated with cytotoxicity.

Further inspection of ^{1}H-NMR spectra showed that treatment of pediatric glioblastoma cells with the PI3K pathway inhibitors PI-103 and GDC-0941 was associated with a marked decrease (> 60%) in lactate levels. In contrast, treatment with TMZ had no effects on lactate levels. These results are in line with recent findings [38–40] showing a decrease in lactate levels following treatment with various inhibitors of the PI3K/AKT/mTOR

signaling pathway *in vitro* and *in vivo* using different tumor models including adult glioblastoma.

It is well established that cancer cells reprogram their metabolism to facilitate growth and survival, leading to alterations in glucose, glutamine and lipid metabolism [41,42]. These metabolic pathways are regulated by signaling pathways known to be activated in and contributing to cancer development. For example, the PI3K/AKT/mTOR signaling pathway is a master regulator of enzymes involved in glucose, glutamine and lipid metabolism [43,44]. Therefore, it is not surprising that inhibition of the PI3K signaling pathway would impact on levels and/or activities of these enzymes. In the present study, we have explored possible mechanisms underlying NMR-detectable metabolic changes with the focus on SF188 cell line treated with PI-103 as a model. We have shown that the decrease in PC following treatment with PI-103 is associated with a reduction in the protein expression level of CHKA, the enzyme responsible for phosphorylation of choline into PC, confirming our previous findings in

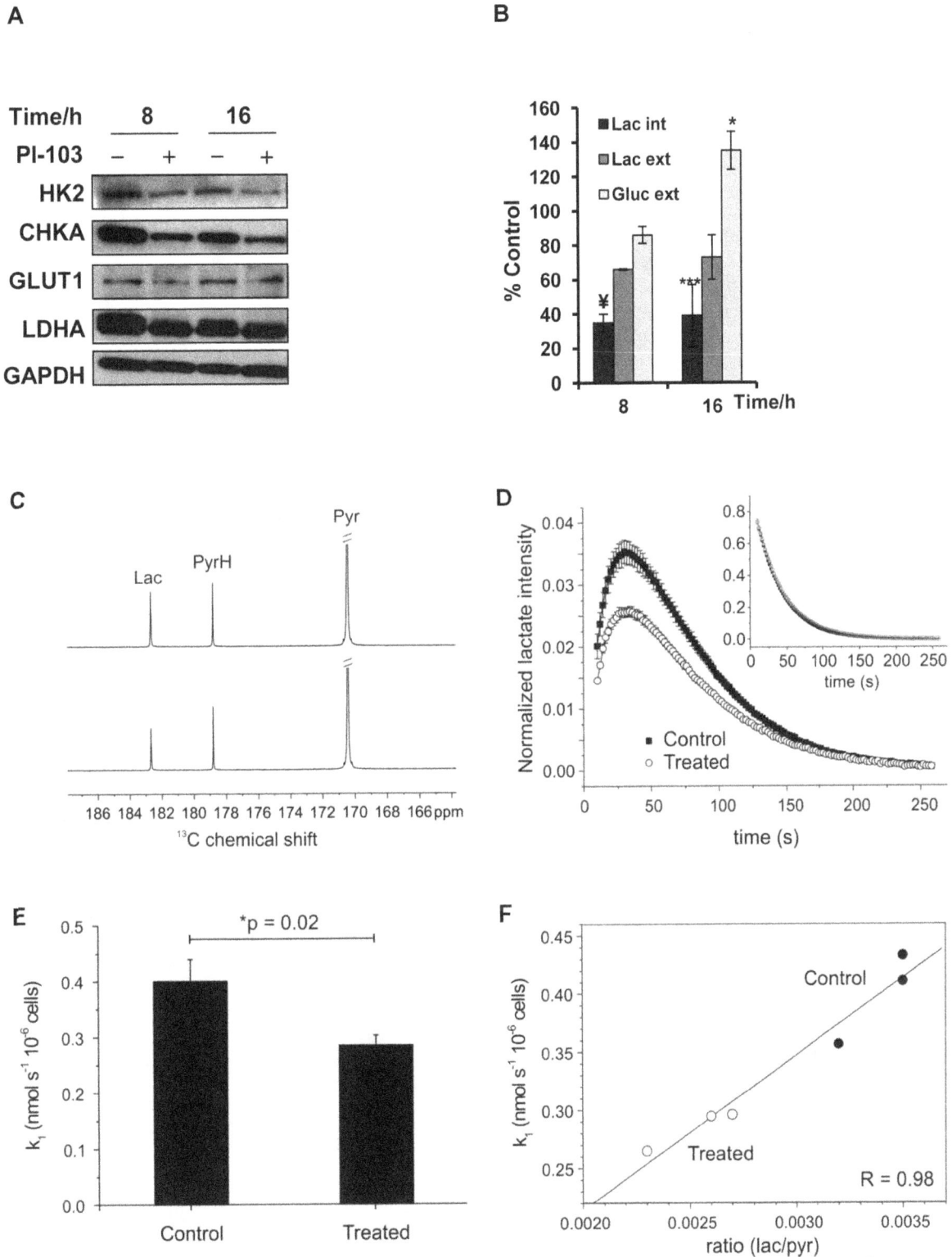

Figure 7. Investigation of mechanisms underlying NMR-detected changes in the levels of choline metabolites and lactate following treatment of SF188 pediatric glioblastoma cells with PI-103 (5×GI$_{50}$). (A) Representative Western blots showing changes in protein expression levels of enzymes involved in choline metabolism (CHKA) and glucose metabolism including: GLUT1, HK2 and LDHA, at selected time points post treatment with PI-103. GAPDH was used as a loading control. (B) Quantitative measurement of ^{1}H-NMR detected percentage changes in the levels of lactate (Lac, internal & external) and glucose (external) at selected time points post treatment with PI-103 relative to controls, 8 hours n = 2. Results are expressed as percentage of treated to control and presented as the mean ± SD (error bars). Statistically significant different from the control *p≤0.05, **p<0.01, †p≤0.005, ‡p<0.0005; two-tailed unpaired t test was used for all comparisons. (C) Sum ^{13}C-NMR spectra over the entire time-series with peaks corresponding to lactate, pyruvate and pyruvate hydrate in either control (top) or PI-103 treated groups (bottom), from which

a decrease in the lactate peak intensity can be appreciated. (D) The time-series of the lactate peak integral normalized to cell number with inset showing the pyruvate time dependence. (E) A decrease in the rate of pyruvate-lactate exchange rate constants was detected in PI-103 treated cells compared to controls. (F) A decrease in the area under the curve was also observed in PI-103 treated cells compared to controls, p = 0.005.

other cancer models [24]. We have also shown that the decrease in lactate levels was associated with a decrease in the protein expression levels of the glycolytic enzymes HK2 and LDHA. Furthermore, we demonstrated that the ^{1}H-NMR-detected higher levels of glucose in the medium of treated cells compared to their controls, is consistent with the decrease in the protein levels of the facilitated glucose transporter GLUT1. A previous report demonstrated that the reduction in LDH expression is mediated by a reduction in HIF1A following inhibition of the PI3K signaling pathway in adult glioblastoma [40]. The possible involvement of HIF1A in the decrease of the expression of several glycolytic enzymes detected in our model, need to be confirmed. Interestingly, the protein expression levels of the glycolytic enzyme GAPDH which we used as a loading control, were not affected by PI3K inhibition, indicating that it is not a general effect on glycolytic enzymes.

Taken together, our findings suggest that PI-103 inhibits glucose uptake and reduces levels of glycolytic enzymes resulting in a decrease in the production of lactate. This supports recent reports [45,46] suggesting the utility [^{18}F]FDG as a tracer for measuring response to PI3K inhibition. Interestingly, decreased [^{18}F]FDG uptake (25%) was observed in 53% of patients following treatment with the PI3K inhibitor BKM120, and it was suggested that this effect may be due to a combination of antitumor activity and direct PI3K inhibition [14,18]. Furthermore, our data are consistent with our previously published genome-wide cDNA microarray profiling, showing altered expression of genes involved in glucose and cholesterol biosynthesis in response to PI-103 in the PTEN null human glioblastoma cells U87MG (ref. [47] and Supplementary data published therein).

The DNP technique has recently been implemented to monitor the exchange of hyperpolarized ^{13}C from pyruvate to lactate [32,40,48]. This novel method provides an enhancement in signal-to-noise ratio of over 10,000-fold when compared with traditional ^{13}C-NMR [49], and has undergone an initial clinical trial [50]. Using DNP, we have demonstrated here a reduction in the rate of hyperpolarized pyruvate to lactate exchange kinetics in PI-103 treated SF188 cells when compared to controls. This is consistent with the decrease in LDHA protein expression levels in PI-103 treated cells. Our findings are in line with a previous report showing a decrease in ^{13}C lactate exchange and LDH expression and activity following PI3K/AKT/mTOR inhibition in adult glioblastoma [40]. This suggests that this novel method could be used to monitor modulation of the PI3K/mTOR pathway in pediatric glioblastoma. However, the mechanisms of drug action leading to changes in pyruvate-lactate exchange are complicated and have been shown to be influenced not only by LDH activity,

but also NAD/NADH ratio, endogenous concentrations of lactate as well as the influence of monocarboxylate transporters MCT1 and 4.

As discussed in our previous publications [24,51], although our NMR-detected metabolic changes may not be specific to the PI3K pathway, they can provide valuable biomarkers of response [17]. Many biomarkers are not specific to a given pathway, nonetheless have considerable clinical value (e.g. [^{18}F]FDG).

In vitro research represents the first approach to testing a drug effect on target pathways, providing a well-defined environment and minimizing the use of animals. The important *in vivo* validation of the potential non-invasive metabolic biomarkers we have identified *in vitro* requires a PI3K inhibitor suitable for clinical studies that, in relation to glioblastoma, would ideally also cross the blood brain barrier. Despite being highly potent and selective inhibitors of PI3K signaling, neither PI-103 nor GDC-0941 fulfill these criteria as PI-103 does not have optimal drug-like properties and is not a clinical candidate, and GDC-0941 does not cross the blood-brain barrier. Having identified potential biomarkers of PI3K inhibition in pediatric glioblastoma cell lines, further validation will be best performed in an orthotopic model using an inhibitor that is a clinical candidate and crosses the blood-brain barrier. Orthotopic models are in the late stages of development in our Centre and will be invaluable for future *in vivo* research.

In conclusion, we have shown that PI3K/mTOR inhibition in pediatric glioblastoma cell lines interferes with glucose and choline metabolism leading to decreases in lactate and choline metabolite levels that are detected by NMR. Alterations in these metabolites may have considerable potential as non-invasive biomarkers for monitoring response to PI3K/mTOR inhibitors in early phase clinical trials in children with glioma, thereby helping to optimize dosing and treatment of this disease which has devastatingly poor prognosis.

Acknowledgments

The authors would like to thank Dr I. Titley and Mrs G. Vijayaraghavan for their help with flow cytometry analyses.

Author Contributions

Conceived and designed the experiments: NMSA LVM AA PAC CJ PW ADJP MOL. Performed the experiments: NMSA LVM LEJ GB TRE AA. Analyzed the data: NMSA LVM LEJ GB TRE AA. Contributed reagents/materials/analysis tools: NMSA LVM LEJ GB TRE AA PAC CJ PW ADJP MOL. Contributed to the writing of the manuscript: NMSA LVM LEJ GB TRE AA PAC CJ PW ADJP MOL.

References

1. Hargrave DR, Zacharoulis S (2007) Pediatric CNS tumors: current treatment and future directions. Expert. Rev. Neurother. 7: 1029–1042.

2. Louis DN, Ohgaki H, Wiestler OD, Cavenee WK, Burger PC, et al. (2007) The 2007 WHO classification of tumours of the central nervous system. Acta Neuropathol. 114: 97–109.

3. Jones C, Perryman L, Hargrave D (2012) Paediatric and adult malignant glioma: close relatives or distant cousins? Nat. Rev. Clin. Oncol. 9: 400–413.

4. Bjerke L, Mackay A, Nandhabalan M, Burford A, Jury A, et al. (2013) Histone H3.3 Mutations Drive Pediatric Glioblastoma through Upregulation of MYCN. Cancer Discov. 3: 512–519.

5. Paugh BS, Qu C, Jones C, Liu Z, Adamowicz-Brice M, et al. (2010) Integrated molecular genetic profiling of pediatric high-grade gliomas reveals key differences with the adult disease. J. Clin. Oncol. 28: 3061–3068.

6. Popov S, Jury A, Laxton R, Doey L, Kandasamy N, et al. (2013) IDH1-associated primary glioblastoma in young adults displays differential patterns of tumour and vascular morphology. PLoS. One. 8: e56328.

7. Schwartzentruber J, Korshunov A, Liu XY, Jones DT, Pfaff E, et al. (2012) Driver mutations in histone H3.3 and chromatin remodelling genes in paediatric glioblastoma. Nature 482: 226–231.

8. Sturm D, Witt H, Hovestadt V, Khuong-Quang DA, Jones DT, et al. (2012) Hotspot mutations in H3F3A and IDH1 define distinct epigenetic and biological subgroups of glioblastoma. Cancer Cell 22: 425–437.

9. Stupp R, Mason WP, van den Bent MJ, Weller M, Fisher B, et al. (2005) Radiotherapy plus concomitant and adjuvant temozolomide for glioblastoma. N. Engl. J. Med. 352: 987–996.

10. Broniscer A, Chintagumpala M, Fouladi M, Krasin MJ, Kocak M, et al. (2006) Temozolomide after radiotherapy for newly diagnosed high-grade glioma and unfavorable low-grade glioma in children. J. Neurooncol. 76: 313–319.

11. Ruggiero A, Cefalo G, Garre ML, Massimino M, Colosimo C, et al. (2006) Phase II trial of temozolomide in children with recurrent high-grade glioma. J. Neurooncol. 77: 89–94.

12. Gallia GL, Rand V, Siu IM, Eberhart CG, James CD, et al. (2006) PIK3CA gene mutations in pediatric and adult glioblastoma multiforme. Molecular Cancer Research 4: 709–714.

13. Gaspar N, Marshall L, Perryman L, Bax DA, Little SE, et al. (2010) MGMT-independent temozolomide resistance in pediatric glioblastoma cells associated with a PI3-kinase-mediated HOX/stem cell gene signature. Cancer Res. 70: 9243–9252.

14. Clarke PA, Workman P (2012) Phosphatidylinositide-3-kinase inhibitors: addressing questions of isoform selectivity and pharmacodynamic/predictive biomarkers in early clinical trials. J. Clin. Oncol. 30: 331–333.

15. Shuttleworth SJ, Silva FA, Cecil AR, Tomassi CD, Hill TJ, et al. (2011) Progress in the preclinical discovery and clinical development of class I and dual class I/IV phosphoinositide 3-kinase (PI3K) inhibitors. Curr. Med. Chem. 18: 2686–2714.

16. Yap TA, Garrett MD, Walton MI, Raynaud F, de Bono JS, et al. (2008) Targeting the PI3K-AKT-mTOR pathway: progress, pitfalls, and promises. Curr. Opin. Pharmacol. 8: 393–412.

17. Workman P, Aboagye EO, Chung YL, Griffiths JR, Hart R, et al. (2006) Minimally invasive pharmacokinetic and pharmacodynamic technologies in hypothesis-testing clinical trials of innovative therapies. Journal Of The National Cancer Institute 98: 580–598.

18. Bendell JC, Rodon J, Burris HA, de Jonge M, Verweij J, et al. (2012) Phase I, dose-escalation study of BKM120, an oral pan-Class I PI3K inhibitor, in patients with advanced solid tumors. J. Clin. Oncol. 30: 282–290.

19. Lucignani G, De Palma D (2011) PET/CT in paediatric oncology: clinical usefulness and dosimetric concerns. Eur. J. Nucl. Med. Mol. Imaging 38: 179–184.

20. Gadian DG (1995) The information available from NMR. In. NMR and its applications to living systems: New York: Oxford University Press Inc. 29–64.

21. Bulik M, Jancalek R, Vanicek J, Skoch A, Mechl M (2013) Potential of MR spectroscopy for assessment of glioma grading. Clin. Neurol. Neurosurg. 115: 146–153.

22. Murphy PS, Viviers L, Abson C, Rowland IJ, Brada M, et al. (2004) Monitoring Temozolomide treatment of low-grade glioma with proton magnetic resonance spectroscopy. British Journal Of Cancer 90: 781–786.

23. Nelson SJ (2011) Assessment of therapeutic response and treatment planning for brain tumors using metabolic and physiological MRI. NMR Biomed. 24: 734–749.

24. Al-Saffar NM, Jackson LE, Raynaud FI, Clarke PA, Ramírez de Molina A, et al. (2010) The Phosphoinositide 3-Kinase Inhibitor PI-103 Downregulates Choline Kinase {alpha} Leading to Phosphocholine and Total Choline Decrease Detected by Magnetic Resonance Spectroscopy. Cancer Res. 70: 5507–5517.

25. Beloueche-Babari M, Jackson LE, Al-Saffar NMS, Eccles SA, Raynaud FI, et al. (2006) Identification of magnetic resonance detectable metabolic changes associated with inhibition of phosphoinositide 3-kinase signaling in human breast cancer cells. Molecular Cancer Therapeutics 5: 187–196.

26. Haas-Kogan DA, Yount G, Haas M, Levi D, Kogan SS, et al. (1996) p53-dependent G1 arrest and p53-independent apoptosis influence the radiobiologic response of glioblastoma. Int. J. Radiat. Oncol. Biol. Phys. 36: 95–103.

27. Takeshita I, Takaki T, Kuramitsu M, Nagasaka S, Machi T, et al. (1987) Characteristics of an established human glioma cell line, KNS-42. Neurol. Med. Chir (Tokyo) 27: 581–587.

28. Bax DA, Little SE, Gaspar N, Perryman L, Marshall L, et al. (2009) Molecular and phenotypic characterisation of paediatric glioma cell lines as models for preclinical drug development. PLoS. One. 4: e5209.

29. Cory AH, Owen TC, Barltrop JA, Cory JG (1991) Use of an aqueous soluble tetrazolium/formazan assay for cell growth assays in culture. Cancer Commun. 3: 207–212.

30. Al-Saffar NS, Troy H, Ramírez de Molina A, Jackson LE, Madhu B, et al. (2006) Noninvasive magnetic resonance spectroscopic pharmacodynamic markers of the choline kinase inhibitor MN58b in Human Carcinoma models. Cancer Research 66: 427–434.

31. Tyagi RK, Azrad A, Degani H, Salomon Y (1996) Simultaneous extraction of cellular lipids and water-soluble metabolites: Evaluation by NMR spectroscopy. Magnetic Resonance in Medicine 35: 194–200.

32. Hill DK, Orton MR, Mariotti E, Boult JKR, Panek R, et al. (2013) Model Free Approach to Kinetic Analysis of Real-Time Hyperpolarized 13C Magnetic Resonance Spectroscopy Data. PLoS One 8: e71996.

33. Hill DK, Jamin Y, Orton MR, Tardif N, Parkes HG, et al. (2013) 1H NMR and hyperpolarized 13C NMR assays of pyruvate-lactate: a comparative study. NMR Biomed. 26: 1321–1325.

34. Heiss WD, Heindel W, Herholz K, Rudolf J, Bunke J, et al. (1990) Positron emission tomography of fluorine-18-deoxyglucose and image-guided phosphorus-31 magnetic resonance spectroscopy in brain tumors. J. Nucl. Med. 31: 302–310.

35. Peet AC, Arvanitis TN, Leach MO, Waldman AD (2012) Functional imaging in adult and paediatric brain tumours. Nat. Rev. Clin. Oncol. 9: 700–711.

36. Quon H, Brunet B, Alexander A, Murtha A, Abdulkarim B, et al. (2011) Changes in serial magnetic resonance spectroscopy predict outcome in high-grade glioma during and after postoperative radiotherapy. Anticancer Res. 31: 3559–3565.

37. Chung YL, Troy H, Banerji U, Jackson LE, Walton MI, et al. (2003) Magnetic resonance spectroscopic pharmacodynamic markers of the heat shock protein 90 inhibitor 17-allylamino,17- demethoxygeldanamycin (17AAG) in human colon cancer models. Journal Of The National Cancer Institute 95: 1624–1633.

38. Lee SC, Marzec M, Liu X, Wehrli S, Kantekure K, et al. (2013) Decreased lactate concentration and glycolytic enzyme expression reflect inhibition of mTOR signal transduction pathway in B-cell lymphoma. NMR Biomed. 26: 106–114.

39. Su JS, Woods SM, Ronen SM (2012) Metabolic consequences of treatment with AKT inhibitor perifosine in breast cancer cells. NMR Biomed. 25: 379–388.

40. Venkatesh HS, Chaumeil MM, Ward CS, Haas-Kogan DA, James CD, et al. (2012) Reduced phosphocholine and hyperpolarized lactate provide magnetic resonance biomarkers of PI3K/Akt/mTOR inhibition in glioblastoma. Neuro. Oncol. 14: 315–325.

41. Cairns RA, Harris IS, Mak TW (2011) Regulation of cancer cell metabolism. Nat. Rev. Cancer 11: 85–95.

42. Dang CV (2012) Links between metabolism and cancer. Genes Dev. 26: 877–890.

43. Braccini L, Ciraolo E, Martini M, Pirali T, Germena G, et al. (2012) PI3K keeps the balance between metabolism and cancer. Adv. Biol. Regul. 52: 389–405.

44. Yecies JL, Manning BD (2011) mTOR links oncogenic signaling to tumor cell metabolism. J. Mol. Med. (Berl) 89: 221–228.

45. Kelly CJ, Hussien K, Muschel RJ (2012) 3D tumour spheroids as a model to assess the suitability of [18F]FDG-PET as an early indicator of response to PI3K inhibition. Nucl. Med. Biol. 39: 986–992.

46. Nguyen QD, Perumal M, Waldman TA, Aboagye EO (2011) Glucose metabolism measured by [18F]fluorodeoxyglucose positron emission tomography is independent of PTEN/AKT status in human colon carcinoma cells. Transl. Oncol. 4: 241–248.

47. Guillard S, Clarke PA, Te-Poele R, Mohri Z, Bjerke L, et al. (2009) Molecular pharmacology of phosphatidylinositol 3-kinase inhibition in human glioma. Cell Cycle 8: 443–453.

48. Kurhanewicz J, Vigneron DB, Brindle K, Chekmenev EY, Comment A, et al. (2011) Analysis of cancer metabolism by imaging hyperpolarized nuclei: prospects for translation to clinical research. Neoplasia. 13: 81–97.

49. Ardenkjaer-Larsen JH, Fridlund B, Gram A, Hansson G, Hansson L, et al. (2003) Increase in signal-to-noise ratio of >10,000 times in liquid-state NMR. Proc. Natl. Acad. Sci. U. S. A 100: 10158–10163.

50. Nelson SJ, Kurhanewicz J, Vigneron DB, Larson PE, Harzstark AL, et al. (2013) Metabolic Imaging of Patients with Prostate Cancer Using Hyperpolarized [1-13C]Pyruvate. Sci. Transl. Med. 5: 198ra108.

51. Beloueche-Babari M, Chung YL, Al-Saffar NM, Falck-Miniotis M, Leach MO (2010) Metabolic assessment of the action of targeted cancer therapeutics using magnetic resonance spectroscopy. Br. J. Cancer 102: 1–7.

23

The Association between Quality of HIV Care, Loss to Follow-Up and Mortality in Pediatric and Adolescent Patients Receiving Antiretroviral Therapy in Nigeria

Bisola Ojikutu[1,2]*, Molly Higgins-Biddle[1], Dana Greeson[3], Benjamin R. Phelps[4], Anouk Amzel[4], Emeka Okechukwu[5], Usman Kolapo[6], Howard Cabral[7], Ellen Cooper[8], Lisa R. Hirschhorn[9]

1 John Snow Inc., Boston, Massachusetts, United States of America, 2 Massachusetts General Hospital, Infectious Disease Division, Boston, Massachusetts, United States of America, 3 Columbia University, Department of Epidemiology, New York, New York, United States of America, 4 United States Agency for International Development (USAID), Washington, D. C., United States of America, 5 United States Agency for International Development (USAID), Abuja, Nigeria, 6 Indepth Precision, Abuja, Nigeria, 7 Boston University School of Public Health, Department of Biostatistics, Boston, Massachusetts, United States of America, 8 Boston University School of Medicine, Boston, Massachusetts, United States of America, 9 Harvard Medical School, Department of Global Health and Social Medicine, Harvard Medical School, Boston, Massachusetts, United States of America

Abstract

Access to pediatric HIV treatment in resource-limited settings has risen significantly. However, little is known about the quality of care that pediatric or adolescent patients receive. The objective of this study is to explore quality of HIV care and treatment in Nigeria and to determine the association between quality of care, loss-to-follow-up and mortality. A retrospective cohort study was conducted including patients ≤18 years of age who initiated ART between November 2002 and December 2011 at 23 sites across 10 states. 1,516 patients were included. A quality score comprised of 6 process indicators was calculated for each patient. More than half of patients (55.5%) were found to have a high quality score, using the median score as the cut-off. Most patients were screened for tuberculosis at entry into care (81.3%), had adherence measurement and counseling at their last visit (88.7% and 89.7% respectively), and were prescribed co-trimoxazole at some point during enrollment in care (98.8%). Thirty-seven percent received a CD4 count in the six months prior to chart review. Mortality within 90 days of ART initiation was 1.9%. A total of 4.2% of patients died during the period of follow-up (mean: 27 months) with 19.0% lost to follow-up. In multivariate regression analyses, weight for age z-score (Adjusted Hazard Ratio (AHR): 0.90; 95% CI: 0.85, 0.95) and high quality indicator score (compared a low score, AHR: 0.43; 95% CI: 0.26, 0.73) had a protective effect on mortality. Patients with a high quality score were less likely to be lost to follow-up (Adjusted Odds Ratio (AOR): 0.42; 95% CI: 0.32, 0.56), compared to those with low score. These findings indicate that providing high quality care to children and adolescents living with HIV is important to improve outcomes, including lowering loss to follow-up and decreasing mortality in this age group.

Editor: Antonio Carlos Seguro, University of São Paulo School of Medicine, Brazil

Funding: This research has been supported by the President's Emergency Plan for AIDS Relief (PEPFAR) through the U.S. Agency for International Development under the terms of contract no. GHH-I-00–07–00059–00. Bisola Ojikutu and Molly-Higgins Biddle are employed by John Snow Inc. Usman Kolapo is employed by Indepth Precision. The funders had no role in study design, data collection and analysis, decision to publish, or preparation of the manuscript.

Competing Interests: Bisola Ojikutu and Molly-Higgins Biddle are employed by John Snow Inc. Usman Kolapo is employed by Indepth Precision. Benjamin R. Phelps and Anouk Amzel, are employed by the U.S. Agency for International Development. There are no patents, products in development or marketed products to declare.

* Email: bojikutu@jsi.com

Introduction

Though numerous challenges have limited scale-up of pediatric antiretroviral therapy (ART), significant progress has been made. [1–3] Access to pediatric ART in resource limited settings has risen more than 7-fold from 75,000 children receiving ART in low and middle income countries in 2005 to 562,000 by the end of 2011. [4] As pediatric treatment becomes more widely available, determining standards for and measuring the quality of HIV care and treatment that children receive has become a high priority. In order to derive the full benefit of ART, children and adolescents must be provided with high quality care and treatment that addresses their multifaceted needs, including adherence counsel-ing, disclosure support, laboratory monitoring, and opportunistic infection screening along with other critical services.

The Institute of Medicine defines health care quality as the extent to which health services provided to individuals and populations improve desired health outcomes and are consistent with current professional knowledge. [5] Performance indicators are measurement tools that may be used to assess health care quality. [6] These indicators fall into three categories: (1) structure (characteristics of the health care setting such as human resource availability); (2) process (aspects of the encounter with the patient such as which tests are ordered); or (3) outcome (the patient's subsequent health status). [7–10] Structure and process may influence outcome, indirectly or directly. [11] Understanding this relationship is essential for quality improvement efforts, particularly in settings where resources to institute structural or procedural change are limited. Numerous studies conducted in sub-Saharan Africa have assessed the impact of selected structural changes, such as task-shifting and decentralization of services, on HIV treatment outcomes. [12–17] Process indicators capturing key services, such as semi-annual CD4 count monitoring, routine opportunistic infection screening and regular adherence support, are frequently collected for programmatic monitoring and evaluation. However, the correlation between process indicators such as these and clinical outcomes of HIV care and treatment has not been well explored in resource limited settings. [18,19]

Moreover, quality assessment of pediatric HIV care and treatment lags far behind that of adults internationally. Several national programs have identified process and outcomes indicators to guide improvement efforts. However, few reports of HIV care quality that focus on pediatric or adolescent services have been published. [20–22] Reports describing clinical outcomes in this age group have documented significant challenges, with numerous studies noting high rates of loss to follow-up and early mortality. [23–28] Many factors—including late presentation, malnutrition, lack of caregiver involvement, nondisclosure, and HIV-related stigma—contribute to these findings. [27,29,30] Whether the quality of care received by children and young adults is associated with loss to follow-up or mortality has not been assessed. As pediatric and adolescent ART becomes more widely available globally, identifying appropriate measures of quality and determining their association with outcomes is critical and should help guide future programmatic planning.

Nigeria is home to the second largest number of people living with HIV in the world after South Africa. In 2012, approximately 3,400,000 people in Nigeria were living with HIV, including 430,000 children. [31] Though coordinated efforts have been underway in Nigeria to increase access to ART for pediatric patients since 2005, a significant disparity exists between pediatric and adult ART coverage (7% versus 26%, respectively). [32] Limited data exist describing clinical outcomes or quality of care in pediatric or adolescent patients on ART in Nigeria. [33,34] The objective of this study is to explore quality of care received by pediatric and adolescent patients receiving ART in Nigeria and to determine the association between quality of care and loss to follow-up and mortality.

Methods

Ethical Review

The study protocol and assessment tools were submitted to the National Health Research Ethics Committee of Nigeria (NHREC) and approved on April 9th, 2011. Individual signed, written informed consent from participants was waived by NHREC. Patient information was de-identified prior to analysis. Unique patient identifiers were assigned to each patient to protect patient confidentiality.

Study design

A retrospective cohort study was conducted including patients enrolled in care between November 2002 and December 2011. This chart review was a component of a larger assessment of access to pediatric and adolescent treatment services funded by the United States Government/PEPFAR Nigeria Program. [File S1] Purposive sampling was used to select 23 sites providing antiretroviral therapy from 10 states across the 6 geopolitical zones of Nigeria. At the time of this assessment, all pediatric HIV care and treatment in Nigeria was provided at hospitals that offered secondary and tertiary-level specialty services. The criteria

guiding site selection included geographic location and setting (i.e., urban, peri-urban, or rural). Safety concerns limited inclusion of sites in certain states. All treatment sites are monitored by the Federal Ministry of Health and supported by a variety of US government funded implementing partners (IPs).

Charts representing 10% of the total number of patients 0–18 years of age receiving antiretroviral therapy (ART) in the 10 states chosen were selected using random sampling. Each site was asked to provide a list of all enrolled patients 0–18 years of age meeting the inclusion criteria by medical record number. Chart design and contents were standardized in 2008 to include the same variables across all sites throughout the country, and sites maintained either paper or electronic records.

Patients were eligible for inclusion in the study if they were 0–18 years of age and initiated ART during the study period. Follow-up was censored either at the time of the loss to follow-up (as defined below), death or the end of the study period.

Outcomes

The two main outcomes were lost to follow-up and death. Loss to follow-up was defined as no evidence of a visit to the clinic or drug pick up for 90 days following the last scheduled appointment as documented in the chart. Death was only counted if verified by the patient's family or if death occurred within the hospital.

Independent variables including quality of care indicators

The primary independent variable of interest was a quality score comprised of six process indicators: (1) screening for tuberculosis at entry into care, (2) adherence measurement at last visit, (3) adherence counseling at last visit, (4) prescription of co-trimoxazole at any time since enrollment, (5) at least one CD4 count in the last six months, and (6) documented weight at last visit. These indicators are recommended by the World Health Organization and should be standard components of clinical practice as outlined by the 2005 and 2010 National Guidelines on Paediatric HIV and AIDS Treatment and Care in Nigeria. [35,36] Recommendations regarding these process indicators did not change over time. Similar indicators have been used to assess pediatric HIV care and treatment quality in other studies conducted in resource limited settings. [22] Screening for tuberculosis in pediatric and adolescent patients includes symptom assessment (poor weight gain, fever, and cough), determination of contact history with a known TB case, clinical examination and radiology followed by sputum induction, if warranted. The standard procedure for adherence assessment in HIV clinics in Nigeria is to ask the patient or the caregiver the number of ART doses missed within the last three days. Review of pharmacy records, returned syrup measurement and pill counting are not routinely conducted. Adherence counseling should be offered at every visit. More intensive counseling is provided if the patient or caregiver reports missed ART doses. CD4 count testing and co-trimoxazole are provided free of charge at all sites. A quality score was calculated with one point assigned for each service received and zero points assigned if the service was not received, for a total of six points. For ease of interpretation, the score was categorized into "high quality" versus "low quality" using the median score as a cutoff for bivariate and multivariate regression models.

Additional patient characteristics and clinical variables related to the outcomes of interest were also collected including: gender, age at ART initiation, CD4 count/percentage (baseline and most recent value), baseline weight/height (to determine age-for-weight z-score), current ART regimen, and facility type (rural, peri-urban and urban). Viral load measurement was not standard of care during the study period, and therefore was not included as an outcome measure.

Baseline immunosuppression at entry into care was calculated using patient age and either initial CD4 count or initial CD4 percentage. For patients less than two years of age, "severe immunosuppression" was defined as an initial CD4 count less than 750 cells/mm^3 or a percentage less than 15%, while "moderate immunosuppression" was defined as CD4 count between 750 and 1500 cells/mm^3 or a percentage of between 15% and 25%. "No immunosuppression" was defined as an initial CD4 count of 1500 cells/mm^3 or more or a percentage of 25% or more. For patients between two and five years of age, "severe immunosuppression" was defined as an initial CD4 count less than 500 cells/mm^3 or percentage less than 15%, "moderate immunosuppression" as an initial CD4 count of between 500 and 1000 cells/mm^3 or percentage of between 15% and 25%, and "no immunosuppression" as an initial CD4 count of 1000 cells/mm^3 or more or percentage of 25% or more. For patients five years of age or older, "severe immunosuppression" was defined as an initial CD4 count less than 200 cells/mm^3 or percentage less than 15%, "moderate immunosuppression" as an initial CD4 count of between 200 and 500 cells/mm^3 or percentage of between 15% and 25%, and "no immunosuppression" as an initial CD4 count of 500 cells/mm^3 or more or percentage of 25% or more. [35]

Data Analysis

Means and standard deviations were computed for continuous variables and counts with percentages for categorical variables. Differences in mortality and loss to follow-up by age group and differences in quality indicators by year of initial visit were compared using chi-square statistics. Bivariate methods were used to examine the relationships of individual independent variables with the primary outcomes of survival and loss-to-follow up, including Kaplan-Meier estimation with log rank testing. One predictor Cox proportional hazards regression models were used for survival and one predictor logistic regression models for loss to follow-up.

In survival analyses, associations were estimated using hazard ratios (HR) with 95 percent confidence intervals (CI). In the analysis of loss to follow-up, associations were estimated using odds ratios (OR) with 95 percent CIs. The multivariate logistic regression models included independent variables that were significant in the bivariate models defined as p<0.05 and/or were potential confounders of the relationship between the quality score and the outcomes (e.g., weight for age (z-score) and age at ART initiation). The multivariate Cox regression model was limited to four predictors due to the number of deaths in the sample, using a guide of ten events or deaths required per predictor. [37]

The proportional hazards assumption was checked by graphical methods and by testing interaction terms that included the log of follow-up time. The discrimination ability of the logistic models was measured by c-statistics with calibration assessed using Hosmer-Lemeshow chi-square statistics and their associated p-values. Where data were sufficient, we tested for interactions among the independent variables in these models. Patient-level variability across sites was investigated using the intra-cluster correlation coefficient (ICC). The ICC was close to zero, indicating similarity between within-site variability and variability across sites. We employed an alpha of 0.05 in all statistical tests to determine statistical significance. All data management and statistical analyses were performed using SAS for Windows version 9.2.

Results

Study population

A total of 1,516 patients were sampled from 23 sites. Most patients (73.6%) received care at urban facilities (Table 1). The average human resource distribution for pediatric HIV care and treatment was similar across facilities with an average of 23 full-time clinical staff (including doctors, nurses, pharmacists and counselors) per site. Approximately one-quarter of patients were 24 months old or younger at ART initiation, while 40.0% were between two and six years old, 21.1% were six to nine years old, and 14.9% were 10 to 18 years old (Table 1). Most patients had an initial visit and initiated ART between 2008 and 2011. Approximately one-half of patients were male (52.8%). Almost half of patients were severely immunosuppressed at baseline (46.3%), 32.5% were moderately immunosuppressed, and 21.3% were not immunosuppressed. The mean weight for age (z-score) at baseline was −1.08 (±4.04).

The mean duration of follow-up time was 27.7 months (±19.7). Most patients were on an ART regimen comprised of AZT/3TC/NVP (81.5%) at the time of chart review. For those on regimens containing d4T, the mean length of time on the regimen was 36.7 months (±18.5).

Quality of care

Most patients were screened for tuberculosis at entry into care (81.3%) and had adherence counseling at their last visit (89.7%) (Table 1). Similarly, the majority of patients had their adherence measured at their last visit (88.7%). Almost all patients had been prescribed co-trimoxazole at some point during their enrollment in care (98.8%). Weight for age was documented at the last visit in 72.2% of charts evaluated. However, less than half of patients alive and in care at the time of the chart review had obtained a CD4 count in the six months prior to chart review (37.0%). A higher percentage of patients who were >10 years old were screened for TB compared to those who were <10 years (87.4% vs. 80.3%, p = 0.0148). Over half of patients had a quality score of the median or higher (greater than four points out of six) (55.5%). No significant difference was noted in overall quality score between adolescents (10–18) and younger patients (p = 0.325).

Two quality indicators improved over time. The percentage of patients with a CD4 count in the last six months (p<0.0001) and weight for age documented at the last visit (p = 0.0034) was higher for those with an initial visit in more recent years (2008 to 2011) than for those who enrolled in care prior to 2008.

Outcomes

Documented mortality within 90 days of ART initiation was 1.9% (Table 2). A total of 4.2% of patients died during the period of follow-up. Mortality was highest for those 24 months old or less at ART initiation (35.9%) (p = NS). Loss to follow-up was 19.0% during the follow-up period, with 3.6% of patients lost within six months of ART initiation and 6.9% lost within the first twelve months. Loss to follow-up was highest for those 25 to 71 months old at ART initiation (35.9%), compared to the other age groups (p = 0.0130). No significant difference was noted in mortality or loss to follow-up between adolescents (age 10–18) and younger patients (p = 0.583 and p = 0.565, respectively).

Bivariate results

Patients with a high quality score were more likely to survive over time (p = 0.0011) and less likely to be loss to follow-up (p< 0.0001) than patients with a low quality indicator score (Figures 1 and 2). Gender was not statistically significant in bivariate results

Table 1. Characteristics of sampled pediatric and adolescent patients (age 0 to 18 years).

	All Patients (n = 1516)	
	N	Mean (SD) or %
Demographics		
Age at ART initiation		
0–24 months	363	24.0%
25–71 months	605	40.0%
6–9 years	318	21.1%
10–18 years	225	14.9%
Gender (Male)	799	52.8%
Clinical factors		
Baseline immunosuppression[1]		
Severe	666	46.3%
0–24 months	165	24.8%
25–71 months	256	38.4%
6–9 years	124	18.6%
10–18 years	121	18.2%
Moderate	468	32.5%
0–24 months	106	22.7%
25–71 months	202	43.3%
6–9 years	92	19.7%
10–18 years	67	14.4%
No suppression	306	21.3%
0–24 months	47	15.4%
25–71 months	126	41.3%
6–9 years	97	31.8%
10–18 years	35	11.5%
Weight for age (z-score)	1382	−1.08 ($\pm$4.04)
Most recent CD4 count among those alive		
<350 cells/mm^3	369	27.3%
≥350 cells/mm^3	983	72.7%
Treatment		
Duration of follow-up in months	1511	27.7 ($\pm$19.7)
Current ART regimens		
AZT/3TC/NVP	1236	81.5%
Regimens containing d4T	81	5.3%
Other regimen	196	13.0%
Patients enrolled by facility type		
Rural	199	13.1%
Peri-urban	201	13.3%
Urban	1116	73.6%
Quality indicators		
Screened for tuberculosis at entry into care	1115	81.3%
Adherence counseling documented at last visit	1311	89.7%
Adherence measured at last visit	1296	88.7%
Ever prescribed co-trimoxazole	1482	98.8%
Alive and not lost to follow up with at least one CD4 count in last six months	518	37.0%
Weight documented in chart at patient's last visit	1049	72.2%
High quality indicator score[2]	842	55.5%

[1]For patients less than two years of age, severe immunosuppression was defined as an initial CD4 count less than 750 cells/mm^3 or percentage less than 15%, moderate immunosuppression as an initial CD4 count of between 750 and 1500 cells/mm^3 or percentage of between 15% and 25%, and no immunosuppression as an initial CD4 count of 1500 cells/mm^3 or more, or percentage of 25% or more. For patients between two and five years of age, severe immunosuppression was defined as an initial

CD4 count less than 500 cells/mm³ or percentage less than 15%, moderate immunosuppression as an initial CD4 count of between 500 and 1000 cells/mm³ or percentage of between 15% and 25%, and no immunosuppression as an initial CD4 count of 1000 cells/mm³ or more, or percentage of 25% or more. For patients between five years of age or older, severe immunosuppression was defined as an initial CD4 count less than 200 cells/mm³ or percentage less than 15%, moderate immunosuppression as an initial CD4 count of between 200 and 500 cells/mm³ or percentage of between 15% and 25%, and no immunosuppression as an initial CD4 count of 500 cells/mm³ or more, or percentage of 25% or more.
[2]1 point assigned for each service received (screened for tuberculosis, adherence counseling at last visit, adherence measured by patient/caregiver self-report at last visit, ever prescribed co-trimoxazole, alive and not lost to follow-up with at least one CD4 count in the last six months, and weight documented in chart at patient's last visit, and 0 points assigned if the service was not received, for a total of 6 points. A high score was defined as having the median score or above (>4 points).

for mortality or loss to follow-up. A one-point increase in weight for age z-score had a protective effect on mortality (HR: 0.90; 95% CI: 0.85, 0.95) (Table 3). Patients 24 months or younger at ART initiation had a greater likelihood of death (HR: 1.76; 95% CI: 1.06, 2.94) and loss to follow-up (OR: 1.56; 95% CI: 1.16, 2.09), compared to those older than 24 months at ART initiation. Patients with severe immunosuppression were more likely to die (HR: 6.11; 95% CI: 1.89, 19.76) and be lost to follow-up (OR: 1.48; 95% CI: 1.02, 2.14) than patients with no suppression. Overall, a high quality score had a protective effect on mortality (HR: 0.43; 95% CI: 0.26, 0.73) and loss to follow-up (OR: 0.40; 95% CI: 0.31, 0.53) compared to those with a low score.

Multivariate results

In multivariate Cox regression analyses, adjusting for other factors, weight for age z-score (AHR: 0.92; 95% CI: 0.87, 0.98) and high quality score (compared a low score, AHR: 0.47; 95% CI: 0.26, 0.87) had a protective effect on mortality. Patients with severe baseline immunosuppression were more likely to die than those with no immunosuppression (AHR: 7.21; 95% CI: 1.72, 30.21) (Table 3). Adjusting for other factors in multiple logistic regression analysis, patients with a high quality score were less likely to be lost to follow-up (AOR: 0.42; 95% CI: 0.32, 0.56), compared to those with low score.

Discussion

To our knowledge, this is the first report of a pediatric and adolescent HIV care and treatment quality assessment in Nigeria. Our findings suggest that providing high quality care to children and adolescents living with HIV is associated with lower loss to follow-up and mortality, providing compelling evidence that investing in quality has the potential to retain this age group in care and save lives.

In this study, six process indicators were selected to measure quality. Overall, receipt of services was high. More than 80% of patients were screened for TB at entry into care. However, a higher percentage of adolescents were screened for TB compared to pediatric patients. Though the World Health Organization recommends screening for TB in pediatric patients as described, under-diagnosis and diagnostic delays are common. [38] Intensive training and improved strategies for early TB diagnosis in this age group are needed. Adherence was measured, and adherence counseling was provided to nearly 90% of patients at their last visit. Almost all patients were started on co-trimoxazole at some point since enrollment. Weight for age (z-score) was documented in approximately 70% of charts. The percentage of patients with documented weight for age (z-score) increased in 2008–2011 compared to previous years. Increasing site level experience, improved availability of resources (scales) and training may have contributed to this difference. Low quality scores were largely due to deficits in receipt of CD4 count testing within 6 months of the chart review. The low rates of CD4 count testing may have been due to human resource deficits, dysfunctional equipment, reagent stock-outs, or limited ability to transport samples to a central lab

facility, all common challenges identified in a larger assessment of these sites. [File S1]

The quality score devised for this study was significantly correlated with both loss to follow-up and mortality, with a higher score associated with decreased loss to follow-up and increased survival. This finding correlates with limited data from studies in the US demonstrating the association between quality of HIV care and clinical outcomes. [39,40] In this study, survival may have been lower in patients who did not receive selected process indicators because sub-optimal adherence and treatment failure were missed. Many of the patients who were lost to follow-up may have been too ill to return to the clinic. Higher weight for age z-score had a protective effect on mortality. Numerous studies have also noted this finding. [41–44]

Very limited clinical outcomes data are currently available from the Nigerian pediatric and adolescent HIV treatment program. Though the focus of this study was not solely on clinical outcomes, this study provides a reasonable estimate of loss to follow-up and mortality within the Nigerian national program. Early mortality was 1.9% across all age groups, while mortality during the period of follow-up was noted to be 4.2%. Compared to data from similar pediatric and adolescent cohorts in sub-Saharan Africa, mortality was lower in the Nigerian program. [44,45] Similar to other studies, loss to follow-up was high at 19.0%. [46,47]

This study has several limitations. Sites were not randomly selected because we wanted to include a geographically diverse sample. Furthermore, we were limited to certain states due to safety concerns. We did not measure all site characteristics that may have impacted the process indicators included in the quality score in this study. This was because our goal was to focus on process, not structure. Furthermore, we knew from a larger assessment that all the sites had similar resource availability. [File S1] Though we provided an estimate of pediatric program staffing, we were unable to account for individual provider characteristics

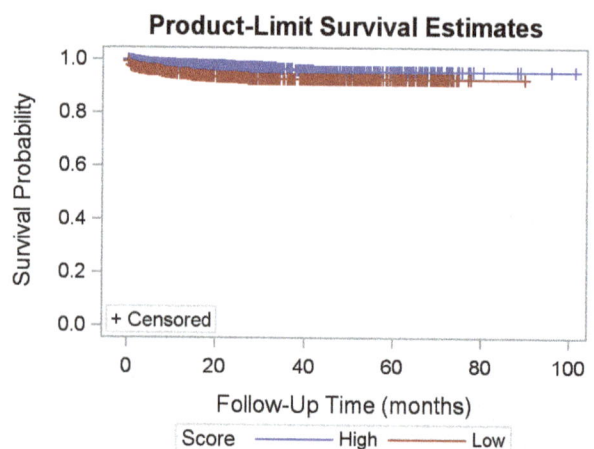

Figure 1. Kaplan-Meier survival by quality indicator score (high vs. low).

Table 2. Mortality and loss to follow-up by age at ART initiation.

Mortality	n	%	p value[1]
Within 90 days of ART Initiation	30	1.9%	
During period of follow-up	64	4.2%	
By age at ART initiation			
0–24 months	23	35.9%	NS
25–71 months	20	31.3%	
6–9 years	13	20.3%	
10–18 years	8	12.5%	
Loss to follow-up			
Within 6 months of ART Initiation	52	3.6%	
Within 12 months of ART Initiation	100	6.9%	
During period of follow-up	276	19.0%	
By age at ART initiation			
0–24 months	83	30.4%	p = 0.0130
25–71 months	98	35.9%	
6–9 years	48	17.6%	
10–18 years	44	16.1%	

[1]Differences between age groups significant at p<0.05.
NS, not significant.

such as years of experience treating pediatric or adolescent patients living with HIV or specialty training which may have impacted performance measures. In addition, as death was only documented in the chart if confirmation was obtained from the patient's family or caregiver or if death occurred in the hospital, it is not possible to know how many patients who were lost to follow up were actually dead. Staff members were trained to contact caregivers when patients were loss to follow-up, but standards regarding the timeliness of this contact were not well defined, and deaths may have been missed. Lastly, accurate measurement of quality is largely dependent upon the accuracy of documentation which is challenging to confirm in a retrospective study.

Pediatric and adolescent access to antiretroviral therapy in Nigeria is expanding. Since 2013, the number of facilities across the country that provide ART to children and adolescents has increased significantly. In order to expedite access to treatment, decentralization or down-referral of pediatric care to primary health clinics has been initiated. Efforts are also underway to standardize services across facilities and to ensure that quality improvement is incorporated into regular in service training. [Federal Ministry of Health of Nigeria, Personal Communication, January 15, 2013] As pediatric and adolescent ART access continues to expand in Nigeria and in similar resource limited settings, ensuring the quality of care that patients receive will be essential to reducing mortality and loss to follow-up. The next logical step toward achieving this goal in the Nigerian treatment program would be to use these data to inform a quality improvement intervention. Quality improvement studies are infrequently published in the medical literature. However, a few studies have demonstrated the efficacy of quality improvement in HIV care and treatment in resource limited settings. [48–50] More broadly, quality improvement methods strengthen health systems and help program planners utilize scarce resources more efficiently. [51] Considering the enormous investment that has been made in expanding access to pediatric and adolescent HIV treatment, assessments of quality followed by the development of appropriate interventions are critically important to maximize the benefits of ART.

Supporting Information

File S1 Greeson D, Ojikutu B, Kolapo U, Higgins Biddle M, Cabral H, et al. (2012) Rapid assessment of pediatric HIV treatment in Nigeria. Arlington, VA: USAID's AIDS Support and Technical Assistance Resources, AIDSTAR-One, Task Order 1.

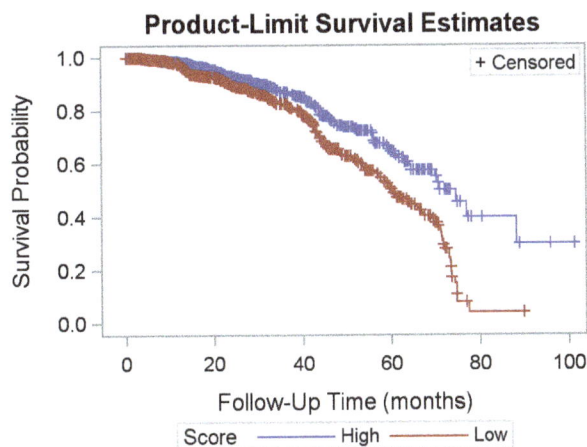

Product-Limit Survival Estimates

+ Censored

Survival Probability

Follow-Up Time (months)

Score — High — Low

Figure 2. Kaplan-Meier loss to follow-up by quality indicator score (high vs. low).

Table 3. Factors associated with mortality and loss to follow-up.

	Mortality (n = 1315)					Loss to Follow-up			Loss to Follow-up (n = 1386)	
	Bivariate			Multivariate		Bivariate			Multivariate	
	N	HR (95% CI)	p-value	AHR (95% CI)	p-value	N	OR (95% CI)	p-value	AOR (95% CI)	p-value
Male (Ref: Female)	1509	1.50 (0.90, 2.49)	NS	—	—	1450	1.00 (0.77, 1.30)	NS	—	—
Weight for age (z-score)	1379	0.90 (0.85, 0.95)	0.0003	0.92 (0.87, 0.98)	0.0121	1328	0.99 (0.96, 1.03)	NS	—	—
Age at ART initiation ≤24 months (Ref: >24)	1506	1.76 (1.06, 2.94)	0.0297	1.00 (0.51, 1.99)	NS	1447	1.56 (1.16, 2.09)	0.0029	1.36 (0.99, 1.87)	NS
Baseline immunosuppression[1]	1435					1388				
Severe		6.11 (1.89, 19.76)	0.0025	7.21 (1.72, 30.21)	0.0068		1.48 (1.02, 2.14)	0.0374	1.45 (0.99, 2.11)	NS
Moderate		1.95 (0.53, 7.19)	NS	2.88 (0.62, 13.39)	NS		1.14 (0.77, 1.70)	NS	1.13 (0.75, 1.70)	NS
No suppression		Ref		Ref			Ref		Ref	
High quality indicator score[2] (Ref: Low)	1511	0.43 (0.26, 0.73)	0.0015	0.47 (0.26, 0.87)	0.0165	1452	0.40 (0.31, 0.53)	<0.0001	0.42 (0.32, 0.56)	<0.0001

HR, hazard ratio; AHR, adjusted hazard ratio; OR, odds ratio; AOR, adjusted odds ratio; CI, confidence interval; NS, not significant.

[1]For patients less than two years of age, severe immunosuppression was defined as an initial CD4 count less than 750 cells/mm^3 or percentage less than 15%, moderate immunosuppression as an initial CD4 count of between 750 and 1500 cells/mm^3 or percentage of between 15% and 25%, and no immunosuppression as an initial CD4 count of 1500 cells/mm^3 or more, or percentage of 25% or more. For patients between two and five years of age, severe immunosuppression was defined as an initial CD4 count less than 500 cells/mm^3 or percentage less than 15%, moderate immunosuppression as an initial CD4 count of between 500 and 1000 cells/mm^3 or percentage of between 15% and 25%, and no immunosuppression as an initial CD4 count of 1000 cells/mm^3 or more, or percentage of 25% or more. For patients between five years of age or older, severe immunosuppression was defined as an initial CD4 count less than 200 cells/mm^3 or percentage less than 15%, moderate immunosuppression as an initial CD4 count of between 200 and 500 cells/mm^3 or percentage of between 15% and 25%, and no immunosuppression as an initial CD4 count of 500 cells/mm^3 or more, or percentage of 25% or more.

[2]1 point assigned for each service received (screened for tuberculosis, adherence counseling at last visit, ever prescribed co-trimoxazole, alive and not lost to follow-up with at least one CD4 count in the last six months, and weight documented in chart at patient's last visit and 0 points assigned if the service was not received, for a total of 6 points. A high score was defined as having the median score or above (>4 points).

Author Contributions

Conceived and designed the experiments: BO MHB DG BRP AA EO UK HC EC LH. Performed the experiments: BO MHB DG UK EC HC.

Analyzed the data: BO MHB DG HC LH. Contributed reagents/materials/analysis tools: BO MHB DG EO UK HC EC LH. Wrote the paper: BO MHB DG EO UK HC LH.

References

1. Kline MW (2006) Perspectives on the pediatric HIV/AIDS pandemic: catalyzing access of children to care and treatment. Pediatrics. 117: 1388–93.

2. Abrams EJ, Simonds RJ, Modi S, Rivadeneira E, Vaz P, et al. (2012) PEPFAR scale-up of pediatric HIV services: innovations, achievements, and challenges. J Acquir Immune Defic Syndr. 60 Suppl 3:S105–12.

3. Meyers T, Moultrie H, Naidoo K, Cotton M, Eley B, et al. (2007) Challenges to pediatric HIV care and treatment in South Africa. J Infect Dis. 196 Suppl 3:S474–81.

4. World Health Organization. Treatment of HIV in Children (2013) Available at: http://www.who.int/hiv/topics/paediatric/en/index.html. Accessed 2014 Jun 1.

5. The Institute of Medicine. Crossing the Quality Chasm: The IOM Health Care Quality Initiative (1998) Available at: http://www.iom.edu/Global/News%20Announcements/Crossing-the-Quality-Chasm-The-IOM-Health-Care-Quality-Initiative.aspx. Accessed 2014 Jun 1.

6. Mainz J (2003) Defining and classifying clinical indicators for quality improvement. Int J Qual Health Care. 15: 523–30.

7. Brook RH, McGlynn EA, Cleary PD (1996) Quality of health care. Part 2: measuring quality of care. N Engl J Med. 335: 966–70.

8. Donabedian A (1988) The quality of care. How can it be assessed? JAMA. 260: 1743–8.

9. Donabedian A (1988) Quality assessment and assurance: unity of purpose, diversity of means. Inquiry. 25: 173–92.

10. Brook RH, Davies Avery A, Greenfield S, Harris LJ, Lelah T, et al. (1977) Assessing the quality of medical care using outcome measures: an overview of the method. Med Care. 15:suppl 1–165.

11. Campbell SM, Roland MO, Buetow SA (2000) Defining quality of care. Soc Sci Med. 51: 1611–25.

12. Emdin CA, Chong NJ, Millson PE (2003) Non-physician clinician provided HIV treatment results in equivalent outcomes as physician-provided care: a meta-analysis. J Int AIDS Soc. 16: 18445.

13. Moon TD, Burlison JR, Blevins M, Shepherd BE, Baptista A, et al. (2011) Enrollment and programmatic trends and predictors of antiretroviral therapy initiation from president's emergency plan for AIDS Relief (PEPFAR)-supported public HIV care and treatment sites in rural Mozambique. Int J STD AIDS. 22: 621–7.

14. Morris MB, Chapula BT, Chi BH, Mwango A, Chi HF, et al. (2009) Use of task-shifting to rapidly scale-up HIV treatment services: experiences from Lusaka, Zambia. BMC Health Serv Res.9: 5.

15. Brennan AT, Long L, Maskew M, Sanne I, Jaffray I, et al. (2011) Outcomes of stable HIV-positive patients down-referred from a doctor-managed antiretroviral therapy clinic to a nurse-managed primary health clinic for monitoring and treatment. AIDS. 25: 2027–36.

16. Sutcliffe CG, Bolton Moore C, van Dijk JH, Cotham M, Tambatamba B, et al. (2010) Secular trends in pediatric antiretroviral treatment programs in rural and urban Zambia: a retrospective cohort study. BMC Pediatr. 29: 849–54.

17. Fayorsey RN, Saito S, Carter RJ, Gusmao E, Frederix K, et al.(2013) Decentralization of pediatric HIV care and treatment in five sub-Saharan African countries. J Acquir Immune Defic Syndr. 62: e124–30.

18. Alemayehu YK, Bushen OY, Muluneh AT (2009) Evaluation of HIV/AIDS clinical care quality: the case of a referral hospital in North West Ethiopia. Int J Qual Health Care. 21: 356–62.

19. Thanprasertsuk S, Supawitkul S, Lolekha R, Ningsanond P, Agins BD, et al. (2012) HIVQUAL-T: monitoring and improving HIV clinical care in Thailand, 2002–08. Int J Qual Health Care. 24: 338–47.

20. Ciampa PJ, Tique JA, Jumá N, Sidat M, Moon TD, et al. (2012) Addressing poor retention of infants exposed to HIV: a quality improvement study in rural Mozambique. J Acquir Immune Defic Syndr. 60: e46–52.

21. Were MC, Nyandiko WM, Huang KT, Slaven JE, Shen C, et al. (2013) Computer-generated reminders and quality of pediatric HIV care in a resource-limited setting. Pediatrics. 131: e789–96.

22. Lolekha R, Chunwimaleung S, Hansudewechakul R, Leawsrisook P, Prasitsuebsai W, et al. (2010) Pediatric HIVQUAL-T: measuring and improving the quality of pediatric HIV care in Thailand, 2005–2007. Jt Comm J Qual Patient Saf. 36: 541–51.

23. Leroy V, Malateste K, Rabie H, Lumbiganon P, Ayaya S, et al. (2013) Outcomes of antiretroviral therapy in children in Asia and Africa: a comparative analysis of the IeDEA pediatric multiregional collaboration. J Acquir Immune Defic Syndr. 62: 208–19.

24. Lamb MR, Fayorsey R, Nuwagaba Birbonwoha H, Viola V, Mutabazi V, et al. (2013) High attrition before and after ART initiation among youth (15–24 years of age) enrolled in HIV care. AIDS. 28: 559–68.

25. George E, Noël F, Bois G, Cassagnol R, Estavien L, et al. (2007) Antiretroviral therapy for HIV-1-infected children in Haiti. J Infect Dis. 195: 1411–8.

26. Nyandiko W, Vreeman R, Liu H, Shangani S, Sang E, et al. (2013) Nonadherence to clinic appointments among HIV-infected children in an ambulatory care program in western Kenya. J Acquir Immune Defic Syndr. 63: e49–55.

27. Walker AS, Prendergast AJ, Mugyenyi P, Munderi P, Hakim J, et al. (2012) Mortality in the year following antiretroviral therapy initiation in HIV-infected adults and children in Uganda and Zimbabwe. Clin Infect Dis. 55: 1707–18.

28. Weigel R, Estill J, Egger M, Harries AD, Makombe S, et al. (2012) Mortality and loss to follow-up in the first year of ART: Malawi national ART programme. AIDS. 26: 365–73.

29. Marazzi MC, De Luca S, Palombi L, Scarcella P, Ciccacci F, et al. (2013) Predictors of adverse outcomes in HIV-1 infected children receiving combination antiretroviral treatment: results from a DREAM Cohort in Sub-Saharan Africa. Pediatr Infect Dis J. 2014 Mar; 33(3):295–300.

30. Braitstein P, Songok J, Vreeman RC, Wools Kaloustian KK, Koskei P, et al. (2011) "Wamepotea" (they have become lost): outcomes of HIV-positive and HIV-exposed children lost to follow-up from a large HIV treatment program in western Kenya. J Acquir Immune Defic Syndr. 57: e40–6.

31. UNAIDS. Country profile: Nigeria. Available: http://www.unaids.org/en/regionscountries/countries/nigeria/. Accessed 2014 Jun 1.

32. UNAIDS (2011) Global HIV/AIDS response: epidemic update and health sector progress towards universal access: progress report 2011. Geneva: WHO. Available at: http://www.who.int/hiv/pub/progress_report2011/en/(Joint publication of WHO, Joint United Nations Programme on HIV/AIDS (UNAIDS), and United Nations Children's Fund (UNICEF). Accessed 2014 Jun 1.

33. Mukhtar Yola M, Adeleke S, Gwarzo D, Ladan ZF (2006) Preliminary investigation of adherence to antiretroviral therapy among children in Aminu Kano Teaching Hospital, Nigeria. Afr J AIDS Res. 5: 141–144.

34. Anigilaje EA, Olutola A (2013) Prevalence and clinical and immunoviralogical profile of human immunodeficiency virus-Hepatitis B co-infection among children in an antiretroviral therapy programme in Benue State, Nigeria. ISRN Pediatr. 932697.

35. World Health Organization (2010) Antiretroviral therapy for HIV infection in infants and children: towards universal access. Available at: http://whqlibdoc.who.int/publications/2010/9789241599801_eng.pdf. Accessed 2013 Dec 14.

36. Federal Ministry of Health of Nigeria (2010) National guidelines on pediatric HIV and AIDS treatment and care. Available at: http://www.aidstar-one.com/sites/default/files/treatment/national_treatment_guidelines/Nigeria_peds_2010_tagged.pdf. Accessed 2013 Dec 14.

37. Peduzzi P, Concato J, Feinstein AR, Holford TR (1995) Importance of events per independent variable in proportional hazards regression analysis II. Accuracy and precision of regression estimates. J Clin Epidemiol. 48: 1503–10.

38. World Health Organization (2011) Guidelines for intensified case finding for people living with HIV in resource constrained settings. Available at: http://whqlibdoc.who.int/publications/2011/9789241500708_eng.pdf?ua = 1. Accessed 2014 May 18.

39. Virga PH, Jin B, Thomas J, Virodov S (2012) Electronic health information technology as a tool for improving quality of care and health outcomes for HIV/AIDS patients. Int J Med Inform. 81: e39–45.

40. Horberg M, Hurley L, Towner W, Gambatese R, Klein D, et al. (2011) HIV quality performance measures in a large integrated health care system. AIDS Patient Care STDS. 25: 21–8.

41. Davies MA, May M, Bolton Moore C, Chimbetete C, Eley B, et al. (2013) Prognosis of Children with HIV-1 Infection Starting Antiretroviral Therapy in Southern Africa: A Collaborative Analysis of Treatment Programs. Pediatr Infect Dis J.

42. Zhao Y, Li C, Sun X, Mu W, McGoogan JM, et al. (2013) Mortality and treatment outcomes of China's National Pediatric antiretroviral therapy program. Clin Infect Dis. 56: 735–44.

43. Zanoni BC, Phungula T, Zanoni HM, France H, Feeney ME (2011) Risk factors associated with increased mortality among HIV infected children initiating antiretroviral therapy (ART) in South Africa. PLoS One. 6: e22706.

44. Ekouevi DK, Azondekon A, Dicko F, Malateste K, Touré P, et al. (2011) 12-month mortality and loss-to-program in antiretroviral-treated children: the IeDEA pediatric West African database to evaluate AIDS (pWADA), 2000–2008. BMC Public Health. 11: 519.

45. KIDS-ART-LINC Collaboration (2008) Low risk of death, but substantial program attrition, in pediatric HIV treatment cohorts in Sub-Saharan Africa. J Acquir Immune Defic Syndr. 49: 523–31.

46. Bygrave H, Mtangirwa J, Ncube K, Ford N, Kranzer K, et al. (2012) Antiretroviral therapy outcomes among adolescents and youth in rural Zimbabwe. PLoS One. 7: e52856.

47. Evans D, Menezes C, Mahomed K, Macdonald P, Untiedt S, et al. (2013) Treatment outcomes of HIV-infected adolescents attending public-sector HIV clinics across Gauteng and Mpumalanga, South Africa. AIDS Res Hum Retroviruses. 29: 892–900.

48. Ciampa PJ, Tique JA, Jumá N, Sidat M, Moon TD, et al. (2012) Addressing poor retention of infants exposed to HIV: a quality improvement study in rural Mozambique. J Acquir Immune Defic Syndr. 60: e46–52.

49. Sripipatana T, Spensley A, Miller A, McIntyre J, Sangiwa G, et al. (2007) Site-specific interventions to improve prevention of mother-to-child transmission of human immunodeficiency virus programs in less developed settings. Am J Obstet Gynecol. 197: S107–S112.

50. Doherty T, Chopra M, Nsibande D, Mngoma D (2009) Improving the coverage of the PMTCT programme through a participatory quality improvement intervention in South Africa. BMC Public Health. 9: 406.

51. Leatherman S, Ferris TG, Berwick D, Omaswa F, Crisp N (2010) The role of quality improvement in strengthening health systems in developing countries. Int J Qual Health Care. 22: 237–243.

Permissions

The contributors of this book come from diverse backgrounds, making this book a truly international effort. This book will bring forth new frontiers with its revolutionizing research information and detailed analysis of the nascent developments around the world.

We would like to thank all the contributing authors for lending their expertise to make the book truly unique. They have played a crucial role in the development of this book. Without their invaluable contributions this book wouldn't have been possible. They have made vital efforts to compile up to date information on the varied aspects of this subject to make this book a valuable addition to the collection of many professionals and students.

This book was conceptualized with the vision of imparting up-to-date information and advanced data in this field. To ensure the same, a matchless editorial board was set up. Every individual on the board went through rigorous rounds of assessment to prove their worth. After which they invested a large part of their time researching and compiling the most relevant data for our readers.

The editorial board has been involved in producing this book since its inception. They have spent rigorous hours researching and exploring the diverse topics which have resulted in the successful publishing of this book. They have passed on their knowledge of decades through this book. To expedite this challenging task, the publisher supported the team at every step. A small team of assistant editors was also appointed to further simplify the editing procedure and attain best results for the readers.

Apart from the editorial board, the designing team has also invested a significant amount of their time in understanding the subject and creating the most relevant covers. They scrutinized every image to scout for the most suitable representation of the subject and create an appropriate cover for the book.

The publishing team has been an ardent support to the editorial, designing and production team. Their endless efforts to recruit the best for this project, has resulted in the accomplishment of this book. They are a veteran in the field of academics and their pool of knowledge is as vast as their experience in printing. Their expertise and guidance has proved useful at every step. Their uncompromising quality standards have made this book an exceptional effort. Their encouragement from time to time has been an inspiration for everyone.

The publisher and the editorial board hope that this book will prove to be a valuable piece of knowledge for researchers, students, practitioners and scholars across the globe.

List of Contributors

Ivana Milovanovic, Falucar Njuieyon, Samia Deghmoun and Claire Levy-Marchal
INSERM CIE 05 – Unité d'épidémiologie clinique, Hôpital Robert Debré, Paris, France

Didier Chevenne
Service de biochimie et hormonologie, Hôpital Robert Debré, Paris, France

Jacques Beltrand
Endocrinologie et diabétologie pédiatrique, Hôpital Necker, Paris, France
Université Paris 5, René Descartes, Paris, France
INSERM U845, Imagine Affiliated, Paris, France

Germán Iñiguez, Juan José Castro, M. Cecilia Johnson, Fernando Cassorla and Verónica Mericq
Institute of Maternal and Child Research, University of Chile, Santiago, Chile

Mirna Garcia and Elena Kakarieka
Hospital Clínico San Borja-Arriarán, University of Chile, Santiago, Chile

Sonia Prot-Labarthe
Pharmacie, AP-HP Hô pital Robert-Debré, Paris, France

Thomas Weil
Pharmacie, AP-HP Hô pital Robert-Debré, Paris, France
Pharmacie Clinique, Université Paris Descartes, Paris, France

François Angoulvant
Service d'Accueil des Urgences, AP-HP Hô pital Robert-Debré, Paris, France

Rym Boulkedid
Unité d'Epidémiologie Clinique, AP-HP Hô pital Robert Debré, Paris, France
Inserm U 1123 et CIC 1426, Paris, France

Corinne Alberti
Unité d'Epidémiologie Clinique, AP-HP Hôpital Robert Debré, Paris, France
Inserm U 1123 et CIC 1426, Paris, France
Sorbonne Paris Cité UMRS 1123, Université Paris Diderot, Paris, France

Olivier Bourdon
Pharmacie, AP-HP Hô pital Robert-Debré, Paris, France
Pharmacie Clinique, Université Paris Descartes, Paris, France
Laboratoire Educations et Pratiques de Santé, Université Paris XIII, Bobigny, France

Corinna Vossius
SAFER (Stavanger Acute Medicine Foundation for Education and Research), Stavanger University Hospital, Stavanger, Norway

Hege L. Ersdal
SAFER (Stavanger Acute Medicine Foundation for Education and Research), Stavanger University Hospital, Stavanger, Norway
Research Institute, Haydom Lutheran Hospital, Haydom, Tanzania

Editha Lotto, Sara Lyanga and Estomih Mduma
Research Institute, Haydom Lutheran Hospital, Haydom, Tanzania

Georgina Msemo
Ministry of Health and Social Welfare, Dar es Salaam, Tanzania

Jeffrey Perlman
Department of Pediatrics, Weill Cornell Medical College, New York, New York, United States of America

Lauren Elizabeth Veit, Jay Fong and Benjamin Udoka Nwosu
Department of Pediatrics, University of Massachusetts Medical School, Worcester, Massachusetts, United States of America

Louise Maranda
Department of Quantitative Health Sciences, University of Massachusetts Medical School, Worcester, Massachusetts, United States of America

Micheá l de Barra and Val Curtis
Environmental Health Group, London School of Hygiene and Tropical Medicine, London, United Kingdom

M. Sirajul Islam
Environmental Microbiology Lab, ICDDR,B, Dhaka, Bangladesh

Wenhua Yu, Changping Li, Xiaomeng Fu, Zhuang Cui, Xiaoqian Liu, Linlin Fan, Guan Zhang and Jun Ma
Department of Health Statistics, College of Public Health, Tianjin Medical University, Tianjin, China

Yan Wang, Jing Xue, Jingzhi He, Xuedong Zhou, Meng You, Qin Du, Lei Cheng, Mingyun Li, Yuqing Li, Jiyao Li and Xin Xu
State Key Laboratory of Oral Diseases, West China Hospital of Stomatology, Sichuan University, Chengdu, China

Xue Yang and Yiping Zhu
Department of Pediatric Hematology and Oncology, West China Second University Hospital, Sichuan University, Chengdu, China

Jing Zou
Department of Pediatric Dentistry, West China Hospital of Stomatology, Sichuan University, Chengdu, China

Wenyuan Shi
UCLA School of Dentistry, Los Angeles, California, United States of America

Penelope M. Enarson and Donald A. Enarson
Child Lung Health Division, International Union Against Tuberculosis and Lung Disease, Paris, France
Desmond Tutu TB Centre, Department of Paediatrics and Child Health, Faculty of Medicine and Health Sciences, Stellenbosch University, Tygerberg, South Africa

Robert P. Gie
Department of Paediatrics and Child Health, Faculty of Medicine and Health Sciences, University of Stellenbosch, Tygerberg, South Africa

Charles C. Mwansambo
Ministry of Health, Lilongwe, Malawi

Ellubey R. Maganga
UNICEF Malawi, Lilongwe, Malawi

Carl J. Lombard
Biostatistics Unit, South Africa Medical Research Council (MRC), Cape Town, South Africa

Stephen M. Graham
Child Lung Health Division, International Union Against Tuberculosis and Lung Disease, Paris, France
Centre for International Child Health, University of Melbourne Department of Paediatrics and Murdoch Children's Research Institute, Royal Children's Hospital, Melbourne, Australia

Günther Fink, Christopher R. Sudfeld, Goodarz Danaei and Wafaie W. Fawzi
Harvard School of Public Health, Boston, Massachusetts, United States of America

Majid Ezzati
MRC-PHE Centre for Environment and Health, Departments of Epidemiology and Biostatistics, Imperial College London, London, United Kingdom

Stephanie M. Perkins and Todd DeWees
Department of Radiation Oncology, Washington University School of Medicine, Saint Louis, Missouri, United States of America

Eric T. Shinohara
Department of Radiation Oncology, Vanderbilt University School of Medicine, Nashville, Tennessee, United States of America

Haydar Frangoul
Department of Pediatrics, Vanderbilt University School of Medicine, Nashville, Tennessee, United States of America

Azzurra Ruggeri
Max Planck Institute for Human Development, Berlin, Germany

Michaela Gummerum and Yaniv Hanoch
University of Plymouth, Plymouth, England

Ashley Di Battista
School of Behavioural Science, University of Melbourne, Melbourne, Australia
Department of Psychology, The Hospital for Sick Children, Toronto, Ontario, Canada
Clinical Sciences, Murdoch Children's Research Institute, Royal Children's Hospital, Melbourne, Australia

Celia Godfrey and Cheryl Soo
Clinical Sciences, Murdoch Children's Research Institute, Royal Children's Hospital, Melbourne, Australia

Cathy Catroppa
School of Behavioural Science, University of Melbourne, Melbourne, Australia
Clinical Sciences, Murdoch Children's Research Institute, Royal Children's Hospital, Melbourne, Australia
Department of Paediatrics, University of Melbourne, Melbourne, Australia

Vicki Anderson
School of Behavioural Science, University of Melbourne, Melbourne, Australia
Clinical Sciences, Murdoch Children's Research Institute, Royal Children's Hospital, Melbourne, Australia
Psychology, Royal Children's Hospital, Melbourne, Australia
Department of Paediatrics, University of Melbourne, Melbourne, Australia

Michael DeKlerk
Directorate of Special Programmes, Republic of Namibia Ministry of Health and Social Services, Windhoek, Namibia
Anna Jonas, Victor Sumbi, Samson Mwinga and Francina Tjituka
Strengthening Pharmaceutical Systems, Management Sciences for Health, Windhoek, Namibia

Scott Penney and Alice M. Tang
Department of Public Health and Community Medicine, Tufts University School of Medicine, Boston, Massachusetts, United States of America

Michael R. Jordan and Steven Y. Hong
Department of Public Health and Community Medicine, Tufts University School of Medicine, Boston, Massachusetts, United States of America
Division of Geographic Medicine and Infectious Diseases, Tufts Medical Center, Boston, Massachusetts, United States of America

Tiruneh Desta
World Health Organization Namibia, Klein Windhoek, Namibia

Bach Xuan Tran, Arto Ohinmaa, Jeffrey A. Johnson and Paul J. Veugelers
School of Public Health, University of Alberta, Edmonton, Alberta, Canada

Stefan Kuhle
Department of Pediatrics, Obstetrics & Gynecology, Dalhousie University, Halifax, NS, Canada

Valentin A. Schriever, Wenke Petters, Carolin Boerner and Thomas Hummel
Smell & Taste Clinic, Department of Otorhinolaryngology, University Hospital Carl Gustav Carus, Technische Universität (TU) Dresden, Dresden, Germany

Eri Mor
Department of Otorhinolaryngology, Jikei University, School of Medicine, Tokyo, Japan

Martin Smitka
Department of Neuropediatrics, University Hospital Carl Gustav Carus, Technische Universita¨t (TU) Dresden, Dresden, Germany

Sheila Xinxuan Soh and John W. J. Huang
Cancer and Stem Cell Biology Program, Duke-NUS Graduate Medical School, Singapore, Singapore

Joshua Yew Suang Lim and Nan Jiang
Department of Paediatrics, Yong Loo Lin School of Medicine, National University of Singapore, Singapore, Singapore

Allen Eng Juh Yeoh
Department of Paediatrics, Yong Loo Lin School of Medicine, National University of Singapore, Singapore, Singapore
National University Cancer Institute, National University Health System, Singapore, Singapore
Viva-University Children's Cancer Centre, University Children's Medical Institute, National University Health System, Singapore, Singapore
Cancer Science Institute, National University of Singapore, Singapore, Singapore

S. Tiong Ong
Department of Haematology, Singapore General Hospital, Singapore, Singapore
Department of Medical Oncology, National Cancer Centre, Singapore, Singapore
Division of Medical Oncology, Duke University Medical Center, Durham, North Carolina, United States of America

Chia-Huei Chu, Tzong-Yang Tu and An-Suey Shiao
Department of Otolaryngology Head Neck Surgery, Taipei Veterans General Hospital, Taipei, Taiwan and School of Medicine, National Yang-Ming University, Taipei, Taiwan

Pesus Chou
Institute of Public Health and Community Medicine Research Center, National Yang-Ming University, Taipei, Taiwan

Mao-Che Wang
Department of Otolaryngology Head Neck Surgery, Taipei Veterans General Hospital, Taipei, Taiwan and School of Medicine, National Yang-Ming University, Taipei, Taiwan
Institute of Public Health and Community Medicine Research Center, National Yang-Ming University, Taipei, Taiwan

Ying-Piao Wang
Institute of Public Health and Community Medicine Research Center, National Yang-Ming University, Taipei, Taiwan
Department of Otolaryngology Head Neck Surgery, Mackay Memorial Hospital, Taipei, Taiwan and Department of Audiology and Speech Language Pathology and School of Medicine, Mackay Medical College, New Taipei City, Taiwan

Maren Johanne Heilskov Rytter and Henrik Friis
Department of Nutrition, Exercise and Sports, Faculty of Science, University of Copenhagen, Frederiksberg, Denmark

Lilian Kolte
Department of Infectious Diseases, Copenhagen University Hospital, Hvidovre, Denmark

André Briend
Department of Nutrition, Exercise and Sports, Faculty of Science, University of Copenhagen, Frederiksberg, Denmark
Department for International Health, University of Tampere, School of Medicine, Tampere, Finland

Vibeke Brix Christensen
Department of Paediatrics, Copenhagen University Hospital Rigshospitalet, Copenhagen, Denmark

Eirin Krüger Skaftun and Ole Frithjof Norheim
Department of Global Public Health and Primary Care, University of Bergen, Bergen, Norway

Merima Ali
Chr. Michelsen Institute, Bergen, Norway

Marko Wilke
Department of Pediatric Neurology and Developmental Medicine, Children's Hospital, University of Tübingen, Tübingen, Germany
Experimental Pediatric Neuroimaging group, Pediatric Neurology & Department of Neuroradiology, University Hospital, Tübingen, Germany

Nada M. S. Al-Saffar, L. Elizabeth Jackson, Geetha Balarajah, Alice Agliano and Martin O. Leach
Cancer Research UK and EPSRC Cancer Imaging Centre, Division of Radiotherapy and Imaging, The Institute of Cancer Research and The Royal Marsden NHS Foundation Trust, London, United Kingdom

Andrew D. J. Pearson
Division of Cancer Therapeutics, The Institute of Cancer Research and The Royal Marsden NHS Foundation Trust, London, United Kingdom
Division of Clinical Studies. The Institute of Cancer Research and The Royal Marsden NHS Foundation Trust, London, United Kingdom

Lynley V. Marshall
Division of Molecular Pathology, The Institute of Cancer Research and The Royal Marsden NHS Foundation Trust, London, United Kingdom
Division of Cancer Therapeutics, The Institute of Cancer Research and The Royal Marsden NHS Foundation Trust, London, United Kingdom
Division of Clinical Studies. The Institute of Cancer Research and The Royal Marsden NHS Foundation Trust, London, United Kingdom

Thomas R. Eykyn
Cancer Research UK and EPSRC Cancer Imaging Centre, Division of Radiotherapy and Imaging, The Institute of Cancer Research and The Royal Marsden NHS Foundation Trust, London, United Kingdom
Division of Imaging Sciences and Biomedical Engineering, King's College London, St Thomas' Hospital, London, United Kingdom

Paul A. Clarke and Paul Workman
Division of Cancer Therapeutics, The Institute of Cancer Research and The Royal Marsden NHS Foundation Trust, London, United Kingdom
Cancer Research UK Cancer Therapeutics Unit, The Institute of Cancer Research, London, United Kingdom

Chris Jones
Division of Molecular Pathology, The Institute of Cancer Research and The Royal Marsden NHS Foundation Trust, London, United Kingdom

Division of Cancer Therapeutics, The Institute of Cancer Research and The Royal Marsden NHS Foundation Trust, London, United Kingdom

Bisola Ojikutu
John Snow Inc., Boston, Massachusetts, United States of America
Massachusetts General Hospital, Infectious Disease Division, Boston, Massachusetts, United States of America

Molly Higgins-Biddle
John Snow Inc., Boston, Massachusetts, United States of America

Dana Greeson
Columbia University, Department of Epidemiology, New York, New York, United States of America

Benjamin R. Phelps and Anouk Amzel
United States Agency for International Development (USAID), Washington, D. C., United States of America

Emeka Okechukwu
United States Agency for International Development (USAID), Abuja, Nigeria

Usman Kolapo
Indepth Precision, Abuja, Nigeria

Howard Cabral
Boston University School of Public Health, Department of Biostatistics, Boston, Massachusetts, United States of America

Ellen Cooper
Boston University School of Medicine, Boston, Massachusetts, United States of America

Lisa R. Hirschhorn
Harvard Medical School, Department of Global Health and Social Medicine, Harvard Medical School, Boston, Massachusetts, United States of America

Index

www.ingramcontent.com/pod-product-compliance
Lightning Source LLC
Chambersburg PA
CBHW082101190326
41458CB00010B/3539